RECENT DEVELOPMENTS IN

ALCOHOLISM

VOLUME 17

ALCOHOL PROBLEMS IN ADOLESCENTS AND YOUNG ADULTS

RECENT DEVELOPMENTS IN

Edited by

MARC GALANTER

New York University School of Medicine
New York, New York

Section Editors

CHERRY LOWMAN,
ASSOCIATE EDITOR
GAYLE M. BOYD
VIVIAN B. FADEN
ELLEN WITT

Assistant Editor

DOLLY LAGRESSA

An Official Publication of the American Society of Addiction Medicine and the Research Society on Alcoholism.
This series was founded by the National Council on Alcoholism.

ALCOHOLISM

VOLUME 17
ALCOHOL PROBLEMS IN ADOLESCENTS AND YOUNG ADULTS

Epidemiology
Neurobiology
Prevention
Treatment

Springer

Library of Congress Cataloging-in-Publication Data

Recent developments in alcohollism: an official publication of the American Medical Society on Alcoholism, and the Research Society on Alcoholism, and the National Council on Alcoholism—Vol. 1—New York: Plenum Press, c 1983–

v.: ill.; 25 cm.

Cataloging in publication

Editor: Marc Galanter.

ISSN 0738-422X = Recent developments in alcoholism

1. Alcoholism—Periodicals. I. Galanter, Marc. II. American Medical Society on Alcoholism. III. Research Society on Alcohol (U.S.) IV. National Council on Alcoholism [DNLM:

1. Alcoholism—periodicals. W1 RE106AH(P)]

HV5001.R4 616.861'1'05—dc19 83-643791

Library of Congress [8311] AACR 3 MARC-S

ISBN 0-306-48625-3

Printed in the United States of America. (SPI)

10 9 8 7 6 5 4 3

springer.com

Contributors

Richard L. Bell, Indiana University School of Medicine, Institute of Psychiatric Research, Indianapolis, Indiana 46202-4887

Gayle Boyd, Health Scientist Administrator, Prevention Research Branch, NIAAA Division of Clinical and Prevention Research, Bethesda, Maryland 20892-7003

Kristen G. Anderson, University of California San Diego, LaJolla, California 92093-0109

Sandra A. Brown, University of California San Diego, Department of Psychology, Veterans Affairs San Diego Healthcare System, LaJolla, California 92093-0109

Oscar G. Bukstein, University of Pittsburgh School of Medicine, Pittsburgh, Pennsylvania 15213-2593

Tammy Chung, Assistant Professor of Psychiatry, University of Pittsburgh Medical Center, Western Psychiatric Institute and Clinic, Pittsburgh, Pennsylvania 15213

Duncan B. Clark, University of Pittsburgh School of Medicine, Pittsburgh, Pennsylvania 15213-2593

Jack R. Cornelius, Professor of Psychiatry and Pharmacological Sciences, University of Pittsburgh, Pittsburgh, Pennsylvania 15213-2593

Vivian B. Faden, National Institute on Alcohol Abuse and Alcoholism, Chief Epidemiology Branch, Division of Biometry and Epidemiology, Bethesda, Maryland 20892-7003

Tamara Fahnhorst, Center for Adolescent Substance Research, University of Minnesota, Minneapolis, Minnesota 55455

Marc Galanter, New York University School of Medicine, Department of Psychiatry, Division of Alcoholism and Drug Abuse, New York, New York 10016

Mark D. Godley, Chestnut Health Systems, Bloomington, Illinois 61701

Kristina Jackson, University of Missouri, Columbia and the Midwest Alcoholism Research Center, Columbia, Missouri 65211-0001

Yifrah Kaminer, University of Connecticut Health Center, Alcohol Research Center and Department of Psychiatry, Farmington, CT 06030-2103

Kelli A. Komro, University of Minnesota, School of Public Health-Division of Epidemiology, Minneapolis, Minnesota 55454

Kathleen M. Lenk, Alcohol Epidemiology Program, University of Minnesota, School of Public Health, Minneapolis, Minnesota 55454-1015

Cherry Lowman, National Institute on Alcohol Abuse and Alcoholism, Treatment Research Branch, Bethesda, Maryland 20892-7003

Jennifer L. Maggs, Pennsylvania State University, Human Development and Family Studies, University Park, Pennsylvania 16802

Christopher S. Martin, University of Pittsburgh Medical Center, Western Psychiatric Institute and Clinic, Pittsburgh, Pennsylvania 15213

William J. McBride, Indiana University School of Medicine, Institute of Psychiatric Research, Indianapolis, Indiana 46202-4887

Brooke S. G. Molina, University of Pittsburgh School of Medicine, Western Psychiatric Institute and Clinic, Pittsburgh, Pennsylvania 15213

James M. Murphy, Indiana University School of Medicine, Institute of Psychiatric Research, Indianapolis, Indiana 46202-4887

Aesoon Park, University of Missouri, Columbia and the Midwest Alcoholism Research Center, Columbia, Missouri 65211-0001

Cheryl L. Perry, University of Minnesota, School of Public Health-Division of Epidemiology, Minneapolis, Minnesota 55454

Danielle E. Ramo, San Diego State University/University of California, San Diego Joint Doctoral Program in Clinical Psychology, La Jolla, California 92093-0109

Zachary A. Rodd, Indiana University School of Medicine, Institute of Psychiatric Research, Indianapolis, Indiana 46202-4887

Ihsan M. Salloum, University of Pittsburgh School of Medicine, Pittsburgh, Pennsylvania 15213-2593

Robert F. Saltz, Pacific Institute for Research and Evaluation Prevention Research Center, Berkeley, California 94704

John E. Schulenberg, University of Michigan, Institute for Social Research and Department of Psychology, Ann Arbor, Michigan 48109

Alecia D. Schweinsburg, VA San Diego, Healthcare System and University of California San Diego, Department of Psychology, San Diego, California 92161

Kenneth Sher, University of Missouri, Columbia, and the Midwest Alcoholism Research Center, Columbia, Missouri 65211-0001

Natasha Slesnick, Department of Psychology, University of New Mexico, Albuquerque, New Mexico 87131

Linda Patia Spear, Distinguished Professor, Binghamton University, Department of Psychology and Center for Developmental Psychobiology, Binghamton, New York 13902-6000

Melissa H. Stigler, University of Minnesota, School of Public Health-Division of Epidemiology, Minneapolis, Minnesota 55454

Wendy N. Strother, Indiana University School of Medicine, Institute of Psychiatric Research, Indianapolis, Indiana 46202-4887

Steve Sussman, University of Southern California, Departments of Preventive Medicine and Psychology, Alhambra, California 91803

H. Scott Swartzwelder, University Medical Center, Neurobiology Research Labs, Veterans Affairs Medical Center, Durham, North Carolina 27710/27705

Susan F. Tapert, University of California San Diego, VA San Diego Healthcare System, San Diego, California 92093

Kristin L. Tomlinson, University of California, San Diego, LaJolla, California 92093-1019

Traci L. Toomey, Alcohol Epidemiology Program, University of Minnesota, School of Public Health, Minneapolis, Minnesota 55454-1015

Elena I. Varlinskaya, Binghamton University, Department of Psychology and Center for Developmental Psychobiology, Binghamton, New York 13902-6000

Alexander C. Wagenaar, Department of Epidemiology and Health Policy Rsearch, University of Florida School of Medicine, Gainesville, Florida 32608

Aaron M. White, Duke University Medical Center, Neurobiology Research Labs, Veterans Affairs Medical Center, Durham, North Carolina 27710

William L. White, Chestnut Health Systems, Bloomington, Illinois 61701

Michael Windle, University of Alabama at Birmingham, Center for the Advancement of Youth Health, Birmingham, Alabama 35294-1200

Rebecca C. Windle, University of Alabama at Birmingham, Center for the Advancement of Youth Health, Birmingham, Alabama 35294-1200

Ken C. Winters, Center for Adolescent Substance Abuse Research, University of Minnesota, Minneapolis, Minnesota 55455

Ellen Witt, National Institute on Alcohol Abuse and Alcoholism, Neuroscience and Behavior Research Branch, Division of Basic Research, Bethesda, Maryland 20892-7003

Maria M. Wong, Addiction Research Center, Department of Psychiatry, University of Michigan, Ann Arbor, Michigan 48105-2194

Robert A. Zucker, Addiction Research Center, Department of Psychiatry, University of Michigan, Ann Arbor, Michigan 48105-2194

Preface

From the President of the American Society for Addiction Medicine

Even after stepping through the doorway into the 21st century, alcoholism remains a major contributor to the excess morbidity and mortality experienced by Americans. No where is this unmet need more dramatic than its impact on adolescents.

In this edition, the authors cover the wide spectrum of epidemiologic, prevention, neurobiological, behavioral and clinical issues related to alcohol use and adolescents. The wide range of topical areas mirrors the prominence of alcoholism and alcohol abuse in the American landscape. Each of these areas alone presents significant challenges and opportunities to assist in understanding the fundamental issues and crafting effective remedies.

Aside from the obvious value of contributing to the scientific portfolio of what is known, the value of this edition is meaningful beyond the eloquent study designs and erudite principles presented by the superb cadre of authors. Adolescence is already challenging. The addition of alcohol has only made it more so.

It makes sense that effective remedies to this major public health and societal challenge would be multifaceted, comprehensive, and guided by scientific evidence. The scientific information in this edition provides ample contributions to this effort.

Lawrence S. Brown., Jr., MD, MPH, FASAM
President, American Society on Addiction Medicine

Contents

I

Epidemiology

Vivian B. Faden, *Section Editor*

Alcohol is the substance most frequently used by youth. According to 2002 data from Monitoring the Future (MTF), a nationally representative survey of youth, 78% of 12th graders, 67th of 10th graders and 47% of 8th graders reported consuming alcohol in their lives. Furthermore, 62% of 12th graders, 44% of 10th graders and 21% of 8th graders reported having been drunk. In 2002, the 30-day prevalence of alcohol consumption was 20% for 8th graders, 35% for 10th graders and 49% for 12 graders. The prevalence of heavy episodic drinking (5 or more drinks in a row in the past 2 weeks) was 12% among 8th graders, 22% among 10th graders and 29% among 12th graders (Johnston et al, 2003). And youth who drink may experience a range of adverse short and long-term consequences including academic problems such as lower grades or school failure, social problems, physical problems such as hangovers or medical illnesses, unwanted or unintended sexual activity, physical and sexual assault, memory problems, increased risk for suicide and homicide, alcohol-related car crashes and death from alcohol poisoning. Clearly, drinking by young people and its consequences presents a significant public health problem which must command our attention. This volume of *Recent Developments in Alcoholism* focusing on alcohol consumption by adolescents and young adults is therefore extremely timely.

The first section of the volume is comprised of five chapters which address the epidemiology of alcohol consumption by and alcohol-related problems among adolescents. Epidemiology is defined as the study of how a disease or problem is distributed in the population and of the characteristics that influence that distribution. As such epidemiology informs us about the severity of a problem, its natural history, and its prognosis. From epidemiologic studies (e.g. MTF cited above) we can learn how widespread a problem is, dis-

Vivian B. Faden • National Institute on Alcohol Abuse and Alcoholism, Associate Director, Division of Epidemiology and Prevention Research, Bethesda, Maryland 20892. This introduction was written in a personal capacity and does not represent the opinions of the NIH, DHHS, or the Federal Government.

cover which groups suffer most from it and identify its short and long term consequences. Such studies also serve to identify associated risk and protective factors which in turn help to identify those individuals who may be at increased risk due to neurobiological, environmental and individual factors. These factors include family history and genetic vulnerability, comorbid conditions, socio-demographic characteristics, social stressors such as poverty and lack of social support, family characteristics, alcohol availability and personality and other personal factors to mention just a few. But the ultimate goal of epidemiology goes beyond description; ultimately, a better understanding of what leads to underage use of alcohol at different developmental stages can inform prevention and treatment. For example, knowledge of protective factors may guide the design of interventions to increase resilience and identification of high risk groups may stimulate the design of interventions specifically for these groups.

The first chapter in this section summarizes what we know about the epidemiology of alcohol consumption by adolescents in the general population. In the chapter entitled "Alcohol Consumption and its Consequences Among Adolescents and Young Adults," Michael Windle and Rebecca Windle discuss the high prevalence of drinking among young people and describe its many consequences, some very serious. General population surveys (e.g. National Survey on Drug Use and Health, MTF) as well as smaller more localized studies have uniformly found high rates of alcohol consumption among young people aged 12 to 20. As already mentioned those youth who drink may experience a range of adverse academic, social, legal and medical consequences. The authors indicate that available data consistently show rates of drinking are highest among White and American Indian or Alaskan Native youth, followed by Hispanic youth, African Americans, and Asians. The authors also indicate that alcohol consumption generally increases with increasing age. Prevalence rates for boys and girls are similar in the younger age groups; however among older adolescents, the prevalence for boys is greater than for girls for more frequent and heavier use. The authors also discuss alcohol's association with other health-compromising behaviors such as other substance use and risky sex and the prevalence of alcohol use disorders among youth. Thus, this chapter serves to provide a broad understanding of the prevalence of alcohol consumption and its consequences among youth in general.

In the second chapter in this section entitled "High Risk Adolescent and Young Adult Populations—Consumption and Consequences," Brooke Molina looks more specifically at certain groups of adolescents at increased risk: those with comorbid psychiatric conditions; those with a positive family history of alcohol problems; gay and lesbian youth; homeless and throwaway youth; and those who belong to ethnic and racial groups with greater vulnerability. Studies indicate that at least some youth in each of these categories experience heightened vulnerability and therefore may benefit from targeted interventions. For example, as described in this chapter, there is convergence in the literature that there is a strong association of conduct problems and alcohol consumption, and according to a national survey, youth who identify themselves as gay, lesbian or bisexual are at elevated risk for heavy alcohol consumption. However as the authors of this chapter aptly point out, the same youth are likely to be vulnerable for a number of reasons, as risk factors tend to cluster in individuals. Underage alcohol consumption should therefore be studied in a conceptual framework which addresses the full constellation of risk and protective factors from early childhood through adolescence and into young adulthood.

In the next chapter, "Drinking among College Students—Consumption and Consequences," Kristina Jackson, Kenneth Sher and Aesoon Park consider alcohol consumption, alcohol-related consequences and problems, and alcohol dependence among a specific group of youth who consume alcohol at high levels, college students. Studies consistently indicate that about 4 out of 5 college students drink alcohol, about 2 out of 5 engage in excessive heavy consumption (5 or more drinks in a row for men and 4 or more in a row for women in the past two weeks or 30 days, depending on the survey) and about 1 in 5 engages in frequent episodic heavy consumption (3 or more times in the past two weeks) (NIAAA, 2002). The consequences of this consumption may include academic problems, social problems, legal problems, involvement in physical or sexual assault or risky sex, and even death. The authors of this chapter carefully review available information about levels and patterns of consumption in this population, consider individual, intra-campus and inter-campus factors which relate to drinking in college, and discuss what is currently known about the long-term negative outcomes of drinking by college students. They identify the need for prospective information to establish causality, however, and the need for more information about long-term outcomes, particularly in the area of academic achievement. The authors also highlight the need to consider the developmental course of alcohol involvement among college drinkers and the roles in their drinking of individual and institutional factors, as well as their interactions.

The fourth chapter, "The Initiation and Course of Alcohol Use among Adolescents and Young Adults" by Jennifer Maggs and John Schulenberg, looks within and across individuals to study the initiation of alcohol consumption and its escalation and/or de-escalation over time. In the case of alcohol consumption by adolescents, studying the developmental trajectory of drinking behavior and the roles of various risk and protective factors in influencing those trajectories at different points in development is critical to understanding the complexity of the problem we face as we work to reduce underage alcohol consumption. This chapter discusses research on the initiation of drinking and the significance of the age of initiation for future alcohol-related outcomes. This is very important since national surveys indicate that half of 8th graders have already initiated alcohol use. The chapter goes on to discuss the course of alcohol use during adolescence and early adulthood using both variable centered and pattern centered approaches for understanding drinking trajectories in individuals and populations.

Finally, the last chapter deals with the identification of alcohol abuse and alcohol dependence among youth. Accurate measurement of the problem under consideration is essential to accurate epidemiologic study and reaching appropriate conclusions. One very important part of the epidemiology of alcohol consumption among adolescents and young adults involves estimating the prevalence of alcohol use disorders in this population. In their chapter entitled, "Diagnosis, Course, and Assessment of Alcohol Abuse and Dependence in Adolescents," Tammy Chung, Christopher Martin and Ken Winters discuss the problems with applying the Diagnostic and Statistical Manual of Mental Disorders (DSM) criteria, which were developed for adults, to children and adolescents. For example, the symptoms of tolerance and drinking more or longer than intended may not be appropriate for the developmental period of adolescence. The authors underscore the need for a developmental perspective in studying the manifestation of symptoms among youth and understanding the significance of those symptoms. Although included in this section, this chapter is also pertinent to the study of treatment which involves making appropriate diagnostic inferences and therefore is also relevant to the section of the volume concerning treatment.

In summary, this section provides a great deal of very important information about alcohol consumption among adolescents and young adults. It provides information about how much and about which youth drink, describes the risk and protective factors for this behavior, discusses the initiation and course of alcohol consumption among youth, details its consequences and discusses diagnostic issues particular to youth. But in addition and equally important, each chapter also points out critical conceptual challenges which must be faced as we seek to better understand alcohol consumption and alcohol-related problems among youth in a developmental context.

1. Johnston, L. D., O'Malley, P. M., & Bachman, J. G. (2003). Monitoring the Future national survey results on drug use, 1975–2002. Volume I: Secondary school students (NIH Publication No. 03–5375). Bethesda, MD: National Institute on Drug Abuse, 520 pp.

2. National Institute on Alcohol Abuse and Alcoholism (2002). High-Risk Drinking in College: What We Know and What We Need To Learn, Final Report of the Panel on Contexts and Consequences, Task Force of the National Advisory Council on Alcohol Abuse and Alcoholism, National Institutes of Health, U. S. Department of Health and Human Services.

1

Diagnosis, Course, and Assessment of Alcohol Abuse and Dependence in Adolescents

Tammy Chung, Christopher S. Martin, and Ken C. Winters

Abstract. Risk for the onset of an alcohol use disorder (AUD) peaks during adolescence and the transition to young adulthood, highlighting the public health significance of alcohol use by adolescents. This chapter summarizes recent research on the diagnosis, course, and assessment of adolescent AUDs. This review focuses on developmental considerations in assessment of AUD criteria, the prevalence of DSM-IV AUDs among adolescents, typical alcohol symptom profiles in youth, and limitations of DSM-IV AUD criteria when applied to adolescents. In addition, studies of AUD course in adolescents, as well as factors influencing the course of AUDs are summarized. The chapter also provides an overview of brief alcohol screening instruments and other measures used in more comprehensive assessment of AUDs in adolescents.

1. Diagnosis, Course, and Assessment of Alcohol Abuse and Dependence in Adolescents

Adolescence is a period of dramatic change, involving numerous biological, cognitive, and social transitions. These changes have a significant impact on adolescent functioning, including the development of drinking behavior and alcohol-related problems. Therefore, it is important to take a developmental perspective when studying the diagnosis, course, and assessment of adolescent alcohol use disorders (AUDs). When applied to diagnosis, a developmental perspective requires consideration of how AUD symptoms

Tammy Chung and Christopher S. Martin • University of Pittsburgh Medical Center, Western Psychiatric Institute and Clinic, Pittsburgh, Pennsylvania 15213
Ken C. Winters • Center for Adolescent Substance Abuse Research, University of Minnesota, Minneapolis, Minnesota 55455

manifest differently across the lifespan, reflecting age-related differences in areas such as physical maturation, context of use, and major role obligations (e.g., school vs work). In studies of AUD course, a developmental perspective involves understanding how alcohol use and problems, and maturational and contextual variables unfold and reciprocally influence each other over time. A developmental perspective applied to AUD assessment emphasizes the need to scale measures to an individual's stage of maturation to ensure that the equivalence of a symptom's meaning and clinical significance are maintained across different developmental periods.

In youthful samples, alcohol use and episodic heavy drinking show increasing prevalence with age (Johnston et al., 2003). Adolescents typically engage in a pattern of episodic heavy drinking (Deas et al., 2000), a particularly risky pattern of use that has been associated with the occurrence of alcohol-related problems (Wechsler et al., 1995). A national school-based survey indicated that consumption of five or more drinks in a row in the past two weeks was reported by 12% of eighth graders, 22% of 10th graders, and 29% of high school seniors (Johnston et al., 2003). In this context, risk for the onset of an AUD peaks between the ages of 15 to 20 (Kessler et al., 1994; Helzer et al., 1991). Further, some data suggest an increasing prevalence of adolescent-onset AUDs in recent years (e.g., Nelson et al., 1998). These findings highlight the public health significance of adolescent alcohol use and related problems.

This chapter summarizes recent research on the diagnosis, course, and assessment of AUDs in adolescents. The chapter begins with a review of DSM-IV and ICD-10 criteria for AUDs, developmental considerations in assessment of AUD criteria, the prevalence of DSM-IV AUDs in epidemiologic surveys of adolescents, typical alcohol symptom profiles in youth, and limitations of DSM-IV AUD criteria. Next, studies of predictors and pathways in the course of adolescent AUDs are summarized, including reports on the time course of alcohol symptom development in teens, and the course of AUDs in community and clinical samples of youth. Finally, the section on assessment reviews instruments commonly used in screening for alcohol problems, and more comprehensive methods of evaluating AUDs in adolescents.

2. Diagnosis of AUDs in Adolescents

2.1. *DSM-IV and ICD-10 Alcohol Diagnoses*

Valid diagnosis is essential to advancing treatment and research on the etiology and course of mental disorders. Diagnostic categories represent evolving constructs that organize and describe a cluster of associated symptoms and behaviors. Ideally, the features that define a diagnostic category occur as a result of shared underlying core pathological processes, and thus show a distinctive course (Millon, 1991). Psychiatric diagnoses serve multiple functions, such as facilitating communication among clinicians and researchers, identifying cases for clinical intervention, increasing homogeneity of research samples, providing phenotypes for genetics research, and conveying information about prognosis (Robins & Barrett, 1989; McGue, 1999). Although alcohol problems appear to define a continuum of severity (e.g., Heath et al., 1994), diagnostic categories complement dimensional approaches by providing categorical groupings that are ultimately necessary to guide research and treatment.

DSM-IV (APA, 2000) includes two AUDs, alcohol abuse and alcohol dependence, which are defined by non-overlapping criterion sets (Table 1). DSM-IV abuse focuses on negative psychosocial consequences resulting from alcohol use, as well as hazardous use, and requires the presence of at least 1 of 4 criteria. Abuse is generally considered a milder AUD relative to dependence due to its one symptom threshold for diagnosis (APA, 2000). DSM-IV dependence, based in part on the Alcohol Dependence Syndrome concept (Edwards & Gross, 1976), is diagnosed when at least 3 of 7 criteria are met within the same 12-month period. Dependence criteria relate to addiction constructs such as

Table 1. DSM-IV Alcohol Abuse and Dependence Criteria

	Alcohol Abuse	
Brief Identifier		Abstracted DSM-IV criterion
A1	Role Impairment	Frequent intoxication leading to failure to fulfill obligations at school, work, home
A2	Hazardous Use	Recurrent use when physically hazardous (e.g., drinking and driving)
A3	Legal Problems	Recurrent alcohol-related legal problems
A4	Social Problems	Continued use despite social or interpersonal problems caused or exacerbated by use
	Alcohol Dependence	
Brief Identifier		Abstracted DSM-IV criterion
D1	Tolerance	Need to consume more to obtain the same effect; decreased effect at the same dose
D2	Withdrawal	Withdrawal symptoms; drinking to avoid or relieve withdrawal
D3	Larger/Longer	Drinking more or longer than intended
D4	Quit/Cut Down	Persistent desire or repeated unsuccessful attempts to quit or cut down on alcohol use
D5	Much Time	Much time spent obtaining, using, or recovering from the effects of alcohol
D6	Reduced Activities	Reduce or stop important activities in order to drink
D7	Physical/ Psychological Problems	Continued use despite physical or psychological problems caused or exacerbated by use

physical dependence (i.e., tolerance or withdrawal), salience of alcohol use (e.g., lot of time spent drinking), and impaired control over alcohol use (e.g., drinking more or longer than intended). Although no single criterion is necessary or sufficient for a dependence diagnosis, DSM-IV alcohol dependence can be subtyped as with "physiological features," if criteria for tolerance or withdrawal have been met. A diagnosis of dependence precludes abuse, suggesting a hierarchical relation between the two AUDs. Both DSM-IV AUDs require evidence of clinically significant impairment or subjective distress resulting from alcohol use for diagnosis. DSM-IV criteria for alcohol diagnoses are similar to criteria used to diagnose other drug use disorders, although some important differences exist. Due to the high rate of poly-substance use among youth (e.g., Martin et al., 1996a), both alcohol and other drug use behaviors should be assessed in research and clinical settings.

Other classification systems for AUDs, such as ICD-10 (WHO, 1992), have been less well researched in adolescents compared to DSM-IV. ICD-10, like DSM-IV, includes two AUDs: harmful use and dependence. The harmful use diagnosis is represented by a single criterion that specifies a pattern of alcohol use that is causing damage to physical or psychological health. Dependence in ICD-10 requires that 3 or more of 6 symptoms co-occur within a 12-month period: harmful use, tolerance, withdrawal, strong desire to use, impaired control over alcohol use, and preoccupation with use (e.g., giving up activities to drink instead). As in DSM-IV, an ICD-10 diagnosis of dependence precludes harmful use. However, in contrast to DSM-IV, ICD-10 diagnoses of abuse and dependence have overlapping criterion sets. Diagnostic concordance between DSM-IV and ICD-10 AUDs in adolescent drinkers indicated high agreement for the distinction between dependence and no dependence groups (kappa=.81), but poor agreement for the distinction between abuse/harmful use and no diagnosis groups (kappa=.10) (Pollock et al., 2000). These findings reveal a substantial limitation of the abuse/harmful use diagnosis that results from inconsistency in the definition of the abuse/harmful use category across the DSM-IV and ICD-10 classification systems. Other, alternative AUD classification schemes developed specifically for youth also have been proposed (e.g., Wolraich et al., 1996). However, recent diagnostic research on teens has focused almost exclusively on the application of DSM-IV AUDs.

2.2. *Developmental Considerations in AUD Assessment*

Diagnostic criteria for AUDs were derived largely from clinical and research experience with adults, and have been applied to adolescents with no modification of the criteria or diagnostic thresholds. However, numerous developmental differences between adolescents and adults may affect the applicability of AUD criteria to youth. For example, adolescent drinkers have shorter histories of alcohol use compared to adults; and adolescents tend to drink less often, but typically consume a similar quantity per occasion (i.e., heavy episodic drinking) (Bailey et al., 2000; Deas et al., 2000). Developmental differences in alcohol use patterns emphasize the need to adapt constructs and criteria to make them relevant to and properly scaled for an adolescent's stage of maturation (Brown, 1999). Further, assessment that includes expanded descriptions of symptoms such as "blackout" and "passing out," and specific examples of the phenomenon of interest, can facilitate shared understanding between respondent and interviewer regarding the symptom being queried. Because a construct may manifest differently in adolescents and adults (e.g., role impairment at school vs work), a developmental perspective that takes maturational factors and contextual influences into account is essential for valid assessment of AUDs across the life span.

2.3. *Prevalence of Adolescent AUDs*

The prevalence of adolescent AUDs increases with age, and is generally higher among males compared to females (Martin & Winters, 1998). Using DSM-III-R criteria, AUD prevalence increased from 3.5% among 14 to 16 year olds to 14.6% of 17 to 20 year olds (Cohen et al., 1993). Among 15 to 18 year olds in the National Comorbidity Survey, 13.5% met criteria for a lifetime DSM-IV AUD (Warner et al., 2001). In addition to teens who meet criteria for an alcohol diagnosis, a substantial proportion of youth have AUD symptoms (i.e., 1–2 dependence symptoms), but do not meet criteria for an alcohol diagnosis. These symptomatic teens without an alcohol diagnosis are known as "diagnostic orphans" (Pollock & Martin, 1999), and account for up to an additional 17% of adolescents in community surveys (Chung et al., 2002).

A review of cross-study consistency in DSM-IV AUD prevalence across 4 community surveys in the United States noted lifetime prevalence estimates ranging widely from 1.0 to 13.5% (Chung et al., 2002). In these 4 surveys, lifetime prevalence of DSM-IV alcohol abuse ranged from 0.4 to 9.6%, while alcohol dependence ranged from 0.6 to 4.3%. Variability in the estimated prevalence of AUDs across surveys may be explained, in part, by differences in factors such as sampling strategy (i.e., household vs school-based survey), sample age range, time frame for diagnosis (e.g., past year vs lifetime), and other methodological factors. However, although absolute proportions of cases with an AUD diagnosis may vary due to methodological factors, the relative prevalence of abuse and dependence diagnoses, that is, the ratio of abuse to dependence diagnoses should be relatively consistent across community surveys. DSM-IV does not specify an expected ratio of abuse to dependence in the general population. In the general population, however, milder cases of illness (i.e., abuse) usually outnumber more severe cases (i.e., dependence) (Skinner, 1986). Across 5 community surveys, the abuse-to-dependence ratio ranged from 0.4:1.0 to 4.5:1.0 with a mean ratio of 2.2:1.0 (Chung et al., 2002). Two of the 5 community surveys reported higher rates of the more severe dependence diagnosis relative to the milder abuse diagnosis, and in both surveys, several alcohol dependence symptoms had higher absolute prevalence than the most frequently assigned abuse symptom. These findings point to a major limitation of DSM-IV AUDs in adolescents, because if abuse and dependence diagnoses are to provide clinically meaningful information, the diagnostic criteria should produce a consistent ratio of the two diagnoses across community samples. Some problems in the assignment of alcohol diagnoses in teens appear to be due to the prevalence of certain dependence symptoms, such as tolerance and drinking more or longer than intended (Chung et al., 2001; Chung & Martin, 2002), emphasizing the importance of valid symptom assessment in youth.

Certain adolescent populations, such as homeless youth, teens involved in the juvenile justice system, and youth seen in psychiatric and some medical settings, have elevated rates of AUD. In a convenience sample of homeless youth, 45% met criteria for alcohol dependence in the past year, 22% for abuse, and 13% were alcohol orphans (Baer et al., 2003). Overall, the majority (80%) of homeless youth in that study reported at least one AUD symptom. Among teens involved with the juvenile justice system, almost one-third (32%) are estimated to meet criteria for an AUD, although the prevalence of AUDs in this high-risk population is largely unknown (Bilchik, 1998). Among adolescent psychiatric inpatients, one study found that 41% met criteria for a current DSM-III-R AUD (Grilo et al., 1996). In an adolescent emergency department sample, 18% of 14 to 19 year olds presenting for treatment of a non-alcohol related injury met criteria for a current DSM-IV AUD (Chung et al., 2000). The high rate of AUDs in certain adolescent populations indicates the utility of alcohol screening among at-risk teens to efficiently identify those who may benefit from alcohol treatment.

Little is known about cross-cultural differences in adolescent AUD prevalence. The literature indicates higher AUD prevalence among teens in the United States compared to Puerto Rico (Warner et al., 2001), and slightly higher AUD prevalence among German youth (Nelson & Wittchen, 1998) compared to teens in the National Comorbidity Survey.

2.4. *Alcohol Symptom Profiles in Youth*

A review of the relative prevalence of DSM-IV AUD symptoms in 5 community and 4 clinical samples of adolescents found only a modest level of agreement (mean Spearman rho=0.47) across studies (Chung et al., 2002). The AUD symptoms assigned to teens most often were two dependence criteria: tolerance and drinking more or longer than intended. Importantly, cross-study variation in the high prevalence of these two common dependence symptoms strongly affect the ratio of abuse to dependence diagnoses, the prevalence of the physiological dependence subtype, and the proportion of subthreshold cases of dependence.

Another method of characterizing adolescents' alcohol symptom profiles, latent class analysis (LCA), assumes that a small number of mutually exclusive latent classes or subtypes can be used to represent the symptom profiles of individuals in a sample. LCA of adolescents' alcohol symptoms does not support the distinct categories of abuse and dependence defined by DSM-IV (Bucholz et al., 2000; Chung & Martin, 2001). Instead, LCA suggests that DSM-IV alcohol symptoms represent classes arranged along a gradient of illness severity that represent milder and more severe problems, such that the total number of symptoms, rather than type of symptom (i.e., abuse or dependence) distinguishes the classes (Chung & Martin, 2001). In the milder severity class, alcohol-related social problems, an abuse symptom, and tolerance, a dependence symptom had high probability of endorsement. The more severe class was characterized by symptoms that were elevated in the mild class, as well as by higher rates of endorsement for symptoms of alcohol-related role impairment, drinking more or longer than intended, and much time spent drinking. Across all classes, withdrawal was endorsed least often. Some research suggests that withdrawal, in addition to its relatively low prevalence in youth (Langenbucher et al., 2000), may manifest differently in teens compared to adults (Stewart & Brown, 1995). Although LCA produces severity-based profiles of alcohol symptoms in both adolescent and adult samples (e.g., Heath et al., 1994), important developmental differences have been identified with regard to rate of progression from use to problems, severity of alcohol problems and dependence, and the types of alcohol-related problems most likely to be experienced (Deas et al., 2000).

2.5. *Limitations of DSM-IV AUDs in Adolescents*

Although DSM-IV AUDs have shown some validity when used with adolescents in that teens classified as having alcohol dependence, abuse, and no diagnosis differ on external measures of alcohol involvement (e.g., Lewinsohn et al., 1996; Winters et al., 1999), DSM-IV AUDs have limitations, some of which are particularly evident when the criteria are applied to teens. In particular, the abuse and dependence criterion sets are not well distinguished conceptually, and research does not support the distinction between the two criterion sets in severity, age of symptom onset, or symptom profiles identified by latent class analysis or factor analysis. Specific limitations of the abuse diagnosis include its low concordance across different diagnostic systems (Pollock et al., 2000; Mikulich et al., 2001). Abuse criteria also appear to cover problems that are more severe compared to some dependence criteria (Bailey, 1999; Pollock & Martin, 1999). Further, because abuse is generally considered a milder illness category than dependence, the onset of abuse is expected to precede dependence, however, dependence symptoms of tolerance and drinking more or longer than intended typically precede the onset of most abuse symptoms (Martin et al., 1996b; Wagner et al., 2002). In addition, some community surveys report higher prevalence of the more severe dependence diagnosis relative to the milder abuse diagnosis (Chung et al., 2002), a situation that does not conform to most disorders in medicine in which milder conditions are more prevalent than severe conditions. Another limitation of DSM-IV AUDs more generally is the existence of "diagnostic orphans" (i.e., those who have 1–2 dependence symptoms, but do not meet criteria for a DSM-IV AUD). Orphans receive no alcohol diagnosis, but do not differ from those with DSM-IV alcohol abuse on various external validators and outcomes (Pollock & Martin, 1999).

At the criterion level, certain symptoms (e.g., withdrawal) tend to occur only after years of heavy drinking, and have low prevalence and limited utility when applied to teens. In contrast, many adolescents who engage in relatively low levels of alcohol use meet criteria for an abuse diagnosis merely due to alcohol-related arguments with family members, and may be considered to constitute a group termed "diagnostic impostors" (Martin, 1999). Other DSM-IV AUD symptoms appear to be more relevant to specific adolescent subgroups. For example, hazardous use and legal problems have been associated with male gender, increased age, ethnic background, and presence of conduct disorder symptoms in teens (Langenbucher & Martin, 1996; Wagner et al., 2002). Ethnicity and gender have been found to influence whether and when certain DSM-IV AUD symptoms tend to occur in teen drinkers (Wagner et al., 2002).

In addition, some symptoms appear to be poorly defined or scaled for the developmental period of adolescence (Martin & Winters, 1998; Winters et al., 1999). Specifically, symptoms with high prevalence among adolescent drinkers, such as tolerance and drinking more or longer than intended, tend to identify a substantial proportion of adolescents with relatively low levels of consumption and problem severity. For example, because some level of tolerance may occur as a normative developmental phenomenon, better guidelines regarding the identification of a clinically significant level of tolerance need to be developed for use with adolescents. Research has demonstrated limitations of DSM's tolerance criterion when operationally defined as a "marked increase to obtain the same effect" by pointing out how large individual differences in initial quantity to become intoxicated affect whether or not the tolerance symptom is assigned (Chung et al., 2001). Using DSM's change-based definition of tolerance (i.e., a marked increase in quantity), individuals who report low initial quantities to become intoxicated are more likely to report larger increases to obtain the same effect (e.g., increase from 2 drinks to 8), while those with high initial quantities tend to report smaller increases to obtain the same effect (e.g. increase from 6 drinks to 8). Thus, in rating the presence of tolerance based on a "marked increase" as defined by DSM, the tolerance symptom may be overassigned to those who report low initial quantities and underassigned to those who report high initial quantities. To improve validity of symptom assessment in youth, developmentally appropriate operational definitions of AUD criteria, such as tolerance, need to be developed and tested.

Another limitation regarding symptom assessment in adolescents is that some AUD criteria may be interpreted differently or have different meaning when used with adolescents. Specifically, the high prevalence symptom of drinking more or longer than intended may be susceptible to false positive assignments in youth (i.e., assignment of the symptom in the true absence of the phenomenon). Despite some evidence for the concurrent validity of the symptom in adolescent drinkers (Chung & Martin, 2002), "drinking more than intended" may occur in teens due to poor judgment, inexperience with alcohol's effects, or social pressures to drink, rather than a compulsive pattern of alcohol use. Development of more specific interview probes that query contextual factors, such as adolescents' motivations for drinking, reasons for limiting alcohol use, and perceived ability to control alcohol use within a drinking episode is needed to better identify the clinical phenomenon of impaired control over alcohol use in adolescents.

3. Course of Adolescent AUDs

Clinical course refers to changes and trends in the manifestation of disorders and associated functioning over time (Brown, 1993). Studies of the course of adolescent AUDs are critical to understanding prognosis and etiology, and determining the predictive validity of diagnostic categories. Whereas some adolescent alcohol use may reflect experimentation that occurs as a normative developmental transition (Kandel, 1975), early initiation of drinking (i.e., before age 20) has been associated with greater risk for alcohol problems in adulthood (Nelson & Wittchen, 1998; Rhode et al., 2001). Many adolescent drinkers, particularly those with less severe alcohol problems, tend to mature out of problem drinking (Labouvie, 1996; Maisto et al., 2001), while others show a more chronic course through adulthood (Abrantes et al., 2002). Multiple developmental trajectories of adolescent-onset alcohol use and problems exist (e.g., Schulenberg et al., 2001), and have been characterized as developmentally-limited or persistent, with problems that may be relatively continuous or intermittent (Zucker et al., 1994). Developmental changes in areas such as co-occurring psychopathology and other drug use, social relationships, and role transitions have been found to affect AUD course in adolescents.

3.1. *Development of Alcohol Symptoms in Youth*

Compared to adults, adolescents tend to show more rapid progression from use to problems (Deas et al., 2000). In one community survey, females had earlier onset of AUD compared to males (14.6 vs 16.1 years old; Lewinsohn et al., 1996). However, males developed alcohol-related problems at a faster rate between the ages of 18–19 (Lewinsohn et al., 1996). Research using survival analysis to examine the sequential emergence of DSM-IV alcohol symptoms in youth suggests that AUD symptoms tend to emerge in three stages: heavy and heedless use, dependence, and withdrawal (Martin et al., 1996b; Wagner et al., 2002). Within the first two years after the start of regular drinking, the first stage of heavy and heedless use tends to emerge, as indicated by the onset of drinking more or longer than intended and interpersonal problems due to drinking. Through the third and fourth years of regular drinking, dependence symptoms of tolerance and much time spent using tend to onset. The third stage, represented by the emergence of alcohol withdrawal, does not occur for most teens. Although several stages of symptom development appear to exist, progression from one stage to another is not inevitable.

3.2. *Course in Community and Clinical Samples of Adolescents*

3.2.1. Community Samples. Few community studies have described the course of adolescent-onset AUDs. In longitudinal epidemiologic studies, alcohol problems that occur in adolescence and young adulthood are only modestly associated (e.g., Baer et al., 1995; Rohde et al., 2001). The average duration of an AUD was about 52 weeks in community adolescents (Lewinsohn et al., 1996). The alcohol abuse diagnosis appears to be particularly transient, with a high rate of transitions into and out of this category during adolescence (Nelson & Wittchen, 1998). In a school-based sample followed through age 24, the annual rate of AUD recurrence was 8% among those with an AUD at the initial assessment (Rohde et al., 2001). Compared to teens with no AUD symptoms at initial assessment, teens with symptoms but no alcohol diagnosis (i.e., diagnostic orphans) were more likely to have an AUD by age 24 than those with no symptoms (Rohde et al., 2001).

3.2.2. Clinical Samples. At least 4 years of follow-up have been recommended to describe the clinical course of AUDs (Nathan & Skinstad, 1987). However, most studies of treated adolescents report outcomes through one year follow-up or less (Catalano & Hawkins, 1990–91; Williams & Chang, 2000). Much of the existing clinical literature on adolescents has focused on the high rates of relapse following treatment, which are similar to those for treated adults, although differences in reasons for initial relapse and continuing alcohol use have been identified, with teens typically reporting social, rather than negative affect, reasons as factors motivating their alcohol use behavior (Brown, 1993; Cornelius et al., 2003). Sustained abstinence from alcohol among treated youth occurs as a relatively rare outcome across studies (Winters, 1999). However, some research suggests that a substantial proportion of treated youth change to moderate drinking without apparent associated problems and show concurrent improvements in psychosocial functioning over follow-up (Maisto et al., 2002). Apparent non-problem drinking among treated youth suggests the need to consider different definitions of relapse and successful treatment outcomes.

Treated adolescents generally show reductions in alcohol use and problems over both short and longer-term follow-up (Chung et al., 2003; Williams & Chang, 2000). In an adolescent clinical sample followed over 3 years, transitions in AUD status suggested particular patterns of diagnosing: dependent adolescents were equally likely to remain dependent or remit to no diagnosis; adolescents with abuse were most likely to remain abusers or remit to no diagnosis; and those with no AUD at baseline had a high likelihood of maintaining this status (Martin et al., 2000a). Transition probabilities were fairly stable across 1- and 3-year follow-ups. Other data also suggest that the longer-term course of adolescent AUDs is highly variable (Brown et al, 2001; Chung et al., 2003). For example, among adolescent inpatients followed over 8 years, 4 alcohol involvement trajectories were identified: abstainers (22%), infrequent users (24%), worse with time (36%), and frequent users (18%) (Abrantes et al., 2002;

Brown et al., 2001). Teens in the low alcohol use trajectories tended to use fewer drugs during follow-up, and had better psychosocial functioning. Changes in different domains of psychosocial functioning occurred at different rates: school functioning improved relatively quickly, but improvements in family functioning only became evident after 2-years (Brown et al., 1994; Abrantes et al., 2002).

Pretreatment, during treatment, and post-treatment variables have been examined as predictors of course in treated teens. *Pretreatment* patient characteristics typically associated with better teen substance use outcomes include lower substance use severity at admission (e.g., Maisto et al., 2001), greater readiness to change (e.g., Kelly et al., 2000), and fewer conduct problems and other co-occurring psychopathology (e.g., Grella et al., 2001; Winters et al., 2000). *During treatment* factors generally found to predict better substance use outcomes include longer length of treatment (e.g., Hser et al., 2001) and family involvement in treatment (Liddle & Dakof, 1995). *Posttreatment* factors consistently associated with better youth outcomes include participation in aftercare (e.g., Winters et al., 2000b), low levels of peer substance use during follow-up (e.g., Winters et al., 2000b), use of substance-coping (Myers et al., 1993), and continued commitment to abstain (Kelly et al., 2000). Overall, posttreatment factors accounted for more of the variance in teens' clinical outcomes through 1-year than pre- and during-treatment factors (e.g., Hsieh et al., 1998). Importantly, the impact of a predictor on course may vary as a function of the length of follow-up, and the predictor itself may change over time. For example, sibling drug use was associated with more frequent drug use in the first 6 months posttreatment, however, as follow-up continued, peer use became a more important predictor of outcome than family environment variables such as sibling substance use (Latimer et al., 2000).

3.2.3. Co-occurring Psychopathology and AUD Course. AUD course needs to be considered in the broader context of co-occurring psychopathology. In a school-based sample, more than 80% of teens with an AUD had a co-occurring lifetime conduct, mood, substance or tobacco use disorder (Rohde et al., 1996). Similarly, the majority of youth (63%) in the Drug Abuse Treatment Outcome Studies for Adolescents had a co-occurring non-substance related mental disorder (Hser et al., 2001). Increased understanding of the temporal relationships between the onset of AUD and other psychopathology has implications for determining the extent to which co-occurring disorders share a common etiologic diathesis (e.g., AUD and disruptive behavior disorders) or reciprocally influence illness course (e.g., AUD and negative affect disorder) (e.g., Sher & Gotham, 1999). With regard to the sequential emergence of disorders over time in youth, other non-substance-related psychopathology often precedes the onset of AUD (Armstrong & Costello, 2002; Clark et al., 1999; Myers et al., 1998). Of particular concern, disruptive behavior disorders have been associated with more rapid progression from use to problems in adolescents (Costello et al., 1999; Rohde et al., 1996). Further, conduct disorder that precedes AUD onset predicts poorer outcomes among treated adolescents (Myers et al., 1995; Whitmore et al., 1997). Although antisocial behavior may be exacerbated by alcohol and other drug use (e.g., Myers et al., 1998), retrospective research with adults suggests that a developmental trajectory of persistent antisociality and alcohol problems may reflect shared etiologic factors (e.g., Hopfer et al., 2003; Slutske et al., 1998).

4. Assessment of AUDs in Adolescents

Depending on the purpose of the evaluation, the assessment of adolescent alcohol use, associated problems, and AUDs can range from brief alcohol screening to in-depth evaluation that involves multidimensional measures of substance use severity and psychosocial functioning. This section reviews selected measures used to screen adolescents for AUDs; diagnostic interviews used to determine the presence of substance use disorders, along with data on the reliability and validity of diagnostic interviews; and selected questionnaire measures used to assess adolescent alcohol involvement. Review articles and sourcebooks provide more detailed guidelines for the selection of interview and questionnaire measures to meet specific assessment needs (e.g., Allen & Columbus, 1995; Center for Substance Abuse Treatment, 1999; Leccese & Waldron, 1994; Meyers et al., 1999; Winters, 2001).

4.1. *Screening Adolescents for AUDs*

Alcohol screening efficiently identifies youth who may have alcohol problems or an AUD, and who would benefit from more in-depth assessment and possible intervention. The American Medical Association recommends that health care providers routinely screen all adolescents seen in medical settings for AUDs (Elster & Kuznets, 1994). Screening also plays an important role in identifying youth at high-risk for AUDs in settings where assessment time and resources may be limited, such as schools, juvenile justice and psychiatric settings, and homeless shelters. Although screening can quickly identify youth who may have an AUD, screening results need to be interpreted with caution. A score above a screen's designated cut-off does not necessarily indicate the presence of an AUD, only that more in-depth assessment should be conducted to determine the nature and severity of alcohol involvement. Similarly, a score below the screening cut-off does not signify the absence of an AUD, only that its presence is not likely. Research comparing the performance of brief screens (i.e., $\leq$10 items) in identifying AUDs in adolescents suggests the superior utility of two screens: the Alcohol Use Disorders Identification Test (AUDIT; Babor et al., 1989) and CRAFFT (Knight et al., 2003). Although the CAGE (Ewing, 1984) is used widely with adults, its coverage of later occurring alcohol problems limits its utility when used to screen adolescents (Chung et al., 2000; Knight et al., 2003).

The AUDIT is a 10-item questionnaire developed for use with adults that queries level of consumption (3 items) and alcohol-related problems (7 items). In adolescent medical patients, the AUDIT performed best at a cut-score of 3 (sensitivity=.76, specificity=.97; Knight et al., 2003) or at a cut-score of 4 (sensitivity=.94, specificity=.80; Chung et al., 2000). Of note, suggested scores for use with teens are lower than the recommended cut-score of 8 typically used with adults. A particular strength of the AUDIT is its inclusion of items querying level of alcohol consumption. In one study, a teen's score on the AUDIT's three consumption items, at a cut-score of 3, had similar overall performance compared to the AUDIT total score in identifying youth with an AUD, highlighting the importance of querying level of alcohol consumption when screening youth (Chung et al., 2002). Despite the AUDIT's better performance compared to other screens (e.g., CAGE), its length and relatively complicated scoring limit its use as a screen that a clinician can administer verbally and from memory.

CRAFFT is an acronym for a 6-item screen that was designed specifically for use with adolescents to detect both alcohol and drug problems. The screen's brevity and ease of verbal administration and scoring provide distinct advantages, and its overall performance in identifying youth with an AUD did not differ significantly from the AUDIT (Knight et al., 2003). CRAFFT cues the following questions: Have you ridden in a *C*ar driven by someone (including yourself) who had been drinking or using drugs? Do you use alcohol or drugs to *R*elax, feel better about yourself, or fit in? Do you use alcohol or drugs while you are by yourself, *A*lone? Do you *F*orget things you did while using alcohol or drugs? Do your family or *F*riends tell you that you should cut down on your drinking or drug use? Have you gotten into *T*rouble while using alcohol or drugs? The CRAFFT, which assumes that level of consumption has been queried separately, performed best at a cut-score of 2 (sensitivity=.71, specificity=.94) when used to identify teens with a DSM-IV substance use disorder in a medical clinic setting (Knight et al., 2003).

4.2. *Comprehensive AUD Assessment*

Comprehensive substance use assessment is usually conducted in clinical settings to determine need for treatment and appropriate level of care, or for research purposes. In-depth assessment typically reviews a teen's pattern of alcohol and other drug use, reasons for substance use (e.g., social, coping motives), readiness to change substance use behavior, the frequency and persistence of substance-related problems, extent of family and peer substance use, prior episodes of mental health and medical treatment, legal history (e.g., arrests, probation), co-occurring psychopathology, and psychosocial functioning (e.g., school achievement, peer relations). With regard to pattern of use, specific information on age at initiation of alcohol and other drug use, and onset of regular use pattern (i.e., weekly or more frequent use), including changes in level of consumption (i.e., frequency, quantity consumed per occasion, duration at specific use levels) over time, is needed to determine need for any treatment, and the most appropriate level of care. Determination of ages of symptom onset and offset is useful in tracking illness course, as well as monitoring treatment effects over time.

4.2.1. Diagnostic Interviews. To determine the presence of DSM-based alcohol and other substance use disorder diagnoses, a number of structured and semi-structured interviews have been developed that use standardized symptom definitions and question formats (Table 2). Symptom probes and thresholds used to determine the presence of a diagnosis have been designed to correspond directly to DSM criteria. Some interviews were developed specifically to assess level of substance involvement and substance use disorders in adolescents (e.g., Adolescent Diagnostic Interview). Whereas structured interviews require that questions are asked verbatim, semi-structured interviews provide a highly trained interviewer with greater flexibility in asking follow-up questions and determining the clinical significance of reported symptoms. Both types of interview use a decision tree format to determine the nature, persistence, duration, and clinical significance of reported symptoms. Although structured interviews may provide more consistency in results across interviewers, many researchers believe that semi-structured interviews provide for more comprehensive assessment because the interviewer can use follow-up questions to obtain a better understanding of symptom severity and factors influencing its occurrence. Selection of the type of interview to use depends on consideration of the goals of assessment, the setting in which assessment will occur, interviewer training requirements, and time allotted for the assessment.

4.2.2. Reliability and Validity of Diagnostic Interview Measures. Studies of interrater and re-test reliability of both structured and semi-structured diagnostic interview measures typically report estimates in the good to excellent range for alcohol diagnoses and criteria (e.g., Winters & Henly, 1993; Brown et al., 1998; Martin et al., 2000b). In some studies, interviewer training required that a minimum level of interrater reliability with an experienced diagnostician (i.e., kappa >.80) be obtained to ensure satisfactory levels of diagnostic reliability (e.g., Lewinsohn et al., 1996).

Certain interview measures also have demonstrated some concurrent validity of DSM-IV AUDs in adolescents. That is, teens diagnosed with DSM-IV alcohol dependence, abuse, and no diagnosis have been found to differ when compared against external validators such as quantity and frequency of alcohol use, and severity of alcohol problems (e.g., ADI: Winters & Henly, 1993; SCID: Baer et al., 2003; Martin et al., 1995; K-SADS: Lewinsohn et al., 1996). Other measures, such as the CDDR, have been shown to discriminate between youth in the general population and those in treatment, and produce results that are consistent with other diagnostic measures (Brown et al., 1998).

Table 2. Interviews for Assessing DSM-IV Alcohol Use Disorders in Adolescents

Measure	Abbreviation	Author and Supporting References	Time frame
Semi-Structured Interviews			
Child and Adolescent Psychiatric Assessment	CAPA	Angold et al., 2000	Life/3-mos
Kiddie-Schedule for Affective Disorders and Schizophrenia	K-SADS	Orvaschel et al., 1995	Life/last yr
Child Semi-structured Interview for Genetics of Alcoholism, derived in part from the DICA	C-SSAGA	Bucholz et al., 1994; Kuperman et al., 2001	Life/last yr
Structured Clinical Interview for DSM-IV	SCID	First et al., 1995; Martin et al., 1995, 2000	Life/last yr
Longitudinal Interval Follow-up Evaluation	LIFE	Keller et al., 1987; Lewinsohn et al., 1996	Length of follow-up interval
Structured Interviews			
Diagnostic Interview for Children and Adolescents	DICA	Herjanic et al., 1977; Reich et al., 1992	Life/6-mos
Diagnostic Interview Schedule-Children	DIS-C	Costello et al., 1985; Shaffer et al., 1996	Life/6-mos
Composite International Diagnostic Interview	CIDI	WHO, 1998; Andrews & Peters, 1998; Perkonigg et al., 1999	Life/6-mos
Diagnostic Interview Schedule for DSM-IV	DIS-IV	Robins et al., 2000	Life/6-mos/1-mo
Substance Involvement and Substance Use Disorder Interviews			
Adolescent Diagnostic Interview	ADI	Winters & Henly, 1993; Winters et al., 1993	Life/last yr
Customary Drinking and Drug Use Record	CDDR	Brown et al., 1998	Life/past 3 mos
Global Appraisal of Individual Needs	GAIN	Dennis et al., 2000	Life/last yr

4.2.3. Questionnaire Measures of Alcohol Involvement. Compared to interviews, questionnaires can provide a less threatening means for teens to provide information on the severity of their alcohol and other drug involvement. However, questionnaires are used primarily to gauge level of alcohol involvement, and typically are not administered to determine AUD status because they usually do not provide full coverage of DSM-IV AUD criteria. Questionnaires range in length, and can bridge the gap between brief alcohol screening and more comprehensive interview assessment, while also providing complementary information about level of use and associated problems when included as part of a comprehensive substance use assessment battery. Questionnaires commonly used to assess adolescent alcohol involvement that have good psychometric properties and that correlate with the presence of AUD diagnoses include, for example, the Adolescent Alcohol Involvement Scale (14 items; Mayer & Filstead, 1979), Rutgers Alcohol Problems Inventory (23 items; White & Labouvie, 1989), Personal Experiences Screening Questionnaire (40 items; Winters, 1992), and Personal Experiences Inventory (PEI, 276 items; Winters & Henly, 1989). Longer measures, such as the PEI, include subscales that assess personal and environmental risk factors, screen for other problem behaviors (e.g., eating disorders), and detect response bias. More information about these measures and others may be obtained in review articles (e.g., Winters, 2001) and sourcebooks (e.g., Allen & Columbus, 1995).

4.3. *Validity of Self- and Collateral Reports*

4.3.1. Validity of Self-Reports. Self-reports provide the most direct information about a teen's substance use and related problems. However, the validity of teens' self-reports remains controversial. Teen self-reports can be subject to intentional distortion of information (i.e., minimization, exaggeration). Some adolescents also may be delayed in cognitive development, which can affect their perception of problems and their willingness or ability to provide valid reports (Winters, 2001). Further, factors such as inattention, lack of motivation, and misunderstanding of questions can contribute to biased reporting by adolescents (Martin & Winters, 1998). The method of data collection also may affect the teen's willingness to provide sensitive information. Questionnaires may provide a less threatening method of reporting substance use compared to interviews, and often include scales to assess response bias. When using interviews with youth, valid self-reporting can be maximized through development of rapport, use of follow-up questions to clarify responses and inconsistencies, and comparison of self-report data with information from other sources (e.g., urine drug screen, medical record, collateral report) (Maisto et al., 1995). Despite potential challenges in obtaining valid teen self-report of sensitive information, support for the validity of youth self-reports exists (e.g., Brown et al., 1998; Winters et al., 1991). Specifically, a large proportion of youth in treatment disclose histories of substance use and related problems, information provided by the teen tends to agree with reports from other sources (e.g., parents, medical records), and reports of lifetime substance use patterns generally remain consistent over time (Stinchfield, 1997; Winters, 2001).

4.3.2. Validity of Collateral Informant Reports. Information provided by the teen's parent or guardian, sibling, and peers have been used to supplement teen self-reports of substance use and problems. Many parents and other collaterals, however, cannot provide details about their child's substance use, resulting in modest associations between mother and teen reports of the adolescent's alcohol and other drug use (Winters et al., 1996). Mothers tend to underreport the teen's level of substance use compared to the teen (Winters et al., 2000b). Similarly, peers and siblings may have limited information about the teen's actual use patterns. In one study, correlations of reports by parent and sibling informants with teen self-report of substance use were low to moderate (Waldron et al., 2001). Collateral informants may be most useful when providing data on the timing or occurrence of certain types of events, such as substance-related legal problems or episodes of hospitalization and treatment.

5. Summary

Assessment of AUDs in adolescents requires a developmental perspective that takes into account maturational and contextual factors that may affect the way in which syndromes and symptoms are manifested, as well as their potential clinical significance. Existing screening and diagnostic interviews show some utility identifying youth with AUDs, and research generally supports the reliability and validity of diagnostic interviews. Much work remains, however, to improve the validity of AUD assessment in youth. Research indicates that certain symptoms, particularly tolerance and drinking more or longer than intended, may not be appropriately scaled or operationally defined for the developmental period of adolescence. Importantly, the high, yet variable, prevalence of these dependence symptoms has had a significant impact on estimates of AUD prevalence in teens. To address the need for a better national estimate of the prevalence of DSM-IV AUDs in teens, the National Comorbidity Survey of Adolescents, which will survey 10,000 youth, was put into the field in 2001. Extending findings from cross-sectional research on adolescent AUD prevalence, longitudinal follow-up of community and clinical adolescents indicates that multiple developmental trajectories of alcohol use and problems exist, refuting the notion of an inevitable progression of alcohol symptoms in youth. A key issue for future research involves increased understanding of the course of AUDs in the context of developmental transitions, and other substance use and co-occurring psychopathology.

ACKNOWLEDGMENTS: Preparation of this chapter was supported by National Institute on Alcohol Abuse and Alcoholism K01 AA00324 and K02 AA00249, and National Institute on Drug Abuse R01 DA04434 and R01 DA05104.

References

Abrantes, A, McCarthy, DM, Aarons, GA, & Brown, SA. (July 2002). *Trajectories of alcohol involvement following addiction treatment through 8-year follow-up in adolescents.* Paper presented at the 2003 Research Society on Alcoholism meeting, San Francisco, CA.

Allen, JP & Columbus, M (Eds). (1995). *Assessing alcohol problems: A guide for clinicians and researchers* (NIAAA Treatment Handbook Series 4). Bethesda, MD: National Institute on Alcohol Abuse and Alcoholism.

American Psychiatric Association. (2000). *Diagnostic and Statistical Manual of Mental Disorders, Fourth Edition (DSM-IV), text revision.* Washington, DC: Author.

Andrews, G & Peters, L. (1998). The psychometric properties of the Composite International Diagnostic Interview. *Social Psychiatry and Psychiatric Epidemiology, 33,* 80–88.

Angold A & Costello EJ (2000) The Child and Adolescent Psychiatric Assessment (CAPA). *Journal of the American Academy of Child & Adolescent Psychiatry, 39,* 39–48.

Armstrong, TD & Costello, EJ. (2002). Community studies of adolescent substance use, abuse, or dependence and psychiatric comorbidity. *Journal of Consulting and Clinical Psychology, 70,* 1224–1239.

Babor, TF, De LaFuente, JR, Saunders, J & Grant, M. (1989). AUDIT: The alcohol use disorders identification test: Guidelines for use in primary health care. WHO Publication No 89.4. Geneva: World Health Organization.

Baer, JS, Ginzler, JA, & Peterson, PL (2003). DSM-IV alcohol and substance abuse and dependence in homeless youth. *Journal of Studies on Alcohol, 64,* 5–14.

Baer, JS, Kivlahan, DR & Marlatt, GA. (1995). High risk drinking across the transition from high school to college. *Alcoholism: Clinical and Experimental Research, 19,* 54–61.

Bailey, SL. (1999). The measurement of problem drinking in young adulthood. *Journal of Studies on Alcohol, 60,* 234–244.

Bailey, SL, Martin, CS, Lynch, KG, & Pollock, NK. (2000). Reliability and concurrent validity of DSM-IV subclinical symptom ratings for alcohol use disorders among adolescents. *Alcoholism: Clinical and Experimental Research, 24,* 1795–1802.

Bilchik, S. 1998. *Mental Health Disorders and Substance Abuse Problems Among Juveniles.* Fact Sheet. Washington, DC: U.S. Department of Justice, Office of Justice Programs, Office of Juvenile Justice and Delinquency Prevention.

Brown, SA (1993). Recovery patterns in adolescent substance abuse. In JS Barr, GA Marlatt & RJ Mahon (Eds), *Addictive behaviors across the life span* (pp. 161–183).

Brown, SA. (1999, July). A double-developmental model of adolescent substance abuse. Presented at the annual meeting of the Research Society on Alcoholism, Santa Barbara, CA.

Brown, SA, D'Amico, EJ, McCarthy, DM, & Tapert, SF. (2001). Four-year outcomes from adolescent alcohol and drug treatment. *Journal of Studies on Alcohol, 62,* 381–388.

Brown, S.A., Myers, M.G., Lippke, L., Tapert, S.F., Stewart, D.G., & Vik, P.W. (1998). Psychometric evaluation of the customary drinking and drug use record (CDDR): A measure of adolescent alcohol and drug use involvement. *Journal of Studies on Alcohol, 59,* 427–438.

Brown, SA, Myers, MG, Mott, MA & Vik, PW. (1994). Correlates of success following treatment for adolescent substance abuse. *Applied Preventive Psychology, 3,* 61–73.

Bucholz KK, Cadoret R, Cloninger CR. (1994). A new, semi-structured psychiatric interview for use in genetic linkage studies: a report on the reliability, of the SSAGA. *Journal of Studies on Alcohol, 55:*149–158

Bucholz, KK, Heath, AC, & Madden, PAF. (2000). Transitions in drinking in adolescent females: Evidence from the Missouri Adolescent Female Twin Study. *Alcoholism: Clinical and Experimental Research, 24,* 914–923.

Catalano, RF, Hawkins, JD, Wells, EA, & Miller, JL (1990–91) Evaluation of the effectiveness of adolescent drug abuse treatment, assessment of risks for relapse, and promising approaches for relapse prevention. *International Journal of the Addictions, 25,* 1085–1140.

Center for Substance Abuse Treatment. (1999). *Screening and assessing adolescents for substance use disorders* (Treatment Improvement Protocol Series 31). Rockville, MD: Substance Abuse Mental Health Services Administration.

Chung, T, Colby, SM, Barnett, NP, & Monti, PM. (2002). Alcohol Use Disorders Identification Test: Factor structure in an adolescent emergency department sample. *Alcoholism: Clinical and Experimental Research, 26,* 223–231.

Chung, T., Colby, S., Barnett, N., Rohsenow, D., Spirito, A., & Monti, P. (2000). Screening adolescents for problem drinking in a hospital setting. *Journal of Studies on Alcohol, 61,* 579–587.

Chung, T & Martin, CS. (2001). Classification and course of alcohol problems among adolescents in addictions treatment programs. *Alcoholism: Clinical and Experimental Research, 25,* 1734–1742.

Chung, T & Martin, CS (2002). Concurrent and discriminant validity of DSM-IV symptoms of impaired control over alcohol consumption in adolescents. *Alcoholism: Clinical and Experimental Research, 26,* 485–492.

Chung, T, Martin, CS, Armstrong, TD & Labouvie, EW (2002). Prevalence of DSM-IV alcohol diagnoses and symptoms in adolescent community and clinical samples. *Journal of the American Academy of Child and Adolescent Psychiatry, 41,* 546–554.

Chung T, Martin CS, Grella C, Winters KC, & Abrantes AM (2003). Course of alcohol problems in treated adolescents: Symposium proceedings of 2002 Research Society on Alcoholism Meeting. *Alcoholism: Clinical and Experimental Research, 27,* 253–261.

Chung, T., Martin, CS, Winters, KC & Langenbucher, JW. (2001). Assessment of alcohol tolerance in adolescents. *Journal of Studies on Alcohol, 62,* 687–695.

Clark, DB, Parker, AM & Lynch, KG. (1999). Psychopathology and substance-related problems during early adolescence: A survival analysis. *Journal of Clinical Child Psychology, 28,* 333–341.

Cohen, P., Cohen, J., Kasen, S., Velez, C.M., Hartmark, C., Johnson, J., Rojas, M., Brook, J., & Streuning, E.L. (1993) An epidemiological study of disorders in late childhood and adolescence, I. Age- and gender-specific prevalence. *Journal of Child Psychology and Psychiatry, 34,* 851–867.

Cornelius, JR, Maisto, SA, Pollock, NK, Martin, CS, Salloum, IM, Lynch, KG & Clark, DB. (2003). Rapid relapse generally follows treatment for substance use disorders among adolescents. *Addictive Behaviors, 28,* 381–386.

Costello, EJ, Edelbrock, C & Costello, AJ. (1985). Validity of the NIMH Diagnostic Interview Schedule for Children: A comparison between psychiatric and pediatric referrals. *Journal of Abnormal Child Psychology, 13,* 570–595.

Costello, EJ, Erkanli, A, Federman, E, & Angold, A. (1999). Development of psychiatric comorbidity with substance abuse in adolescents: Effects of timing and sex. *Journal of Clinical Child Psychology, 28,* 298–311.

Deas, D., Riggs, P., Langenbucher, J., Goldman, M., & Brown, S. (2000). Adolescents are not adults: Developmental considerations in alcohol users. *Alcoholism: Clinical and Experimental Research, 24,* 232–237.

Dennis, ML, Titus, JC, White, MK, Unsicker, JI & Hodgkins, D. (2002). *Global Appraisal of Individual Needs (GAIN): Administration guide for the GAIN and related measures.* Bloomington, IL: Chestnut Health Systems. [Online] Available at: www.chestnut.org/li/gain.

Edwards, G., & Gross, M. (1976). Alcohol dependence: provisional description of a clinical syndrome. *British Medical Journal, 1,* 1058–1061.

Elster, AB & Kuznets, NJ (Eds). (1994). *American Medical Association Guidelines for Adolescent Preventive Service (GAPS).* Baltimore, MD: Williams & Wilkins.

Ewing, JA (1984). Detecting alcoholism: The CAGE questionnaire. *JAMA, 252:* 1905–1907.

First, MB, Spitzer, RL, Gibbon, M & Williams, JBW. (1997). *Structured clinical interview for DSM-IV Axis I Disorders, Research Version, Non-patient edition. (SCID-I/NP).* New York: Biometrics Research, New York State Psychiatric Institute.

Grella, C, Hser, Y-I, Joshi, V, & Rounds-Bryant, J. (2001). Drug treatment outcomes for adolescents with comorbid mental and substance use disorders. *Journal of Nervous and Mental Disease, 189,* 384–392.

Grilo, CM, Becker, DF, Fehon, DC, Edell, WC, & McGlashan, TH. (1996). Conduct disorder, substance use disorders, and co-existing conduct and substance use disorders in adolescent inpatients. *The American Journal of Psychiatry, 153,* 914–920.

Heath, AC, Bucholz, KK, Slutske, WS, Madden, PAF, Dinwiddie, SH, Dunne, MP, Statham, DB, Whitfield, JB, Martin, NG, & Eaves, LJ. (1994). The assessment of alcoholism in surveys of the general community: What are we measuring? Some insights from the Australian twin panel interview survey. *International Review of Psychiatry, 6,* 295–307.

Helzer, JE, Burnam, A, & McEvoy, LT. (1991). Alcohol abuse and dependence. In L Robins and D Regier (Eds), *Psychiatric disorders in America: The Epidemiologic Catchment Area Study.* New York: MacMillan, pp 81–115.

Herjanic, B & Campbell, W. (1977). Differentiating psychiatrically disturbed children on the basis of a structured interview. *Journal of Abnormal Child Psychology, 5,* 127–134.

Hopfer, CJ, Crowley, TJ, & Hewitt, JK. (2003). Review of twin and adoption studies of adolescent substance use. *Journal of the American Academy of Child and Adolescent Psychiatry, 42,* 710–719.

Hser, YI, Grella, CE, Hubbard, RL, Hsieh, SC, Fletcher, BW, Brown, BS, & Anglin, MD. (2001). An evaluation of drug treatments for adolescents in 4 US cities. *Archives of General Psychiatry, 58,* 689–695.

Hsieh, S, Hoffman, NG, & Hollister, CD. (1998). The relationship between pre-, during-, posttreatment factors, and adolescent substance abuse behaviors. *Addictive Behaviors, 23,* 477–488.

Johnston, L. D., O'Malley, P. M., & Bachman, J. G. (2003). *Monitoring the Future national survey results on drug use, 1975–2002. Volume I: Secondary school students* (NIH Publication No. 03–5375). Bethesda, MD: National Institute on Drug Abuse, 520 pp.

Kandel, DB. (1975). Stages in adolescent involvement in drug use. *Science, 90,* 912–914.

Keller, MB, Lavori, PW, Friedman, B, Nielsen, E, Endicott, J, McDonald-Scott, P, & Andreason, NC. (1987). The Longitudinal Interval Follow-up Evaluation: A comprehensive method for assessing outcome in prospective longitudinal studies. *Archives of General Psychiatry, 44,* 540–548.

Kelly, JF, Myers, MG, & Brown, SA. (2000). A multivariate process model of adolescent 12-step attendance and substance use outcome following inpatient treatment. *Psychology of Addictive Behaviors, 4,* 376–389.

Kessler, RC, McGonagle, KA, Zhao, S, Nelson, CB, Hughes, M, Eshleman, S, Wittchen, H-U, & Kendler, KS. (1994). Lifetime and 12-month prevalence of DSM-III-R psychiatric disorders in the United States: Results from the National Comorbidity Survey. *Archives of General Psychiatry, 51,* 8–19.

Knight, JR, Sherritt, L, Harris, SK, Gates, EC, & Chang, G. (2003). Validity of brief alcohol screening tests among adolescents: A comparison of the AUDIT, POSIT, CAGE, and CRAFFT. *Alcoholism: Clinical and Experimental Research, 27,* 67–73.

Kuperman, S, Schlosser, SS, Kramer, JR, Bucholz, K, Hesselbrock, V, Reich, T & Reich, W. (2001). Risk domains associated with an adolescent alcohol dependence diagnosis. *Addiction, 96,* 629–636.

Labouvie, E. (1996). Maturing out of substance use: Selection and self-correction. *Journal of Drug Issues, 26,* 455–474.

Langenbucher, JW & Martin, CS. (1996). Alcohol abuse: adding content to category. *Alcoholism: Clinical and Experimental Research, 20(Suppl),* 270A-275A.

Langenbucher, JW, Martin, CS, Labouvie, E, San Juan, PM, Bavly, L, & Pollock, NK. (2000). Toward the DSM-V: The withdrawal-gate model versus the DSM-IV in the diagnosis of alcohol abuse and dependence. *Journal of Consulting and Clinical Psychology, 68,* 799–809.

Latimer, WW, Newcomb, M, Winters, KC, & Stinchfield, RD. (2000). Adolescent substance abuse treatment outcome: The role of substance abuse problem severity, psychosocial, treatment factors. *Journal of Consulting and Clinical Psychology, 68,* 684–696.

Leccese, M & Waldron, HB (1994). Assessing adolescent substance use: A critique of current measurement instruments. *Journal of Substance Abuse Treatment, 11,* 553–563.

Lewinsohn, P.M., Rohde, P., & Seeley, J.R. (1996). Alcohol consumption in high school adolescents: Frequency of use and dimensional structure of associated problems. *Addiction, 91,* 375–390.

Liddle, HA & Dakof, GA. (1995). Family-based treatment for adolescent drug use: State of the science. In ERD Czechowicz (Ed), *Adolescent Drug Abuse: Clinical Assessment and Therapeutic Interventions.* Rockville, MD: National Institute on Drug Abuse.

Maisto, SA, Connors, GJ & Allen, JP. (1995). Contrasting self-report screens for alcohol problems: A review. *Alcoholism: Clinical and Experimental Research, 19,* 1510–1516.

Maisto, SA, Martin, CS, Cornelius, JR, Pollock, NK & Chung, T. (2002). Non-problem drinking outcomes in adolescents treated for alcohol use disorders. *Experimental and Clinical Psychopharmacology, 10,* 324–331.

Maisto, SA, Pollock, NK, Lynch, KG, Martin, CS, & Ammerman, R. (2001). Course of functioning in adolescents 1-year after alcohol and other drug treatment. *Psychology of Addictive Behaviors, 15,* 68–76.

Martin, CS. (1999, June). Contrasting alternative diagnostic criteria for adolescent alcohol use disorders. Paper presented at the annual meeting of the Research Society on Alcoholism, Santa Barbara, CA.

Martin, CS, Kaczynski, NA, Maisto, SA, & Tarter, RE. (1996a). Polydrug use in adolescent drinkers with and without DSM-IV alcohol abuse and dependence. *Alcoholism: Clinical and Experimental Research, 20,* 1099–1108.

Martin, C.S., Kaczynski, N.A., Maisto, S.A., Bukstein, O.M., & Moss, H.B. (1995). Patterns of DSM-IV alcohol abuse and dependence symptoms in adolescent drinkers. *Journal of Studies on Alcohol, 56,* 672–680.

Martin, C.S., Langenbucher, J.W., Kaczynski, N.A., & Chung, T. (1996b). Staging in the onset of DSM-IV alcohol abuse and dependence symptoms in adolescent drinkers. *Journal of Studies on Alcohol, 57,* 549–558.

Martin, CS, Maisto, SA, Pollock, NK, & Cornelius, JR. (2000a). Changes in DSM-IV alcohol diagnostic status across three years in adolescent drinkers. *Alcoholism: Clinical and Experimental Research, 24* (Supplement), 138A, Abstract #792.

Martin, CS, Pollock, NK, Bukstein, OG, & Lynch, KG. (2000b). Inter-rater reliability of the SCID alcohol and substance use disorders section among adolescents. *Drug and Alcohol Dependence, 59,* 173–176.

Martin, CS & Winters, KC. (1998). Diagnosis and assessment of alcohol use disorders among adolescents. *Alcohol Health and Research World, 22,* 95–105.

Mayer, J & Filstead, WJ. (1979). The adolescent alcohol involvement scale: An instrument for measuring adolescent use and misuse of alcohol. *Journal of Studies on Alcohol, 40,* 291–300.

McGue, M. (1999). The behavioral genetics of alcoholism. *Current Directions in Psychological Science, 8,* 109–115.

Meyers, K, Hagan, TA, Zanis, D, Webb, A, Frantz, J, Ring-Kurtz, S, Rutherford, M, & McLellan, AT. (1999). Critical issues in adolescent substance use assessment. *Drug and Alcohol Dependence, 55,* 235–246.

Mikulich, SK, Hall, SK, Whitmore, EA & Crowley, TJ. (2001). Concordance between DSM-III-R and DSM-IV diagnoses of substance use disorders in adolescents. *Drug and Alcohol Dependence, 61,* 237–248.

Millon, T. (1991). Classification in psychopathology: Rationale, alternatives, and standards. *Journal of Abnormal Psychology, 100,* 245–261.

Myers, MG, Brown, SA & Mott, MA. (1993). Coping as a predictor of adolescent substance abuse treatment outcome. *Journal of Substance Abuse, 5,* 15–29.

Myers, MG, Brown, SA & Mott, MA. (1995). Preadolescent conduct disorder behaviors predict relapse and progression of addiction for adolescent alcohol and drug abusers. *Alcoholism: Clinical and Experimental Research, 19,* 1528–1536.

Myers, MG, Stewart, DG & Brown, SA. (1998). Progression from conduct disorder to antisocial personality disorder following treatment for adolescent substance abuse. *American Journal of Psychiatry, 155,* 479–485.

Nathan, P & Skinstad, A. (1987). Outcomes of treatment for alcohol problems: Current methods, problems, and results. *Journal of Consulting and Clinical Psychology, 55,* 332–340.

Nelson, CB, Heath, AC, & Kessler, RC. (1998). Temporal progression of alcohol dependence symptoms in the U.S. household population: Results from the National Comorbidity Survey. *Journal of Consulting and Clinical Psychology, 66,* 474–483.

Nelson, CB & Wittchen, H-U. (1998). DSM-IV alcohol disorders in a general population sample of adolescents and young adults. *Addiction, 93,* 1065–1077.

Orvaschel, H. (1995). *Schedule for Affective Disorders and Schizophrenia for School Age Children-Epidemiologic Version-5, (K-SADS-E-5).* Fort Lauderdale, FL: Nova Southeast University.

Perkonigg, A, Lieb, R, Hoefler, M, Schuster, P, Sonntag, H & Wittchen, H-U. (1999). Patterns of cannabis use, abuse and dependence over time: Incidence, progression and stability in a sample of 1,228 adolescents. *Addiction, 94,* 1663–1678.

Pollock, N.K. & Martin, C.S. (1999). Diagnostic orphans: Adolescents with alcohol symptoms who do not qualify for DSM-IV abuse or dependence diagnoses. *American Journal of Psychiatry, 156,* 897–901.

Pollock, NK, Martin, CS & Langenbucher, JW. (2000). Diagnostic concordance of DSM-III, DSM-III-R, DSM-IV and ICD-10 alcohol diagnoses in adolescents. *Journal of Studies on Alcohol, 61,* 439–446.

Reich, W, Shayla, JJ & Taibelson, C. (1992). *The Diagnostic Interview for Children and Adolescents-Revised (DICA-R).* St Louis, MO: Washington University.

Robins, LN, Cottler, LB, Bucholz, KK & Compton, W. (2000). Diagnostic Interview Schedule for DSM-IV. St Louis, MO: Washington University.

Robins, LN & Barrett, JE (Eds). (1989). *The validity of psychiatric diagnosis.* New York: Raven Press.

Rohde, P, Lewinsohn, PM, Kahler, CW, Seeley, JR, & Brown, RA. (2001). Natural course of alcohol use disorders from adolescence to young adulthood. *Journal of the American Academy of Child and Adolescent Psychiatry, 40,* 83–90.

Rohde, P, Lewinsohn, PM & Seeley, JR. (1996). Psychiatric comorbidity with problematic alcohol use in high school students. *Journal of the American Academy of Child and Adolescent Psychiatry, 35,* 101–109.

Schulenberg, J, Maggs, JL, Steinman, KJ, & Zucker, RA. (2001). Development matters: Taking the long view on substance abuse etiology and intervention during adolescence. In PM Monti, SM Colby & TA O'Leary (Eds), *Adolescents, alcohol, and substance use: Reaching teens through brief interventions,* pp 19–57. New York: Guilford Press.

Shaffer, D, Fisher, P & Dulcan, M. (1996). The NIMH Diagnostic Interview Schedule for Children (DISC 2.3): Description, acceptability, prevalences, and performance in the MECA study. *Journal of the Academy of Child and Adolescent Psychiatry, 35,* 865–877.

Sher, KJ & Gotham, HJ (1999). Pathological alcohol involvement: A developmental disorder of young adulthood. *Development and Psychopathology, 11,* 933–956.

Skinner, H (1986). Construct validation approach to psychiatric classification. In Millon, T & Klerman, G (Eds), *Contemporary directions in psychopathology: Toward the DSM-IV,* New York: Guilford Press, pp 307–330.

Slutske, WS, Heath, AC, Dinwiddie, SH, Madden, PAF, Bucholz, KK, Dunne, MP, Statham, DH & Martin, NG. (1998). Common genetic risk factors for conduct disorder and alcohol dependence. *Journal of Abnormal Psychology, 107,* 363–374.

Stewart, D., & Brown, S. (1995). Withdrawal and dependency symptoms among adolescent alcohol and drug abusers. *Addiction, 90,* 627–635.

Stinchfield, RD. (1997). Reliability of adolescent self-reported pretreatment alcohol and other drug use. *Substance use and Misuse, 32,* 63–76.

Wagner, EF, Lloyd, DA, & Gil, AG. (2002). Racial/ethnic and gender differences in the incidence and onset age of DSM-IV alcohol use disorder symptoms among adolescents. *Journal of Studies on Alcohol, 63,* 609–619.

Waldron, HB, Slesnick, N, Brody, JL, Turner, CW, & Peterson, TR. (2001). Treatment outcomes for adolescent substance abuse at 4- and 7-month assessments. *Journal of Consulting and Clinical Psychology, 69,* 802–813.

Warner, LA, Canino, G, & Colon, HM (2001). Prevalence and correlates of substance use disorders among older adolescents in Puerto Rico and the United States: A cross-cultural comparison. *Drug and Alcohol Dependence, 63,* 229–243.

Wechsler, H., Dowdall, G.W., Davenport, A., & Castillo, S. (1995). Correlates of college student binge drinking. *American Journal of Public Health, 85,* 921–926.

White, HR & Labouvie, EW. (1989). Towards the assessment of adolescent problem drinking. *Journal of Studies on Alcohol, 50,* 30–37.

Whitmore, EA, Mikulich, SK, Thompson, LL, Riggs, PD, Aarons, GA & Crowley, TJ. (1997). Influences on adolescent substance dependence: Conduct disorder, depression, attention deficit hyperactivity disorder, and gender. *Drug and Alcohol Dependence, 47,* 87–97.

Williams, RJ, Chang, SY & Addiction Centre Adolescent Research Group (2000) A comprehensive and comparative review of adolescent substance abuse treatment outcome. *Clinical Psychology: Science and Practice, 7,* 138–166.

Winters, KC (1992). Development of an adolescent alcohol and other drug abuse screening scale: Personal Experiences Screening Questionnaire. *Addictive Behaviors, 17,* 479–490.

Winters, KC (1999). Treating adolescents with substance use disorders: An overview of practice issues and treatment outcome. *Substance Abuse, 20,* 203–225.

Winters, K.C. (2001). Assessing adolescent substance use problems and other areas of functioning: State of the art. In PM Monti, SM Colby, TA O'Leary (Eds), *Adolescents, alcohol and substance use.* New York: Guilford Press, pp 80–108.

Winters, KC, Anderson, N, Bengston, P, Stinchfield, RD & Latimer, WW (2000a). Development of a parent questionnaire for use in assessing adolescent drug abuse. *Journal of Psychoactive Drugs, 32,* 3–13.

Winters, KC & Henly, GA (1989). *Personal Experience Inventory and Manual.* Los Angeles, CA: Western Psychological Services.

Winters, KC & Henly, GA (1993). *Adolescent Diagnostic Interview Schedule and Manual.* Los Angeles: Western Psychological Services.

Winters, KC, Latimer, WW & Stinchfield, RD. (1999). DSM-IV criteria for adolescent alcohol and cannabis use disorders. *Journal of Studies on Alcohol, 60,* 337–344.

Winters, KC, Stinchfield, RD & Henly, GA. (1996). Convergent and predictive validity of scales measuring adolescent substance abuse. *Journal of Child and Adolescent Substance Abuse, 5,* 37–55.

Winters, KC, Stinchfield, RD, Henly, GA & Schwartz, RH (1991). Validity of adolescent self-report of alcohol and other drug involvement. *International Journal of Addictions, 25,* 1379–1395.

Winters, KC, Stinchfield, RD, Opland, E, Weller, C, & Latimer, WW. (2000b). The effectiveness of the Minnesota Model approach in the treatment of adolescent drug abusers. *Addiction, 95,* 601–612.

Wolraich, ML, Felice, ME, Drotar, D (Eds). (1996). *The classification of child and adolescent mental diagnoses in primary care: Diagnostic and Statistical Manual for Primary Care (DSM-PC) Child and Adolescent Version.* Elk Grove Village, IL: American Academy of Pediatrics.

World Health Organization. (1992). *International Classification of Mental and Behavioural Disorders, 10th edition.* Geneva, Switzerland: World Health Organization.

World Health Organization. (1998). Composite International Diagnostic Interview for DSM-IV. Geneva, Switzerland: Author. [Online] Available at: http://www3.who.int/cidi.

Zucker, RA, Fitzgerald, HE, & Moses, HD. (1994). Emergence of alcohol problems and the several alcoholisms: A developmental perspective on etiologic theory and life course trajectory. In D. Cichetti (Eds), *Advanced Developmental Psychopathology, Vol 2,* New York: Wiley.

2

Initiation and Course of Alcohol Consumption among Adolescents and Young Adults

Jennifer L. Maggs and John E. Schulenberg

Abstract. This chapter takes a normative developmental perspective on the etiology of alcohol use, focusing on the initiation and course of alcohol use (rather than alcohol use disorders) during adolescence and early adulthood. We review evidence regarding the sequelae and meaning of the age of initiation of alcohol use, consider variable- and pattern-centered approaches to modeling trajectories describing the course of alcohol use across adolescence and young adulthood, and offer developmental conceptualizations of risk and protective factors for alcohol use and related problems.

The initiation and subsequent course of alcohol use represent key developmental phenomena that are as important to the etiology of alcohol use as they are to broader psychosocial development during adolescence and the transition to adulthood. The adolescent years are characterized by an increased willingness to engage in behaviors considered by society to be risky, harmful, or even antisocial (Elliott *et al.*, 1985; Moffitt, 1993; Johnston *et al.*, 2002). For the majority of individuals, the likelihood of engaging in many forms of misbehavior, including alcohol and other drug use, reaches its lifetime peak roughly during the decade following the start of high school. The high prevalence of alcohol use suggests that it is a normative behavior, at least in the statistical sense, for older adolescents and young adults. Of course, what is statistically common is not necessarily ideal. Fortunately, however, for the majority of individuals, heavy alcohol use tends to subside with the acquisition of adult roles, particularly the roles of spouse, parent, and worker (Bachman *et al.*, 1997; Gotham *et al.*, 2003).

Jennifer L. Maggs • Pennsylvania State University, Human Development and Family Studies, University Park, Pennsylvania 16802
John E. Schulenberg • University of Michigan, Institute for Social Research and Department of Psychology, Ann Arbor, Michigan 48109

For an important minority of individuals, however, heavy alcohol use continues through early adulthood and beyond, setting the stage for continuing problems with alcohol and often with life in general.

This chapter is organized into three sections. First, research on the sequelae of the initiation of drinking alcohol is summarized, with a focus on the etiological significance of the age of initiation. Second, the course of alcohol use across adolescence is described, distinguishing variable- and pattern-centered approaches for modeling normative trajectories and important subgroup variations. Third, we argue for the benefits of taking a developmental perspective to the study of the complex relationships linking risk and protective factors with alcohol and other drug use.

1. The Initiation of Alcohol Use

1.1. *Defining the Age of Initiation*

Initiating alcohol use early in adolescence or in childhood is a clear indicator or marker for later problems, including heavier use of alcohol and other drugs during adolescence (e.g., Robins and Przybeck, 1985; Hawkins *et al.*, 1997). Age of initiation, or onset, of alcohol use has been defined variously, from the age at which the first drink of alcohol is consumed (e.g., Vega *et al.*, 2002)—sometimes with sips or tastes excluded (e.g., Grant, 1998; Dewit *et al.*, 2000)—to the age of first regular use (e.g., Grant *et al.*, 2001) or weekly use (e.g., Gruber *et al.*, 1996). In this paper our focus is primarily on the initiation and course of alcohol use in adolescents and young adults, rather than on alcohol abuse and dependence. We use the term *initiation* of alcohol use rather than the more clinical term *onset* to distinguish it clearly from the onset of alcohol use disorders (AUDs).

Operationally, *early* initiation has often been defined categorically as use beginning prior to a certain age. The cutoff age defined as "early" varies greatly between studies—for example, as use before age 13 (Gruber *et al.*, 1996), 14 (Muthén and Muthén, 2000b), 15 (Chou and Pickering, 1992), or 18 (Dawson, 2000). Many studies have collected retrospective data to reconstruct alcohol use histories including the age alcohol was first consumed (e.g., Vega *et al.*, 2002) or the age diagnostic criteria were first reached (e.g., Nelson and Wittchen, 1998). Regardless of how initiation has been defined, starting to drink at an early age appears to be a consistent predictor (or at least correlate) of later problems with alcohol. When continuous age data are coded categorically, use earlier in adolescence (e.g., prior to age 14–16) predicts a greater risk for later development of various alcohol problems (Grant *et al.*, 2001), with the risk appearing greatest when use is initiated particularly early (Robins and Przybeck, 1985; Dawson, 2000; DeWit *et al.*, 2000; Hingson *et al.*, 2000). In studies that use dummy codes to distinguish comparisons of multiple age cutoffs, beginning alcohol use at every age prior to 19 (Dewit *et al.*, 2000) or 21 (Hingson *et al.*, 2000) is associated with a greater risk for subsequent problems with alcohol relative to beginning use later.

1.2. *Sequelae of Early Initiation*

An earlier age of initiation of alcohol use predicts heavier use throughout adolescence and emerging adulthood (Humphrey and Friedman, 1986; Hawkins *et al.*, 1997; Labouvie *et al.*, 1997); more problems, including blackouts, abuse, tolerance, and dependence (Robins and Przybeck, 1985; Gruber *et al.*, 1996; Grant and Dawson, 1997); and a greater incidence of driving after drinking and motor vehicle accidents (Hingson *et al.*, 2000).

1.3. *Ages of Higher Risk for Alcohol Use Initiation*

In the United States, based on the nationally representative Monitoring the Future surveys, nearly half (47%) of the 8th graders in 2002 had already initiated alcohol use (more than just a few sips); this lifetime prevalence rate was similar for boys (47.2%) and girls (46.8%), higher among Hispanic youth (57.4%) than among African American (48.0%) and White (48.4%) youth, and inversely related to parent education level (ranging from 56.9% for lowest parent education level to 37.7% for highest parent education level) (Johnston *et al.*, 2003). Lifetime prevalence rates among 8th graders for alcohol use have dropped over the past decade and especially over the past few years (Johnston *et al.*, 2003), suggesting that adolescents are initiating alcohol use later. Based on retrospective accounts from the 2002 cohort of 8th grade students, 13.2% reported that they first used alcohol (more than just a few sips) before or during 5th grade, and 24.9% reported first use during 6th or 7th grade. Over the past decade, and particularly over the past few years, fewer 8th graders have reported first use at earlier grade levels (Johnston *et al.*, 2003).

In an international comparison of epidemiological data from six Western countries, Vega *et al.* (2002) found very similar patterns in the average ages of alcohol use initiation across countries despite significant variation in legal purchase ages and adult prevalence rates. The likelihood of first use increased by age 11, with the curve accelerating through mid adolescence to a peak at age 18, followed by a rapid decrease in the likelihood of first use occurring in early adulthood. Similarly, Chen and Kandel (1995) showed that the major risk periods for initiation of alcohol use increased through adolescence, peaked at age 18, and were essentially over by age 20. In these and other studies (e.g., Nelson and Wittchen, 1998), men and women evidenced similarly shaped curves, though men had consistently higher rates of use and abuse.

Despite significant inter-country variation in the prevalence of use among adults, age of initiation is remarkably similar across diverse countries (Vega *et al.*, 2002). This similarity suggests the important influences of social factors—including the major developmental transitions of adolescence and early adulthood, which are relatively similar among Western countries (Schulenberg *et al.*, 1997; Schulenberg and Maggs, 2002; Ferri *et al.*, 2003).

1.4. *Normative Reductions in the Third Decade of Life*

Many adolescents drink heavily through late adolescence and emerging adulthood, thereby risking acute consequences and the development of AUDs. However, only a small percentage of alcohol users, as with other drug users, go on to meet diagnostic criteria of abuse or dependence (Robins and Pryzbeck, 1985). The majority of adolescents mature out of their heavy drinking (Jessor *et al.*, 1991; Chen and Kandel, 1995; Bachman *et al.*, 1997). In the clinical realm as well, there is not inevitable escalation or even maintenance of alcohol problems. Even the majority of those with AUDs mature out of their alcohol problems (Nelson and Wittchen, 1998), evidencing developmentally limited alcoholism (Zucker, 1994; Sher and Gotham, 1999).

As described by Zucker (1987, 1994), developmentally limited alcoholism involves the presence of significant externalizing behavior but is different than antisocial alcoholism in that the deviant behavior is specific to the adolescent life phase and is tightly connected to normative developmental tasks, including shifting relationships from parents to peers (see also Sher and Gotham, 1999). This normative decline among developmentally limited alcoholics and among non-problematic drinkers appears to be tightly connected to the assumption of traditional adulthood roles, particularly marriage and, to a lesser extent, full-time employment and parenthood (Bachman *et al.*, 1997; Leonard and Rothbard, 1999). Most important, in developmentally limited alcoholism both the alcoholic symptomatology and the characteristic externalizing behavior disappear with the adoption of adult social roles. This decline is in contrast to continued and escalating problems with alcohol that are characteristic of other types of alcoholism, such as antisocial alcoholism and negative affect alcoholism (Zucker, 1994; Sher and Gotham, 1999).

1.5. *Rival Hypotheses About the Meaning of Early Initiation*

As reviewed above, many studies have documented consistent negative associations between age of initiation and subsequent heavy drinking and AUDs. However, it remains controversial how this relationship should be interpreted (Grant, 1998; Grant *et al.*, 2001; Prescott and Kendler, 1999, 2001). The debate centers around whether early initiation *causes* alcohol problems or is simply an early sign of more or less inevitable alcohol problems caused by, for example, genetic, family, or personality characteristics. Relatedly, there is disagreement whether delaying the age of initiation would be an effective method of reducing alcohol-related problems and disorders. At least two major hypotheses or models of the meaning of this relationship can be distinguished.

1.5.1. The General Vulnerability or Selection Hypothesis. The *General Vulnerability* (Prescott and Kendler, 1999) or *Selection* (Gotham *et al.*, 2003) hypothesis states that earlier drinking and later problematic drinking are manifestations of the same underlying susceptibility to alcohol problems rather than earlier initiation causing problems *per se* (Legrand *et al.*, 1999; Prescott and Kendler, 1999). Genetic risk, inadequate parenting and family environment, personality, or psychopathology are possible third variables that may explain the relationship between age of initiation and later alcohol use (Zucker, 1994; Legrand *et al.*, 1999; Prescott and Kendler, 1999; Tarter *et al.*, 1999). In this view, delaying initiation would not lead to a reduction in problems if the root causes remained unchanged. Instead, a more successful intervention approach might be to disrupt the progression from early use to later problematic use (Prescott and Kendler, 1999).

1.5.2. The Causation or Risk Factor Hypothesis. The *Causation* (Gotham *et al.*, 2003) or *Risk Factor* hypothesis, in contrast, views early alcohol use as placing adolescents on a trajectory toward heavier and more frequent use that has its own direct and indirect negative effects. In addition to the immediate risks of alcohol misuse common to all ages (e.g., risky driving, alcohol poisoning), individuals who begin use earlier than their age cohort face additional risks such as negative labeling, segregation into older and more deviant peer groups, and legal sanctions. A variant of this hypothesis focuses on alcohol's interference with the achievement of normative developmental tasks. For example, Newcomb (1987) highlights potential costs of being *off time* developmentally by beginning to drink early (see also Tarter *et al.*, 1999). In particular, alcohol use may interfere with the acquisition of effective coping strategies or healthy relationships (Baumrind and Moselle, 1985; Gotham *et al.*, 2003) or may lead to a premature truncation of adolescence and may lower academic and occupational achievement if earlier transitions are made to the work force, partnering, and parenthood (Newcomb and Bentler, 1988; see also Sher and Gotham, 1999). Viewed from an alternative perspective, beginning to drink *on time* rather than early may be indicative of normal social functioning rather than of underlying psychopathology; thus its predictors may lie more in youth culture, situational factors, and normative developmental processes than in genetic or environmental deficits (Robins and Przybeck, 1985; Chen and Kandel, 1995; Schulenberg and Maggs, 2002). If true, the Risk Factor hypothesis would suggest that prevention efforts to delay the initiation of alcohol use, if successful, would reduce the negative consequences of alcohol use in the long term, even if individuals initiated alcohol use later in adolescence or emerging adulthood.

1.6. Disentangling Evidence for Effects of Early Initiation

It is difficult to compare the plausibility of these competing hypotheses with cross-sectional, retrospective, or even prospective longitudinal designs.

Age of initiation and continued use are undoubtedly predicted by similar factors and influences; thus it becomes very difficult to disentangle whether starting to drink early increases the risk for alcohol problems independent of the individual's pre-existing liability for such problems (Robins and Pryzbeck, 1985). In contrast to correlational designs, genetically informed designs such as twin studies (e.g., Prescott and Kendler, 1999) or adoption studies (e.g., Cadoret *et al.*, 1986) can provide some answers to these important basic and applied research questions. Grant and Dawson (1997) showed that an earlier age of initiation predicted increased odds of abuse and dependence, even after controlling for family history of alcoholism. This result was replicated by Prescott and Kendler (1999) in a large twin sample. However, twin pair analyses suggested that most of this co-variation was due to shared family genetic and environmental variation. This latter study concluded that the evidence did not support age of initiation as a direct risk factor for alcoholism but rather supported the shared vulnerability hypothesis.

Randomized prevention trials could also help to answer the question of whether age of initiation of alcohol use is a direct risk factor for subsequent problems (Coie *et al.*, 1993; Kellam and Rebok, 1992; Maggs and Schulenberg, 2001). If the age of initiation were delayed among participants in the treatment condition and other risk factors remained unchanged, it would be possible to test whether a later age of initiation alone reduced later difficulties with alcohol or in other domains.

Though unequivocal evidence for a causal association between early initiation and later alcohol problems may be lacking, the consistency of the relationship has led many researchers to recommend that prevention efforts aim to delay the initiation of alcohol and other drug use (e.g., Robins and Pryzbeck, 1985; Hingson *et al.*, 2000; Kosterman *et al.*, 2000). Consistent with this view is the goal of the U.S. Public Health Service to increase by 2010 the average age of initiation of alcohol use by 3 years from 13.1 to 16.1 years of age (U.S. Department of Health and Human Services, 2000). Though not disputing the serious risks associated with adolescent alcohol use, some authors have cautiously questioned the practicality of delaying initiation indefinitely, given the central place of experimentation with alcohol in youth culture and the keen ability of older adolescents to challenge inconsistencies in laws and norms (Newcomb, 1987; Zucker, 1994; Schulenberg and Maggs, 2002).

2. The Course of Alcohol Use across Adolescence and Young Adulthood

An important reason for interest in the age of initiation of alcohol use is that it marks the beginning of what may become a harmful or risky pattern of *continued* use. This leads to the second focus of this review, which is the course or pattern of alcohol use across adolescence and early adulthood. In general, based on the national ongoing surveys from the Monitoring the Future study, alcohol use tends to peak at about age 21–22, and this is true for a variety of indicators of alcohol use, including annual use, 30-day use, and heavy episodic drinking (sometimes known as binge drinking) (Johnston *et al.*, 2002, 2003). The actual rates vary from year to year as a function of historic trends, but this pattern of increasing use through adolescence until early adulthood, followed by a decline, is consistent. Based on the 2001 surveys, the 30-day prevalence rates of alcohol use for 8th, 10th, and 12th graders were 22%, 39%, and 50%; for those of modal ages 19–20, 21–22, 23–24, 25–26, and 27–28, prevalence rates were 59%, 72%, 71%, 69%, and 67%; for heavy episodic drinking over the past two weeks, corresponding prevalence rates were 13%, 25%, 30%, 36%, 42%, 38%, 34%, and 29%. These cross-sectional age-based trends are useful, suggesting a developmental function that corresponds to other developmental functions of adolescence and early adulthood related to independence, social relations, and personal responsibility. Still, several questions remain open about how specifically the courses of alcohol and other drug use are embedded in young people's lives, a topic to be considered later.

Over the past decade, there has been an important change in how many researchers think about and study the courses of alcohol and other drug use during adolescence and into adulthood. This change has been stimulated in part by the closer connection between the study of substance use and developmental science (e.g., Zucker, 1994; Windle and Davies, 1999; Bennett *et al.*, 1999; Schulenberg *et al.*, 2001; Schulenberg and Maggs, 2002), as well as by statistical advances for understanding change that move beyond two-wave considerations of change (Curran and Muthén, 1999; Bates, 2000; Jackson *et al.*, 2000; Muthén and Muthén, 2000a, b; Schulenberg and Maggs, 2001). By tying considerations of substance use etiology to developmental conceptualizations, it is possible to connect the course of substance use with psychosocial development; similarly, by considering trajectories of alcohol and other drug use across multiple waves, it is possible to examine how the courses of substance use relate to other developmental phenomena as dynamic predictors, correlates, and consequences.

There are a variety of approaches to conceptualize and study trajectories of alcohol use during adolescence and early adulthood, including retrospective accounts and prospective studies. Prospective studies offer several advantages, especially when they include multiple waves of assessment over time.* In prospective studies involving repeated observations per respondent, it is possible to consider trajectories or patterns of alcohol use that include such characteristics as level, escalation, peak, and decline. In the relevant literature, such studies generally have taken one of two routes, focusing either on the normative group trajectory (and considering individual deviations from the normative trajectory in terms of variations around the intercept and slope[s]) or on

---

* Retrospective accounts have advantages as well, particularly in terms of minimizing respondent and investigator burden; but major disadvantages are problems with selective recall and sample coverage.

prototypes or common trajectories (e.g., chronically high use, escalation across adolescence, low/no use across adolescence, escalation/decline). These two approaches, which are sometimes referred to as variable- and pattern-centered approaches, respectively, are not mutually exclusive, and newer analytic techniques such as growth mixture modeling combine the two (e.g., Muthén and Muthén, 2000a; Li *et al.*, 2001). However, they tend to have various assumptions about the extent to which a sample/population normative trajectory usefully describes the important features of individual trajectories of alcohol use across adolescence and young adulthood.

2.1. *Variable-Centered Approaches: Normative Trajectories and Variations*

An individual's course of alcohol use across the adolescent and young adult years can be characterized mathematically as a developmental trajectory describing the pattern of growth and/or decline in alcohol use over a series of measurement occasions. Quantitatively, trajectories can be defined as slopes that take any mathematical function, with linear (and often quadratic) trajectories perhaps being the most commonly estimated shapes. Growth functions are defined by two or more parameters, the first indicating an intercept, which represents the individual's level of a variable at a particular researcher-selected time point (e.g., initial, average, or endpoint level), and others representing the slope for the individual over time (Bryk and Raudenbush, 1987; Muthén and Curran, 1997). Depending on the specificity of the theory and the breadth of the data, the growth function can be parameterized in more complex ways—for example, a higher-order polynomial that represents acceleration and/or deceleration in change.

Whereas repeated measures analyses of variance examine mean-level developmental trajectories for entire groups (e.g., males vs. females, treatment vs. control), the newer generations of growth modeling procedures (e.g., hierarchical linear and latent curve analyses) simultaneously estimate developmental trajectories at the individual level *and* examine whether variation in the parameters of these trajectories (e.g., initial level, linear rate of change) is systematically predicted by time-invariant (e.g., gender) and time-varying (e.g., marital status) predictors (Bryk and Raudenbush, 1987; Muthén and Curran, 1997).

Across early adolescence there are normative increases in drinking as indexed by measures of frequency-quantity and misuse (e.g., Maggs and Schulenberg, 1998; Schulenberg and Maggs, 2001). Chen and Kandel (1995) used reconstructed drug histories from four waves of data spanning ages 15–16 to 34–35 to model normative trends in alcohol use across the 19 years. Monthly alcohol use increased sharply in adolescence, stabilized in the late teens, and declined slightly in the late 20s. The periods of most intense use were in late adolescence and the early 20s. Similarly, in an analysis of longitudinal data from the National Longitudinal Survey of Youth, Muthén and Muthén (2000b) observed a peak in heavy drinking in the early 20s, with slow but steady declines through age 37.

2.2. *Pattern-Centered Approaches: Distinguishing Prototypes or Subgroups*

Pattern- or person-centered approaches to trajectories of change typically group people by how they change or do not change over time. Thus, rather than assuming that everyone, more or less, follows a similar developmental trajectory (as is the case with typical variable-centered approaches), this approach aggregates individuals into multiple, relatively homogenous groups according to their common trajectories. This disaggregation approach has revealed a great diversity of patterns of change in heavy drinking during adolescence and early adulthood (e.g., Schulenberg, O'Malley *et al.*, 1996; Bates and Labouvie, 1997; Schulenberg *et al.*, 2001; Zucker, 2000).

For example, across early adolescence, based on five waves of panel data from 6th grade through 10th grade, Steinman and Schulenberg (2003) used a pattern-centered approach to derive six trajectory groups reflecting distinct courses of alcohol use (frequency-quantity) during early and middle adolescence: abstinence, rare use, high school onset, early but non-escalating use, early and gradually escalating use, and consistently high use. In the emerging adult years, based on nationally representative panel data drawn from the Monitoring the Future (MTF) project, Schulenberg, O'Malley *et al.* (1996) used conceptual groupings and cluster analyses to distinguish six distinct trajectories of change in heavy drinking across ages 18 to 24 (see figure 1): chronic heavy drinkers, decreased, increased, fling (i.e., low, high, low), rare, and never. Similarly, Sher's longitudinal study of AUDs among college students

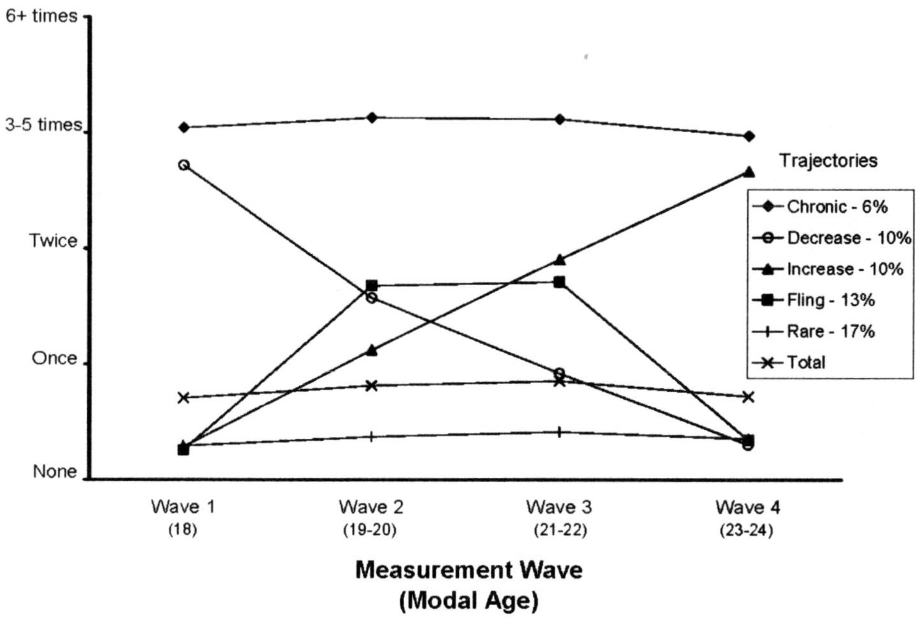

Figure 1. Mean Score for 5+ Drinks in a Row in Past 2 Weeks by Binge Drinking Trajectory

followed into young adulthood identified three subgroups using configural frequency analyses: those chronically meeting diagnostic criteria, those recovering (labeled developmentally limited), and those never diagnosed (Sher and Gotham, 1999). Similar groups of distinct trajectories have also been identified using mixture modeling in normal (e.g., Hill *et al.*, 2000) and high-risk (e.g., Chassin *et al.*, 2002) samples. Together, these and related findings (e.g., Casswell *et al.*, 1997; Li *et al.*, 2001) suggest that a single normative trajectory does not describe the course of alcohol use for all or even most young people. Such analyses identify potentially qualitative differences in the course, antecedents, and sequelae between groups or profiles of drinkers that would not be revealed if only the sample mean trajectory were modeled.

Long-term developmental trajectories of alcohol and other drug use are useful in many ways, but it is important to keep in mind that these trajectories, whether defined by normative slopes or group patterns over time, are more descriptive than explanatory or prognostic. In addition, the relatively long periods between waves (in most studies, several months to years) and the use of analytic techniques that assume off-trajectory values represent measurement error can lead to overgeneralizations about the smoothness of developmental curves. Future analyses should also use age-specific, time-varying predictors to explain further within-person variations in alcohol use (Maggs and Schulenberg, 1998; Muthén and Muthén, 2000b; Schulenberg and Maggs, 2001).

3. Risk Factors for and Protective Factors against Alcohol Use: A Developmental Perspective

As a science, our current knowledge of the vast array of potential risk and protective factors is extensive. At the same time, our understanding of how various risk and protective factors interrelate over time and how they are embedded in the course of an individual's life remains limited (Schulenberg *et al.*, 2001). In this section, we take a step back from the extensive literature on risk and protective factors and consider conceptual issues related to defining risk and protective factors in order to embed them within the life course and contexts of young people and to consider them in terms of multifinality, equifinality, and developmental timing.

3.1. *Definition and Relationship of Risk and Protective Factors*

Simply stated, risk factors are variables that predict a higher likelihood of a negative outcome, and protective factors are variables that predict a higher likelihood of a positive outcome. However, the relationship between risk and protective factors can be conceptualized in different ways (Luthar *et al.*, 2000; Schulenberg and Maggs, 2002). In one approach, risk and protective factors are viewed as independent main effects or as representing opposite ends of the same continuum (e.g., Werner and Smith, 1992). Alternatively, protective factors can be viewed as potential moderators or buffers that may reduce the effects of risk factors (Garmezy *et al.*, 1984; Rutter, 1990; Brook *et al.*, 1992; Hawkins *et al.*, 1992; Johnson and Johnson, 1999). In this latter view, protective factors are believed to operate only in the presence of existing risk factors, either by diluting or reversing the risk factor's impact (statistical interaction). Thus, the concept of protection is invoked to explain more positive outcomes among individuals exposed to similar levels of risk (Hawkins *et al.*, 1992).

3.2. *Risk and Protective Factors for Alcohol Use*

A wide variety of risk and protective factors for the initiation, escalation, and maintenance of alcohol use has been identified from decades of research. In a major review of evidence regarding risk factors for alcohol and other drug problems in adolescence, Hawkins *et al.* (1992) grouped these into 17 categories. These included contextual factors such as laws, availability of substances, and extreme economic deprivation; family factors such as conflict and management; academic failure; peer rejection; early onset of problem behavior and drug use; and physiological factors such as genetic background. Petraitis *et al.* (1995) summarized 14 theoretical models for understanding experimental substance use during adolescence. These models ranged from sociological theories focusing on more distal socio-structural factors (e.g., an absence of commitments to conventional society) to cognitive-affective theories emphasizing proximal processes (e.g., decision-making) and predictors (e.g., substance-specific expectancies). Thinking about risk and protective factors developmentally can help situate the myriad of risk/protective factors and probabilistic theoretical models into the context of normative developmental changes of adolescence and emerging adulthood (Zucker, 1994; Maggs *et al.*, 1997; Sher and Gotham, 1999; Schulenberg and Maggs, 2001, 2002).

3.3. *Developmental Perspective on Normative Developmental Transitions and Psychopathology*

An interdisciplinary developmental perspective draws attention to multidimensional and multidirectional change across the life span, normative and non-normative transitions and life events that structure and shape development, and complex interactions of biological, psychological, and contextual influences on behavior and adjustment (Bronfenbrenner, 1979; Baltes, 1987; Elder, 1998). Humans are considered to play a strong, active role in their own development, and social and physical environments are viewed as also playing strong, active roles (Caspi & Moffitt, 1993; Brandtstädter and Lerner, 1999). Through a process of niche selection, individuals sort themselves into environments and activities from differing ranges of options based on personal characteristics, beliefs, interests, and competencies. Selected ecological niches then afford various opportunities (Plomin *et al.*, 1977). This progressive accommodation of individuals and environments can foster the qualities of coherence and continuity that appear to describe much of human development. But consistent with an emphasis on dynamic person-context interactions and multi-directional change, development is not necessarily expected to exhibit a smooth and progressive function, and early experiences may not always have strong or lasting effects (e.g., Lewis, 1998; Cairns, 2000; Schulenberg *et al.*, 2003). Thus, both continuity and discontinuity are anticipated across the life course.

Developmental perspectives draw attention to normative transitions that occur across the life course for many individuals within a given society. Commonly experienced transitions in biological, cognitive, affiliative, and achievement domains during adolescence and emerging adulthood provide a structure and backdrop for initiating and experimenting with alcohol use.* For example, in the affiliative domain of interpersonal relationships, the adolescent and emerging adult years bring major transformations in relationships with peers. The increased importance of peer relations and sensitivity to peer culture during adolescence (Berndt, 1992) raises exposure to norms and influences that may encourage experimentation with alcohol. Although most adolescent alcohol use occurs in the company of peers in a shared social experience, peer influences are not monolithic in their power or direction of influence (e.g., Brown *et al.*, 1997). Rather, individuals tend to seek out and be selected by peers who have similar goals, values, and behaviors (Kandel *et al.*, 1990; Dishion and Owen, 2002). Thus peer influences, depending on their nature and direction, can both encourage or discourage alcohol use.

A developmental perspective on risk and protective factors can also bring insights to the understanding of clinical disorders. For example, developmental psychopathology views all clinical disorders as arising from difficulties in or failures of healthy development (Cicchetti, 1999). From this perspective, normative developmental transitions and changes may be related to risk or protective factors for alcohol use problems, or they may modify the expression of disorders (Sher and Gotham, 1999). Moreover, it is clear that some risk factors have more impact at particular periods of the life span—for example, peer influences during adolescence, as described above.

3.4. *Equifinality and Multifinality*

Risk and protective factors are not static over the life course, nor does a given risk or protective factor act similarly for all people or at all times. Longitudinal panel studies from early childhood to young adulthood suggest that some risk and protective factors first appear during childhood or earlier, well before the initiation of any substance use. While such factors as early antisocial behavior or genetic susceptibility to substance use increase one's vulnerability to negative outcomes, they do not necessarily doom a child to a life of substance

---

* For reviews of major developmental transitions as they relate to health behaviors, see Schulenberg, Maggs and Hurrelmann, 1997; Schulenberg and Maggs, 2001, 2002.

abuse problems (O'Connor and Rutter, 1996). Longitudinal studies on substance use are needed to identify why great numbers of individuals do not develop serious substance abuse problems despite exposure to significant risk factors, and likewise why many individuals do develop problems despite little exposure to risk factors (Rutter, 1989; Cicchetti, 1999; Zucker, 2000).

The concepts of equifinality and multifinality are of particular importance in this regard (e.g., Gottlieb, 1991; Cicchetti and Rogosch, 1996). Equifinality refers to the process by which several different types of risk/protective factors may lead to the same outcome. For example, among older adolescents who engage in frequent heavy drinking with accompanying concurrent alcohol-related symptoms (the outcome), there may be a group that initiated alcohol use early, evidenced childhood antisociality, and has a greater family history of alcoholism, and another group that initiated later in response to age-graded social influences (Zucker, 1994; see also Moffitt, 1993; Sher and Gotham, 1999).

Multifinality refers to the fact that any given risk or protective factor can lead to a multitude of different outcomes. For example, a family history of alcoholism predicts both a heightened and a reduced likelihood of alcohol problems. That is, children of alcoholics are more likely to develop alcohol abuse and dependence but also are more likely to become abstainers (Rutter, 1996; Sher, 1991; Zucker, 2000).

3.5. *Timing Matters*

The developmental timing of risk and protective factors is also key (Schulenberg *et al.*, 2001). Although early experiences are important (Hawkins *et al.*, 1992; Petraitis *et al.*, 1995), the influence of earlier experiences may be mediated, erased, or even reversed by later experiences (cf. Bandura, 1982; Lewis, 1998), especially when major transitions are involved. In particular, the transition from adolescence to adulthood is a time of widespread change that can engender considerable discontinuity in ongoing trajectories of health and well-being (Schulenberg *et al.*, 2003).

These concepts and examples highlight the probabilistic nature of risk and protective factors (Zucker, 1994). Among the many identified potential risk and protective factors, none is sufficient or necessary for particular outcomes, thus requiring conceptualizations of explanatory processes that focus on the diversity of causal connections (Cloninger *et al.*, 1997; Magnusson, 1997; Newcomb, 1997; Cairns *et al.*, 1998; Wachs, 2000; Schulenberg *et al.*, 2003).

4. Summary and Conclusion

Initiating alcohol use earlier in adolescence is of concern because of its association with heavier and more persistent alcohol use and related problems, although it remains unclear how early initiation causally relates to future difficulties. From a developmental perspective, early initiation can be viewed as an early sign of or risk factor for an escalating trajectory of alcohol use and problem behaviors. However, in light of the multifinality of early signs and risk factors regarding various problematic and salutary outcomes, as well as the equifinality of problematic outcomes following from the same risk factors, unhealthy behaviors at one point in time do not imply an inevitable and enduring problematic trajectory. Moreover, while there are normative age trends in alcohol use across adolescence and early adulthood, it is important to remember that such normative trends can hide significant interindividual differences in the shape of alcohol use trajectories for large segments of the population.

ACKNOWLEDGEMENTS: Preparation of this manuscript was facilitated by NIAAA grant AA13763 to Jennifer Maggs; John Schulenberg's efforts were made possible in part by NIDA grant DA01411 and NIMH grant MH59396.

References

Bachman, J. G., Wadsworth, K. N., O'Malley, P. M., Johnston, L. D., and Schulenberg, J. E. (1997). *Smoking, Drinking, and Drug Use in Young Adulthood: The Impact of New Freedoms and New Responsibilities.* Mahwah, NJ: Lawrence Erlbaum.

Baltes, P. B. (1987). Theoretical propositions of life-span developmental psychology: On the dynamics between growth and decline. *Developmental Psychology, 23*:611–626.

Bandura, A. (1982). The psychology of chance encounters and life paths. *American Psychologist, 37*:747–755.

Bates, M. E. (2000). Integrating person-centered and variable-centered approaches in the study of developmental courses and transitions in alcohol use: Introduction to the special section. *Alcoholism: Clinical and Experimental Research, 24*:878–881.

Bates, M. E., and Labouvie, E. W. (1997). Adolescent risk factors and the prediction of persistent alcohol and drug use into adulthood. *Alcoholism: Clinical and Experimental Research, 21*:944–950.

Baumrind, D., and Moselle, K. A. (1985). A developmental perspective on adolescent drug abuse. *Advances in Alcohol and Substance Abuse, 4*:41–67.

Bennett, M. E., McCrady, B. S., Johnson, V., and Pandina, R. J. (1999). Problem drinking from young adulthood to adulthood: Patterns, predictors and outcomes. *Journal of Studies on Alcohol, 60*:605–614.

Berndt, T. J. (1992). Friendship and friends' influence in adolescence. *Current Directions in Psychological Science, 1*:156–159.

Brandtstädter, J. and Lerner, R. M. (eds.) (1999). *Action and Self-Development: Theory and Research through the Life Span.* Thousand Oaks: Sage.

Bronfenbrenner, U. (1979). *The Ecology of Human Development: Experiments by Nature and Design.* Cambridge, MA: Harvard University Press.

Brook, J. S., Cohen, P., Whiteman, M., and Gordon, A. S. (1992). Psychosocial risk factors in the transition from moderate to heavy use or abuse of drugs. In: Glantz, M., and Pickens, R. (eds.), *Vulnerability to Drug Abuse.* Washington, DC: American Psychological Association, pp. 359–388.

Brown, B. B., Dolcini, M. M., and Leventhal, A. (1997). Transformations in peer relationships at adolescence: Implications for health-related behavior. In: Schulenberg, J., Maggs, J. L., and Hurrelmann, K. (eds.), *Health Risks and Developmental Transitions during Adolescence.* New York: Cambridge University Press, pp. 161–189.

Bryk, A. S., and Raudenbush, S. W. (1987). Application of hierarchical linear models to assessing change. *Psychological Bulletin, 101*:147–158.

Cadoret, R. J., Troughton, E., O'Gorman, T. W., and Heywood, T. (1986). An adoption study of genetic and environmental factors in drug abuse. *Archives of General Psychiatry, 43*:1131–1136.

Cairns, R. B. (2000). Developmental science: Three audacious implications. In: Bergman, L. R., Cairns, R. B., Nilsson, L.-G. and Nystedt, L. (eds.), *Developmental Science and the Holistic Approach.* Mahwah, NJ: Lawrence Erlbaum, pp. 49–62.

Cairns, R. B., Cairns, B. D., Rodkin, P., and Xie, H. (1998). New directions in developmental research: Models and methods. In: Jessor, R. (ed.), *New Perspectives on Adolescent Risk Behavior.* Cambridge, UK: Cambridge University Press, pp. 13–40.

Caspi, A., and Moffitt, T. E. (1993). When do individual differences matter? A paradoxical theory of personality coherence. *Psychological Inquiry, 4*:247–271.

Casswell, S., Pledger, M., and Pratap, S. (2002). Trajectories of drinking from 18 to 26 years: Identification and prediction. *Addiction,* 97:1427–1437.

Chassin, L., Pitts, S. C., and Prost, J. (2002). Binge drinking trajectories from adolescence to emerging adulthood in a high-risk sample: Predictors and substance abuse outcomes. *Journal of Consulting and Clinical Psychology, 70*:67–78.

Chen, K., and Kandel, D. B. (1995). The natural history of drug use from adolescence to the mid-thirties in a general population sample. *American Journal of Public Health, 85*:41–47.

Chou, S. P., and Pickering, R. P. (1992). Early onset of drinking as a risk factor for lifetime alcohol-related problems. *British Journal of Addiction, 87*:1199–1204.

Cicchetti, D. (1999). A developmental psychopathology perspective on drug abuse. In: Glantz, M. D., and Hartel, C. R. (eds.), *Drug Abuse: Origins and Interventions.* Washington DC: American Psychological Association, pp. 97–117.

Cicchetti, D., and Rogosch, F. A. (1996). Equifinality and multifinality in developmental psychopathology. *Development and Psychopathology, 8*:597–600.

Cloninger, C. R., Svrakic, N. M., and Svrakic, D. M. (1997). Role of personality self-organization in development of mental order and disorder. *Development and Psychopathology, 9*:881–906.

Coie, J. D., Watt, N. F., West, S. G., Hawkins, J. D., Asarnow, J. R., Markman, H. J., Ramey, S. L., Shure, M. B., and Long, B. (1993). The science of prevention: A conceptual framework and some directions for a national research program. *American Psychologist, 48*:1013–1022.

Curran, P. J., and Muthén, B. O. (1999). The application of latent curve analysis to testing developmental theories in intervention research. *American Journal of Community Psychology, 27*:567–595.

Dawson, D. A. (2000). The link between family history and early onset alcoholism: Earlier initiation of drinking or more rapid development of dependence? *Journal of Studies on Alcohol, 61*:637–646.

DeWit, D. J., Adlaf, E. M., Offord, D. R., and Ogborne, A. C. (2000). Age at first alcohol use: A risk factor for the development of alcohol disorders. *American Journal of Psychiatry, 157*:745–750.

Dishion, T. J., and Owen, L. D. (2002). A longitudinal analysis of friendships and substance use: Bidirectional influence from adolescence to adulthood. *Developmental Psychology, 38*:480–491.

Elder, G. H., Jr. (1998). The life course and human development. In Damon, W. (Series Ed.), and Lerner, R. M. (Vol. Ed.), *Handbook of Child Psychology: Vol. 1. Theoretical Models of Human Development.* New York: Wiley, pp. 939–991.

Elliott, D. S., Huizinga, D., and Ageton, S. S. (1985). *Explaining Delinquency and Drug Use.* Newbury Park, CA: Sage.

Ferri, E., Bynner, J., and Wadsworth, M. (2003). Changing lives. In: Ferri, E., Bynner, J., and Wadsworth, M. (eds.), *Changing Britain, Changing Lives.* London: Institute of Education.

Garmezy, N., Masten, A. S., and Tellegen, A. (1984). The study of stress and competence in children: A building block for developmental psychopathology. *Child Development, 55*:97–111.

Gotham, H. J., Sher, K. J., and Wood, P. K. (2003). Alcohol involvement and developmental task completion during young adulthood. *Journal of Studies on Alcohol, 64*:32–42.

Gottlieb, G. (1991). Experiential canalization of behavioral development: Theory. *Developmental Psychology, 27*:4–13.
Grant, B. (1998). The impact of family history of alcoholism on the relationship between age at onset of alcohol use and DSM-III alcohol dependence. *Alcohol Health and Research World, 22*:144–147.
Grant, B. F., and Dawson, D. A. (1997). Age at onset of alcohol use and its association with DSM-IV alcohol abuse and dependence: Results from the National Longitudinal Alcohol Epidemiologic Survey. *Journal of Substance Abuse, 9*:103–110.
Grant, B. F., Stinson, F. S., and Harford, T. C. (2001). Age at onset of alcohol use and DSM-IV alcohol abuse and dependence: A 12-year follow-up. *Journal of Substance Abuse, 13*:493–504.
Gruber, E., DiClemente, R. J., Anderson, M. M., and Lodico, M. (1996). Early drinking onset and its association with alcohol use and problem behavior in late adolescence. *Preventive Medicine, 25*:293–300.
Hawkins, J. D., Catalano, R. F., and Miller, J. Y. (1992). Risk and protective factors for alcohol and other drug problems in adolescence and early adulthood: Implications for substance abuse prevention. *Psychological Bulletin, 112*:64–105.
Hawkins, J. D., Graham, J. W., Maguin, E., Abbott, R., Hill, K. G., and Catalano, R. F. (1997). Exploring the effects of age of alcohol use initiation and psychosocial risk factors on subsequent alcohol misuse. *Journal of Studies on Alcohol, 58*:280–290.
Hill, K. G., White, H. R., Chung, I. J., Hawkins, J. D., and Catalano, R. F. (2000). Early adult outcomes of adolescent binge drinking: Person- and variable-centered analyses of binge drinking trajectories. *Alcoholism: Clinical and Experimental Research, 24*:892–901.
Hingson, R. W., Heeren, T., Jamanka, A., and Howland, J. (2000). Age of drinking onset and unintentional injury involvement after drinking. *Journal of the American Medical Association, 284*:1527–1533.
Humphrey, J. A., and Friedman, J. (1986). The onset of drinking and intoxication among university students. *Journal of Studies on Alcohol, 47*:455–458.
Jackson, K. M., Sher, K. J., and Wood, P. K. (2000). Trajectories of conjoint substance use disorders: A developmental, typological approach to comorbidity. *Alcoholism: Clinical and Experimental Research, 24*:902–913.
Jessor, R., Donovan, J. E., and Costa, F. (1991). *Beyond Adolescence: Problem Behavior and Young Adult Development.* New York: Cambridge University Press.
Johnson, P. B., and Johnson, H. L. (1999). Cultural and familial influences that maintain the negative meaning of alcohol. *Journal of Studies on Alcohol, 13*:79-83.
Johnston, L. D., O'Malley, P. M. and Bachman, J. G. (2002). *Monitoring the Future National Survey Results on Drug Use 1975–2001, Volume II: College Students and Adults Ages 19–40.* NIH publication no. 03–5376. Bethesda, MD: National Institute on Drug Abuse.
Johnston, L. D., O'Malley, P. M., and Bachman, J. G. (2003). *Monitoring the Future National Survey of Results on Drug Use, 1975–2002, Volume I: Secondary School Students.* NIH publication no. 03–5375. Bethesda, MD: National Institute on Drug Abuse.
Kandel, D., Davies, M., and Baydar, N. (1990). The creation of interpersonal contexts: Homophily in dyadic relationships in adolescence and young adulthood. In: Robins, L., and Rutter, M. (eds.), *Straight and Devious Pathways from Childhood to Adulthood.* Cambridge, UK: Cambridge University Press, pp. 221–241.
Kellam, S. G., and Rebok, G. W. (1992). Building developmental and etiological theory through epidemiologically based preventive intervention trials. In: McCord, J., and Tremblay, R. (eds.), *Preventing Antisocial Behavior: Interventions from Birth through Adolescence.* New York: Guilford, pp. 162–195.
Kosterman, R., Hawkins, J. D., Guo, J., Catalano, R. F., and Abbott, R. D. (2000). The dynamics of alcohol and marijuana initiation: Patterns and predictors of first use in adolescence. *American Journal of Public Health, 90*:360–366.
Labouvie, E., Bates, K. E., and Pandina, R. J. (1997). Age of first use: Its reliability and predictive utility. *Journal of Studies on Alcohol, 58*:638–643.

Legrand, L. N., McGue, M., and Iacono, W. G. (1999). Searching for interactive effects in the etiology of early-onset substance use. *Behavior Genetics, 29*:433–443.

Leonard, K. E., and Rothbard, J. C. (1999). Alcohol and the marriage effect. *Journal of Studies on Alcohol, 13*:139–146.

Lewis, M. (1998). *Altering Fate: Why the Past Does not Predict the Future.* New York: Guilford.

Li, F., Duncan, T. E., and Hops, H. (2001). Examining developmental trajectories in adolescent alcohol use using piecewise growth mixture modeling analysis. *Journal of Studies on Alcohol, 62*:199–210.

Luthar, S. S., Cicchetti, D. and Becker, B. (2000). The construct of resilience: A critical evaluation and guidelines for future work. *Child Development, 71*:543–562.

Maggs, J. L., and Schulenberg, J. (1998). Reasons to drink and not to drink: Altering trajectories of drinking through an alcohol misuse prevention program. *Applied Developmental Science, 2*:48–60

Maggs, J. L., and Schulenberg, J. (2001). Editors' introduction: Prevention as altering the course of development and the complementary purposes of developmental and prevention sciences. *Applied Developmental Science, 5*:196–200.

Maggs, J. L., Schulenberg, J., and Hurrelmann, K. (1997). Developmental transitions during adolescence: Health promotion implications. In: Schulenberg, J., Maggs, J. L., and Hurrelmann, K. (eds.), *Health Risks and Developmental Transitions during Adolescence.* New York: Cambridge University Press, pp. 522–546.

Magnusson, D. (ed.). (1997). *The Lifespan Development of Individuals: Behavioral, Neurobiological, and Psychosocial Perspectives: A Synthesis.* New York: Cambridge University Press.

Moffitt, T. E. (1993). Adolescence-limited and life-course-persistent antisocial behavior: A developmental taxonomy. *Psychological Review, 100*:674–701.

Muthén, B. O., and Curran, P. J. (1997). General longitudinal modeling of individual differences in experimental designs: A latent variable framework for analysis and power estimation. *Psychological Methods, 2*:371–402.

Muthén, B. O., and Muthén, L. K. (2000a). Integrating person-centered and variable-centered analyses: Growth mixture modeling with latent trajectory classes. *Alcoholism: Clinical and Experimental Research, 24*:882–891.

Muthén, B. O., and Muthén, L. K. (2000b). The development of heavy drinking and alcohol-related problems from ages 18 to 37 in a U. S. national sample. *Journal of Studies on Alcohol, 61*:290–300.

Nelson, C. B., and Wittchen, H.-U. (1998). DSM-IV alcohol disorders in a general population sample of adolescents and young adults. *Addiction, 93*:1065–1077.

Newcomb, M. D. (1987). Consequences of teenage drug use: The transition from adolescence to young adulthood. *Drugs and Society, 1*:25–60.

Newcomb, M. D. (1997). Psychosocial predictors and consequences of drug use: A developmental perspective within a prospective study. *Journal of Addictive Diseases, 16*: 51–89.

Newcomb, M. D., and Bentler, P. M. (1988). Impact of adolescent drug use and social support on problems of young adults: A longitudinal study. *Journal of Abnormal Psychology, 97*: 64–75.

O'Connor, T. G., and Rutter, M. (1996). Risk mechanisms in development: Some conceptual and methodological considerations. *Developmental Psychology, 32*:787–795.

Petraitis, J., Flay, B. R., and Miller, T.Q. (1995). Reviewing theories of adolescent substance use: Organizing pieces of the puzzle. *Psychological Bulletin, 117*:67–86.

Plomin, R., DeFries, J. C., and Loehlin, J. C. (1977). Genotype-environment interaction and correlation in the analysis of human behavior. *Psychological Bulletin, 84*:309–322.

Prescott, C. A., and Kendler, K. S. (1999). Age at first drink and risk for alcoholism: A noncausal association. *Alcoholism: Clinical and Experimental Research, 23*:101–107.

Prescott, C. A., and Kendler, K. S. (2001). Age at first alcohol use: A risk factor for the development of alcohol disorders": Comment. *American Journal of Psychiatry, 158*:1530.

Robins, L. N., and Przybeck, T. R. (1985). Age of onset of drug use as a factor in drug and other disorders. In: Jones, C. L., and Battjes, R. J. (eds.), *Etiology of Drug Abuse.* Rockville, MD: National Institute on Drug Abuse, pp. 178–192.

Rutter, M. (1989). Isle of Wight revisited: Twenty-five years of child psychiatric epidemiology. *Journal of the American Academy of Child and Adolescent Psychiatry, 28:*633–653.

Rutter, M. (1990). Psychosocial resilience and protective mechanisms. In: Rolf, J., Masten, A., Cicchetti, D., Nuechterlein, K. H., and Weintraub, S. (eds.), *Risk and Protective Factors in the Development of Psychopathology.* Cambridge, UK: Cambridge University Press, pp. 181–214.

Rutter, M. (1996). Transitions and turning points in developmental psychopathology: As applied to the age span between childhood and mid-adulthood. *International Journal of Behavioral Development, 19:*603–626.

Schulenberg, J., and Maggs, J. L. (2001). Moving targets: Comparison of alternative strategies for examining prevention effects on trajectories of alcohol misuse and related risk factors during adolescence. *Applied Developmental Science, 5:*237–253.

Schulenberg, J., and Maggs, J. L. (2002). A developmental perspective on alcohol use and heavy drinking during adolescence and the transition to young adulthood. *Journal of Studies on Alcohol, Supplement No. 14:*54–70.

Schulenberg, J., O'Malley, P. M., Bachman, J. G., Wadsworth, K. N., and Johnston, L. D. (1996). Getting drunk and growing up: Trajectories of frequent binge drinking during the transition to young adulthood. *Journal of Studies on Alcohol, 57:*289–304.

Schulenberg, J., Maggs, J. L., and Hurrelmann, K. (eds.) (1997). *Health Risks and Developmental Transitions during Adolescence.* New York: Cambridge University Press, pp. 1–19.

Schulenberg, J., Maggs, J. L., Steinman, K., and Zucker, R. A. (2001). Development matters: Taking the long view on substance abuse etiology and intervention during adolescence. In: Monti, P. M., Colby, S. M., and O'Leary, T. A. (eds.), *Adolescents, Alcohol, and Substance Abuse: Reaching Teens through Brief Interventions.* New York: Guilford Press, pp. 19–57.

Schulenberg, J., Maggs, J. L., and O'Malley, P. M. (2003). How and why the understanding of developmental continuity and discontinuity is important: The sample case of long-term consequences of adolescent substance use. In: Mortimer, J. T., and Shanahan, M. (eds.), *Handbook of the Life Course.* Kluwer Academic/Plenum Publishers, pp. 413–436.

Sher, K. J. (1991). *Children of Alcoholics: A Critical Appraisal of Theory and Research.* Chicago: University of Chicago Press.

Sher, K. J., and Gotham, H. J. (1999). Pathological alcohol involvement: A developmental disorder of young adulthood. *Development and Psychopathology, 11:*933–956.

Steinman, K. J., and Schulenberg, J. (2003). A pattern-centered approach to evaluating substance use prevention programs. In: Damon, W. (Series Ed.), Peck, S. C., and Roeser, R. W. (Vol. Eds.), *New Directions for Child and Adolescent Development: Vol. 101. Person-Centered Approaches to Studying Development in Context.* San Francisco: Jossey Bass, pp. 87–98.

Tarter, R., Vanyukov, M., Giancola, P., Dawes, M., Blackson, T., Mezzich, A., and Clark, D. B. (1999). Etiology of early age onset substance use disorder: a maturational perspective. *Development and Psychopathology, 11:*657–683.

U.S. Department of Health and Human Services. (2000, November). *Healthy People 2010: Tracking Healthy People.* Retrieved September 15, 2003, from http://www.healthypeople.gov/document/html/objectives/26–09.htm

Vega, William A., Aguilar-Gaxiola, S., Andrade, L., Bijl, R., Borges, G., Caraveo-Anduaga, J. J., DeWit, D. J., Heeringa, S., G., Kessler, R. C., Kolody, B., Merikangas, K. R., Molnar, B. E., Walters, E. E., Warner, L. A., and Wittchen, H.-U. (2002). Prevalence and age of onset for drug use in seven international sites: Results from the International Consortium of Psychiatric Epidemiology. *Drug and Alcohol Dependence, 68:* 285–297.

Wachs, T. D. (2000). *Necessary but Not Sufficient: The Respective Roles of Single and Multiple Influences on Individual Development.* Washington DC: American Psychological Association.

Werner, E. E., and Smith, R. S. (eds.). (1992). *Overcoming the Odds: High Risk Children from Birth to Adulthood.* Ithaca, NY: Cornell University Press.

Windle, M., and Davies, P. T. (1999). Developmental theory and research. In: Leonard, K. E., and Blane, H. T. (eds.), *Psychological Theories of Drinking and Alcoholism,* 2nd ed. . New York: Guilford Press, pp. 164–202.

Zucker, R. A. (1987). The four alcoholisms: A developmental account of the etiologic process. In: Rivers, P. C. (ed.), *Nebraska Symposium on Motivation, 1987: Alcohol and Addictive Behavior.* Lincoln: University of Nebraska Press, pp. 27–83.

Zucker, R. A. (1994). Pathways to alcohol problems and alcoholism: A developmental account of the evidence for multiple alcoholisms and for contextual contributions to risk. In: Zucker, R. A., Howard, J., and Boyd, G. M. (eds.), *The Development of Alcohol Problems: Exploring the Biopsychosocial Matrix of Risk.* Rockville, MD: National Institute on Alcohol Abuse and Alcoholism, pp. 255–289.

Zucker, R. A. (2000). Alcohol involvement over the life course. In: National Institute on Alcohol Abuse and Alcoholism, *Tenth Special Report to the U.S. Congress on Alcohol and Health.* Bethesda, MD: Department of Health and Human Services, pp. 25–53.

3

High Risk Adolescent and Young Adult Populations: Consumption and Consequences

Brooke S. G. Molina

1. Introduction

Conceptualization of risk for alcoholism is complicated, with a number of unique factors having been theorized and demonstrated to be important in the development of alcohol problems among youth. These include individual characteristics such as personality or temperament, inherited vulnerability based on familial risk, environmental vulnerability (e.g., socioeconomic disadvantage, exposure to modeling influences, etc.), and the interplay among all of these risk factors (e.g., (Sher, 1991). Among youth, it is sometimes helpful to consider alcoholism risk by virtue of variables that identify group membership; such group membership typically intersects with the constructs implicated in alcoholism theory. Consideration of these risk groups (e.g., psychiatric comorbidities) can inform research and treatment efforts, and without question can assist with policy and funding decisions. In recent decades, a proliferation of studies have accumulated to test hypotheses regarding the contribution of a number of risk variables to alcoholism development in youth. To this end, a number of these risk variables (i.e., risk groups) are considered below for their possible role in alcoholism vulnerability among youth.

2. Adolescents with Comorbid Conditions

Rohde and colleagues reported in their diagnostic interview study of high school students in Oregon (large representative sample) that over 80% of

Brooke S. G. Molina • University of Pittsburgh School of Medicine, Western Psychiatric Institute and Clinic, Pittsburgh, Pennsylvania 15213.

students with an alcohol disorder had another psychiatric disorder (Rohde, Lewinsohn, & Seeley, 1996). Indeed, psychiatric comorbidity among adolescents with alcohol or other substance abuse problems is more common than not (Bukstein, Brent, & Kaminer, 1989). In a recent review of community sample studies, comorbidity between a substance disorder and another psychiatric disorder was estimated at 60% of youths with a substance disorder (Armstrong & Costello, 2002). Yet, the confidence with which conclusions can be drawn regarding the putative causal role of certain conditions is variable.

Without question, the condition most prominently featured in the literature in alcoholism and substance abuse comorbidity is Conduct Disorder (CD). The salience of this construct in etiological models of alcoholism follows from epidemiologic studies of adults finding antisocial personality (ASP) to be the most common psychiatric comorbidity with alcoholism (Robins & Regier, 1991), with 29.6% of alcoholic women and 12.0% of alcoholic men meeting diagnostic criteria for ASP. Conduct problems are significantly associated concurrently and prospectively with alcohol and/or substance use among youth (Chassin et al., 2004; Weinberg & Glantz, 1999). Thus, deviant behavior and deviance-proneness play a central role in theoretical models of alcoholism and substance abuse among youth (Jessor & Jessor, 1977; Sher, 1991). Although the specific terms have somewhat different conceptual implications, this common comorbidity is also referred to as aggression, defiance, or behavioral undercontrol in childhood, CD, conduct problems, delinquency, or antisocial behavior in adolescence, and antisocial personality in adulthood.

Definitional issues aside, among youth there is a strong and robust literature documenting the prospective association between conduct problems and alcohol consumption. For example, teachers' ratings of defiant and aggressive behavior among first grade boys predicted heavier use of alcohol as well as marijuana and cigarettes by the teenage years (Kellam, Brown, Rubin, & Ensminger, 1983). Loeber and colleagues tested whether persistent delinquency and substance use were associated in the Pittsburgh Youth Study of boys, and found significant associations in each of the three age cohorts of the sample (Loeber, Stouthamer-Loeber, & White, 1999). In a large sample of boys recruited in kindergarten, stable disruptive behavior over seven years predicted a composite substance use score that included alcohol use by age 12 (Dobkin, Tremblay, & Sacchitelle, 1997). Among adolescents, early occurring delinquent behavior (i.e., occurring before the age of twelve) was associated with a rapid development of substance dependence symptoms among adolescents (Taylor, Malone, Iacono, & McGue, 2002). In the Great Smoky Mountains study, behavior disorders (principally Conduct Disorder) were significantly associated with alcohol use, as well as use of other substances, among boys and girls (Costello, Erkanli, Federman, & Angold, 1999). Interestingly, the association was stronger among girls, which is consistent with the Epidemiologic Catchment Area Study (ECA) report of higher rates of ASP among female adult alcoholics (Robins & Regier, 1991). These longitudinal studies, as well as studies examining age of onset of comorbid psychiatric and alcohol disorders, strongly suggest the temporal precedence of conduct problems prior to the development of alcohol problems (Rohde et al., 1996), supporting deviance-proneness theories of alcohol disorder (e.g., Jessor & Jessor, 1977; Sher, 1991). Interestingly, however, there does not appear to be a 1:1 correspondence between serious conduct problems and development of alcohol or other substance disorder. For example, among youth in the Great Smoky Mountains study, only 26.2% of girls and 11.3% of boys with substance abuse or dependence met diagnostic criteria for a behavior disorder (Costello et al., 1999). Similarly, in the Oregon study, only 25.5% of youth with alcohol abuse or dependence had a disruptive behavior disorder (Rohde et al., 1996). Although in the latter study disruptive behavior disorders were probably underestimated (parent report was not available), these studies and others (Mason & Windle, 2002) suggest the utility of maintaining a distinction between these outcomes for youth.

There is significant comorbidity between CD and Attention-Deficit/Hyperactivity Disorder (ADHD; Hinshaw, 1987; Waschbusch, 2002). The extent to which underlying temperamental vulnerability consistent with the core symptoms of ADHD (inattention, hyperactivity, and impulsivity) is responsible for the CD-alcoholism link remains an open and interesting question. For example, in the Montreal study, persistent disruptive behavior predicted early substance use (Dobkin et al., 1997), but in the same study boys with high teacher ratings of restlessness, running or jumping up and down, not keeping still, and squirmy and fidgety reported earlier ages of drunkenness at follow-up (Masse & Tremblay, 1997). Caspi and colleagues reported that 3-year old boys observed to be impulsive, restless, and distractible were at increased risk for alcohol dependence by age 21 (Caspi, Moffitt, Newman, & Silva, 1996). Similar findings exist in other longitudinal studies (e.g., (Block, Block, & Keyes, 1988), suggesting that well before conduct problems develop, a temperamental style characterized by behavioral undercontrol and dysregulation increases vulnerability to alcoholism and substance abuse (Chassin & Ritter, 2001).

Although there have been some inconsistencies across studies, children diagnosed with ADHD in clinic settings appear to be at risk for elevated alcohol consumption. Most recently, Molina and Pelham reported more frequent drunkenness, a slightly younger age when first drunk, and more alcohol problems that included subclinical symptomatology, among adolescents with childhood ADHD than among demographically similar adolescents without ADHD (Molina & Pelham, 2003). However, among epidemiologic/community samples, associations with ADHD are generally rendered nonsignificant once the comorbidity with CD is controlled (e.g., Armstrong & Costello, 2002; Boyle et al., 1993; Costello et al., 1999). This result is not surprising if CD serves to mediate alcohol risk among children with ADHD, especially given findings that children with comorbid ADHD and CD begin their antisocial careers at earlier ages and have more persistent delinquent behavior (Moffitt, 1990). In a public middle school sample, students with high teacher ratings of ADHD symptoms and high self-ratings of conduct disorder symptoms reported the highest rates of drunkenness (73% of those with both ADHD and CD versus 36% of students with CD only), indirectly suggesting the viability of a pathway from ADHD to alcoholism through CD (Molina, Smith, & Pelham, 1999). Whether elevated drinking and drinking-related problems among adolescents with ADHD persist into adulthood, or newly appear in adulthood, is a matter for continued longitudinal research.

Finally, internalizing disorders have received much attention in the alcoholism literature for their possible role as contributors to risk. A negative affect pathway of vulnerability, in which adolescents turn to alcohol or other drugs to alleviate psychological distress, is commonly seen in theoretical models. However, the support for depressive or anxious symptomatology as a unique predictor of vulnerability has been inconsistent (Chassin, Hussong, Barrera, Molina, Trim, & Ritter, 2004). Co-occurrence between alcohol use or abuse with depression is common (Armstrong & Costello, 2002). For example, Rohde and colleagues reported a 47.9% depression rate among high school students with alcohol abuse or dependence compared to about 20% in abstainers, experimenters, or social drinkers (Rohde et al., 1996). However, only 17% of the youth with an alcohol disorder had a "pure" internalizing disorder (i.e., an externalizing disorder was not also present), indicating that disruptive behavior vulnerability may underlie much of the alcohol-internalizing comorbidity. Kandel reported a rate of 23.8% with depression among youth drinking alcohol at least weekly compared to 5.0% in abstaining youth (Kandel et al., 1997), and Deykin reported a prevalence of 22.8% for depression with alcohol abuse (Deykin, Levy, & Wells, 1987). Thus, approximately one fifth of youth with an alcohol disorder may suffer from major depression, but a significant number of these youth may also have externalizing behavior problems. The comorbidity with anxiety disorder is much less impressive (Armstrong & Costello, 2002).

Attempts to sort out the temporal ordering, or unique predictive effects of internalizing symptomatology on drinking outcomes have not yielded consistent results. In a number of cases, no significant prediction was found. For example, in a community sample of adolescents, externalizing symptoms but not internalizing symptoms were found to mediate parental alcoholism effects on adolescents' increased heavy drinking over time (Hussong, Curran, & Chassin, 1998). In the same sample, adolescent internalizing symptoms did not predict alcohol or drug diagnoses in adulthood (Chassin, Pitts, DeLucia, & Todd, 1999). However, Hussong has argued that it might be premature to dismiss the role of negative affect in alcoholism vulnerability before research is conducted that assesses affective vulnerability proximal in time to the drinking experience (Hussong, Hicks, Levy, & Curran, 2001). Previous research may have underestimated the role of negative internal states due to the long assessment windows common in survey research (i.e., interviews once a year or less).

3. Adolescents with Positive Family Histories of Alcohol Problems

Alcoholism runs in families. Though by no means a perfect correlation, there is solid empirical evidence for at least a moderate association between parental alcohol disorder and risk for the same in their offspring. Studies that have generated the most convincing data on this matter have directly interviewed parents and offspring recruited from community settings and prospectively followed the children into adolescence and early adulthood.

In an ongoing longitudinal study of children of alcoholics recruited from the community, Chassin and colleagues reported a significant association between parental alcohol disorder and binge drinking in offspring followed through adolescence into early adulthood (Chassin, Pitts, & Prost, 2002). Specifically, after controlling for comorbid parental psychopathology, parental alcohol disorder was associated with binge drinking behavior that included a late-moderate pattern, an infrequent (but present) pattern, and an early-heavy pattern of binge drinking. Moreover, adolescents who were in the early-heavy binge drinking trajectory group were significantly more likely to meet diagnostic criteria for alcohol abuse, drug abuse, and ASP when they were 18–23 years of age (Chassin et al., 2002), indicating the prognostic importance of early binge drinking among adolescents, as well as the significance of a positive family history above and beyond the commonly occurring psychiatric disorders that often occur in adults with alcoholism.

Other research has shown strong familial associations for substance disorder above and beyond antisociality. Merikangas and colleagues reported that among clinic-recruited adults with substance disorders, odds ratios adjusted for antisocial personality ranged from 4.4 to 10.2 for first degree relatives to have a similar drug disorder (i.e., opioids, cocaine, cannabis). Although this specific test was not conducted for alcohol disorder, 35.5% of alcoholics' first degree relatives also had alcohol disorder (vs. 14.9% of controls' relatives), indicating a strong familial pattern (Merikangas et al., 1998). In general for drug disorders, there was an 8-fold increased risk of drug disorders among the relatives of these adult probands.

In the Great Smoky Mountains Study, an epidemiologic study of psychiatric disorder in rural southeast youth, parental report of treatment for substance-related problems was associated with an earlier onset of drinking alcohol. The ages at which these children first began drinking was quite young, with exposed children (parent received treatment) beginning to drink an average of two years earlier than non-exposed children (7.7 years of age versus 9.1 in non-exposed children) (Costello et al., 1999).

Heritability estimates for "alcoholism" variously defined are in the range of 43% to 67% for adults (Heath, 2003). For example, among adult twins, controlling for a variety of confounding variables that includes Conduct Disorder, heritability is still 68% for both men and women (Heath et al., 1997). Among youth, heritability appears to be comparable. A heritability estimate of 60% was reported by Han and colleagues using the Minnesota Twin Family Study

(Han, McGue, & Iacono, 1999). These heritability estimates are consistent with research by Hill and colleagues finding significant effects of familial density of alcoholism on adolescent drinking (Hill, Shen, Lowers, & Locke, 2000; Hill & Yuan, 1999), and indicate that the familial loading for alcoholism may be a particularly important moderator of risk beyond parental disorder alone.

The importance of heritability is underscored by research showing that, above and beyond diagnosis of alcohol disorder in parents, maximum number of drinks by fathers may be even more useful as a predictor of vulnerability in their children. In the Minnesota Twin Family Study, father's maximum number of drinks consumed predicted his childs's use of a range of substances including alcohol, alcohol intoxication, and alcohol disorder symptoms by age fourteen. These findings are important given the well-established link between early drinking and risk for later alcohol disorder (Grant & Dawson, 1997), and findings that neurophysiologic vulnerability to alcoholism (reduced P300 amplitude) is associated with heavy paternal drinking (Iacono, Carlson, Malone, & McGue, 2002). However, the strong familiality and potential genetic underpinnings of alcoholism risk do not negate the importance of environmental factors and their potential interactive effects on alcoholism heritability (Heath, 2003).

Finally, in the University of Michigan-Michigan State University Longitudinal Study (UM-MSU), parental alcoholism was associated with increasing teacher-rated attention problems through childhood, which was subsequently associated with early alcohol consumption and first drunkenness by the age of 14 (Jester et al., 2003). This finding is consistent with other reports by this group pointing to early behavioral undercontrol in the children in these families, especially when antisocial personality is present (Wong, Zucker, Puttler, & Fitzgerald, 1999). The UM-MSU study is uniquely positioned to study the onset and course of cognitive and behavioral difficulties from early childhood into adolescence, and to test whether early temperamental and cognitive difficulties predate antisocial behaviors known for their strong comorbid association with alcohol disorder. Research such as this may help to address some of the confusion regarding the role of temperamental vulnerability, ADHD, and conduct problems in the development of alcohol disorder among youth.

4. Gay and Lesbian Youth

Research on gay, lesbian, and bisexual youth (GLB) and their associated risk for alcohol problems has increased since the 1980s. Concern has arisen regarding mental health vulnerability in this population (Remafedi, Farrow, & Deisher, 1991), with a recent emphasis on need for definitional and methodologic improvements in research with this population (e.g., Institute of Medicine, 1999). Studies addressing increased risk for substance use and abuse among GLB youth have been mostly focused on males and selected self-identified populations (e.g., Jordan, 2000; Rotheram-Borus & Rosario, 1994;

Rotheram-Borus, Rosario, Rossem, Redi, & Gillis, 1995), although recent research has begun to correct this methodologic limitation (Russell, Driscoll, & Truong, 2002).

Using data from the 1995 Youth Risk Behavior Survey in Massachusetts (high school students), Garofalo and colleagues reported a 2.5% prevalence rate of self-identified sexual orientation as gay/lesbian or bisexual (0.6% gay/lesbian, 1.9% bisexual) (Garofalo, Wolf, Kessel, Palfrey, & DuRant, 1998). Among these youth, elevations compared to heterosexual youth were found for a wide range of health risk behaviors (e.g., sexual intercourse) that included alcohol consumption before age 13, lifetime (86.8% vs. 79.0%) and recent (past 30 days) alcohol use (89.4% vs. 52.8%), recent binge drinking (46.2% vs. 33.0%), alcohol use at school (25.0% vs. 6.2%), and alcohol or drug use at last sexual episode (34.7% vs. 13.3%). Group differences were also found for a number of other drug use behaviors (e.g., marijuana use before age 13, inhalant use, etc.), supporting the hypothesis that youth who identify themselves as GLB in high school are at significantly elevated risk for a range of health risk behaviors that include excessive use of alcohol. A limitation of this study was that students who had not yet self-identified as GLB were excluded, which may have resulted in an over-estimate of risk.

In a recent attempt to correct previous methodological limitations of studies in this area, Russell and colleagues examined the association between several alcohol consumption variables and other substance use variables with same-sex romantic attractions and relationships in the ADD Health Study (Russell et al., 2002). Group differences were found, but at more modest rates than had been suggested by prior studies. Youth with romantic attraction to both sexes (bisexual attraction experienced) reported more times drunk, drinking alone, and problems associated with drinking. However, these differences were limited to cross-sectional correlations and same-sex attraction was not predictive of increases in these variables one year later. In contrast, males reporting same-sex relationships experienced increases in drinking alone and in problems caused by drinking (but not drunkenness) by the subsequent year. There were some group differences for marijuana and for other drug use, but these differences were generally cross-sectional, and suggest that GLB alcohol vulnerability may be moderated by early identification with the GLB role. Especially elevated risk among self-identified youth may explain why studies of self-selected samples (e.g., youth seeking services at gay-identified community agencies) report high rates of alcohol and drug use (Rotheram-Borus & Rosario, 1994; Rotheram-Borus et al., 1995). Taken together, the studies to date suggest that moderate risk for early drinking and drinking-related problems is apparent among youth with GLB attractions, but there is significantly elevated risk for a range of mental health problems that includes drug and alcohol use among self-identified GLB youth. Given the social stressors associated with such identification (Savin-Williams, 1994), and the young age at which male GLB individuals begin to recognize their sexual identity (on average, 14; Remafedi, 1987), these studies suggest a need for continued research on this population. Furthermore, longitudinal research is needed to determine whether early problem behaviors that include alcohol use in this population lead to long-term difficulties with drinking and use of other drugs into adulthood, which has been suggested by research on GLB adults (Skinner, 1994).

5. Homeless and Runaway Youth

Runaway, "throwaway," or otherwise homeless youth are, by definition, a hidden population difficult to enumerate, and under-represented in national surveys of substance use among youth (Kral, Molnar, Booth, & Watters, 1997). The Second National Incidence Studies of Missing, Abducted, Runaway, and Thrownaway Children (NISMART-2), a 1999 survey of households and juvenile facilities, estimated that 1,682,900 youths in the United States had a runaway (at least one night away) or throwaway episode (Hammer, Finkelhor, & Sedlak, 2002), with a throwaway episode defined as being told to leave home by a caretaker for at least one night, without adequate alternative care arranged. This represents a slight decrease since NISMART-1 conducted a decade earlier, suggesting that this population is at least stable if not declining in size slightly. Most runaway/throwaway youth (two-thirds) were between the ages of 15 and 17, boys and girls were equally represented, and most (77%) were gone from home less than one week. Three characteristics were prominent among roughly one-fifth of the youth; these included a prior history of physical or sexual abuse (21%), being substance dependent (19%), and using hard drugs (17%). It was not reported whether rates of substance use or disorder were higher in the subset of youth gone from home for extended periods of time, which may be important because research has shown that total time away is correlated, at least for boys, to frequency of substance use (Whitbeck, Hoyt, & Yoder, 1999).

Ennett, Bailey and colleagues interviewed 327 runaway and homeless youth in Washington, D.C. (Ennett, Bailey, & Federman, 1999), two-thirds of whom were identified on the streets (as opposed to shelters, etc.). Most were African-American (80.4%), average age was 17.4, and males and females were equally represented. A third (31.3%) reported three or more drinks at a time, two-thirds (61.5%) also reported marijuana use, and 25.9% reported illicit drug use in the past month. Illicit drug use was more common among youth without any social network (38.5% vs. 21.7% of youth with at least one contact), and presence of alcohol or drug use in the social network was strongly correlated with self-reported substance use, as has also been reported in other studies of this population (Whitbeck et al., 1999).

In the Urban Health Study, an interview study of 775 runaway/homeless adolescents in San Francisco, Denver, and New York City, 11% reported crack use and 15% shared needles in the past three months in 1992 (Kral et al., 1997). These rates were highest in San Francisco (17% and 35%, respectively). Unfortunately, measures of alcohol consumption did not include frequency or quantity of use, but roughly 70% of youth reported having sex while drunk or high, suggesting very high rates of heavy drinking with health risk consequences. Because youth were required to have been away from home at least three months, and the average length of time these youth (mostly 15–19 years old) had been away from home was nearly two years, these statistics are not watered down by the inclusion of youth displaced for brief periods of time.

Among 190 adolescent runaways in New York City shelters, 18.9% reported drinking once a week or more in the past three months, 15.3% reported drug use once a week or more, and use of both was common, with 24.3% reporting any substance use once a week or more (Rotheram-Borus, Mahler, Koopman, & Langabeer, 1996). Youth with a history of sexual abuse were more likely to report weekly drinking, drug use, or both. In addition, Koopman, Rosario, and Rotheram-Borus (1994) reported that more sexual partners and less frequent condom use were associated with substance use.

Taken together, these studies suggest that runaway or otherwise homeless youth report potentially concerning levels of alcohol consumption and other drug use. Most worrisome is the dangerous combination of alcohol consumption and sexual activity reported by Kral and colleagues (1997), yet it is valuable information that most of these studies failed to support the notion that homeless youth are universally addicted to drugs or alcohol. Rather, their circumstances appear to be the result of histories that include a range of variables that are in and of themselves risk factors for alcohol exposure, as well as other adverse outcomes including premature independence from home. For example, Whitbeck reported that a history of family physical or sexual abuse was associated with substance use among runaway and homeless females (Whitbeck et al., 1999). Methodologic complexities are rampant in this research area, including difficulty in the identification of youth, difficulty with tracking them in longitudinal study, and problems with obtaining multiple reporter data. Future research would benefit from identifying the subgroup of adolescents who successfully negotiate the transition from homeless living to successful independent functioning that includes responsible levels of alcohol consumption.

6. Ethnic and Racial Minority Group Vulnerability

Alcohol consumption, as well as use of other drugs, among ethnic and racial minority youth has been reported, at least since the 1970s, to be lower than that of the Caucasian majority (Kandel, Single, & Kessler, 1976; Welte & Barnes, 1987). An exception has been Native American youth, who usually report the highest use of most substances (Kandel et al., 1976; Welte & Barnes, 1987). This finding has also been reported repeatedly by Beauvais and colleagues from their longstanding biennial surveys of American Indian youth (Beauvais, 1992, 1996). In the most recent results of the National Survey on Drug Use and Health (formerly National Household Survey on Drug Abuse), this pattern of group differences among the most prominent minority groups has remained strikingly constant, with American Indian youth (including Alaska Natives) reporting the highest use of a range of substances that includes alcohol. Rates of self-reported binge drinking (five or more drinks on the same occasion at least once in the past 30 days) are highest for American-Indians (18.2%), lowest for African-Americans (4.9%), Asian-Indians (4.0%) and Filipinos (0.9%), with Whites and Hispanic/Latinos in between. White or Caucasian youth report the highest rates after American-Indians (12.5%) and Hispanic/Latino levels fall in between Whites and African-Americans, at 10.5%. This pattern of group differences is also revealed for use of cigarettes, marijuana, and illicit drugs by youth (SAMHSA, 2003), and has been reported in the literature for quite some time, although sometimes differences in alcohol behaviors between Whites and American Indians are not found (Welte & Barnes, 1987).

Rate of alcohol disorder (i.e., alcohol abuse or dependence) was conservatively estimated at 11.0% among American Indian students in the Northern Plains (Beals et al., 1997), a figure significantly higher than the comparative 4.6% reported by Lewinsohn and colleagues (Lewinsohn, Hops, Roberts, Seeley, & Andrews, 1993). Among American Indian youth who present for residential substance abuse treatment, use of alcohol and marijuana is most common (over 90% use alcohol; over 75% use marijuana), over 80% use more than one substance, and first alcohol intoxication occurs very early in life (mean age of first alcohol intoxication is 11.9 years) (Novins, Beals, Shore, & Manson, 1996). Although at the time they were quite young, 9 to 13 year old American-Indians in the Great Smoky Mountains Study were found to have significantly higher rates of substance use disorder, at 1.2% versus 0.1% of Whites (Costello, Farmer, Angold, Burns, & Erkanli, 1997). Alcohol was the most commonly reported substance used.

There are a number of methodologic issues in studying prevalence rates of alcohol consumption and alcohol problems among minority youth that include recognition of regional differences, sociocultural diversity within prominent minority groups, as well as accommodating corrections in sampling techniques to reflect adequate representation of populations in national or epidemiologic surveys. Some attempts have been made to address regional differences in alcohol disorder risk among American Indians, which is an attempt to recognize the diversity of socio-cultural histories among different American-Indian subgroups. For example, Plunkett and Mitchell (2000) found that American Indians in high school were more likely to report alcohol, marijuana, and cocaine use, but less likely to report inhalant and stimulant use, compared to regionally similar estimates from the 1993 Monitoring the Future (MTF) study data (Johnston, Bachman, & O'Malley, 1995). Rates of alcohol use for American Indians were 65.5% of North-Central American-Indian youth versus 51.8% of MTF youth, and 55.8% of Western American-Indian youth versus 48.6% of MTF youth (Plunkett & Mitchell, 2000). Differences in rates of alcohol consumption were not as dramatic as for use of other substances, but measurement of this variable was limited to any alcohol consumption in the past 30 days, which may have obscured power to detect group differences in more concerning levels of use (i.e., repetitive binge drinking, or drinking leading to negative consequences). Other research with this population has found regional differences in whether alcohol, versus marijuana, is first used by American-Indian youth (Novins, Beals, & Mitchell, 2001).

Among Hispanics, there have been pleas to recognize the potential diversities among minorities of different geographic origination, such as Puerto Ricans, Cubans, Mexicans, etc. However, in the most recent report from the National Survey on Drug Use and Health, rates of binge drinking do not differ dramatically, with 10.6% of Mexicans, 10.0% of Puerto Ricans, and 9% of Central or South American youth reporting binge drinking (SAMHSA, 2003). Similarly, rates of binge drinking and heavy drinking do not differ appreciably among these groups at ages 18–25, although heavy drinking does appear to decrease appreciably to 2.8% from 8.0% for Central/South Americans after age 25 (SAMHSA, 2003). Even through group differences within Hispanic ethnicity subgroups may not be substantial, contextual factors affecting binge drinking rates may still vary across these groups and lead to heavy drinking for different reasons (Gordon, 1981).

School drop-out rates are dramatically higher among ethnic and racial minority youth, and school-based surveys such as the MTF study tend to miss these participants. Research suggests that corrections for the high dropout rates of Mexican-Americans (46%) and American-Indians (50%) relative to White non-Hispanics (11%) reveals that school-based surveys may disproportionately underestimate alcohol consumption as well as use of other drugs among minorities (Swaim, Beauvais, Chavez, & Oetting, 1997). For example, in a nationally representative sample of 7th–12th grade American Indian students, corrections for school dropout resulted in an estimate of 55%, instead of 51%, of youth experiencing alcohol intoxication (Beauvais, 1996). Although this statistic does not reflect chronic problems with drinking, nearly one in five American Indian youth are reported to have such problems with drugs in general (Beauvais, 1996), which probably includes alcohol because of the pervasive manner in which alcohol permeates the daily life of many American Indian youth (O'Nell & Mitchell, 1996). Rates of recent alcohol intoxication by youth, corrected after interviewing 774 school drop-outs, increased by only 2.1% for White Non-Hispanics, but by 8.9% for American-Indians, and by 9.3% for Mexican-Americans (Swaim et al., 1997), indicating the importance of considering differential attrition from school for both American-Indians and Mexican-Americans.

Socioeconomic background factors (e.g., parental education, urbanicity) and lifestyle factors (e.g., college plans, truancy, religiosity, evenings out) may be important variables in explaining minority group differences in alcohol and other drug use. Socioeconomic disadvantage among American Indians may elevate risk. Educational aspirations and decreased social influence among Asians, and strong religious affiliation among African-Americans, may decrease risk, relative to Whites (Au & Donaldson, 2000; Wallace & Bachman, 1991). However, these risk and protective factors in and of themselves are not surprising, and have been found at some level to be important in the prediction of substance use and other problem behaviors among all youth regardless of ethnic affiliation. For example, a number of studies specifically focused on comparing explanatory models of substance use among ethnic and racial minority subgroups have failed to find substantial group differences in the suggested processes leading to alcohol or drug use vulnerability (Barrera, Biglan, Ary, & Li, 2001; Brook, Brook, Arencibia-Mireles, Richter, & Whiteman, 2001; Costa, Jessor, & Turbin, 1999; Flannery, Vazsonyi, & Rowe, 1996; Gottfredson & Koper, 1996; Rowe, Vazsonyi, & Flannery, 1994; Swaim, Oetting, Thurman, Beauvais, & Edwards, 1993). For example, Barrera and colleagues found similarities between Hispanics (mostly Mexican), American Indians, and Caucasian students in family and peer influences on substance use, problem behavior, and academic performance (Barrera et al., 2001). Furthermore, substance use prevention programs aimed at competence enhancement have resulted in beneficial effects not only for suburban White samples but also for urban minority samples (e.g., Botvin, Griffin, Diaz, & Ifill-Williams, 2001). Even though factors such as these may relate similarly to substance use across minority groups, such as close-knit family relationships being associated with decreased vulnerability, there may still be socio-contextual differences between groups that underlie distinctions between normative and pathological definitions of drinking, that are not revealed in these models and which warrant further study (O'Nell & Mitchell, 1996).

7. Youth with Multiple Risk Factors

Psychiatric comorbidities, economic and educational disadvantage, and other types of vulnerabilities (positive family history) for early problem drinking behavior are more likely to co-occur than to exist in isolation. In fact, models of alcoholism vulnerability recognize this confluence of factors by their inclusion of multiple non-independent pathways to disorder (e.g., Sher, 1991). Examples of multiple risk factors abound. For example, among teenage girls (mostly African-American) presenting to an adolescent medicine clinic in metropolitan Atlanta, 38% reported drinking alcohol at least once in the past month, and alcohol or other substance use was correlated with number of sexual partners, STD history, pregnancy history, and decreased condom use (Bachanas et al., 2002), illustrating the co-occurrence of alcohol consumption with other health risk behaviors. Among youth surveyed in the 1995 Youth Risk Behavior Survey in Massachusetts, 22% of the American Indians self-identified as gay, lesbian, or bisexual (Garofalo et al., 1998). Thus, among these youth, two separate risk factors are present, notwithstanding other vulnerabilities in this group (e.g., increased risk for school drop-out). As reviewed above, studies of homeless and runaway youth find frequent admixtures of psychiatric disorder, conflict with parents, educational underachievement, and a range of variables all considered to be vulnerability factors for the development of alcohol disorder (and in some cases, consequences). Most studies of youth vulnerability to alcohol disorder report that such behavior does not occur in isolation, which points to the importance of comprehensive assessment of youth suspected of having alcohol problems, and also to the need to address behavioral, psychological, and academic risk factors early in childhood and adolescence before problematic drinking takes hold.

References

Armstrong, T. D., & Costello, E. J. (2002). Community studies on adolescent substance use, abuse, or dependence and psychiatric comorbidity. *Journal of Consulting and Clinical Psychology, 70*(6), 1224–1239.

Au, J. G., & Donaldson, S. I. (2000). Social influences as explanations for substance use differences among Asian-American and European-American adolescents. *Journal of Psychoactive Drugs, 32*(1), 15–23.

Bachanas, P. J., Morris, M. K., Lewis-Gess, J. K., Sarett-Cuasay, E. J., Flores, A. L., Sirl, K. A., & Sawyer, M. K. (2002). Psychological adjustment, substance use, HIV knowledge, and risky sexual behavior in at-risk minority females: Developmental differences during adolescence. *Journal of Pediatric Psychology, 27*(4), 373–384.

Barrera, M., Jr., Biglan, A., Ary, D., & Li, F. (2001). Replication of a problem behavior model with American Indian, Hispanic, and Caucasian youth. *Journal of Early Adolescence, 21*(2), 133–157.

Beals, J., Piasecki, J., Nelson, S., Jones, M., Keane, E., Dauphinais, P., Red Shirt, R., Sack, W. H., & Manson, S. M. (1997). Psychiatric disorder among American Indian Adolescents: Prevalence in Northern Plains Youth. *Journal of the American Academy of Child and Adolescent Psychiatry, 36*(9), 1252–1259.

Beauvais, F. (1992). Indian adolescent drug and alcohol use: Recent patterns and consequences. *American Indian Alaska Native Mental Health Research, 5*(Special Issue), v-78.

Beauvais, F. (1996). Trends in drug use among American Indian students and dropouts, 1975–1994. *American Journal of Public Health, 86*(11), 1594–1598.

Block, J., Block, J. H., & Keyes, S. (1988). Longitudinally foretelling drug usage in adolescence: Early childhood personaligy and environmental precursors. *Child Development, 59*, 336–355.

Botvin, G. J., Griffin, K. W., Diaz, T., & Ifill-Williams, M. (2001). Drug abuse prevention among minority adolescents: One-year follow-up of a school-based prevention intervention. *Prevention Science, 2*, 1–13.

Boyle, M. H., Offord, D. R., Racine, Y. A., Fleming, J. E., Szatmari, P., & Links, P. S. (1993). Predicting substance use in early adolescence based on parent and teacher assessments of childhood psychiatric disorder: Results from the Ontario child health study follow-up. *J. Child Psychol. Psychiat., 34*(4), 535–544.

Brook, J. S., Brook, D. W., Arencibia-Mireles, O., Richter, L., & Whiteman, M. (2001). RIsk factors for adolescent marijuana use across cultures and across time. *The Journal of Genetic Psychology, 162*(3), 357–374.

Bukstein, O. G., Brent, D. A., & Kaminer, Y. (1989). Comorbidity of substance abuse and other psychiatric disorders in adolescents. *American Journal of Psychiatry, 146*, 1131–1141.

Caspi, A., Moffitt, T. E., Newman, D., & Silva, P. (1996). Behavioral observations at age 3 predict adult psychiatric disorders. *Archives of General Psychiatry, 53*, 1033–1039.

Chassin, L., Hussong, A., Barrera, M., Jr., Molina, B. S. G., Trim, R., & Ritter, J. (2004). Adolescent substance use. In R. M. Lerner & L. Steinberg (Eds.), *Handbook of Adolescent Psychology* (Second ed.). Hoboken, NJ: John Wiley & Sons, Inc.

Chassin, L., Pitts, S. C., DeLucia, C., & Todd, M. (1999). A longitudinal study of children of alcoholics: Predicting young adult substance use disorders, anxiety, and depression. *Journal of Abnormal Psychology, 108,* 106–119.

Chassin, L., Pitts, S. C., & Prost, J. (2002). Binge drinking trajectories from adolescence to emerging adulthood in a high-risk sample: Predictors and substance abuse outcomes. *Journal of Consulting and Clinical Psychology, 70*(1), 67–78.

Chassin, L., & Ritter, J. (2001). Vulnerability to substance use disorders in childhood and adolescence. In R. E. Ingram & J. M. Price (Eds.), *Vulnerability to psychopathology. Risk across the lifespan.* (pp. 107–134). New York: The Guilford Press.

Costa, F. M., Jessor, R., & Turbin, M. S. (1999). Transition into adolescent problem drinking: The role of psychosocial risk and protective factors. *Journal of Studies on Alcohol, 60,* 480–490.

Costello, E. J., Erkanli, A., Federman, E. B., & Angold, A. (1999). Development of psychiatric comorbidity with substance abuse in adolescents: Effects of timing and sex. *Journal of Clinical Child Psychology, 28,* 298–311.

Costello, E. J., Farmer, E. M. Z., Angold, A., Burns, B. J., & Erkanli, A. (1997). Psychiatric disorders among American Indian and white youth in Appalachia: The Great Smoky Mountains Study. *American Journal of Public Health, 87,* 827–832.

Deykin, E. Y., Levy, J. C., & Wells, V. (1987). Adolescent depression, alcohol and drug abuse. *American Journal of Public Health, 77,* 178–181.

Dobkin, P. L., Tremblay, R. E., & Sacchitelle, C. (1997). Predicting boys' early onset substance abuse from father's alcoholism, son's disruptiveness, and mother's parenting behavior. *Journal of Consulting and Clinical Psychology, 65*(1), 86–92.

Ennett, S. T., Bailey, S. L., & Federman, E. B. (1999). Social network characteristics associated with risky behaviors among runaway and homeless youth. *Journal of Health and Social Behavior, 40*(March), 63–78.

Flannery, D. J., Vazsonyi, A. T., & Rowe, D. C. (1996). Caucasian and Hispanic early adolescent substance use: Parenting, personality, and school adjustment. *Journal of Early Adolescence, 16,* 71–89.

Garofalo, R., Wolf, R. C., Kessel, S., Palfrey, J., & DuRant, R. H. (1998). The association between health risk behaviors and sexual orientation among a school-based sample of adolescents. *Pediatrics, 101*(5), 859–902.

Gordon, A. J. (1981). The cultural context of drinking and indigenous therapy for alcohol problems in three migrant Hispanic cultures: An ethnographic report. In D. Heath & J. Waddell & M. Topper (Eds.), *Cultural factors in alcohol research and treatment of alcohol problems.* (Vol. Supplement 9, pp. 217–240). New Brunswick, NJ.

Gottfredson, D. C., & Koper, C. S. (1996). Race and sex differences in the prediction of drug use. *Journal of Consulting and Clinical Psychology, 64*(2), 305–313.

Grant, B. F., & Dawson, D. A. (1997). Age at onset of alcohol use and its association with DSM-IV alcohol abuse and dependence: Results from the National Longitudinal Alcohol Epidemiological Survey. *Journal of Substance Abuse, 9,* 103–110.

Hammer, H., Finkelhor, D., & Sedlak, A. J. (2002). *Runaway/thrownaway children: National estimates and characteristics. National Incidence studies of missing, abducted, runaway, and thrownaway children.* Washington, D.C.: U.S. Department of Justice, Office of Justice Programs, Office of Juvenile Justice and Delinquency Prevention.

Han, C., McGue, M., & Iacono, W. (1999). Lifetime tobacco, alcohol, and other substance use in adolescent Minnesota twins: Univariate and multivariate behavior genetic analyses. *Addiction, 94,* 981–983.

Heath, A. C. (2003). *Investigating the interplay of genetic and environmental risk factors in alcoholism.* Paper presented at the Annual Meeting of the Research Society on Alcoholism, Fort Lauderdale, FL.

Heath, A. C., Bucholz, K. K., Madden, P. A. F., Dinwiddie, S. H., Slutske, W. S., Bierut, L. J., Statham, D. J., Dunne, M. P., Whitfield, J. B., & Martin, N. G. (1997). Genetic and environmental contributions to alcohol dependence risk in a national twin sample: Consistency of findings in women and men. *Psychological Medicine, 27*(6), 1381–1396.

Hill, S. Y., Shen, S., Lowers, L., & Locke, J. (2000). Factors predicting the onset of adolescent drinking in families at high risk for developing alcoholism. *Society of Biological Psychiatry, 48*, 265–275.

Hill, S. Y., & Yuan, H. (1999). Familial density of alcoholism and onset of adolescent drinking. *Journal of Studies on Alcohol, 60*, 7–17.

Hinshaw, S. P. (1987). On the distinction between attentional deficits/hyperactivity and conduct problems/aggression in child psychopathology. *Psychological Bulletin, 101*(3), 443–463.

Hussong, A. M., Curran, P. J., & Chassin, L. (1998). Pathways of risk for accelerated heavy alcohol use among adolescent children of alcoholics. *Journal of Abnormal Child Psychology, 26*(6), 453–466.

Hussong, A. M., Hicks, R. E., Levy, S. A., & Curran, P. J. (2001). Specifying the relations between affect and heavy alcohol use among young adults. *Journal of Abnormal Psychology, 110*(3), 449–461.

Iacono, W., Carlson, S. R., Malone, S. M., & McGue, M. (2002). P3 event-related potential amplitude and the risk for disinhibitory disorders in adolescent boys. *Archives of General Psychiatry, 59*, 750–757.

Institute of Medicine (Ed.). 1999. *Lesbian health: Current assessment and directions for the future*. Washington, D.C.: National Academy Press.

Institute of Medicine (Ed.). (1999). *Lesbian health: Current assessment and directions for the future.* Washington, D.C.: National Academy Press.

Jessor, R., & Jessor, S. L. (1977). *Problem behavior and psychosocial development: A longitudinal study of youth.* New York: Academic Press.

Jester, J. M., Nigg, J. T., Fitzgerald, H. E., Puttler, L. I., Wong, M. M., & Zucker, R. A. (2003, June). Developmental trajectories of attention problems in children of alcoholics. In B.S.G. Molina (Chair), *Alcohol and other drug use outcomes among children with attention and impulse control problems: Latest findings from four prospective longitudinal studies.* Symposium conducted at the Annual Meeting of the Research Society on Alcoholism, Fort Lauderdale, FL.

Jordan, K. M. (2000). Substance abuse among gay, lesbian, bisexual, transgender, and questioning adolescents. *School Psychology Review, 29*(2), 201–206.

Kandel, D. B., Johnson, J. G., Bird, H. R., Canino, G., Goodman, S. H., Lahey, B. B., & al., e. (1997). Psychiatric disorders associated with substance use among children and adolescents: Findings from the Methods for the Epidemiology of Child and Adolescent mental disorders (MECA) study. *Journal of Abnormal Child Psychology, 25*, 121–132.

Kandel, D. B., Single, E., & Kessler, R. (1976). The epidemiology of drug use among New York state high school students: Distribution, trends, and change in rates of use. *American Journal of Public Health, 66*, 43–53.

Kellam, S., Brown, C., Rubin, B., & Ensminger, M. (1983). Paths leading to teenage psychiatric symptoms and substance use: developmental epidemiological studies in Woodlawn. In S. B. Guze & F. J. Earls & J. E. Barrett (Eds.), *Childhood psychopathology and development.* New York: Raven Press.

Koopman, C., Rosario, M., & Rotheram-Borus, M. J. (1994). Alcohol and drug use and sexual behaviors placing runaways at risk for HIV infection. *Addictive Behaviors, 19*(1), 95–103.

Kral, A. H., Molnar, B. E., Booth, R. E., & Watters, J. K. (1997). Prevalence of sexual risk behavior and substance use among runaway and homeless adolescents in San Francisco, Denver and New York City. *International Journal of STD & AIDS, 8*(2), 109–117.

Lewinsohn, P. M., Hops, H., Roberts, R. E., Seeley, J. R., & Andrews, J. A. (1993). Adolescent psychopathology, I: Prevalence and incidence of depression and other DSM-III-R disorders in high school students. *Journal of Abnormal Psychology, 102*, 133–144.

Loeber, R., Stouthamer-Loeber, M., & White, H. R. (1999). Developmental aspects of delinquency and internalizing problems and their association with persistent juvenile substance use between ages 7 and 18. *Journal of Clinical Child Psychology, 28*(3), 322–332.

Mason, W. A., & Windle, M. (2002). Reciprocal relations between adolescent substance use and delinquency: A longitudinal latent variable analysis. *Journal of Abnormal Psychology, 111*(1), 63–76.

Masse, L. C., & Tremblay, R. E. (1997). Behavior of boys in kindergarten and the onset of substance use during adolescence. *Archives of General Psychiatry, 54*(1), 62–68.
Merikangas, K., Stolar, M., Stevens, D., Goulet, J., Preisig, M., Fenton, B., Zhang, J., O'Malley, S., & Rounsaville, B. (1998). Familial transmission of substance use disorders. *Archives of General Psychiatry, 55*, 973–979.
Moffitt, T. E. (1990). Juvenile delinquency and attention deficit disorder: Boys' developmental trajectories from age 3 to age 15. *Child Development, 61*, 893–910.
Molina, B. S. G., & Pelham, W. E. J. (2003). Childhood predictors of adolescent substance use in a longitudinal study of children with ADHD. *Journal of Abnormal Psychology, 112*(3), 497–507.
Molina, B. S. G., Smith, B. H., & Pelham, W. E. (1999). Interactive effects of Attention-Defict/Hyperactivity Disorder and Conduct Disorder on early adolescent substance use. *Psychology of Addictive Behaviors, 13*(4), 348–358.
Novins, D. K., Beals, J., & Mitchell, C. (2001). Sequences of substance use among American Indian adolescents. *Journal of the American Academy of Child and Adolescent Psychiatry, 40*(10), 1168–1174.
Novins, D. K., Beals, J., Shore, J. H., & Manson, S. M. (1996). Substance abuse treatment of American Indian adolescents: Comorbid symptomatology, gender differences, and treatment patterns. *Journal of the American Academy of Child and Adolescent Psychiatry, 35*(12), 1593–1601.
O'Nell, T. D., & Mitchell, C. M. (1996). Alcohol use among American Indian adolescents: The role of culture in pathological drinking. *Soc. Sci.Med., 42*(4), 565–578.
Plunkett, M., & Mitchell, C. (2000). Substance use rates among American Indian adolescents: Regional comparisons with Monitoring the Future High School Seniors. *Journal of Drug Issues, 30*, 593–620.
Remafedi, G. (1987). Male homosexuality: The adolescent's perspective. *Pediatrics, 79*, 326–330.
Remafedi, G., Farrow, J., & Deisher, R. (1991). Risk factors for attempted suicide in gay and bisexual youth. *Pediatrics, 87*, 869–875.
Robins, L. N., & Regier, D. A. (1991). *Psychiatric disorders in America. The Epidemiologic Catchment Area Study.* New York: The Free Press.
Rohde, P., Lewinsohn, P. M., & Seeley, J. R. (1996). Psychiatric comorbidity with problematic alcohol use in high school students. *Journal of the American Academy of Child and Adolescent Psychiatry, 35*, 101–109.
Rotheram-Borus, M. J., Mahler, K. A., Koopman, C., & Langabeer, K. (1996). Sexual abuse history and associated multiple risk behavior in adolescent runaways. *American Journal of Orthopsychiatry, 66*(3), 390–400.
Rotheram-Borus, M. J., & Rosario, M. (1994). Sexual and substance use acts of gay and bisexual male adolescents in New York City. *Journal of Sex Research, 31*(1), 47–57.
Rotheram-Borus, M. J., Rosario, M., Rossem, R. V., Redi, H., & Gillis, R. (1995). Prevalence, course, and predictors of multiple problem behaviors among gay and bisexual male adolescents. *Developmental Psychology, 31*(1), 75–85.
Rowe, D. C., Vazsonyi, A. T., & Flannery, D. J. (1994). No more than skin deep: Ethnic and racial similarity in developmental processes. *Psychological Review, 101*, 396–413.
Russell, S. T., Driscoll, A. K., & Truong, N. (2002). Adolescent same-sex romantic attractions and relationships: Implications for substance use and abuse. *American Journal of Public Health, 92*(2), 198–202.
SAMHSA (2003). *Results from the 2002 National Survey on Drug Use and Health: Detailed Tables*, [electronic]. Department of Health and Human Services, Substance Abuse and Mental Health Services Administration, Office of Applied Studies. Available: http://www.DrugAbuseStatistics.SAMHSA.gov [2003, 09/10/2003].
Savin-Williams, R. C. (1994). Verbal and physical abuse as stressors in the lives of lesbian, gay male, and bisexual youths: Associations with school problems, running away, substance abuse, prostitution, and suicide. *Journal of Consulting and Clinical Psychology, 62*(2), 261–269.
Sher, K. J. (1991). *Children of alcoholics. A critical appraisal of theory and research.* Chicago: The University of Chicago Press.

Skinner, W. F. (1994). The prevalence and demographic predictors of illicit and licit drug use among lesbians and gay men. *American Journal of Public Health, 84,* 1307–1310.

Swaim, R. C., Beauvais, F., Chavez, E. L., & Oetting, E. R. (1997). The effect of school dropout rates on estimates of adolescent substance use among three racial/ethnic groups. *American Journal of Public Health, 87*(1), 51–55.

Swaim, R. C., Oetting, E. R., Thurman, P. J., Beauvais, F., & Edwards, R. W. (1993). American Indian adolescent drug use and socialization characteristics: A cross-cultural comparison. *Journal of Cross-Cultural Psychology, 24,* 53–70.

Taylor, J., Malone, S., Iacono, W. G., & McGue, M. (2002). Development of substance dependence in two delinquency subgroups and nondelinquents from a male twin sample. *Journal of the American Academy of Child and Adolescent Psychiatry, 41*(4), 386–393.

Wallace, J. M., & Bachman, J. G. (1991). Explaining racial/ethnic differences in adolescent drug use: The impact of background and lifestyle. *Social Problems, 38*(3), 333–355.

Waschbusch, D. A. (2002). A meta-analytic examination of comorbid hyperactive-impulsive-attention problems and conduct problems. *Psychological Bulletin, 128*(1), 118–150.

Weinberg, N. Z., & Glantz, M. D. (1999). Child psychopathology risk factors for drug abuse: Overview. *Journal of Clinical Child Psychology, 28,* 290–297.

Welte, J. W., & Barnes, G. (1987). Alcohol use among adolescent minority groups. *Journal of Studies on Alcohol, 48,* 329–336.

Whitbeck, L. B., Hoyt, D. R., & Yoder, K. A. (1999). A risk-amplification model of victimization and depressive symptoms among runaway and homeless adolescents. *American Journal of Community Psychology, 27*(2), 273–296.

Wong, M. M., Zucker, R. A., Puttler, L. I., & Fitzgerald, H. E. (1999). Heterogeneity of risk aggregation for alcohol problems between early and middle childhood: Nesting structure variations. *Development and Psychopathology, 11,* 727–744.

4

Alcohol Consumption and Its Consequences among Adolescents and Young Adults

Michael Windle and Rebecca C. Windle

Alcohol consumption among adolescents and young adults occurs at high rates, with such use resulting in potentially adverse consequences in many critical domains of life, such as academic and occupational achievement, family and peer relationships, and physical and mental health. A recent economic analysis of alcohol consumption estimated that underage drinkers (aged 12–20 years) account for 19.7% of consumer expenditures for alcohol in the United States.[1] This quite high rate is a conservative estimate because the national survey data of alcohol consumption on which the economic analyses were based excluded a number of high risk groups such as school dropouts, those in the military, those institutionalized, and homeless youth. A report by Levy et al.[2] indicated that underage drinking costs the United States approximately $53 billion annually due to a broad range of adverse consequences, including alcohol-related traffic crashes, violent crime, suicide attempts, and alcohol poisonings. In response to concerns over the high rates of binge drinking on college campuses and the adverse consequences of heavy drinking, the National Institute on Alcohol Abuse and Alcoholism convened a special council and charged it with evaluating the extent of the problem and making recommendations for effective interventions[3] (also, see the *Journal of Studies on Alcoholism*, Supplement No. 14, 2002). Hence, there is ample evidence that the pervasiveness of alcohol consumption and its adverse consequences among youth are quite costly in terms of psychological, social, and health functioning.

Michael Windle and Rebecca C. Windle • University of Alabama at Birmingham, Center for the Advancement of Youth Health, Birmingham, Alabama 35294-1200.

A number of different indexes have been used to measure alcohol consumption and alcohol-related consequences among adolescents and young adults. For example, there are several common indicators of alcohol use, such as lifetime use, past year use, past 30-day use, and age of initiation. Findings from these indicators provide useful surveillance data about alcohol use for different time windows and are particularly helpful in monitoring historical trends in the age of onset and prevalence of alcohol and other substance use across time.[4] In addition to these indicators of use or non-use of alcohol for specific time windows, there are indicators of more severe alcohol use, such as heavy episodic, or binge, drinking in the last two weeks or last 30 days, having been drunk in the last 30 days, and the daily use of alcohol, which is typically defined for adolescents as having consumed alcohol on 20 or more of the last 30 days. There is some variation across studies in the definition of binge drinking, but for teens, this is currently defined as having five or more drinks on a single occasion at least one time within the past two weeks or past 30 days. Some investigators[5] of college populations have proposed a criterion of five or more drinks on a single occasion as a definition of binge drinking for men, and a criterion of four or more drinks on a single occasion as a definition of binge drinking for women. Adverse physical (e.g., hangover, medical illnesses) and social (missing classes or work, alcohol-related aggression) consequences associated with alcohol use have provided yet another index to evaluate the impact of alcohol use on health-compromising outcomes. Finally, indicators of clinical diagnostic levels of alcohol abuse and dependence provide insight into the tertiary healthcare needs of youth by the healthcare system.

In this chapter, we provide an overview of current epidemiologic findings on alcohol consumption and its consequences among adolescents and young adults. In doing so, we provided data on the different alcohol consumption and consequences indexes described previously, often with subgroup breakdowns along important demographic dimensions such as age, gender, and racial/ethnic group. The chapter has five sections. First, prevalence data were provided for several alcohol consumption indexes, including use for various time intervals (e.g., lifetime, last 30-days) and heavy episodic, or binge, drinking. Second, data were presented on the prevalence of alcohol problems reported by adolescents and young adults and on the secondhand effects (e.g., study or sleep interrupted, property damaged) of alcohol use on non-drinkers by drinkers on college campuses. Third, data were provided on the prevalence of lifetime and current (last year) alcohol disorders. The fourth section focused on some important correlates of alcohol consumption and alcohol-related problems among youth that impact mortality and morbidity, including associations with the three leading causes of death among young people—accidental deaths, homicides, and suicides. A summary section is then provided to describe succinctly the central themes that emerged from these epidemiological findings.

Prevalence of Alcohol Consumption. The prevalence of several indicators of alcohol consumption by age, sex, and race/ethnicity are presented in Tables 1–4. The data presented in these tables are from three national surveys that collect information on alcohol and substance use among U.S. adolescents and young adults: the Monitoring the Future Survey (MFS)[4,6] the National Survey on Drug Use and Health (NSDUH)[7] (prior to the 2002 data collection, the NSDUH was known as the National Household Survey on Drug Abuse), and the Youth Risk Behavior Surveillance (YRBS).[8] Although prevalence estimates vary somewhat across these national studies in part due to differences in data collection procedures (e.g., in-school surveys, in-home personal interviews), findings from each indicate that alcohol consumption—as measured by lifetime and recent (e.g., past 30-day) use, and binge drinking—begins increasing in early adolescence and continues to become more prevalent throughout the teen years and into young adulthood when it peaks and then begins to decline. While rates of alcohol use increase with increasing age, alcohol consumption, including *heavy* consumption, is substantial even among younger teens. For example, data from the MFS (see Table 1) indicate that approximately one in five eighth graders reported consuming alcohol in the past 30 days, and approximately 12% reported at least one episode of binge drinking (i.e., 5+ drinks in a row) in the past two weeks. The YRBS (see Table 3) found that nearly 25% of ninth graders reported binge drinking in the past month.

In addition to age, rates of alcohol consumption also vary by sex and race/ethnicity. As the data in Tables 1–3 indicate, similar percentages of males and females in all age groups have consumed alcohol at sometime in their life. However, these data also show that gender differences in more *frequent* and *heavier* alcohol use patterns emerge with increasing age. For example, MFS data indicate that males and females in all age groups are similar on their rates of

Table 1. Prevalence of Various Indicators of Alcohol Consumption for Eighth, Tenth, and Twelfth Graders, Full-Time College Students, and Other Respondents 1–4 Years Beyond High School by Gender, 2002

Gender	Prevalence of Lifetime Alcohol Use	Prevalence of Past Year Alcohol Use	Prevalence of Past 30-Day Alcohol Use	Prevalence of Past 30-Day Daily Alcohol Use	5+ Drinks in a Row in Last Two Weeks
Male					
8th Graders	47.2	38.1	19.1	0.8	12.5
10th Graders	65.5	58.4	35.3	2.6	23.8
12th Graders	77.9	71.6	52.3	5.3	34.2
College	85.9	83.6	70.2	7.0	50.7
Non-College	84.2	80.8	65.5	5.3	43.8
Female					
8th Graders	46.8	39.2	20.0	0.4	12.1
10th Graders	68.5	61.8	35.7	1.0	21.0
12th Graders	78.5	71.2	45.1	1.7	23.0
College	86.1	82.4	68.0	3.7	33.4
Non-College	88.1	79.6	56.1	3.5	29.0

Source: National Institute on Drug Abuse and University of Michigan, Monitoring the Future Survey[4,6]

lifetime and past year alcohol use. Gender differences begin to emerge in rates of past 30-day alcohol use among older adolescent (i.e., twelfth graders) and young adult males and females, and these gender disparities become more pronounced for past 30-day daily use and binge drinking. Similarly, data from the NSDUH survey found that the rates of drinking among 12–17 year-old males and females are quite similar, but that 18–25 year-old males have a much higher prevalence of past 30-day alcohol use and binge drinking relative to their same-aged female peers.

Disparities in alcohol use by race/ethnicity have been found in YRBS, MFS, and NSDUH data (see Tables 2–4). In Table 2, the NSDUH data indicate that, in general, White and American Indian or Alaska Native teens and young adults have the highest rates of alcohol consumption, followed (in decreasing order of use) by Hispanics, African Americans, and Asians. The YRBS data indicate that Non-Hispanic White and Hispanic teens were roughly equal in their rates of alcohol use, while Non-Hispanic Black adolescents consumed less alcohol relative to these two groups. The MFS data in Table 4 show that White teens have somewhat higher rates of alcohol use compared with Hispanics (especially among tenth and twelfth graders), and that Black teens consume substantially less alcohol than both Whites and Hispanics.

Table 2. Prevalence of Various Indicators of Alcohol Consumption by Age, Gender, and Race/Ethnicity, 2002

Age in Years, Gender, Race/Ethnicity	Prevalence of Lifetime Alcohol Use	Prevalence of Past Year Alcohol Use	Prevalence of Past 30-Day Alcohol Use	5+ Drinks in a Row at Least One Day in Past 30 Days	5+ Drinks in a Row at Least Five Days in Past 30 Days
12–17 year-old males	43.4	33.3	17.4	11.4	3.1
12–17 year-old females	43.4	36.0	17.9	9.9	1.9
18–25 year-old males	88.0	80.1	65.2	50.2	21.1
18–25 year-old females	85.4	75.6	55.7	31.7	8.7
12–17 year-olds					
White	45.8	37.9	20.1	12.5	3.2
Black or African American	35.9	24.7	10.9	4.9	0.6
Hispanic or Latino	44.7	34.0	16.6	10.5	2.2
American Indian or Alaska Native	50.8	41.0	22.6	18.2	2.9
Asian	29.0	21.7	7.4	3.2	0.1
18–25 year-olds					
White	90.1	83.1	66.8	46.8	19.0
Black or African American	81.2	69.2	48.3	26.2	5.9
Hispanic or Latino	81.2	68.7	49.8	34.8	9.1
American Indian or Alaska Native	89.8	*	60.0	44.1	10.6
Asian	74.6	66.2	49.9	24.6	7.0

*Low precision; no estimate reported
Source: SAMHSA, Office of Applied Studies, National Survey on Drug Use and Health[7]

Table 3. Prevalence of Various Indicators of Alcohol Consumption by Gender, Race/Ethnicity, and School Grade, 2001

	Prevalence of Lifetime Alcohol Use			Prevalence of Past 30-Day Alcohol Use			5+ Drinks in a Row at Least One Day in Past 30 Days		
Race/Ethnicity and Grade	Female	Male	Total	Female	Male	Total	Female	Male	Total
Race/Ethnicity									
White, Non-Hispanic	79.6	80.7	80.1	48.3	52.6	50.4	30.5	37.7	34.0
Black, Non-Hispanic	69.7	68.4	69.1	30.6	35.0	32.7	7.5	15.1	11.1
Hispanic	80.1	81.6	80.8	48.8	49.5	49.2	28.7	31.4	30.1
Grade									
9	72.0	74.5	73.1	40.0	42.2	41.1	23.0	26.2	24.5
10	76.9	75.6	76.3	43.5	46.9	45.2	26.3	30.1	28.2
11	79.3	81.4	80.4	45.1	53.6	49.3	26.1	38.5	32.2
12	85.5	84.7	85.1	53.9	56.6	55.2	31.8	42.0	36.7

Source: Centers for Disease Control and Prevention, Youth Risk Behavior Surveillance—United States, 2001[8]

Table 4. Prevalence of Various Indicators of Alcohol Consumption by Race/Ethnicity and School Grade, 2002

	Prevalence of Past 30-Day Alcohol Use			Prevalence of Having Been Drunk in Past 30 Days			5+ Drinks in a Row in Past 2 Weeks		
Race/Ethnicity	Eighth	Tenth	Twelfth	Eighth	Tenth	Twelfth	Eighth	Tenth	Twelfth
White	23.2	40.0	54.0	8.0	23.2	36.6	12.7	25.5	33.7
Black	15.0	24.3	30.1	4.0	8.6	12.1	9.4	12.4	11.5
Hispanic	25.7	37.9	47.5	8.4	17.4	23.5	17.8	26.5	26.4

Source: National Institute on Drug Abuse and University of Michigan, Monitoring the Future Survey[4]

The above discussion illustrates variations in alcohol use based on the three important demographic characteristics of age, sex, and race/ethnicity. A less salient, but nevertheless important, discriminator of alcohol use among teens and young adults is the region of the country in which they reside. Findings from the NSDUH[7] found that, on various indexes of alcohol use, a higher rate of adolescents (12–17 year-olds) and young adults (18–25 year-olds) from the Northeast and Midwest consumed alcohol relative to youth in the South and West. Smaller variations in the prevalence of alcohol use were manifested by the younger age group, whereas larger variations in prevalence were evident for the older age group. For example, the rate of past month alcohol use by 12–17 year-olds in the Northeast and Midwest was approximately 19%; this rate was close to 16% for the same age group in the South and West (a 3% difference). In contrast, the rate of past month alcohol use by 18–25 year-olds in the Northeast and Midwest was about 66% with a rate of approximately 56% among young adults in the South and West (a 10% difference).

Prevalence of Alcohol Problems. Adverse social and health consequences occurring in conjunction with alcohol use, and especially heavy use, are quite prevalent among adolescents and young adults. In addition to the negative alcohol-related effects for the alcohol user, other individuals in the drinker's environment may likewise be adversely affected. Data from two large national surveys of college students' drinking and substance use behaviors—The Harvard School of Public Health College Alcohol Study (CAS)[9] and Southern Illinois University's (SIUs) Core Institute[10]—suggest that substantial percentages of adolescent and young adult drinkers experience a broad range of alcohol-related problems, including difficulties with peers, problems in school, negative physical consequences, and encounters with the law. For example, SIUs Core Institute[10] found that 64.5% of students who drank alcohol during the past year experienced a hangover, 55.3% got nauseated or vomited, 34.7% had a memory loss, and 16.5% had been hurt or injured. Similarly, Wechsler et al.[9] reported that, among college students who drank alcohol in the past year, 36.5% reported doing something they regretted, 22.5% engaged in unplanned sexual activity, and 35.8% drove after drinking. They also found that one in five college students (19.8%) reported *five or more* alcohol-related negative consequences over the past year.

Table 5 presents data from a community-based longitudinal study conducted by the first author of this chapter. The study, referred to as Lives Across Time: A Prospective Study of Adolescent and Adult Development (LAT),[11] has been ongoing since 1988 and has been funded by the National Institute on Alcohol Abuse and Alcoholism since its inception. The sample is comprised of predominantly White, middle-class participants. An important focus of the study has been to identify salient risk factors for the development of alcohol problems and disorders among adolescents and young adults. Data for two different ages are presented: older adolescents who were juniors and seniors in high school at the time of data collection, and young adults whose data were collected in a 5–7 year follow-up. Findings from the LAT show that 75% of older adolescent drinkers and 66% of young adult drinkers reported experiencing at least one alcohol-related consequence in the past 6 months, and that nearly 20%–25% reported five or more problems. In both the Wechsler et al.[9] survey and the LAT,[11] a higher percentage of males experienced negative alcohol-related consequences relative to females. Wechsler et al.[9] found a dose-response relationship between the frequency and quantity of alcohol use and the number of alcohol-related consequences. That is, non-binge drinkers were the least likely to report alcohol-related problems, frequent binge drinkers were the most likely to report these problems, and occasional binge drinkers were intermediate between the two groups in their reports of problems. Both Wechsler et al.[9] and the SIUs Core Institute[10] collected information on students'

Table 5. Prevalence of Alcohol-Related Problems from a Community-Based Longitudinal Study of Older Adolescents/Young Adults

	Percent Reporting Alcohol Consequences					
	Older Adolescents (Mean Age=16.96; SD=0.76)			Young Adults (Mean Age=23.81; SD=1.35)		
Adverse Alcohol-Related Consequences Occurring in Past 6 Months	All (n=832)	Males (n=378)	Females (n=454)	All (n=733)	Males (n=313)	Females (n=420)
Drank before or during work or school	12.3	16.9	8.4	10.4	16.6	5.7
Missed work or school because of drinking	9.4	11.9	7.3	13.6	18.2	10.2
Had a fight with members of my family about my drinking	16.2	19.6	13.4	8.8	10.5	6.7
Did things while I was drinking that I regretted the next day	47.7	49.7	46.0	39.8	46.3	34.8
Thought about cutting down on my drinking	24.5	31.0	19.2	26.9	38.7	18.1
Got drunk or high from alcohol several days in a row	28.9	37.3	21.9	24.0	33.9	16.7
Passed out from drinking	29.6	33.7	26.2	21.4	26.5	17.6
Had fight with my significant other about my drinking	16.6	17.2	16.1	11.2	14.7	8.6
Got into a fight or heated argument with someone I didn't know while drinking	16.6	25.7	9.0	12.2	19.2	6.9
Got into trouble with the law (other than driving-related) while drinking	6.5	11.4	2.4	2.2	4.2	0.7
Drank alone	21.5	25.2	18.5	27.6	34.8	22.1
Drank alcohol to get rid of a hangover	7.6	9.3	6.2	7.8	11.5	5.0
Drank to forget my troubles	37.3	35.4	38.8	22.0	24.0	20.5
Received a ticket for drinking and driving	1.3	2.0	0.7	1.5	2.9	0.5
Had a drinking-driving related accident	1.4	1.8	1.1	1.0	1.9	0.2
Percent Reporting:						
0 consequences	24.9	20.6	28.4	33.6	21.7	42.4
1–2 consequences	31.1	27.2	34.4	31.1	30.4	31.7
3–4 consequences	20.0	20.6	19.4	16.0	18.2	14.3
5–6 consequences	13.5	17.2	10.4	9.7	15.0	5.7
7+ consequences	10.6	14.3	7.5	9.7	14.7	6.0

Note: N's include only those study participants who reported drinking alcohol in the past 6 months.
Source: Data from Lives Across Time: A Prospective Study of Adolescent and Adult Development1.[11]

second-hand experiences of others' drinking. The second-hand experiences ranged in severity from less serious (e.g., interruption of study time) to more serious (e.g., experiencing unwanted sexual advances, being pushed, hit, or assaulted). Wechsler reported that close to 80% of students who were non-binge drinkers or abstainers and who lived in dormitories or fraternity or sorority residences reported having experienced at least one (of eight) adverse consequence related to someone else's drinking.

Prevalence of Alcohol Disorders. Rates of Alcohol Abuse and Alcohol Dependence, as defined by the Diagnostic and Statistical Manual of Mental Disorders, Fourth Edition (DSM-IV),[12] are quite prevalent within the U.S. population, and this is especially true among younger Americans. Because of the high rates of alcohol problems and disorders among young people, such problematic alcohol involvement has been referred to as a "developmental disorder of young adulthood."[13] Findings from the 1992 National Longitudinal Alcohol Epidemiologic Survey (NLAES) illustrate the higher rates of alcohol disorders among adolescents and younger adults relative to older adults. Using NLAES data, Grant[14] estimated that 19.32% of 18–24 year-olds met DSM-IV criteria for a lifetime diagnosis of Alcohol Dependence, while 18.98% of 25–34 year-olds, 14.66% of 35–44 year-olds, 12.05% of 45–55 year-olds, and 4.95% of 55 year-olds and older met diagnostic criteria. The higher rates of lifetime Alcohol Dependence among the younger cohorts might have been due to biased retrospective recall by the older cohorts (i.e., biased recall over longer time periods). However, rates of past[12] month Alcohol Dependence diagnoses manifested a similar pattern as lifetime diagnoses: 18–24 year-olds=11.06%, 25–34 year-olds=6.35%, 35–44 year-olds=3.57%, 45–54 year-olds=2.58%, and 55 and above=0.85%. The strong inverse relationship between age and past 12 month diagnosis for Alcohol Dependence suggests that biased retrospective recall did not impact diagnostic rates (because of the shorter recall time period); rather, this relationship suggests that rates of Alcohol Dependence are indeed higher among younger cohorts.

Table 6 presents data from the NSDUH for past year DSM-IV Alcohol Abuse and Dependence by age, gender, and race/ethnicity. The rates of abuse and dependence were quite similar for 12–17 year-old males and females, but were substantially higher for 18–25 year-old males relative to females. Whites in both age groups tended to have the highest rate of alcohol disorders, followed (in decreasing order) by Hispanics, African Americans, and Asians. Finally, data from the LAT study (see Figure 1) provide rates of DSM-IV Alcohol Abuse and Alcohol Dependence for young adult males and females by lifetime and past 12 month disorders. These data indicate that 17.2% met diagnostic criteria for a lifetime Alcohol Abuse disorder and that 17.1% met diagnostic criteria for a lifetime Alcohol Dependence disorder. Among those with a lifetime Alcohol Dependence disorder, 23.0% were males and 12.6% were females. Rates of past 12 month disorders were lower, with 6.1% meeting criteria for Alcohol Abuse and 2.9% meeting criteria for Alcohol Dependence. Gender differences were also evident for the past 12 month diagnoses.

Table 6. Prevalence of Past Year DSM-IV Alcohol Abuse and Dependence by Age, Gender, and Race/Ethnicity, 2002

Age in Years, Gender, Race/Ethnicity	Prevalence of Past Year DSM-IV Alcohol Abuse	Prevalence of Past Year DSM-IV Alcohol Dependence	Prevalence of Past Year DSM-IV Alcohol Abuse or Dependence
12–17 year-old males	3.8	2.1	5.9
12–17 year-old females	3.7	2.2	5.9
18–25 year-old males	14.1	8.8	22.9
18–25 year-old females	7.2	5.2	12.4
12–17 year-olds			
White	4.5	2.4	6.9
Black or African American	1.5	0.8	2.3
Hispanic or Latino	3.3	2.4	5.7
Asian	1.7	0.3	1.9
18–25 year-olds			
White	12.5	7.8	20.2
Black or African American	6.5	4.8	11.2
Hispanic or Latino	8.2	6.4	14.6
Asian	7.5	2.2	9.7

Source: SAMHSA, Office of Applied Studies, National Survey on Drug Use and Health[7]

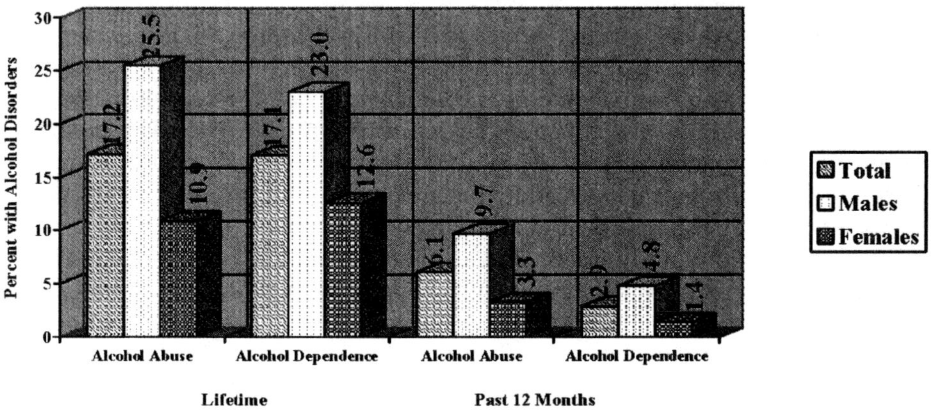

Figure 1. Prevalence of Lifetime and Past 12 Month DSM-IV Alcohol Disorders by Gender in a Community-Based Longitudinal Study of Young Adults

Note: The age range of study participants when these data were collected was 21 to 28 years, with a mean age of 23.81 years (S.D. = 1.35). The study participant Ns were: Total=760, Males=330, Females=430. The data presented here include both alcohol users and non-users.

Source: Data from Lives Across Time: A Prospective Study of Adolescent and Adult Development[11]

Alcohol's Association With Other Health-Compromising Behaviors. Alcohol consumption among adolescents and young adults is associated with a number of other health-compromising, and potentially life-threatening, behaviors. In this section, we provide an overview of the association between alcohol use and rates of accidental death, homicide, and suicide, and then briefly discuss alcohol's relationship to five health-compromising behaviors: dangerous driving, violence, suicidal behaviors, other substance use, and sexual activity. It is important to note that, in subsequent pages, we present epidemiologic data that indicate an *association* between alcohol use and health compromising behaviors. However, these associations are not intended to imply *causal* links between alcohol use and these behaviors. Rather, the relationships between alcohol use and other health-compromising behaviors are quite complex, and research suggests that alcohol interacts with biological, psychological, cognitive, and contextual factors to increase the *probability* of adverse health outcomes (see Cooper[15] for a thoughtful discussion of the relationship between alcohol use and sexual behavior).

According to the Centers for Disease Control and Prevention,[16] the three leading causes of death among young people 15–19 and 20–24 years of age are (in order) accidents, homicides, and suicides. Nationally, postmortem data do not exist in the U.S. on the number of accidental and violent deaths among young people in which alcohol is involved (an exception to this are data on alcohol involvement in traffic-related fatalities and these data are presented subsequently). In order to address this absence of information, Smith et al.[17] used data reported in 65 U.S. medical examiner studies that reported on non-traffic injury fatalities to estimate the percent of homicides, accidents (not including traffic fatalities), and suicides in which the decedent was positive for alcohol or was intoxicated at the time of death. Their findings indicated that the percent of decedents positive for alcohol were as follows: homicides=47.1%, accidents=38.5%, and suicides=29.0%. In addition, the percent of decedents who were intoxicated at the time of death were as follows: homicides=31.5%, accidents=31.0%, and suicides=22.7%. While these data are useful for providing broad estimates of the decedents' use of alcohol, the authors were unable to disaggregate the data by age or sex.

In contrast to the U.S., Finland collects extensive data on the circumstances of accidental and violent deaths via forensic autopsy and postmortem toxicology tests. As a result, Lunetta et al.[18] were able to report on the percentage of accidental deaths, suicides, and homicides associated with alcohol use that occurred in Finland from 1987–1996. These percentages were disaggregated by age and sex and are presented in Table 7. The highest rates of death associated with alcohol use by the deceased were among the youngest cohorts, with these rates decreasing with increasing age. In addition, the rates of alcohol-associated death were substantially higher among males relative to females in all age groups. The findings presented by both Smith et al.[17] and Lunetta et al.[18] indicate that alcohol use is strongly associated with mortality and that this is especially true for males and for younger cohorts.

Table 7. Age-Distribution of Alcohol-Related Accidental Deaths, Suicides, and Victims of Homicides by Age and Sex in Finland, 1987–1996

	% of Accidental Deaths Associated With Alcohol		% of Suicides Associated With Alcohol		% of Alcohol-Positive Victims of Homicide	
Ages	Males	Females	Males	Females	Males	Females
15–24	32.0	15.9	45.8	22.4	52.2	25.4
25–44	32.4	19.0	37.0	14.8	66.8	43.5
45–64	28.2	16.3	25.2	10.4	49.8	31.8
65+	6.6	1.4	10.9	3.3	11.4	7.1

Source: Lunetta, Penttilä, and Sarna[18]

Alcohol Use and Driving. Drinking and driving among youth under the age of 21 has decreased substantially during the past two decades. Hedlund et al.[19] reported that from 1982 to 1998 there was a 61% decrease in the number of drinking drivers under the age of 21 involved in fatal crashes. Despite these encouraging statistics, rates of drinking and driving among young people remain high. Data from the YRBS indicated that 22% of twelfth graders reported drinking and driving at least once in the past 30 days, and 32.8% reported riding with a driver who had been drinking at least once in the past 30 days.[8] Recent data from the NSDUH's 2002 survey[7] showed that almost one-third (32.4%) of 21-year-olds drove under the influence of alcohol during the past year. Data from the 1996 NHSDA[20] found that, among drivers who reported driving within two hours after alcohol use, 8.7% were 16–18 years old, 14.9% were 19–20 years old, and 29.1% were 21–25 years old. Adolescent and young adult males were more likely to drive within two hours after drinking than were females, and Non-Hispanic White teens and young adults were more likely to engage in this driving behavior than were Non-Hispanic Blacks and Hispanics. In addition to these high rates of DUI, Yi et al.[21] reported on the rates of alcohol-involved drivers in fatal traffic crashes during 2000. As shown in Table 8, 25.5% of alcohol-involved drivers in fatal crashes were between the ages of 16 and 24, and the highest rate of all alcohol-involved drivers was among the 21–24 year-old age group (32.2%). In addition, rates among males were much higher than among females.

Alcohol Use and Violence. Data presented in a report by the U.S. Department of Justice, Bureau of Justice Statistics (BJS)[22] indicated a substantial association between alcohol use and violent crime (e.g., murder, rape/sexual assault, robbery, assault). For example, the report found that between 30%–40% of violent offenders self-reported the use of alcohol at the time they committed the offense. In addition, in violent incidents in which alcohol was recorded as a factor by the police, 19% of *offenders* were 15–24 years old, and 25% of *victims* were in this age group. A section of the BJS report focused on alcohol and crime among U.S. college students. In 1995, 1.5 million college students (out of

Table 8. Percent of Drivers' Alcohol Involvement in Fatal Traffic Crashes by Age and Sex in the United States, 2000

Age and Sex	Percent of Alcohol-Involved Drivers
Both Sexes, 16–24	25.5
16–20	20.6
21–24	32.2
25–29	28.8
30–34	25.2
Males, 16–24	29.7
16–20	24.4
21–24	36.4
25–29	32.4
30–34	27.8
Females, 16–24	13.8
16–20	11.2
21–24	18.2
25–29	17.4
30–34	17.3

Source: National Institute on Alcohol Abuse and Alcoholism, Yi, Williams, and Dufour[21]

a population of 15.4 million students) experienced a violent crime; it was estimated that 463,000 of these violent victimizations involved alcohol use by the offender. SIUs Core Institute[10] collected data on the percent of college students who reported experiencing acts of violence and those who were under the influence of alcohol and/or other drugs when the victimization occurred. Among those students who were the victims of actual physical violence, 68.3% were using alcohol and/or other substances when they were victimized. Likewise, among those who experienced unwanted sexual intercourse, 82.6% were using substances at the time of their victimization.

Alcohol Use and Suicidal Behaviors. Alcohol use among adolescents and young adults is associated with a range of suicidal behaviors, including ideation, attempts, and completions.[23,24] In a study using data from the National Adolescent Student Health Survey, Windle et al.[25] investigated the prevalence of lifetime suicidal ideation and suicide attempts among male and female adolescents characterized as "abstainers" (i.e., did not drink in the last 30 days), "light drinkers" (i.e., drank on 1 to 5 occasions in the last 30 days), and "moderate/heavy drinkers" (i.e., drank on 6 or more occasions in the last 30 days). For both males and females, and 8th and 10th graders, a linear relationship was found between alcohol use and suicidal ideation and attempts. For example, among 10th grade female abstainers, 33.5% had thought about committing suicide and 12.3% had attempted suicide. Among light drinkers, 52.0% had thought about suicide and 21.4% had made an attempt. Finally, 63.1% of heavy drinkers had thought about committing suicide and 38.8% had attempted suicide. Powell et al.[24] reported that, in a sample of 13–34 year olds, the strongest predictor of a nearly lethal suicide attempt was drinking within three hours of the attempt, and this was after controlling for a range of other significant predictors. In the Finnish study cited previously,[18] 45.8% of completed suicides among 15–24 year-old males and 22.4% of completed suicides among 15–24 year-old females involved the use of alcohol (see Table 7).

Alcohol Use and Other Substance Use. Adolescents and young adults combine alcohol use with other substance use at high rates,[26,27] and heavier and more frequent alcohol use, relative to lower levels of use or no use, is more likely to co-occur with illicit substance use.[7] Utilizing data from the National Household Survey on Drug Abuse (NHSDA) and the National Comorbidity Survey (NCS), Anthony and Echeagaray-Wagner[29] reported population estimates on the co-occurrence of alcohol and tobacco *use* (from the NHSDA), and DSM-III-R co-morbid alcohol and tobacco *dependence* among recent users (from the NCS). For both males and females, the co-occurrence of alcohol and tobacco use began increasing in early adolescence and continued increasing until it reached a peak in the early- to mid-20s, at which time the use of both substances began to decline. For young adult males, approximately 45% reported concurrent alcohol and tobacco use at the peak of use; for young adult females, this peak rate was approximately 35%. As with alcohol and tobacco use, co-morbid alcohol and tobacco dependence reached a peak in young adulthood and began to decline thereafter. Among 15–18 year-old users, approximately 5% met criteria for co-morbid alcohol and tobacco dependence. This rate increased to 10% among 21–25 year old users. Young adult males had a somewhat higher rate of co-morbid alcohol and tobacco dependence (14%) relative to young adult females (8–10%). Using data from the National Longitudinal Survey of Youth, Shillington and Clapp[29] selected study participants 15–21 years of age who reported using either alcohol or marijuana during the past year. They then divided the sample into Alcohol-Only (n=382) and Alcohol + Marijuana (n=294) groups. A higher percentage of females (52.36%) reported alcohol use only whereas more males (53.40%) reported both alcohol and marijuana use. The two groups were compared on a range of past year alcohol and behavior problems, and for each problem (except for *problem with teacher* and *problem with gambling*), a significantly higher percentage of individuals using both alcohol and marijuana had experienced the problem relative to individuals using alcohol only.

Alcohol Use and Sexual Activity. Alcohol consumption among adolescents and young adults increases the probability that they will engage in sexual intercourse and also will engage in risky sex (e.g., having multiple sexual partners).[15,30] Data from the YRBS[8] presented in Table 9 indicate that, among sexually active teens, 27.8% of White teens, 17.8% of Black teens, and 24.1% of Hispanic teens reported alcohol or drug use at last sexual intercourse. Approximately equal numbers of male and female ninth graders reported substance use at last sexual intercourse, but by twelfth grade, 32.0% of males reported substance use during last intercourse whereas only 19.9% of females reported

Table 9. Use of Alcohol or Drugs at Last Sexual Intercourse among Sexually Active Adolescents by Gender, Race/Ethnicity, and School Grade, 2001

	Alcohol or Drug Use at Last Sexual Intercourse		
Race/Ethnicity and Grade	Female	Male	Total
Race/Ethnicity			
White	22.9	33.6	27.8
Black	10.4	24.2	17.8
Hispanic	21.9	26.2	24.1
Grade			
9	24.5	23.8	24.0
10	20.8	35.7	27.7
11	18.4	31.3	24.7
12	19.9	32.0	25.4

Source: Centers for Disease Control and Prevention, Youth Risk Behavior Surveillance—United States, 2001[8]

the co-occurrence of these behaviors. Using data collected from the 1999 Harvard College Alcohol Study,[31] Hingson et al.[32] evaluated the association between an earlier age of onset of first intoxication and college students' reports that drinking caused unplanned sex and unprotected sex. In the overall sample, 20% reported having *unplanned* sex because of drinking and 10% reported having *unprotected* sex because of drinking. With regard to the age of first intoxication, the data showed that students who reported a younger age of intoxication, relative to those who reported a later age of intoxication or never being intoxicated, were more likely to report that drinking caused unplanned sex and unprotected sex. For example, 31.2% of students who were 12 years-old or younger at first intoxication reported that alcohol caused them to engage in unplanned sex; in contrast, less than 5% of those who reported never having been intoxicated believed alcohol caused them to engage in unplanned sex.

Summary. Findings from national, college, and community studies indicate high rates of alcohol use (as measured by a number of different indexes), alcohol-related adverse consequences, and alcohol disorders among adolescents and young adults. Alcohol use and alcohol disorders increase with age and peak in young adulthood (generally around 21 years of age).[7] Among younger and middle-aged adolescents, the rates of more frequent and heavier alcohol use, and of alcohol disorders, are fairly equal among males and females; however, during older adolescence and young adulthood, gender disparities emerge, with males, relative to females, drinking more frequently and in greater quantity, experiencing more adverse alcohol-related problems, and meeting diagnostic criteria for alcohol disorders. Racial and ethnic group comparisons for alcohol use, binge drinking, and alcohol disorders indicate the highest rates for White and American Indian or Alaska Native teens and young adults, followed by Hispanics, African Americans, and Asians.

National and international studies have indicated a strong association between alcohol use and the three leading causes of mortality among adolescents and young adults: accidental injuries, homicides, and suicides.[17,18] Studies investigating the association between alcohol use and other health-compromising behaviors have indicated that alcohol use by adolescents and young adults is associated with fatal traffic crashes, violent or aggressive incidents as either the perpetrator or victim, suicidal behaviors (including ideation, attempts, and completions), other licit (e.g., cigarettes) and illicit (e.g., marijuana) substance use, and unplanned and unprotected sexual activity. Collectively, these findings support the need for comprehensive intervention programs that target alcohol use reduction as a key element to address morbidity and mortality issues among youth.

ACKNOWLEDGMENTS: This research was supported by National Institute on Alcohol Abuse and Alcoholism Grant R37-AA07861 awarded to Michael Windle. Correspondence concerning the article should be sent to Michael Windle, UAB Center for the Advancement of Youth Health, 912 Building, 1530 3rd Avenue S., Birmingham, AL 35294–1200.

References

1. Foster SE, Vaughan RD, Foster WH, Califano Jr., JA: Alcohol consumption and expenditures for underage drinking and adult excessive drinking. JAMA 289:989–995, 2003.
2. Levy DT, Miller TR, Cox, K: Costs of underage drinking. Calverton, MD, Pacific Institute for Research and Evaluation, 1999.
3. Task Force of the National Advisory Council on Alcohol Abuse and Alcoholism: *A call to action: Changing the culture of drinking at U.S. colleges (NIH Publication No. 02–5010).* Rockville, MD, National Institute on Alcohol Abuse and Alcoholism, 2002. Retrieved September 18, 2003 from http://www.collegedrinkingprevention.gov/images/TaskForce/TaskForceReport.pdf
4. Johnston LD, O'Malley PM, Bachman JG: *Monitoring the Future national survey results on drug use, 1975–2002. Volume I: Secondary school students* (NIH Publication No. 03–5375). Bethesda, MD, National Institute on Drug Abuse, 2003a. Retrieved September 16, 2003, from http://www.monitoringthefuture.org/pubs/monographs/vol1_2002.pdf
5. Wechsler H, Dowdall GW, Davenport A, Rimm EB: A gender-specific measure of binge drinking among college students. *Am J Public Health* 85:982–985, 1995.
6. Johnston LD, O'Malley PM, Bachman JG: *Monitoring the Future national survey results on drug use, 1975–2002. Volume II: College students and adults ages 19–40* (NIH Publication No. 03–537). Bethesda, MD, National Institute on Drug Abuse, 2003b. Retrieved September 16, 2003, from http://www.monitoringthefuture.org/pubs/monographs/vol2_2002.pdf
7. Substance Abuse and Mental Health Services Administration: *Overview of findings from the 2002 National Survey on Drug Use and Health* (Office of Applied Studies, NHSDA Series H-21, DHHS Publication No. SMA 03–3774). Rockville, MD, 2003. Retrieved September 24, 2003, from http://www.DrugAbuseStatistics.SAMHSA.gov
8. Grunbaum JA, Kann L, Kinchen SA, Williams B, Ross, JG, Lowry, R, Kolbe, L: Youth Risk Behavior Surveillance—United States, 2001. In: *Surveillance Summaries,* June 28, 2002. MMWR 51 (No. SS-4):1–62.
9. Wechsler H, Dowdall GW, Maenner G, Gledhill-Hoyt J, Lee H: Changes in binge drinking and related problems among American college students between 1993 and 1997: Results of the Harvard School of Public Health College Alcohol Study. *J Am Coll Health* 47:57–68, 1998.

10. Southern Illinois University, Core Institute: American campuses: 2001 statistics on alcohol and other drug use. Retrieved August 28, 2003, from http://www.siu.edu/departments/coreinst/public_html/recent.html
11. Windle M: *Vulnerability factors and adolescent drinking*. National Institute on Alcohol Abuse and Alcoholism, Grant No. R37–07861, 2003.
12. American Psychiatric Association: *Diagnostic and statistical manual of mental disorders*, Fourth Edition. Washington, DC, American Psychiatric Association, 1994.
13. Sher KJ, Gotham HJ: Pathological alcohol involvement: A developmental disorder of young adulthood. *Dev Psychopathol* 11:933–956, 1999.
14. Grant BF: Prevalence and correlates of alcohol use and DSM-IV alcohol dependence in the United States: Results of the National Longitudinal Alcohol Epidemiologic Survey. *J Stud Alcohol* 58:464–473, 1997.
15. Cooper ML: Alcohol use and risky sexual behavior among college students and youth: Evaluating the evidence. *J Stud Alcohol* Supplement No. 14:101–117, 2002.
16. Anderson, RN: Deaths: Leading causes for 2000. *Natl Vital Stat Rep* 50:1–88, 2002. Retrieved September 2, 2003 from http://www.cdc.gov/nchs/data/nvsr/nvsr50/nvsr50_16.pdf
17. Smith GS, Branas CC, Miller T: Fatal nontraffic injuries involving alcohol: A metaanalysis. *Ann Emerg Med* 33:659–668, 1999.
18. Lunetta P, Penttilä A, Sarna S: The role of alcohol in accident and violent deaths in Finland. *Alcohol Clin Exp Res* 25:1654–1661, 2001.
19. Hedlund JH, Ulmer RG, Preusser DF: *Determine why there are fewer young alcohol-impaired drivers*. Washington, D.C., Department of Transportation, National Highway Traffic Safety Administration, 2001. Retrieved August 26, 2003 from http://www.nhtsa.dot.gov/ people/injury/research/FewerYoungDrivers/tech_doc.htm
20. Townsend TN, Lane J, Dewa CS, Brittingham AM: *Driving after drug or alcohol use: Findings from the 1996 National Household Survey on Drug Abuse*. Rockville, MD, Substance Abuse and Mental Health Services Administration, Office of Applied Studies, 1998. Retrieved August 28, 2003 from http://drugabusestatistics.samhsa.gov
21. Yi H-Y, Williams GD, Dufour MC: *Trends in alcohol-related fatal traffic crashes, United States, 1977–2000 (Surveillance Report #61)*. Bethesda, MD, National Institute on Alcohol Abuse and Alcoholism, 2003. Retrieved September 2, 2003 from http://www.niaaa.nih.gov/publications/surveillance61/fars00.htm
22. Greenfeld LA: *Alcohol and crime: An analysis of national data on the prevalence of alcohol involvement in crime*. Washington, D.C., U.S. Department of Justice, 1998. Retrieved September 2, 2003 from http://www.ojp.usdoj.gov/bjs/pub/pdf/ac.pdf
23. Powell KE, Kresnow M, Mercy JA, Potter LB, Swann AC, Frankowski RF, Lee RK, Bayer TL: Alcohol consumption and nearly lethal suicide attempts. *Suicide Life Threat Behav* 32:30–41, 2001.
24. Windle RC, Windle M: An investigation of adolescents' substance use behaviors, depressed affect, and suicidal behaviors. *J Child Psychol Psychiat* 38: 921–929, 1997.
25. Windle M, Miller-Tutzauer C, Domenico D: Alcohol use, suicidal behavior, and risky activities among adolescents. *J Res Adolesc* 2:317–330, 1992.
26. Hoffman JH, Welte JW, Barnes GM: Co-occurrence of alcohol and cigarette use among adolescents. *Addict Behav* 26:63–78, 2001.
27. Jackson KM, Sher KJ, Cooper ML, Wood PK: Adolescent alcohol and tobacco use: Onset, persistence and trajectories of use across two samples. *Addiction* 97:517–531, 2002.
28. Anthony JC, Echeagaray-Wagner F: Epidemiologic analysis of alcohol and tobacco use: Patterns of co-occurring consumption and dependence in the United States. *Alcohol Res Health* 24:201–208, 2000.
29. Shillington AM, Clapp JD: Beer and bongs: Differential problems experienced by older adolescents using alcohol only compared to combined alcohol and marijuana use. *Am J Drug Alcohol Abuse* 28:379–397, 2002.
30. Sen B: Does alcohol-use increase the risk of sexual intercourse among adolescents? Evidence from the NLSY97. *J Health Econ* 21:1085–1093, 2002.

31. Wechsler H, Lee JE, Kuo M., Lee H: College binge drinking in the 1990s: A continuing problem. Results of the Harvard School of Public Health 1999 College Alcohol Study. *J Am College Health* 48:199–210, 2000.
32. Hingson R, Heeren T, Winter MR, Wechsler H: Early age of first drunkenness as a factor in college students' unplanned and unprotected sex attributable to drinking. *Pediatrics* 111:34–41, 2003.

5

Drinking among College Students
Consumption and Consequences

Kristina M. Jackson, Kenneth J. Sher, and Aesoon Park

For most of the American population, the college years represent the period of life associated with the highest levels of alcohol consumption and, most likely, the highest prevalence of alcohol use disorders during the lifespan (Grant, 1997). Recent research has focused increasingly on college student drinking. For example, a combined PsycINFO/Medline search of abstracts containing the words "alcohol or drink or drinking" shows a dramatic increase in the percentage of scholarly articles that contain the term "college" over the past four decades; 0.7% (1963–1972), 1.9% (1973–1982), 2.5% (1983–1992), and 2.7% (1993–2002). In this chapter, we provide a review of what is currently known about the prevalence and patterns of alcohol use and associated problems in college students; how individual, intra-campus, and inter-campus factors relate to use and problems; and what is currently known regarding the long-term negative consequences of problematic college student drinking.

Most of the prevalence estimates of college student drinking come from a few landmark studies conducted with national datasets in which the data were collected either specifically from college students, such as the College Alcohol Study (CAS; Wechsler, Davenport, Dowdall, Moeykens, & Castillo, 1994; Wechsler, Lee, Kuo, & Lee, 2000), the Core Institute (CORE; Presley, Meilman, & Cashin, 1996), and the National College Health Risk Behavior Survey (NCHRBS; Centers of Disease Control and Prevention, 1997), or more generally from college-aged young adults, including Monitoring the Future (MTF; Johnston, O'Malley, & Bachman, 2002), the National Household Survey on Drug Abuse (NHSDA; Gfroerer, Greenblatt, & Wright, 1997), and the National Longitudinal Study of Youth (NLSY; Center for Human Resource Research, 1993).

Kristina M. Jackson, Kenneth J. Sher, and Aesoon Park • University of Missouri, Columbia and the Midwest Alcoholism Research Center, Columbia, Missouri 65211-0001.

The data obtained in these studies is representative of the populations sampled; all except CORE used probability sampling (although CORE recently completed a national probability study) and none suffered from bias resulting from nonresponse (O'Malley & Johnston, 2002). A number of other studies have collected data at the individual institution level. Although the results of these studies are less generalizable, these studies are important because they are more comprehensive in terms of breadth of measurement and/or assessment of relevant covariates than are the national studies.

1. Drinking in College Student versus Non-Student Populations

Enrolling in college has become a normative experience in the United States. In 2001, 61.7% of students who completed high school enrolled in a college or university (U.S. Department of Commerce; DOC, 2003), and based on data from the National Center for Education Statistics (NCES, 1999) and DOC (2000) the estimated proportion of 18–24 year olds enrolled in college at a given time was 31% (Hingson, Heeren, Zakocs, Kopstein, & Wechsler, 2002). Because college attendance is common, it is valuable to examine how college students differ from their non-collegiate age peers in order to determine the extent to which college-student drinking is closely coupled with college attendance itself versus the extent to which it represents a "stage-of-life" phenomenon largely unrelated to college attendance.

Although certain forms of substance use are much less prevalent in college students than in non-students (e.g., tobacco, cocaine), total alcohol consumption by college students appears to be similar to that of non-students but college students tend to differ in their drinking patterns (i.e., quantity and frequency). Specifically, MTF and NHSDA data indicate that college students have higher prevalence rates of alcohol use and higher rates of heavy use, but lower rates of daily drinking than do their non-student peers (Johnston et al., 2002; O'Malley & Johnston, 2002). Similar findings were reported by Crowley (Crowley, 1991) using NLSY data, who observed higher rates of any drinking by college students but equal frequency and lower quantity than by non-students. Using NHSDA data, Gfroerer, Greenblatt, and Wright (1997) observed that (with the exception of those living at home with their parents), students had higher current rates of frequent heavy drinking than did non-students, even when age, race, and sex were controlled. A similar pattern emerged for past-month alcohol use, although college students who lived with their parents reported higher use than high-school dropouts but lower use than high-school graduates. In general, individuals who dropped out of college had consumption rates similar to college students, suggesting a social class/lifestyle effect (Crowley, 1991).

Using data from the CAS, Knight, Wechsler, Kuo, Seibring, Weitzman, and Schuckit (2002) reported that the percentage of college students (6%) who endorsed criteria for a past-year DSM-IV alcohol dependence diagnosis was lower than the percentage for 18–24 year olds in the U.S. population (13%; Grant, 1997), consistent with Grant's finding that education decreases the odds of being diagnosed with alcohol dependence (although differences in methodology between Knight et al's and Grant's studies make direct comparisons difficult). Slutske et al. (2003) suggested that lower rates of alcohol use disorders (despite higher rates of drinking) among college student women compared to non-student peers may be in part because college provides a buffer against certain symptoms (especially those related to family and vocational adjustment) and in part because other symptoms (e.g., drinking in larger amounts or for longer than intended) may lose relevance against the backdrop of the college environment. Analogously, Hingson et al. (2002) observed that college students were less likely to receive alcohol or drug treatment than were their noncollege peers, and were no more likely to experience alcohol-related health problems than non-students.

Given differences in alcohol involvement between college students and non-students, a critical question is whether or not these differences reflect pre-existing pre-college differences (i.e., a selection effect) or a consequence of college attendance (i.e., an influence effect). A few large-scale studies have addressed this question. First, MTF panel data show that those students who go on to college have lower rates of high school heavy drinking than those who do not go on to college (O'Malley & Johnston, 2002), suggesting that after high school, college students increase their drinking more than and actually surpass their non-college student peers. This suggests that it is the college environment (influence) rather than characteristics of the students themselves (selection) that contributes to heavy drinking on campus. Strong evidence for the role of the college environment in drinking was obtained by Slutske et al (2003) in a study of college-aged female twins. Although most of the association between college attendance and drinking could be attributed to demographic and dispositional/lifestyle factors (e.g., marital status, living situation), getting drunk continued to be associated with college attendance beyond these factors. Further, even after modeling genetic similarity, college attendees reported a greater maximum quantity of alcohol consumed than their non-college attending twins, suggesting that the college experience serves as a risk factor for heavy drinking among women.

These findings suggesting that college attendance is a "situational" risk factor for heavy drinking complement those reported by Muthen and Muthen (2000) who examined heavy drinking and alcohol problems during young adulthood (mid-20s through mid-30s) using NLSY data. They found that individuals who had attended some college by age 22 actually had lower levels of heavy drinking in their late-30s than did those who either completed or dropped out of high school; moreover, the protective effect of college attendance increased with age (up to age 37). Further, the level of alcohol problems for college attendees decreased over time, compared to a sharp increase observed for high-school dropouts. These findings support the idea that there is something situational about the college environment that promotes drinking beyond pre-college background characteristics.

2. Prevalence and Patterns of Alcohol Use in College Students: A Closer Look

Although there is wide variation in how alcohol involvement is defined (Brennan, Walfish, & AuBuchon, 1986b), there are three broad domains to consider when discussing alcohol involvement: (1) alcohol consumption, (2) alcohol-related consequences or problems, and (3) alcohol dependence. While conceptually and empirically related, each refers to a distinct set of phenomena and each has important implications for research on college student drinking. Prior to discussing each of these three domains with reference to college students, we provide a brief introduction to each.

The term *alcohol consumption* refers to the frequency with which alcohol is consumed and/or quantity consumed over a given time. Frequency refers to the number of days or occasions on which someone has consumed alcoholic beverages during a specified interval such as a week, month, or year. Quantity refers to the amount consumed on a given drinking occasion. Most typically, consumption is assessed using number of "standard drinks" (i.e., 5 ounces of wine, 12 ounces of beer, or 1.25 ounces of distilled spirits). Quantity and frequency measures can be combined to form a measure of quantity/frequency (Q-F), which estimates the total volume consumed over a specified time.

For many purposes, the primary concern is the frequency of excessive consumption, often indexed using the frequency of consuming a number of drinks meeting or exceeding a certain threshold. Frequently, excessive- or heavy-drinking occasions are referred to as "binges" in the college student drinking literature. Due to the influential work of Wechsler and colleagues (who define "binge" as five or more drinks in a row for men and four or more drinks in a row for women; see Wechsler, Dowdall, Davenport, & Rimm, 1995), the prevalence of binge drinking has become a key metric in estimating the prevalence of problematic alcohol involvement on college campuses. Because the term "binge drinking" has historically been used to refer to an extended period of heavy drinking by clinicians, some have argued against using this term to describe what is typically a less extreme drinking behavior (Schukit, 1998). However, Wechsler has argued that the criteria of 5 (or 4) drinks "in a row" is a meaningful threshold and that consumption at these levels is associated with a greatly enhanced likelihood of experiencing a range of negative consequences (Wechsler & Nelson, 2001). Whether terms such as "heavy drinking," "binge drinking," or "drinking to intoxication" are used, research has demonstrated that the consumption of large quantities of alcohol on a single drinking occasion is an important variable in assessing college students' alcohol involvement, although the best way of describing excessive drinking remains an open question.

Alcohol-related problems and consequences refer to a variety of negative life events that arise from drinking such as social problems (e.g., physical or verbal aggression, relationship difficulties), legal problems (e.g., arrests for driving while intoxicated, public inebriation), educational/vocational problems (e.g., academic difficulties, termination from employment, failure to achieve career goals), and medical problems (e.g., unintentional injury, liver disease, central nervous system disease). Some would argue that consumption is a major social issue only to the extent that it generates adverse consequences. Consequently, it is possible to conceive of prevention strategies (e.g., designated driver programs) that might not reduce consumption but still reduce consequences.

The term *alcohol dependence* replaces the older term "alcoholism" and refers to a syndrome consisting of signs and symptoms signifying the importance of alcohol consumption in the life of the drinker (Edwards, 1986; Edwards & Gross, 1976) and can include both behavioral and physiological symptoms. Although both alcohol-related consequences and the alcohol dependence syndrome can be viewed as dimensional constructs, psychiatric diagnostic tradition emphasizes categorical distinctions and the fourth edition of the *Diagnostic and Statistical Manual of Mental Disorders* (DSM-IV) describes two major categories of alcohol use disorder, (1) alcohol abuse and (2) alcohol dependence, that roughly correspond to the distinction between alcohol-related disabilities or consequences and the alcohol dependence syndrome (American Psychiatric Association; APA,1994; Edwards & Gross, 1976). In DSM-IV, alcohol dependence is the more severe disorder, and its presence or history excludes the diagnosis of alcohol abuse.

Prevalence of alcohol consumption. There is generally consistency across the major nationally representative studies on college student drinking in terms of prevalence rates for any alcohol use, typical use, and heavy use. Approximately 85% of respondents in the MTF survey report drinking in the past year (Johnston et al., 2002), and the reported thirty-day prevalence of alcohol use among full-time college students is around 70% (O'Malley & Johnston, 2002). Large-scale regional/national studies report modal drinking frequency of a few times per week and modal quantity of 2–4 drinks per occasion, with data from the CORE study indicating that students drink on average 6.6 drinks per week (Core Institute, 1998). A consistent finding is that approximately 40% of college students report heavy drinking in the past two weeks (or 30 days, as in NCHRBS) (O'Malley & Johnston, 2002). In addition, 12% of participants in NHSDA reported *frequent* heavy drinking (defined by heavy drinking on five or more days in the past 30 days).

Prevalence of alcohol problems and consequences. Many surveys indicate that students report relatively high rates of problems from drinking. Although these surveys help to highlight the magnitude of the problem of alcohol on campus, the limitations of these types of data need to be appreciated. Although the causal status of alcohol in some types of problems (e.g., blackouts, hangover, nausea and vomiting) is reasonably clear, the causal role in some other types of problems (e.g., fighting, high risk sex, academic failure) can be difficult to establish. As outlined by Cooper (2002), the mechanisms underlying the relationship between alcohol involvement and a given consequence (e.g., risky sexual behavior) can be distinguished along two dimensions. The first dimension differentiates between three alternative causal mechanisms: (1) alcohol might causally promote some problem; (2) the experience of a given problem might lead to alcohol consumption; or (3) a common third-variable might cause both behaviors. The second dimension classifies the mechanisms in terms of time course, including (1) event-based phenomena (e.g., acute intoxication leads to a violent episode; being victimized leads one to drink; certain bars promote both drinking and fighting) or (2) more global, chronic, and stable processes (e.g., chronic alcohol use might lead to association with a violent subculture; individuals who have been victimized develop a chronic syndrome that leads to heavy drinking; certain types of people like to both drink and fight). Unfortunately, the dearth of both prospective panel data and event-based data on alcohol use and covariates of interest usually makes it difficult to determine which of these families of mechanisms are at work. Much research has relied upon the respondent making the link between drinking behavior and related consequences, a link that he or she may not be able to make validly. We review the results of surveys of consequences in this section, focusing first on academic problems and then discussing problems that college students share with others their own age, and then we revisit the issue of alcohol's role in a select number of problems in the penultimate section of this chapter.

Berkowitz and Perkins (1986), in a review of the literature from 1975–1985, reported a wide range in estimates of prevalence of problem drinking, ranging from 6% to 72%, depending on how problem drinking was defined. Wechsler, Dowdall, Maenner, Gledhill-Hoyt, and Lee (1998a) also reported endorsement of past-year alcohol problems ranging from 1% to 36% in the 1997 CAS.

A particularly important domain of alcohol consequences among college students is *academic performance*. According to data from the CAS and CORE survey, 21% of students report that they have performed poorly on tests/projects, 24–27% report having missed a class, and 19% report getting behind in schoolwork due to drinking in the previous year (Presley et al., 1996; Wechsler et al., 1998a). The negative association between self-reported drinking and grades is a robust one (e.g., Engs, Diebold, & Hanson, 1996; Harford, Wechsler, & Rohman, 1983; Knight et al., 2002; Perkins, 1992; Presley et al., 1996; Pullen, 1994; Schukit, 1998; Wechsler, Dowdall, Davenport, & Castillo, 1995) but it is not clear to what extent it is causal. In a prospective study, Wood, Sher, Erickson, and DeBord (1997) addressed limitations of earlier research by controlling for third variables including conduct problems, precollegiate academic ability and performance, parental education, and other drug use. In addition, this study also addressed limitations in prior self-report research by assessing academic failure with archival data using transcripts from all universities attended. Moderate bivariate associations were observed between freshman alcohol involvement and cumulative academic problems in college; however, the association did not hold when plausible "third-variable" confounds (especially college entrance test scores, high-school class rank, conduct disorder symptoms, gender, other drug use) were statistically controlled. These findings are consistent with those of Paschall and Freisthler (2003) who prospectively examined college academic performance (GPA) and found that neither alcohol use nor problems were associated with college GPA once high-school GPA and other demographic characteristics were controlled for. Given the results of these better-controlled studies, it appears that the effect of alcohol on academic performance may be overstated in the literature; a strong association exists, but the extent to which it is causal is unclear.

Drinking-related health consequences are relatively common in this population. In terms of short-term health consequences, nearly half of all students reported at least one hangover and half reported nausea or vomiting due to alcohol/drug use in the past year (Perkins, 2002b). Data on blackouts (memory loss for events while intoxicated), another index of short-term health, show that blackouts range in frequency from 22% to 26% in the past year in data from the CAS and the CORE studies (Perkins, 2002b). In addition, the prevalence of self-reported personal injuries in the past year due to drinking or other drug use range from 9% to 20% (Perkins, 1992, 2002b). Death resulting from alcohol ingestion (fatal alcohol poisoning) and drinking-related suicide are matters of great concern in the college population, but unfortunately little data exist, and reports tend to be anecdotal and not systematic. Although a small number of alcohol overdose deaths have drawn attention to drinking problems on college campuses, the more critical cause of mortality is unintentional fatal injuries (Hingson et al., 2002). Using data from the Centers for Disease Control (CDC) and the NHSDA, Hingson et al. estimated that among college students, 1,400 unintentional alcohol-related fatal injuries occur each year, 1,100 of which are traffic-related fatalities.

Although many students have limited needs for driving and many institutions restrict automobile use (Toor, 2003), 33% of college students report having *driven under the influence* during the academic year and 1.7% reported being arrested for drunk driving (Presley et al., 1996). Correspondingly, the two most common alcohol-related health risks are (1) driving after drinking and (2) riding with a drunk driver, with 28% of students (over 2 million) driving under the influence and 39% riding with a drunk driver (Hingson et al., 2002). Not surprisingly, heavy drinkers are more likely to drive drunk (56% of men and 43% of women) than light-to-moderate drinkers (17% of men and 10% of women) (Engs et al., 1996).

Alcohol consumption is consistently associated with *high-risk sexual behavior* such as unplanned sex and multiple sexual partners (Desiderato & Crawford, 1995; Santelli, Brener, Lowry, Bhatt, & Zabin, 1998; Wechsler, Dowdall et al., 1995; Wechsler & Isaac, 1992). Rates of risky sexual behavior are quite high in the college population, with about 20 to 25 percent of college students reporting unintended sexual activity due to drinking at least once in the past year (Meilman, 1993; Perkins, 1992; Wechsler et al., 1998a), with many of these individuals doing so on more than one occasion. Rates of unprotected sex are also high, with 10–20% of respondents reporting having had unprotected sex due to drinking (Meilman, 1993; Wechsler et al., 1998a). However, data on the relation between drinking and condom use is somewhat inconsistent (Desiderato & Crawford, 1995; Graves, 1995). In her recent review of the college student risky-sex literature, Cooper (2002) concluded that there exist strong associations between alcohol use and the decision to have sex and to have indiscriminate forms of risky sex (e.g., multiple or casual partners) but an inconsistent association with protective behaviors (e.g., condom use).

Another potential alcohol-related problem is sexual victimization. CORE data show that 12% of students reported having been taken advantage of sexually in the past year due to drinking (Presley et al., 1996), and Frintner and Rubinson (1993) found that 27% of female students at a single institution were victims of sexual assault or abuse or attempted sexual assault. Of these victims, 55% were drinking; of these, 60% reported that their judgment had been impaired due to drinking.

Alcohol-related behavior often has important consequences for other students and for the college environment, so called "*second-hand effects*" of drinking. Rates of property damage due to drinking are high; across multiple studies, past-year property damage committed by students hovers around 8% (Perkins, 1992), with 12% of students sustaining property damage due to others' drinking (Wechsler, Moeykens, Davenport, Castillo, & Hansen, 1995). Second-hand effects of others' drinking such as being interrupted while studying, having to take care of a drunk student, being insulted, or being a victim of unwanted sexual advances are relatively common in college. Wechsler et al. (2000) found that, overall, 77% of students reported having experienced at least one second-hand effect during the current school year in 1999.

One of the most serious types of "second-hand" effects is *sexual assault* In a recent review of the literature, Abbey (2002) concluded that at least half of the sexual assaults among college students involve alcohol use by the perpetrator, the victim, or both. Abbey (1991, 2000) outlined a number of ways that alcohol consumption on the part of the perpetrator or the victim can increase the likelihood of sexual aggression taking place, including misinterpretation of various verbal and nonverbal cues as indicative of sexual interest and gender-based stereotypes that women are supposed to be reluctant to initiate sexual contacts or reciprocate sexual advances, both of which are accentuated when the perpetrator has been drinking, given alcohol's ability to narrow attentional focus (Steele & Josephs, 1990). Additional research shows that, although level of *typical* alcohol use is somewhat associated with sexual assault for both victims and perpetrators (Abbey, Ross, McDuffie, & McAuslan, 1996; Koss & Dinero, 1989; Larimer, Lydum, Anderson, & Turner, 1999; Tyler, Hoyt, & Whitbeck, 1998; Ullman, Karabatsos, & Koss, 1999), level of *pre-assault* alcohol use is the more important factor. Using data from the National Survey of College Women (Koss, Gidycz, & Wisniewski, 1987), Ullman et al. (1999) found that although frequency of intoxication and pre-assault drinking were both positively associated with sexual victimization severity in both perpetrators and victims, the association was stronger for pre-assault drinking. Notably, though, perpetrator aggression was more strongly associated with sexual assault severity in incidents without pre-assault alcohol use, a pattern of results that, as Ullman et al. (1999) noted, is not consistent with the notion of alcohol's disinhibiting effects on offender's aggressive behavior.

The residential environment also leads to high rates of *interpersonal violence.* CORE data show that 30% of students were involved in an argument or fight due to drinking or drug use in the past year (Presley et al., 1996), and CAS data indicate that 13% of students claimed that they had been pushed, hit, or assaulted, 22% had experienced a serious quarrel, and 27% had been insulted or humiliated as result of another student's drinking (Wechsler, Moeykens et al., 1995). Similar rates were observed by Engs & Hanson (1994), who reported that 14% of students reported having gotten into fight due to drinking in the past year. In terms of alcohol's effect on violence in a relationship, although earlier work concludes that alcohol is not an important risk factor for dating violence (Brodbelt, 1983; Laner, 1983; Sugarman & Hotaling, 1989), more recent research has observed positive findings (e.g., Follingstad, Bradley, Laughlin, & Burke, 1999; Stets & Henderson, 1991), although other work has been more inconsistent (Nicholson et al., 1998; Shook, Gerrity, Jurich, & Segrist, 2000). Existing data with college student samples, although sparse, suggest that the relationship between typical alcohol use and dating violence is non-existent, whereas relations between proximal alcohol use and dating violence are modest (Wood & Sher, 2002). It is becoming increasingly recognized that relations between alcohol use and violent behaviors are complex, and that alcohol use is best viewed as operating in combination with a range of other individual and situational factors.

These "second hand" consequences of alcohol that affect others (e.g., assault, disruptive behavior) strongly differ from campus to campus and, within a given campus, from dorm to dorm. Students at colleges with higher heavy drinking rates were more likely to encounter second-hand effects of others' drinking (Wechsler, Lee et al., 2000) and, correspondingly, students at schools that ban alcohol were less likely to experience second-hand effects (Wechsler, Lee, Gledhill-Hoyt, & Nelson, 2001). Finally, the prevalence of second-hand drinking effects was lower in substance (alcohol and tobacco)-free housing than in unrestricted housing (although the prevalence of second-hand consequences were not lower in alcohol-free housing than in unrestricted housing) (Wechsler, Lee, Nelson, & Lee, 2001).

Prevalence of alcohol use disorders. Although rates of specific alcohol-related problems have received a great deal of focus in the research literature, considerably less attention has been devoted to estimating the extent of alcohol use disorders in the college population; however, the limited existing data suggest that alcohol use disorders are prevalent in this population. Knight et al. (2002) documented rates of alcohol abuse and dependence using CAS data and found that 31% of college students endorsed criteria for a past-year DSM-IV alcohol abuse diagnosis and 6% endorsed criteria for DSM-IV alcohol dependence, with over 40% reporting at least one symptom of abuse or dependence. In a high-risk college-aged sample, Sher, Walitzer, Wood, and Brent (1991) showed that 35% of male and 17% of female freshmen met diagnostic criteria for alcohol abuse or dependence according to DSM-III (APA, 1980) criteria. Although they did not explicitly sample college students, the National Comorbidity Survey (NCS; Kessler et al., 1994) and the National Longitudinal Alcohol Epidemiological Survey (NLAES; Grant, 1997; Grant et al., 1994) showed the highest prevalence rates of (past-year) alcohol abuse and dependence in the youngest age strata surveyed (i.e., late adolescence/early young adulthood). The strong age gradient showing the peak prevalence of AUDs in the early 20s implies that AUDs are highly prevalent in college student populations.

Developmental course of alcohol involvement. The prevalence rates discussed above represent normative rates of drinking, but they fail to account for the considerable variability in drinking patterns over time observed across individuals. These mean levels of alcohol involvement actually represent very few individuals in the population. Researchers have attempted to describe the course of drinking as a function of developmental stage, although findings are inconsistent, perhaps due to the restricted age span of college students. A limited body of work has examined alcohol involvement as a function of age. Data from MTF and NLSY reveal that alcohol consumption (particularly heavy drinking) increases up to age 20 or 21 and generally decreases thereafter (Johnston et al., 2002; Muthen & Muthen, 2000). Some researchers have specifically examined the extent to which drinking behavior in those under the legal drinking age of 21 differs from drinking among those over age 21 (e.g., Engs et al., 1996; O'Hare, 1990; Wechsler et al., 1994; Wechsler, Dowdall et al., 1995). Neither O'Hare nor Wechsler and colleagues found an effect for legal drinking age on consumption or alcohol problems. Engs et al. (1996), however, noted that underage drinkers were more likely to be heavy drinkers but reported no difference in weekly total consumption rates. These findings suggest that perhaps underage drinkers are taking more advantage of their limited opportunities to drink (Wechsler, Kuo, Lee, & Dowdall, 2000). Engs et al. (1996) also suggested that those under 21 drink out of reactance to the drinking age (consistent with their finding that freshman have the highest drinking rates).

Some studies of developmental trends in drinking are based on grade level instead of age in years. Age and academic grade level tend to be closely coupled, with a rough correspondence of age 18 with the freshman year and age 21 with the senior year, although there is not complete parallelism in the age and the grade-level research findings. The literature on academic grade level is also inconsistent, with some studies concluding no difference in heavy drinking as a function of year in school (Wechsler et al., 1994; Wechsler, Dowdall et al., 1995) but others observing a monotonic increase in light drinking (Harford et al., 1983) and mean weekly drinking (with the exception of freshman year; Engs, 1990) but a monotonic decrease in heavy drinking (Engs et al., 1996) as a function of year in school.

Recent research has begun charting the developmental course of alcohol involvement for distinct subgroups of drinkers, although only a small portion has specifically focused on college student populations (Jackson & Sher, 2003; Jackson, Sher, & Wood, 2000). Most major college drinking studies, with the exception of MTF, do not prospectively follow individual students and are not capable of resolving individual differences in drinking trajectory. Jackson and Sher examined five indices of alcohol involvement (alcohol use disorder, alcohol consequences, alcohol dependence, alcohol quantity-frequency, and heavy drinking) and identified four prominent groups, including chronic (i.e., high at all measurement occasions although sometimes also exhibiting a decrease post college), which ranged from 3% to 24% of the sample; developmentally limited (i.e., high during the early years of college with low involvement thereafter; 8% to 26%); later-onset (i.e., low in the freshman year but high thereafter; 2% to 14%); and non-drinking or non-problematic drinking; 45% to 74%). The relatively large developmentally limited group is consistent with Baer's (2002) suggestion that developmentally limited drinking may account for much of college student drinking. This is also consistent with research showing a marked decrease in alcohol use and abuse in individuals in their mid- to late-twenties, presumably due to the adoption of a more conventional lifestyle (Fillmore, 1988; Jessor, Donovan, & Costa, 1991) including social roles such as establishing a career, getting married, and becoming a parent.

Although work done by Schulenberg and colleagues (Schulenberg, O'Malley, Bachman, Wadsworth, & Johnston, 1996; Schulenberg, Wadsworth, O'Malley, Bachman, & Johnston, 1996) using MTF was not specific to college students, they were able to predict trajectory membership from college student status. In their work, they identified six drinking trajectories, including Never and Rare (which involved no frequent heavy drinking); Chronic (heavy drinking at all four waves); Decreased (increasingly less heavy drinking over time); Increased (increasingly greater heavy drinking over time); and "Fling" (moderate heavy drinking at Waves 2 and 3). Relative to their non-college attending peers, college students were overrepresented in the Increase and Fling groups and underrepresented in the Decrease group (Schulenberg & Maggs, 2002). Moreover, students who lived on campus were more likely to belong to the Chronic, Increase, or Fling groups and less likely to belong to the Never group. These trajectory-based approaches to studying drinking highlight the considerable variability in the course of collegiate drinking and suggest that focusing on mean group data obscures this important variability.

3. Individual Factors Predicting Drinking

Most college student research has focused on the study of alcohol involvement at the level of the individual (Dowdall & Wechsler, 2002). Given the high variability in drinking among college students—the top 19% of the CAS sample consumed 68% of the alcohol consumed by college students, whereas the 57% of students who do not drink heavily consumed only 9% of the alcohol (Wechsler, Molnar, Davenport, & Baer, 1999)—much research (see Baer, 2002) has attempted to explain individual variability in drinking. Although there are multiple determinants of alcohol involvement, we focus on four broad classes, including demographics (i.e., sex, race, and family history of alcoholism), personality, drinking motives and expectations about the effects of alcohol, and peer use.

Sex. Congruent with sex differences in the general population (Wilsnack & Wilsnack, 1997), nearly all indices of alcohol involvement are consistently higher among male than female students across all nationally representative studies (O'Malley & Johnston, 2002), with the exception of annual consumption rates and alcohol consequences. This sex difference is particularly striking in heavy drinking (O'Malley & Johnston, 2002), even when controlling for other risk factors such as age and race (e.g., (Wechsler, Dowdall et al., 1995). MTF data from 1999 show that 50% of men report heavy drinking in the past two weeks versus 34% of women (O'Malley & Johnston, 2002).

In terms of alcohol problems and consequences, the gender gap was apparent in older literature but is less so in recent studies (although data from CORE and CAS still indicate considerable differences; Presley et al., 1996; Wechsler, Dowdall, Maenner, Gledhill-Hoyt, & Lee, 1998b). In an early review of the literature from 1975–1985, Berkowitz and Perkins (1986) reported that men were more likely to report drinking-related consequences; likewise, in a subsequent review, Engs and Hanson (1990) demonstrated that men experienced more problems than women, but they present evidence that the differences in drinking between the sexes might be narrowing. However, more recent evidence is mixed, with some studies showing no gender difference in problems (e.g., O'Hare, 1990) but others (e.g., Loughlin & Kayson, 1990), including a sample of students from colleges representing every state (Engs et al., 1996), demonstrating elevated rates for men. Perkins (1992) specifically examined the trend in gender patterns in alcohol consequences over four assessments spanning ten years. Despite the research positing a convergence in consequence rates for men and women, presumably due to increasing homogenization of academic and social environments for male and female students, men reported more negative consequences than women, particularly along the domains of public problems, problems that involve legal repercussions, and problems that endanger others. However, little gender difference was observed among more personal consequences and among consequences less prone to public response. Perkins suggests that recent societal norms tend to associate drinking with the male sex role, and society has greater tolerance for male intoxication and male deviant behavior in general. In sum, it may be that a broader array of consequences is now being assessed, and that this, rather than a historical trend, has produced the convergence in rates of alcohol problems among men and women. Consistent with this, studies that failed to find a gender difference (e.g., O'Hare, 1990) still observed a difference for a subset of items.

Race. Racial and ethnic differences in college student drinking have been well documented across various alcohol measures. Recent studies on representative nationwide samples of college students has demonstrated that Caucasian and Native American college students are at highest risk, with African American and Asian students at lowest risk and Hispanic students at intermediate risk, for greater frequency and quantity of drinking, heavy and frequent heavy drinking, and negative consequences (Presley et al., 1996; Wechsler, Lee et al., 2000). Despite different comparison groups and regions of study, the highest risk in Caucasian college students has been found consistently in other studies with non-representative national samples, in terms of prevalence of alcohol use (Akutsu, Sue, Zane, & Nakamura, 1989; Crowley, 1991; Engs et al., 1996; O'Hare, 1990, 1995), quantity of alcohol consumption (Clements, 1999; Crowley, 1991; Engs et al., 1996; Keefe & Newcomb, 1996; Schall, Kemeny, & Maltzman, 1992), frequency of alcohol consumption (Clements, 1999; Crowley, 1991; Keefe & Newcomb, 1996), heavy drinking (Akutsu et al., 1989; Clements, 1999; Engs et al., 1996; O'Hare, 1990, 1995), frequency of drunkenness (Humphrey & Friedman, 1986; Humphrey, Stephens, & Allen, 1983), and adverse consequences (Clements, 1999; Engs et al., 1996; Meilman, Presley, & Lyerla, 1994; O'Hare, 1995; Williams, Newby, & Kanitz, 1993). It is also noteworthy that Caucasian students endorsed about twice as many diagnostic criteria for both abuse and dependence than did African-American students, although the relations between ethnicity and either current diagnosis or lifetime diagnosis were barely significant (Clements, 1999).

Given these consistently observed racial and ethnic differences in college drinking, exploration of potential reasons for these differences is important. Caucasians were more likely to drink if they were college students and had a higher family income, whereas African Americans who were non-college students and who had low incomes were more likely to drink (Crowley, 1991). Thus, social status might influence drinking patterns differently depending on race and ethnicity. Compared with Caucasian college students, African American students may be "even more highly self-selected" (Crowley, 1991, p. 15), more goal-oriented, under greater pressure to succeed, and therefore less likely to engage in risky drinking practices. There also might be environmental/cultural factors operating in drinking among African American students, such as more authority and supervision from parents or community, greater emphasis on spirituality, and adverse socio-systematic factors, such as low financial availability for drinking and non-accessibility to support systems for African American problem drinkers to sustain student status (Meilman, Presley, & Cashin, 1995; Meilman et al., 1994; Schall et al., 1992).

Family history of alcoholism. Individuals with a family history of alcoholism tend to have more academic problems at every level of education and, thus, are less likely to become college students because either academic problems or early alcohol problems interfere with pursuing higher education (Sher, 1991). Still, the question of the role of familial risk for alcohol involvement is an important one given the robustness of this risk factor in the general population. Although highly variable in quality, a number of studies have emerged that investigate the effect of a positive family history of alcoholism on alcohol involvement among college students (Baer, 2002). Findings have thus far been mixed, with a number of studies reporting no difference in daily drinking rates (George, La Marr, Barrett, & McKinnon, 1999), mean weekly alcohol consumption or (nonlinear) drinking patterns (Engs, 1990), alcohol quantity or frequency, frequency of intoxication, alcohol-related symptoms or consequences (Alterman, Searles, & Hall, 1989), or likelihood or severity of problem drinking (Havey & Dodd, 1993).

Other studies, however, report family history effects. Although the effect was small, Perkins and Berkowitz (1991) observed a group difference in alcohol consumption as a function of family history status. Furthermore, differences between family history positive and negative individuals in rates of alcohol problems (Sher et al., 1991) and diagnosable alcohol use disorders (Knight et al., 2002; Pullen, 1994; Sher et al., 1991) have been observed. Knight et al. (2002) found that those who reported being the child of a problem drinker were more likely to be diagnosed with alcohol dependence (but not alcohol abuse), and Rodney and Rodney (1996) found greater drinking for African American male children of alcoholics (COAs) than nonCOAs. In general it appears that those studies that find more problematic alcoholic involvement among college students with a family history of alcoholism have employed more conservative definitions of family history (see Baer, 2002), problem-based (as opposed to consumption-based) measures, and better designs from the perspective of sampling strategy and sample size.

One limitation of most existing research on family history of alcoholism and college drinking is that a majority of studies have simply adopted a cross-sectional perspective and not examined how family history affects the course of drinking over college (and beyond). A prospective study conducted by Jackson, Sher, Gotham, and Wood (2001) found in a primarily college-student sample that individuals with family history of alcoholism were less likely to regress (e.g., mature out) from high-effect (i.e., getting high, getting drunk) to moderate-effect drinking than those without such a family history, but there was no difference in drinking at baseline (age 18). The high normative rates of heavy consumption during the freshman year seemingly obscure individual differences associated with family history, and family history relates to the persistence of more problematic alcohol involvement in early adulthood rather than to the initiation into heavier drinking, which would occur during the college years.

Personality. The association between drinking and personality in college students is largely consistent with the broader literature (see Sher, Trull, Bartholow, & Vieth, 1999 for a review of this literature). Specifically, personality traits related to impulsivity/disinhibition appear to be robust correlates of both drinking and drinking problems and traits related to neuroticism/negative emotionality are often, but inconsistently, associated with problematic alcohol involvement (Baer, 2002; Brennan, Walfish, & AuBuchon, 1986a). For example, measures indexing traits related to impulsivity and disinhibition have consistently been found to relate to higher frequency and quantity of drinking as well as to more negative consequences (Baer, 2002; Baer, Kivlahan, & Marlatt, 1995; Berkowitz & Perkins, 1986; Brennan et al., 1986a; Schall, Weede, & Maltzman, 1991; Sher, Wood, Crews, & Vandiver, 1995). Studies of the relation between neuroticism/negative emotionality and alcohol involvement have provided mixed findings, with some showing an association (Brennan et al., 1986a; Camatta & Nagoshi, 1995; Pullen, 1994) and others not (see Brennan et al., 1986a). Although the relation between normal range neuroticism/negative affectivity and problematic alcohol involvement is variable in existing studies, it appears that extremely high levels of negative affectivity are associated with drinking problems. For example, in our high-risk study of college student drinking, diagnosis with alcohol abuse or dependence was nearly twice as likely among students with an anxiety disorder (Kushner & Sher, 1993). The association between consumption and extraversion/sociability has generally been weak (Baer, 2002). Those who are more sociable may be more likely to drink but are not more likely to experience alcohol-related problems (Baer, 2002).

Although not typically considered a basic dimension of personality, religiosity/conventionality should be noted as a potentially important correlate because it has consistently been shown to relate to drinking frequency and quantity, likelihood of drinking onset, heavy drinking, and problem drinking (Berkowitz & Perkins, 1986; Engs et al., 1996; Patock-Peckman, Hutchinson, Cheong, & Nagoshi, 1998; Wechsler, Dowdall et al., 1995), even after controlling for a range of potential confounding variables (Igra & Moos, 1979). Engs et al. (1996) observed that less religious students drank twice as many drinks and had more alcohol problems than those who were more religious. Igra and Moos (1979) also found that baseline drinking predicted commitment to religious values, suggesting a reciprocal relation.

Drinking motives and expectancies. The college student literature examining the association between alcohol involvement and alcohol expectancies and drinking motives also parallels the general literature (for a review, see Goldman, Darkes, & Del Boca, 1999). In general, research on college students has supported two motives for drinking: drinking for social purposes and drinking for escape or relief (Baer, 2002; Brennan et al., 1986a). Cronin (1997) noted that social motives were more likely to predict consumption whereas mood enhancement motives were more likely to predict alcohol problems and problem drinking. Analogously, Brown (1985) found that social drinkers expect social enhancement from alcohol whereas problem drinkers expect tension reduction.

Regardless of the nature of the outcome expected from alcohol's effects, positive expectancies are more predictive of drinking than negative expectancies (Leigh & Stacy, 1993), and heavier drinkers report more positive effects (Leigh, 1987). Consistent with this, Wood, Sher, and Strathman (1996) found that when college students were asked to generate expectancies about the effects of alcohol, more were generated by those with more alcohol dependence symptoms. Berkowitz and Perkins (1986) suggest that problem drinkers have a wider range of drinking motivations and may use alcohol more versatilely.

Peer use. Social influence variables arguably are the strongest correlates of drinking in adolescence and young adulthood (Borsari & Carey, 2001; Donovan,

Jessor, & Jessor, 1983). Those students who report an active social network (e.g., socialize a certain number of hours per day, live with a roommate, have close friends) are more likely to drink and get drunk (Brennan et al., 1986a), to drink heavily (Igra & Moos, 1979; Wechsler, Dowdall et al., 1995) and to be diagnosed with alcohol abuse or dependence (Knight et al., 2002). In addition to numerous studies showing strong associations between peers' and one's own drinking (Bullers, Cooper, & Russell, 2001; Curran, Stice, & Chassin, 1997), increasing numbers of studies have shown that perceived drinking norms are robust correlates of drinking (Baer & Carney, 1993; Perkins, 2002a). Students believe that other students and the college environment in general have more permissive attitudes about drinking (and consequently, drink in greater quantities) than they themselves do (Baer, 2002). Interestingly, students perceived their friends to be more disapproving of heavy drinking from high school to freshman year in college. Baer suggests that high-school students may have extreme beliefs about campus lifestyles that are attenuated once they enter college.

4. Inter-campus Factors Predicting Drinking

The power of the college environment is strong (Presley, Meilman, & Leichliter, 2002) and as Shore and colleagues (Shore, Rivers, & Berman, 1983) suggest, campus life is so isolated from the "real world" that the campus environment is as important as (or more important than) individual influences. Currently, however, college campuses are not homogeneous, with more nontraditional and ethnic students, more off-campus housing, and more influential local business environments (Presley et al., 2002) than in the past. Additionally, what constitutes a college environment is increasingly difficult to describe (Presley et al., 2002) because of the lack of homogeneity across campuses (inter-campus differences) and because individual campuses are not homogeneous (intra-campus differences). In fact, Wechsler's CAS indicated that rates of heavy episodic drinking at 140 colleges ranged from 1% to 70% in 1993 (Wechsler et al., 1994), suggesting that campuses differ greatly from one another in terms of alcohol involvement and likely differ in terms of risk factors for and consequences of heavy drinking. Unfortunately, much of what we know about college student drinking comes from single-campus studies (Dowdall & Wechsler, 2002), and of nearly 4,000 colleges and universities in existence, fewer than one third are of the type found in the college student drinking literature (Dowdall & Wechsler, 2002). Some multi-campus studies, however, have attempted to identify campuses that have high rates of heavy drinking and to resolve the factors that lead to these inter-campus differences. In understanding inter-campus variables, variables beyond the institutional environment (e.g., alcohol availability in the community) come into play, but here we focus on those characteristics that are intrinsic to the campus environment itself such as region, size, residential/commuter, etc.

Only a small number of national studies are informative with respective to inter-campus variables. Among two national datasets (CAS and MTF), consumption, heavy drinking, and alcohol problem rates tended to be higher in the Northeast and North Central regions and lower in the Southern and Western regions (with Western regions lower than Southern regions in recent years) (Engs et al., 1996; O'Malley & Johnston, 2002; Presley et al., 2002; Wechsler et al., 1994). O'Malley and Johnston suggest that this may be in part because college students in California are generally older, more likely to be married, and less likely to live on campus (Wechsler, Fulop, Padilla, Lee, & Patrick, 1997). In addition, Presley et al. (2002) found that schools that are located in smaller communities had greater consumption rates and more alcohol problems than schools located in large cities. Location is closely tied to characteristics such as availability of alcohol, price and marketing, and local drinking traditions (Dowdall & Wechsler, 2002). Perhaps not surprisingly then, Wechsler et al. (1994) observed that residential campuses tended to have higher heavy drinking rates than commuter schools. Further, smaller institutions tend to have greater rates of weekly drinking than larger institutions (Presley et al., 2002). In addition, the difference in consumption between public and private campuses appears to be minimal. Wechsler et al. (2000) noted little difference in heavy drinking rates for public versus private schools, and Engs, Diebold, and Hanson (1996) observed a (slightly) lower percentage of drinkers and lower rates of alcohol problems in private schools; however, when only drinkers were considered, the trend was reversed: rates of heavy drinking were (slightly) higher in private schools (although they did not observe a difference in drinks per week).

Somewhat surprisingly, no studies to date have determined whether campuses that have Greek organizations are more likely to have high drinking rates (Presley et al., 2002), although CORE data show that schools with higher heavy drinking rates tend to have more fraternity housing and more students belonging to a fraternity or sorority, compared to schools with lower heavy drinking rates (Presley et al., 2002). As with Greek systems, no studies to our knowledge have systematically examined the drinking rates at campuses with and without intercollegiate athletic programs (Presley et al., 2002).

In general, students are more likely to live on campus in schools with higher heavy drinking rates compared to schools with less heavy drinking rates (Presley et al., 2002). In addition, data from CAS indicated that rates of abstinence were higher and rates of heavy drinking were lower in schools (N=19) that banned alcohol than in schools that did not (N=76) (Wechsler, Lee, Gledhill-Hoyt et al., 2001), even when controlling for sex, race, age, year in school, region of the country rural/urbanicity, heavy drinking in high school, and school response rate, although there was no difference in frequency or quantity of drinking, drunkenness, or alcohol problems. However, when only drinkers were considered, no differences in heavy drinking or alcohol problems were observed, and in a related study, Knight et al. (2002) found that those who lived on an alcohol-free campus were not any less likely to be diagnosed with alcohol abuse or dependence than those on traditional campuses.

Consumption and heavy drinking at historically Black institutions are lower than at predominately White institutions (Meilman et al., 1995), even when controlling for sex, proportion of students who are in Greek organizations, and proportion of students living on campus (Presley et al., 2002). Even White students at historically Black schools had lower levels of alcohol consumption and heavy drinking than those in traditional university settings (Meilman et al., 1995), and Debro (1991) observed that Black students at Black institutions drank less than Black students at traditional universities. In addition, Meilman et al. (1995) observed fewer alcohol consequences at the Black institutions. It is unclear whether the protective influence of a historically Black institution is due to aspects of the culture of the Black versus nonBlack institution (e.g., focus on spirituality, disposable income, sense of purpose, pressure to succeed; Crowley, 1991) or whether those who choose to attend Black colleges (including White students) are characteristically less heavy drinkers.

Wechsler et al.(1995) reported that women at women's colleges engaged in heavy drinking less frequently and had fewer alcohol problems than women at co-educational institutions. However, Presley et al. (2002) observed inconsistency in the relation between consumption and attendance at women's colleges versus coeducational colleges using CORE data, noting that the consumption rates for women at women's colleges do not look very different than those for women attending co-educational institutions.

Although much of the interest in college student drinking is centered around traditionally aged students attending four-year colleges, it is worth noting that two-year institutions have lower consumption and lower heavy drinking rates than four-year institutions (Presley et al., 2002). Moreover, as noted by O'Malley and Johnson (2002), most studies of college student drinking exclude part-time students.

Thus, the wide variability across campuses that is associated with multiple institutional variables indicates that "college student drinking" on any single campus is likely to be unique or at least, atypical, in one or more ways. Although these findings should give us pause in generalizing from a single campus to campuses in general (and from full-time to part-time students), we also should be hesitant in applying national statistics to individual campuses. As we next discuss, even within a campus, there are often large differences in drinking as a function of other structural and organizational variables.

5. Intra-campus Factors Predicting Drinking

Although Presley et al. (2002) suggest that students seek out certain environments on campus based on their expectancies of alcohol use, most research on college drinking does not examine intra-campus environmental risk factors (Dowdall & Wechsler, 2002). The environmental risk factors that have received the most research attention include type of college residence, participation in intercollegiate athletics, and membership in Greek organizations.

College residence. The transition from living at home with parents to living in a student residence (e.g., dormitory; off-campus housing without parents) is characteristic of the passage from adolescence into young adulthood (Maggs, 1997) and a corresponding increase in alcohol consumption. As such, although this transition is a time of growth and opportunity, it also is a time of vulnerability to a high-risk environment (Maggs, 1997). According to a number of studies using national data (CAS, NHSDA, NLSY) or data from individual institutions (e.g., Gfroerer et al., 1997; Harford & Muthen, 2001; Harford, Wechsler, & Muthen, 2002; Harford, Wechsler, & Seibring, 2002; O'Hare, 1990; but see Globetti, Stern, Marasco, & Haworth-Hoeppner, 1988), those students living on campus were more likely to drink and to drink heavily, and were least likely abstain than those living off campus with parents, even controlling for age, sex, and race (Gfroerer et al., 1997); those living independently off campus tended to fall somewhere in between but frequently were not statistically different from those living on campus. Analogously, greater alcohol-related problems are observed for those living on campus than those living off campus, with the exception of drinking and driving, which is higher for those living off-campus (with or without parents) (Harford, Wechsler, & Muthen, 2002), even controlling for college lifestyle factors such as socializing and attending parties (although alcohol consequences in the home may not have been sufficiently assessed). Harford et al. (2002) noted that the relation between residence and driving under the influence of alcohol was mediated by frequency of driving.

Harford and Muthen (2001) specifically examined *change* in drinking as a function of change in residence over a three-year period using NLSY data. Students living in residence halls or in independent off-campus living showed elevations in heavy drinking, relative to those who lived off campus with parents who showed no such growth. In addition, a change to a dormitory or independent off-campus living arrangement from living off campus with parents was associated with an increase in subsequent drinking, indicating the powerful influence of the college environment. This finding is consistent with work showing an increase in heavy drinking between high school and college (Baer et al., 1995). Baer (Baer, 1994) suggests that living situations during the first year in college may promote certain social processes; however, his study failed to identify differences in perceptions about drinking between students living in dormitory housing and those living off campus (perhaps because independent off-campus housing was grouped with off-campus housing with parents). Although the above work certainly is consistent with the idea of college environment as a risk factor, Harford et al. (2002) also demonstrated that heavy drinkers in high school were more likely to live in coeducational residence halls or independently off campus, supporting a selection effect as well. However, Harford and Muthen (2001) failed to find support for residence as a mediator of the relation between prior (high school) problem behaviors and college drinking, suggesting the housing effect is not merely indexing a selection effect. Thus, existing data suggest that not only do higher-risk students self-select into residence halls, but there is an additional influence of residence beyond this selection (a finding we also see with membership in Greek organizations as discussed below).

Greek system. Involvement in Greek social organizations has been suggested to be among the strongest risk factors in college drinking. More extensive alcohol use among fraternity and sorority members, compared with other students, has been well documented across various measures of alcohol involvement. A substantial body of recent research on multi-campus samples has reported uniformly that among fraternity and sorority members there was a higher proportion of drinkers (Engs et al., 1996; Wechsler, Kuh, & Davenport, 1996), a higher quantity of alcohol consumption (Alva, 1998; Cashin, Presley, & Meilman, 1998; Engs et al., 1996; Presley, Meilman, & Lyerla, 1993), a higher frequency of drinking (Alva, 1998), a higher proportion of heavy drinkers (Cashin et al., 1998; Engs et al., 1996; Presley et al., 1993; Wechsler, Dowdall et al., 1995; Wechsler et al., 1996), and a higher proportion of frequent heavy drinkers (Presley et al., 1993; Wechsler et al., 1996) than among students who were not involved in Greek organizations. Also, Greek members report more negative consequences from alcohol use (Cashin et al., 1998; Engs et al., 1996; Presley et al., 1993), and higher rates of alcohol abuse and dependence (Knight et al., 2002) than non-Greek members. Wechsler, Lee, Kuo, Seibring, Nelson, and Lee (2002) found that Greek members as well as Greek house residents remained the groups most at risk for heavy drinking compared with other residence groups, despite significant decreases in the proportion of heavy drinkers among these groups over time.

Not all Greek members, however, are involved in risky alcohol use, and there are considerable differences in drinking behaviors among Greek members. Primarily, sorority members are less likely to be involved in risky alcohol use than fraternity members (Alva, 1998; Goodwin, 1992; Harrington, Brigham, & Clayton, 1997). Also, differences in drinking behaviors as a function of other variables have been documented, including residence in a Greek house (Wechsler et al., 1996), house reputation for alcohol consumption (Larimer, Irvine, Kilmer, & Marlatt, 1997), and degree of involvement in Greek activities (Cashin et al., 1998). Finally, it is noteworthy that in one sample, the effect of Greek involvement on heavy drinking during the college years was not observed either three or seven years after college (Bartholow, Sher, & Krull, in press; Sher, Bartholow, & Nanda, 2001).

Interestingly, entering freshmen who reported that they intended to join a fraternity or sorority showed higher levels of several alcohol involvement variables (Cantebury et al., 1992; Werner & Greene, 1992) and higher negative consequences of drinking (Read, Wood, Davidoff, McLacken, & Campbell, 2002), as compared with other students who did not intend to join a fraternity and sorority. Similarly, O'Connor, Cooper, and Thiel (1996) found that freshmen who consumed alcohol in high quantities pledged fraternities more than did students who drank less. These findings suggest a selection effect; that is, those students who are already involved in heavy drinking tend to seek out Greek affiliations. Yet, other researchers have found evidence of a causal effect of Greek affiliation on alcohol involvement. Lo and Globetti (1993) found that involvement in a fraternity and sorority was one of the strongest predictors of initiating drinking during college among those who abstained during the senior year of high school. Several other studies have suggested that both selection and causal effects of Greek affiliation are operating in drinking among Greek members (Baer et al., 1995; Lo & Globetti, 1995; Wechsler et al., 1996).

The factors shown to predict risky drinking among Greek members include cognitive variables, such as higher perceived peer norms for drinking (Baer, 1994; Baer, Stacy, & Larimer, 1991), higher positive alcohol expectancies (Alva, 1998; Cashin et al., 1998; Klein, 1992; Larimer, Anderson, Baer, & Marlatt, 2000; Wechsler et al., 1996), and lower perceived risk of drinking (Tampke, 1990). Also, the environment (Kodman & Sturmak, 1984) and culture (Kuh & Arnold, 1993) of Greek organizations have been suggested as factors which engender and maintain problematic alcohol use among Greek members.

Athletics. We next consider differences between athletes and nonathetes, recognizing that this distinction could be considered either an individual difference variable or an intra-campus variable, depending upon one's frame of reference. Despite lore that athletes might drink less than nonathletes due to health concerns, no studies have found evidence supporting this idea, although many studies have shown no difference between the two groups (Gutgesell, Moreau, & Thompson, 2003; Overman & Terry, 1991). In fact, most research on drinking among athletes has shown the opposite to be true for indices of consumption, heavy drinking, drunkenness, and consequences (Leichliter, Meilman, Presley, & Cashin, 1998; Nattiv & Puffer, 1991; Nelson & Wechsler, 2001). These findings emerge despite athletes' greater motivations to limit their drinking and greater exposure to educational programs on drinking (Nelson & Wechsler, 2001) and remain significant even after controlling for age, sex, and race (Nelson & Wechsler, 2001). Correspondingly, Knight et al. (2002) found that those who played intercollegiate sports more than one hour per day were more likely to meet diagnostic criteria for alcohol abuse or dependence.

A number of studies have attempted to explore the mechanisms underlying this group difference, focusing on personality and social factors. Although Wechsler and Davenport (Wechsler & Davenport, 1997) observed that frequently studied correlates of college drinking (e.g., high school heavy drinking; viewing parties as important) were similar for athletes and college students as a whole, Young (Young, 1990) showed athletes to be higher in sensation seeking and antisocial behavior than nonathletes. Consistent with this, athletes have been shown to engage in more risky/unhealthy behaviors relative to nonathletes (Nattiv & Puffer, 1991). Tombs (2000) suggested that drinking among athletes is a function of a strong social network and showed that perceived norms had a modest effect on drinking status, although they failed to find a stronger effect for the perceived norm specific to the athletic team versus the perceived norm of the entire student body (although both were overestimated). Leichliter and colleagues examined the drinking behavior of athletic leaders and found that, rather than being more responsible in using alcohol than other team members, athletic leaders actually reported more heavy drinking and more consequences, particularly among men (Leichliter et al., 1998). This suggests that members of athletic teams may model their drinking behavior after those who are the most salient figures in their social network. Relatedly, Nelson and Wechsler (2001) demonstrated that athletes have a stronger social network (e.g., more friends, more likely to spend time socializing) and are more likely to have a "party-minded" mentality that serves as a risk factor for excessive alcohol consumption, and that athletes' peers are more likely to drink heavily. This "athletic effect" appears to be independent of Greek membership (Meilman, Leichliter, & Presley, 1999) and is not restricted to drinking during the competitive season (e.g., Selby, Weinstein, & Stewart Bird, 1990). Further, these heavier drinking patterns of athletes appear to be somewhat established prior to college (Hildebrand, Johnson, & Bogle, 2001).

6. Long-term Consequences of College Student Drinking: The Effect of College Drinking on Later Development

The college years represent a critical time of human development with important growth in knowledge, cognitive abilities, and social skills, including the ability to develop intimate relationships. Given the importance of this period, an understanding of the consequences of collegiate alcohol use and abuse is vital. More specifically, it is critical that we determine whether the many acute problems associated with college drinking represent time-limited phenomena with little implications for successful adaptation to the new challenges of early adulthood or if they represent "developmental snares" (Moffitt, 1993) that derail normal development and undermine successful transitions to adult roles and compromise success in those roles.

Post-college heavy drinking and drinking problems. Alcohol involvement during the college years has a lasting effect. In an early study examining problem behavior over young adulthood, Jessor, Donovan, and Costa (1991) reported high stability in problem behavior from college to an eight year follow-up, particularly for times drunk among men (r=.61), although not for times drunk among women (r=.15). O'Neill, Parra, and Sher (2001) observed that, consistent with Fillmore (1974, 1975), problematic alcohol involvement during the college years significantly and substantially predicted alcohol involvement more than a decade later, although a normative age-graded decrease in alcohol involvement was observed over the eleven-year interval. Average college heavy drinking over four years correlated not only with heavy drinking at age 29–30 (r=.29), but also with alcohol consequences (r=.35), symptoms of alcohol dependence (r=.38), and DSM-IV alcohol abuse or dependence (r=.39); these values were obtained after controlling for sex and family history of alcoholism. Fillmore (1974) showed that being classified as a problem drinker in college predicted classification as a problem drinker a full 20 years later, and her 1975 study replicated this finding for measures of college heavy drinking and frequent intoxication.

Educational attainment. Wood, Sher, and McGowan (2000) recently examined the relation between collegiate alcohol involvement and educational attainment seven years post-matriculation. Prior academic achievement in high school moderated the relation between collegiate alcohol involvement and educational attainment such that individuals who had higher secondary school class ranks were more negatively affected by pathologic alcohol involvement than those with lower levels of prior academic achievement. In other words, high-school academic achievers were more likely than their counterparts in the middle or lower end of their high-school class rank to be "derailed" by pathological alcohol involvement during college.

Development of higher-level cognitive abilities. Higher-education researchers have documented that the college years represent a time for growth in higher intellectual functions (e.g., critical thinking, reflective judgment). There are reasons to suspect that collegiate alcohol involvement could interfere with this expected growth either because of neurotoxic effects of alcohol on the brain and/or alcohol interfering with study behaviors and engagement in an academic curriculum that presumably contributes to intellectual growth. Wood, Sher, and Bartholow (2002) examined the effect of alcohol use during the college years on cognitive development, controlling for freshman neuropsychological test performance on a subsample of 68 individuals who were diagnosed with a DSM-III alcohol use disorder at least twice during the college years. At Year 7 (i.e., after college) most of the Year 1 measures were re-administered, along with measures of cognitive outcomes associated with higher education.

Overall, analyses revealed few differences between the alcohol use disordered and control groups, suggesting that the effect of alcohol abuse and dependence during the college years on later cognitive functioning is not pronounced; however, Wood et al. did find some long-term effect on visuospatial functioning in those who show relatively poor performance in this area at baseline. These findings are in seeming contradiction to findings recently reported by others (e.g., Brown, Tapert, Granholm, & Delis, 2000), although it is important to note that there were differences between alcohol use disordered and control participants in the same sample at baseline (Sher, Martin, Wood, & Rutledge, 1997). One possible explanation for this pattern of findings is that there is a period of heightened vulnerability to alcohol-related brain insult during adolescence that decreases in young adulthood. This hypothesis has received some support in basic animal research (e.g., Swartzwelder, Wilson, & Tayyeb, 1995).

Vocational outcomes. Another critical question concerns the effects of alcohol involvement during college on later occupational attainment. Wood, Sher, and McGowan (2000) examined the prospective relationship between alcohol involvement and occupational attainment seven years post-matriculation. They observed somewhat inconsistent evidence for a prospective relation between alcohol involvement and early adult occupational attainment, perhaps in part due to the relatively early stage of career development that characterized the sample three years post-college. Bryant, Samaranayake, and Sher (2003) extended these findings by looking at vocational and economic outcomes 11 years post-matriculation, a time when any effects of earlier alcohol involvement would be expected to be more pronounced. After controlling for various confounds including type of occupation, they found that (broadly defined) alcohol use disorders were not significantly associated with post-college wages. An important exception are those who met DSM-III criteria for (physiological) alcohol dependence during the college years, although this finding was limited to those who continued to be alcohol dependent following college; those who remitted from alcohol dependence were not so affected. These findings are in contrast to college-year drug use disorders which were negatively related to post-college wages regardless of whether former students continued to abuse illicit drugs.

Unfortunately, the area of long-term effects of college student drinking is severely understudied and a full appreciation of the risks of alcohol involvement during college requires an understanding of the extent to which alcohol use and problems during college negatively affect later adult development. Hopefully, as follow-up studies of college student drinking become more common, we will be able to assess the extent that problems during this period have important long-term effects on life-course development.

7. Conclusion

As noted at the outset of this paper, college students represent a very heavy drinking population and incur a large number of problems from their drinking. To a large extent, the alcohol involvement of college students reflects a stage-of-life phenomenon given that nonstudent age peers also show high rates of consumption and problems. Moreover, many of the individual difference variables that are strong correlates of alcohol involvement are not specific to college students and appear to be general risk factors for drinking.

There is good reason to focus on college students as a special, high-risk population, however. First, because of the nature of college campus, there is a concentration of high-risk individuals in a permissive environment, leading to a high concentration of problems not only for the drinker but for others who do not drink and for the larger institution. Additionally, there appear to be certain aspects of the college environment (e.g., the Greek system) that appear to represent a major environmental risk factor. Although our knowledge of college-student drinking has increased dramatically in recent years, there are still a number of questions that require further study. Foremost among these is the effect of drinking on academics, arguably the reason for college attendance. In a related way, there is a shocking paucity of data on the long-term effects of college drinking. Fortunately, these questions are now starting to be addressed and, hopefully, the answers will be more definitive in the coming years.

ACKNOWLEDGMENTS: Supported by grants K01 AA13938, R37 AA007231, R01 AA013987, and P50 AA11998 from the National Institute on Alcohol Abuse and Alcoholism.

References

Abbey, A. (1991). Acquaintance rape and alcohol consumption on college campuses: How are they linked? *Journal of American College Health, 39,* 165–169.

Abbey, A. (2000). *Alcohol-related sexual assault: A common problem among college students:* Paper prepared for the National Institute of Alcohol Abuse and Alcoholism's Advisory Panel on College Student Drinking.

Abbey, A. (2002). Alcohol-Related Sexual Assault: A Common Problem among College Students. *Journal of Studies on Alcohol, Supplement 14,* 118–128.

Abbey, A., Ross, L. T., McDuffie, D., & McAuslan, P. (1996). Alcohol and dating risk factors for sexual assault among college women. *Psychology of Women Quarterly, 20,* 147–169.

Akutsu, P. D., Sue, S., Zane, N. W. S., & Nakamura, C. Y. (1989). Ethnic Differences in Alcohol Consumption among Asians and Caucasians in the United States: An Investigation of Cultural and Physiological Factors. *Journal of Studies on Alcohol, 50*(3), 261–267.

Alterman, A. I., Searles, J. S., & Hall, J. G. (1989). Failure to Find Differences in Drinking Behavior as a Function of Familial Risk for Alcoholism: A Replication. *Journal of Abnormal Psychology, 98*(1), 50–53.

Alva, S. A. (1998). Self-Reported Alcohol Use of College Fraternity and Sorority Members. *Journal of College Student Development, 39*(1), 3–10.

American Psychiatric Association. (1980). Diagnostic and statistical manual of mental disorders (3rd ed.). In. Washington, D.C.: Author.

American Psychiatric Association. (1994). *Diagnostic and statistical manual of mental disorders* (4th ed.). Washington, DC: American Psychiatric Association.

Baer, J. S. (1994). Effects of College Residence on Perceived Norms for Alcohol Consumption: An Examination of the First Year in College. *Psychology of Addictive Behaviors, 8*(1), 43–50.

Baer, J. S. (2002). Student Factors: Understanding Individual Variation in College Drinking. *Journal of Studies on Alcohol, Supplement No. 14, 2002,* 40–53.

Baer, J. S., & Carney, M. M. (1993). Biases in the perceptions of the consequences of alcohol use among college students. *Journal of Studies on Alcohol, 54*(1), 54–60.

Baer, J. S., Kivlahan, D. R., & Marlatt, G. A. (1995). High-Risk Drinking across the Transition From High School to College. *Alcoholism: Clinical and Experimental Research, 19*(1), 54–61.

Baer, J. S., Stacy, A., & Larimer, M. (1991). Biases in the Perception of Drinking Norms among College Students. *Journal of Studies on Alcohol, 52*(6), 580–586.

Bartholow, B. D., Sher, K. J., & Krull, J. L. (In Press: 2002). Changes in Heavy Drinking Over the Third Decade of Life as a Function of Collegiate Fraternity and Sorority Involvement: A Prospective, Multilevel Analysis. *Health Psychology,* 1–31.

Berkowitz, A. D., & Perkins, H. W. (1986). Problem Drinking among College Students: A Review of Recent Research. *Journal of American College Health, 35,* 21–28.

Borsari, B., & Carey, K. B. (2001). Peer influences on college drinking: A review of the research. *Journal of Substance Abuse, 13*(4), 391–424.

Brennan, A. F., Walfish, S., & AuBuchon, P. (1986a). Alcohol Use and Abuse in College Students. I. A Review of Individual and Personality Correlates. *The International Journal of the Addictions, 21*(4&5), 449–474.

Brennan, A. F., Walfish, S., & AuBuchon, P. (1986b). Alcohol Use and Abuse in College Students. II. Social/Environmental Correlates, Methodological Issues, and Implications for Intervention. *The International Journal of the Addictions, 21*(4&5), 475–493.

Brodbelt, S. (1983). College dating and aggression. *College Student Journal, 17,* 283–286.

Brown, S. A. (1985). Expectancies Versus Background in the Prediction of College Drinking Patterns. *Journal of Consulting and Clinical Psychology, 53*(1), 123–130.

Brown, S. A., Tapert, S. F., Granholm, E., & Delis, D. C. (2000). Neurocognitive functioning of adolescents: Effects of protracted alcohol use. *Alcoholism: Clinical & Experimental Research, 24,* 164–171.

Bryant, R. R., Samaranayake, V. A., & Sher, K. J. (2003). *The relationship between wages and drug/alcohol abuse and dependence. Unpublished manuscript.*Unpublished manuscript.

Bullers, S., Cooper, M. L., & Russell, M. (2001). Social networks drinking and adult alcohol involvement: A longitudinal exploration of the direction of influence. *Addictive Behaviors, 26,* 181–199.

Camatta, C. D., & Nagoshi, C. T. (1995). Stress, Depression, Irrational Beliefs, and Alcohol Use and Problems in a College Student Sample. *Alcoholism: Clinical and Experimental Research, 19*(1), 142–146.

Cantebury, R. G., Gressard, C. F., Vieweg, W. V. R., Grossman, S. J., McKelway, R. B., & Westerman, P. S. (1992). Risk-taking Behavior of College Students and Social Forces. *American Journal of Drug and Alcohol Abuse, 18*(2), 213–223.

Cashin, J., R. , Presley, C. A., & Meilman, P. W. (1998). Alcohol Use in the Greek System: Follow the Leader? *Journal of Studies on Alcohol,* 63–70.

Center for Human Resource Research. (1993). *NLS Users Guide.* Columbus, OH: Author, Ohio State University.

Centers of Disease Control and Prevention. (1997). Youth risk behavior surveillance: National College Health Risk Behavior Survey - United States, 1995. *Morbidity and Mortality Weekly Report, 46,* 1–56.

Clements, R. (1999). Prevalence of Alcohol-use Disorders and Alcohol-Related Problems in a College Student Sample. *Journal of American College Health, 48,* 111–118.

Cooper, M. L. (2002). Alcohol Use and Rishky Sexual Behavior among College Students and Youth: Evaluating the Evidence. *Journal of Studies on Alcohol, Supplement No. 14,* 101–117.

Core Institute. (1998). *American Campuses: 2001 Statistics on Alcohol and Other Drug Use.*

Cronin, C. (1997). Reasons for Drinking Versus Outcome Expectancies in the Prediction of College Student Drinking. *Substance Use and Misuse, 32*(10), 1287–1311.

Crowley, J. E. (1991). Educational Status and Drinking Patterns: How Representative Are College Students? *Journal of Studies on Alcohol, 52*(1), 10–16.

Curran, P. J., Stice, E., & Chassin, L. (1997). The relation between adolescent alcohol use and peer alcohol use: A longitudinal random coefficients model. *Journal of Consulting and Clinical Psychology, 65,* 130–140.

Debro, J. (1991). *Drug use and abuse at historically Black colleges.* Paper presented at the Problems of Drug Dependence 1990: Proceedings of the 52nd Annual Scientific Meeting of the Committee on Problems of Drug Dependence, Inc. NIDA Research Monograph 105, Rockville, MD.

Department of Commerce. (2000). *Bureau of the Census (2000),* from http://www.census.gov/

Desiderato, L. L., & Crawford, H. J. (1995). Risky sexual behavior in college students: Relationships between number of sexual partners, disclosure of previous risky behavior, and alcohol use. *Journal of Youth & Adolescence, Vol 24*(1), 55–68.

Donovan, J. E., Jessor, R., & Jessor, L. (1983). Problem drinking in adolescence and young adulthood: A follow-up study. *Journal of Studies on Alcohol, 44,* 109–137.

Dowdall, G. W., & Wechsler, H. (2002). Studying College Alcohol Us: Widening the Lens, Sharpening the Focus. *Journal of Studies on Alcohol, Supplement No. 14,* 14–22.

Edwards, G. (1986). The alcohol dependence syndrome: A concept as stimulus to enquiry. *British Journal of Addiction, 81,* 171–183.

Edwards, G., & Gross, M. (1976). Alcohol dependence: Provisional decription of a clinical syndrome. *British Medical Journal, 1,* 1058–1061.

Engs, R. C. (1990). Family Background of Alcohol Abuse and Its Relationship to Alcohol Consumption among College Students: An Unexpected Finding. *Journal of Studies on Alcohol, 51*(6), 542–547.

Engs, R. C., Diebold, B. A., & Hanson, D. J. (1996). The Drinking Patterns and Problems of a National Sample of College Students, 1994. *Journal of Alcohol & Drug Education, 41*(3), 13–33.

Engs, R. C., & Hanson, D. J. (1990). Gender Differences in Drinking Patterns and Problems Among College Students: A Review of the Literature. *Journal of Alcohol & Drug Education, 35*(2), 36–47.

Engs, R. C., & Hanson, D. J. (1994). The Student Alcohol Questionnaire: An updated reliability of the Drinking Patterns, Problems, Knowledge, and Attitude subscales. *Psychological Reports, 74*(1), 12–14.

Fillmore, K. M. (1974). Drinking and problem drinking in early adulthood and middle age: An exploratory 20-year follow-up study. *Quarterly Journal of Studies on Alcohol, 35*(3-A), 819–840.

Fillmore, K. M. (1975). Relationships between specific drinking problems in early adulthood and middle age: An exploratory 20-year follow-up study. *Journal of Studies on Alcohol, 36*(7), 882–907.

Fillmore, K. M. (1988). *Alcohol Use Across the Life Course.* Toronto: Addiction Research Foundation.

Follingstad, D. R., Bradley, R. G., Laughlin, J. E., & Burke, L. (1999). Risk factors and correlates of dating violence: The relevance of examining frequency and severity levels in a college sample. *Violence and Victims, 14*, 365–380.

Frintner, M. P., & Rubinson, L. (1993). Acquaintance rape: The influence of alcohol, fraternity membership, and sports team membership. *Journal of Sex Education & Therapy, 19*(4), 272–284.

George, W. H., La Marr, J., Barrett, K., & McKinnon, T. (1999). Alcoholic parentage, self-labeling, and endorsement of ACOA-codependent traits. *Psychology of Addictive Behaviors, Vol 13*(1), 39–48.

Gfroerer, J. C., Greenblatt, J. C., & Wright, D. A. (1997). Substance Use in the US College-Age Population: Differences according to Educational Status and Living Arrangement. *American Journal of Public Health, 87*(1), 62–65.

Globetti, G., Stern, J. T., Marasco, F., & Haworth-Hoeppner, S. (1988). Student Residence Arrangements and Alcohol Use and Abuse: A Research Note. *The Journal of College and University Student Housing, 18*(1), 28–33.

Goldman, M. S., Darkes, J., & Del Boca, F. K. (1999). Expectancy mediation of biopsychosocial risk for alcohol use and alcoholism. In E. I. Kirsch (Ed.), *How expectancies shape experience* (pp. 233–262). Washington, DC: American Psychological Association.

Goodwin, L. (1992). Alcohol and Drug Use in Fraternities and Sororities. *Journal of Alcohol and Drug Education, 37*(2), 52–63.

Grant, B. F. (1997). Convergent validity of DSM-III-R and DSM-IV alcohol dependence: Results from the national longitudinal alcohol epidemiologic survey. *Journal of Substance Abuse, 9*, 89–102.

Grant, B. F., Harford, T. C., Dawson, D. A., Chou, P., Dufor, M., & Pickering, R. (1994). Prevalence of DSM-IV alcohol abuse and dependence. *Alcohol Health and Research World, 18*, 243–248.

Graves, K. L. (1995). Risky sexual behavior and alcohol use among young adults: Results from a national survey. *American Journal of Health Promotion, Vol 10*(1), 27–36.

Gutgesell, M. E., Moreau, K. L., & Thompson, D. L. (2003). Weight Concerns, Problem Eating Behaviors, and Problem Drinkig Behaviors in Female Collegiate Athletes. *Journal of Athletic Training, 38*(1), 62–66.

Harford, T. C., & Muthen, B. O. (2001). Alcohol Use among College Students: The Effects of Prior Problem Behaviors and Change of Residence. *Journal of Studies on Alcohol, 62*(3), 306–312.

Harford, T. C., Wechsler, H., & Muthen, B. O. (2002). The Impact of Current Residence and High School Drinking on Alcohol Problems among College Students. *Journal of Studies on Alcohol, 63*(3), 271–279.

Harford, T. C., Wechsler, H., & Rohman, M. (1983). The Structural Context of College Drinking. *Journal of Studies on Alcohol, 44*(4), 722–732.

Harford, T. C., Wechsler, H., & Seibring, M. (2002). Attendance and Alcohol Use at Parties and Bars in College: A National Survey of Current Drinkers. *Journal of Studies on Alcohol, 63*(6), 726–733.

Harrington, N. G., Brigham, N. L., & Clayton, R. R. (1997). Differences in Alcohol Use and alcohol-Related problems among Fraternity and Sorority Members. *Drug and Alcohol Dependence, 47*, 237–246.

Havey, J. M., & Dodd, D. K. (1993). Variables Associated with Alcohol Abuse Among Self-Identified Collegiate COAs and Their Peers. *Addictice Behaviors, 18*, 567–575.

Hildebrand, K. M., Johnson, D. J., & Bogle, K. (2001). Comparison of Patterns of Alcohol Use Between High School and College Athletes and Non-Athletes. *College Student Journal, 35*(3), 358–366.

Hingson, R. W., Heeren, T., Zakocs, R. C., Kopstein, A., & Wechsler, H. (2002). Magnitude of Alcohol-Related Mortality and Morbidity among U.S. College Students Ages 18–24. *Journal of Studies on Alcohol, 63*(2), 136–144.

Humphrey, J. A., & Friedman, J. (1986). The Onset of Drinking and Intoxication among University Students. *Journal of Studies on Alcohol, 47*(6), 455–458.

Humphrey, J. A., Stephens, V., & Allen, D. F. (1983). Race, Sex, Marihuana Use and Alcohol Intoxication in College Students. *Journal of Studies on Alcohol, 44*(4), 733–738.

Igra, A., & Moos, R. H. (1979). Alcohol Use Among College Students: Some Competing Hypotheses. *Journal of Youth and Adolescence, 8*(4), 393–405.

Jackson, K. M., & Sher, K. J. (2003). *Similarities & Differences of Longitudinal Phenotypes Across Alternate Measures of Alcohol Involvement. Manuscript in preparation.*Unpublished manuscript.

Jackson, K. M., Sher, K. J., Gotham, H. J., & Wood, P. K. (2001). Transitioning into and out of large-effect drinking in young adulthood. *Journal of Abnormal Psychology, Vol 110*(3), 378–391.

Jackson, K. M., Sher, K. J., & Wood, P. K. (2000). Trajectories of conjoint substance use disorders: A developmental, typological approach to comorbidity. *Alcoholism: Clinical and Experimental Research, 24*, 902–913.

Jessor, R., Donovan, J. E., & Costa, F. M. (1991). *Beyond adolescence: Problem behavior and young adult development.* Cambridge: Cambridge University Press.

Johnston, L. D., O'Malley, P. M., & Bachman, J. G. (2002). *National survey results on drug use from the Monitoring the Future study, 1975–2001.* (Vol. Volume II: College students and young adults.). Bethesda, MD: National Institute on Drug Abuse.

Keefe, K., & Newcomb, M. D. (1996). Demographic and Psychosocial Risk for Alcohol Use: Ethnic Differences. *Journal of Studies on Alcohol, 57*(7), 521–530.

Kessler, R. C., McGonagle, K. A., Zhao, S., Nelson, C. B., Hughes, M., Eshleman, S., et al. (1994). Lifetime and 12-month prevalence of DSM-III-R psychiatric disorders in the United States: Results from the National Comorbidity Study. *Archives of General Psychiatry, 51*, 8–19.

Klein, H. (1992). College Students' attitudes toward the use of alcoholic beverages. *Journal of Alcohol and Drug Education, 37*, 35–52.

Knight, J. R., Wechsler, H., Kuo, M., Seibring, M., Weitzman, E. R., & Schuckit, M. A. (2002). Alcohol Abuse and Dependence among U.S. College Students. *Journal of Studies on Alcohol, 63*(3), 263–270.

Kodman, F., & Sturmak, M. (1984). Drinking Patterns Among college Fraternities: A Report. *Journal of Alcohol and Drug Education, 29*(3), 65–69.

Koss, M. P., & Dinero, T. E. (1989). Discriminant analysis of risk factors for sexual victimization among a national sample of college women. *Journal of Consulting and Clinical Psychology, 57*, 242–250.

Koss, M. P., Gidycz, C. A., & Wisniewski, N. (1987). The scope of rape: Incidence and prevalence of sexual aggression and victimization in a national sample of higher education students. *Journal of Consulting and Clinical Psychology, 55*, 162–170.

Kuh, G. D., & Arnold, J. C. (1993). Liquid Bonding: A Cultural Analysis of the Role of Alcohol in Fraternity Pledgeship. *Journal of College Student Development, 34*, 327–334.

Kushner, M. G., & Sher, K. J. (1993). Comorbidity of Alcohol and Anxiety Disorders Among College Students: Effects of Gender and Family History of Alcoholism. *Addictice Behaviors, 18*, 543–552.

Laner, M. R. (1983). Courtship abuse and aggression: Contextual aspects. *Sociological Spectrum, 3*, 69–83.

Larimer, M. E., Anderson, B. K., Baer, J. S., & Marlatt, G. A. (2000). An Individual in Context: Predictors of Alcohol Use and Drinking Problems Among Greek and Residence Hall Students. *Journal of Substance Use, 11*(1), 53–68.

Larimer, M. E., Irvine, D. L., Kilmer, J. R., & Marlatt, G. A. (1997). College Drinking and the Greek-System: Examining the Role of Perceived Norms for High-Risk Behavior. *Journal of College Student Development, 38*(6), 589–596.

Larimer, M. E., Lydum, A. R., Anderson, B. K., & Turner, A. P. (1999). Male and female recipients of unwanted sexual contact in a college student sample: Prevalence rates, alcohol use, and depression symptoms. *Sex Roles, 40*, 295–308.

Leichliter, J. S., Meilman, P. W., Presley, C. A., & Cashin, J. R. (1998). Alcohol Use and Related Consequences Among Students with Varying Levels of Involvement in College Athletics. *Journal of American College Health, 46*, 257–262.

Leigh, B. C. (1987). Beliefs About the Effects of Alcohol on Self and Others. *Journal of Studies on Alcohol, 48*(5), 467–475.

Leigh, B. C., & Stacy, A. W. (1993). Alcohol Outcome Expectancies: Scale Construction and Predictive Utility in Higher Order Confirmatory Models. *Psychological Assessment, 5*(2), 216–229.

Lo, C. C., & Globetti, G. (1993). A Partial Analysis of the Campus Influence on Drinking Behavior: Student Who Enter College As Nondrinkers. *The Journal of Drug Issues, 23*(4), 715–725.

Lo, C. C., & Globetti, G. (1995). The Facilitating and Enhancing Roles Greek Associations Play in College Drinking. *The International Journal of the Addictions, 30*(10), 1311–1322.

Loughlin, K. A., & Kayson, W. A. (1990). Alcohol Consumption and Self-Reported Drinking-Related Problem Behaviors as Related to Sex, Work Environment, and Level of Education. *Psychological Reports, 67*, 1323–1328.

Maggs, J. L. (1997). Alcohol use and binge drinking as goal-directed action during the transition to postsecondary education. In J. E. M. Schulenberg, Jennifer L. (Ed); et al. (Ed.), *Health risks and developmental transitions during adolescence* (pp. 345–371).

Meilman, P. W. (1993). Alcohol-induced sexual behavior on campus. *Journal of American College Health, 42*(1), 27–31.

Meilman, P. W., Leichliter, J. S., & Presley, C. A. (1999). Greeks and Athletes: Who Drinks More? *Journal of American College Health, 47*(4), 187–191.

Meilman, P. W., Presley, C. A., & Cashin, J. R. (1995). The Sober Social Life at the Historically Black Colleges. *The Journal of Blacks in Higher Education, 9*, 98–100.

Meilman, P. W., Presley, C. A., & Lyerla, R. (1994). Black College Students and Binge Drinking. *The Journal of Blacks in Higher Education, 4*, 70–71.

Moffitt, T. E. (1993). Adolescence-limited and life-course-persistent antisocial behavior: A developmental taxonomy. *Psychological Review, 100*(4), 674–701.

Muthen, B. O., & Muthen, L. K. (2000). The development of heavy drinking and alcohol-related problems from ages 18 to 37 in a U. S. national sample. *Journal of Studies on Alcohol, Vol 61*(2), 290–300.

National Center for Education Statistics. (1999). *Integrated Post Secondary Education Data System "Fall Enrollment, 1997" Survey.* Washington: Department of Education.

Nattiv, A., & Puffer, J. C. (1991). Lifestyles and Health Risks of Collegiate Athletes. *The Journal of Family Practice, 33*(6).

Nelson, T. F., & Wechsler, H. (2001). Alcohol and College Athletes. *Medicine and Science in Sports and Exercise, 33*(1), 43–47.

Nicholson, M. E., Maney, D. W., Blair, K., Wambold, P. M., Mahoney, B. S., & Yuan, J. (1998). Trends in alcohol-related campus violence: Implications for prevention. *Journal of Alcohol and Drug Education, 43*(3), 34–52.

O'Connor, R. M. J., Copper, S. E., & Thiel, W. S. (1996). Alcohol Use as a Predictor of Potential Fraternity Membership. *Journal of College Student Development, 37*(6), 669–675.

O'Hare, T. M. (1990). Drinking in College: Consumption Patterns, Problems, Sex Differences and Legal Drinking Age. *Journal of Studies on Alcohol, 51*(6), 536–541.

O'Hare, T. M. (1995). Differences in Asian and Whites Drinking: Consumption Level, Drinking Contexts, and Expectancies. *Addictive Behaviors, 20*(2), 261–266.

O'Malley, P. M., & Johnston, L. D. (2002). Epidemiology of Alcohol and Other Drug Use among American College Students. *Journal of Studies on Alcohol, Supplement No. 14*, 23–39.

O'Neill, S. E., Parra, G. R., & Sher, K. J. (2001). Clinical relevance of heavy drinking during the college years: Cross-sectional and prospective perspectives. *Psychology of Addictive Behaviors, 15*(4), 350–359.

Overman, S. J., & Terry, T. (1991). Alcohol Use and Attitudes: A Comparison of College Athletes and Nonathletes. *Journal of Drug Education, 21*(2), 107–117.

Paschall, M. J., & Freisthler, B. (2003). Does heavy drinking affect academic performance in college? Findings from a prospective study of high achievers. *Journal of Studies on Alcohol, 64*(4), 515–519.

Patock-Peckman, J. A., Hutchinson, G. T., Cheong, J., & Nagoshi, C. T. (1998). Effect of religion and religiosity on alcohol use in a college student sample. *Drug and Alcohol Dependence, 49*, 81–88.

Perkins, H. W. (1992). Gender Patterns in Consequences of Collegiate Alcohol Abuse: A 10-Year Study of Trends in an Undergraduate Population. *Journal of Studies on Alcohol, 53*(5), 458–462.

Perkins, H. W. (2002a). Social norms and the prevention of alcohol misuse in collegiate contexts. *Journal of Studies on Alcohol, Supplement 14*, 164–172.

Perkins, H. W. (2002b). Surveying the Damage: A Review of Research on Consequences of Alcohol Misuse in College Populations. *Journal of Studies on Alcohol, Supplement No. 14*, 91–100.

Perkins, H. W., & Berkowitz, A. D. (1991). Collegiate COAs and Alcohol Abuse: Problem Drinking in Relation to Assessments of PArent and Grandparent Alcoholism. *Journal of Counseling and Development, 69*, 237–240.

Presley, C. A., Meilman, P. W., & Cashin, J. R. (1996). *Alcohol and Drugs on America's College Campuses: Use, Consequences, and Perceptions of the Campus Environment* (Vol. Volume IV 1992–1994). Carbondale, IL: Core Institute Student Health Program, Southern Illinois University-Carbondale.

Presley, C. A., Meilman, P. W., & Leichliter, J. S. (2002). College Factors That Influence Drinking. *Journal of Studies on Alcohol, Supplement No. 14*, 82–90.

Presley, C. A., Meilman, P. W., & Lyerla, R. (1993). Alcohol and Drug Use among Residents of Greek Houses. *Discoveries: A Bulletin of the Core Institute.*

Pullen, L. M. (1994). The Relationship Aong Alcohol Abuse in College Students and Selected Psychological/Demographic Variables. *Journal of Alcohol & Drug Education, 40*, 36–50.

Read, J. P., Wood, M. D., Davidoff, O. J., McLacken, J., & Campbell, J. F. (2002). Making the Transition From High School to College: The Role of Alcohol-Related Social Influence Factors in Students' Drinking. *Substance Abuse, 23*(1), 53–65.

Rodney, H. E., & Rodney, L. (1996). An exploratory study of African American collegiate adult children of alcoholics. *Journal of American College Health, 44*(6), 267–272.

Santelli, J. S., Brener, N. D., Lowry, R., Bhatt, A., & Zabin, L. S. (1998). Multiple sexual partners among U.S. adolescents and young adults. *Fam. Plan. Perspect, 30*, 271–275.

Schall, M., Kemeny, A., & Maltzman, I. (1992). Factors Associated with Alcohol Use in University Students. *Journal of Studies on Alcohol, 53*(2), 122–136.

Schall, M., Weede, T. J., & Maltzman, I. (1991). Predictors of Alcohol Consumption by University Students. *Journal of Alcohol & Drug Education, 37*, 72–80.

Schukit, M. A. (1998). Editorial Response to "Correspondence: Binge Drinking: The Five/Four Measure." *Journal of Studies on Alcohol, 59*(1), 123–124.

Schulenberg, J., O'Malley, P. M., Bachman, J. G., Wadsworth, K. M., & Johnston, L. D. (1996). Getting drunk and growing up: Trajectories of frequent binge drinking during the transition to young adulthood. *Journal of Studies on Alcohol, 57*, 289–304.

Schulenberg, J., Wadsworth, K. M., O'Malley, P. M., Bachman, J. G. , & Johnston, L. D. (1996). Adolescent risk factors for binge drinking during the transition to young adulthood: Variable- and pattern-centered approaches to change. *Developmental Psychology, 32*, 659–674.

Schulenberg, J. E., & Maggs, J. L. (2002). A Developmental Perspective on Alcohol Use and Heavy Drinking during Adolescence and the Transition to Young Adulthood. *Journal of Studies on Alcohol, Supplement No. 14,* 54–70.

Selby, R., Weinstein, H. M., & Stewart Bird, T. (1990). The Health of University Athletes: Attitudes, Behaviors, and Stressors. *Journal of American College Health, 39,* 11–18.

Sher, K. J. (1991). *Children of alcoholics: A critical appraisal of theory and research.* Chicago: University of Chicago Press.

Sher, K. J., Bartholow, B. D., & Nanda, S. (2001). Short- and Long-Term Effects of Fraternity and Sorority Membership on Heavy Drinking: A Social Norms Perspective. *Psychology of Addictive Behaviors, 15*(1), 42–51.

Sher, K. J., Martin, E. D., Wood, P. K., & Rutledge, P. C. (1997). Alcohol use disorders and neuropsychological functioning in first-year undergraduates. *Experimental & Clinical Psychopharmacology, 5*(3), 304–315.

Sher, K. J., Trull, T. J., Bartholow, B. D., & Vieth, A. (1999). Personality and alcoholism: Issues, methods, and etiological processes. In K. E. B. Leonard, Howard T. (Ed.), *Psychological theories of drinking and alcoholism (2nd ed.).* (pp. 54–105).

Sher, K. J., Walitzer, K. S., Wood, P. K., & Brent, E. E. (1991). Characteristics of children of alcoholics: Putative risk factors, substance use and abuse, and psychopathology. *Journal of Abnormal Psychology, 100,* 427–448.

Sher, K. J., Wood, M., Crews, T., & Vandiver, T. A. (1995). The Tridimensional Personality Questionnaire: Reliability and validity studies and derivation of a short form. *Psychological Assessment, 7,* 195–208.

Shook, N. J., Gerrity, D. A., Jurich, J., & Segrist, A. E. (2000). Courtship violence among college students: A comparison of verbally and physically abusive couples. *Journal of Family Violence, 15,* 1–22.

Shore, E. R., Rivers, P. C., & Berman, J. J. (1983). Resistance by College Students to Peer Pressure to Drink. *Journal of Studies on Alcohol, 44*(2), 352–361.

Slutske, W. S., Hunt-Carter, E. E., Nabors-Oberg, R. E., Sher, K. J., Anokhin, A., Bucholz, K. K., et al. (2003). Do College Students Drink More Than Their Non-College-Attending Peers? , 1–34.

Steele, C. M., & Josephs, R. A. (1990). Alcohol myopia: Its prized and dangerous effects. *American Psychologist, 45*(8), 921–933.

Stets, J. E., & Henderson, D. A. (1991). Contextual factors surrounding conflict resolution while dating: Results from a national study. *Family Relations, 40,* 29–36.

Sugarman, D. B., & Hotaling, G. T. (1989). Dating violence: Prevalence, context, and risk markers. In M. Pirog-Good & J. Stets (Eds.), *Violence in dating relationships* (pp. 3–32). New York: Prager.

Swartzwelder, H. S., Wilson, W. A., & Tayyeb, M. I. (1995). Age-dependent inhibition of long-term potentiation by ethanol in immature versus mature hippocampus. *Alcoholism: Clinical & Experimental Research, 19,* 1480–1485.

Tampke, D. R. (1990). Alcohol Behavior, Risk Perception, and Fraternitiy and Sorority Membership. *NASPA Journal, 28*(1), 71–77.

Thombs, D. L. (2000). A Test of the Perceived Norms Model to Explain Drinking Patterns Among University Student Athletes. *Journal of American College Health, 49,* 75–83.

Toor, W. (2003). The Road Less Traveled: Sustainable Transportation for Campuses. *Planning for Higher Education, 31*(3), 131–141.

Tyler, K. A., Hoyt, D. R., & Whitbeck, L. B. (1998). Coercive sexual strategies. *Violence and Victims, 13,* 47–60.

U.S. Department of Commerce, B. o. t. C. (2003). *Current Population Survey (CPS) October 1972–2001.*Unpublished manuscript.

Ullman, S. E., Karabatsos, G., & Koss, M. P. (1999). Alcohol and sexual assault in a national sample of college women. *Journal of Interpersonal Violence, 14,* 603–625.

Wechsler, H., & Davenport, A. (1997). Binge Drinking, Tobacco, and Illicit Drug Use and Involvement in College Athletics. *Journal of American College Health, 45*(5), 195–201.

Wechsler, H., Davenport, A., Dowdall, G., Moeykens, B., & Castillo, S. (1994). Health and Behavioral Consequences of Binge Drinking in College: A National Survey of Students at 140 Campuses. *Journal of the American Medical Association, 272*(21), 1672–1677.

Wechsler, H., Dowdall, G. W., Davenport, A., & Castillo, S. (1995). Correlates of College Student Binge Drinking. *American Journal of Public Health, 85*(7), 921–926.

Wechsler, H., Dowdall, G. W., Davenport, A., & Rimm, E. B. (1995). A gender-specific measure of binge drinking among college students. *American Journal of Public Health, 85,* 982–985.

Wechsler, H., Dowdall, G. W., Maenner, G., Gledhill-Hoyt, J., & Lee, H. (1998a). Changes in binge Dinking and related problems among American college students between 1993–1997. *Journal of American College Health, 47*(2), 57–68.

Wechsler, H., Dowdall, G. W., Maenner, G., Gledhill-Hoyt, J., & Lee, H. (1998b). Changes in Binge Drinking and Related Problems Among American College Students Between 1993 and 1997 Results of the HArvard School of Public Health College Alcohol Study. *Journal of American College Health, 47*(2), 57–68.

Wechsler, H., Fulop, M., Padilla, A., Lee, H., & Patrick, K. (1997). Binge Drinking Among College Students: A Comparison of California With Other States. *Journal of American College Health, 45,* 273–277.

Wechsler, H., & Isaac, N. (1992). Binge drinkers at Massachusetts colleges: Prevalence, drinking style, time trends, and associated problems. *JAMA, 267,* 2929–2931.

Wechsler, H., Kuh, G., & Davenport, A. E. (1996). Fraternities, Sororities and Binge Drinking: Results from a National Study of American Colleges. *NASPA Journal, 33,* 260–279.

Wechsler, H., Kuo, M., Lee, H., & Dowdall, G. W. (2000). Environmental Correlates of Underage Alcohol Use and Related Problems of College Students. *American Journal of Preventative Medicine, 19*(1), 24–29.

Wechsler, H., Lee, J. E., Gledhill-Hoyt, J., & Nelson, T. F. (2001). Alcohol Use and Problems at Colleges Banning Alcohol. *Journal of Studies on Alcohol, 62*(2), 133–141.

Wechsler, H., Lee, J. E., Kuo, M., & Lee, H. (2000). College Binge Drinking in the 1990s: A Continuing Problem Results of the Harvard School of Public Health 1999 College Alcohol Study. *Journal of American College Health, 48,* 199–210.

Wechsler, H., Lee, J. E., Kuo, M., Seibring, M., Nelson, T. F., & Lee, H. (2002). Trends in College Binge Drinking During a Period of Invreased Prevention Efforts Findings from 4 Harvard School of Public Health College Alcohol Study Surveys: 1993–2001. *Journal of American College Health, 50*(5), 203–217.

Wechsler, H., Lee, J. E., Nelson, T. F., & Lee, H. (2001). Drinking Levels, Alcohol Problems and Secondhand Effects in Substance-Free College Residences: Results of a National Study. *Journal of Studies on Alcohol, 62*(1), 23–31.

Wechsler, H., Moeykens, B., Davenport, A., Castillo, S., & Hansen, J. (1995). The Adverse Impact of Heavy Episodic Drinkers on Other College Students. *Journal of Studies on Alcohol, 56*(6), 628–634.

Wechsler, H., Molnar, B. E., Davenport, A., & Baer, J. S. (1999). College Alcohol Use: A Fully or Empty Glass? *Journal of American College Health, 47,* 247–252.

Wechsler, H., & Nelson, T. F. (2001). Binge drinking and the American college student: What's five drinks? *Psychology of Addictive Behaviors, 15*(4), 287–291.

Werner, M. J., & Greene, J. W. (1992). Problem Drinking Among College Freshmen. *Journal of Adolescent Health, 13,* 487–492.

Williams, J. E., Newby, R. G., & Kanitz, H. E. (1993). Assessing the need for alcohol abuse programs for African-American college students. *Journal of Multicultural Counseling & Development, 21*(3), 155–167.

Wilsnack, R. W., & Wilsnack, S. C. (Ed.). (1997). *Gender and alcohol: Individual and social perspectives.* New Brunswick, NJ: Rutgers Center of Alcohol Studies.

Wood, M. D., & Sher, K. J. (2002). Sexual assault and relationship violence among college students: Examining the role of alcohol and other drugs. In C. Wekerle & A.-M. Wall (Eds.), *The violence and addiction equation: Theoretical and clinical issues in substance abuse and relationship violence* (pp. 169–193). New York, NY, US: Brunner-Routledge.

Wood, M. D., Sher, K. J., & McGowan, A. K. (2000). Collegiate alcohol involvement and role attainment in early adulthood: Findings from a prospective high-risk study. *Journal of Studies on Alcohol, 61*(2), 278–289.

Wood, M. D., Sher, K. J., & Strathman, A. (1996). Alcohol Outcome Expectancies and Alcohol Use and Problems. *Journal of Studies on Alcohol, 57*(3), 283–288.

Wood, P. K., Sher, K. J., & Bartholow, B. D. (2002). Alcohol Use Disorders and Cognitive Abilities in Young Adulthood: A Prospective Study. *Journal of Consulting and Clinical Psychology, 70*(4), 897–907.

Wood, P. K., Sher, K. J., Erickson, D. J., & DeBord, K. A. (1997). Predicting academic problems in college from freshman alcohol involvement. *Journal of Studies on Alcohol, 58*(2), 200–210.

Young, T. J. (1990). Sensation Seeking and Self-Reported Criminality Among Student-Athletes. *Perceptual and Motor Skills, 70*, 959–962.

II

Neurobiology

Ellen D. Witt, *Section Editor*

Alcohol remains the most commonly abused substance among adolescents. According to data from the most recent Monitoring the Future Survey (2003)[1]—a nationally representative sample of 8th, l0th, and 12th graders—alcohol use is extremely widespread among today's teenagers. Nearly four out of five students (78%) have consumed alcohol (more than a few sips) by the end of their senior year; and nearly half (47%) have done so by 8th grade. Of greater concern is the prevalence of episodes of heavy intake referred to as binge drinking (defined as consuming five or more drinks on a single occasion in the past two weeks). More than one in four (28.6%) high school seniors reported binge drinking. Furthermore, individuals that start drinking before age 15 have a four times greater chance of becoming alcohol-dependent than those who start drinking at 20 or o1der (1997). Given the early onset of drinking and its frequency, it is important that we understand the impact of teenage alcohol exposure on the development of biological, psychological., and social processes, since alterations in these ongoing processes—particularly brain development—may lead to increased alcohol problems later in life.

Evidence is emerging from developmental neuroscience that during the period of late childhood and adolescence maturation of the brain is incomplete. Although final brain size and available neurons are largely fixed early in infancy, plasticity of the brain continues during adolescence through the processes of overproduction and elimination of synapses, progressive myelination, variation in the evolution of neurotransmitter systems, and changes in the rate of brain electrical and metabolic activity. In addition, hormonal levels change dramatically during adolescence as the result of the onset of puberty. At least three hormonal axes are activated during this period (gonadal, andrenal androgens, and growth) which stimulate sexual maturation and rapid physical growth.

Ellen Witt • National Institute on Alcohol Abuse and Alcoholism, Division of Neuroscience and Behavior, Bethesda, Maryland 20892-9034.

Corresponding to the shifts in brain and hormonal status are significant transitions in cognitive, psychological, and social development. Adolescence is marked by the emergence of new thinking skills, reassessment of body image, focus on peer relationships, and a desire to establish self-identity and distance from parents. Sensation seeking and risk taking behaviors also increase in adolescence relative to other ages, which is consistent with the need to establish new social relationships, explore novel domains, and achieve parental independence. Increased life stressors associated with sexual and social maturation could contribute to increased alcohol consumption during the adolescent period. Thus, environmental influences during adolescence, including highly stressful situations or alcohol consumption per se, may interact with unique neurobiological and physiological strengths and vulnerabilities to predispose or protect an individual from alcohol abuse and/or dependence. A better understanding of alcohol's effects during adolescence on the complicated interaction among neurobiological, behavioral, genetic, and social factors could help determine the most effective timing and focus of prevention and treatment strategies, and modify developmental trajectories away from alcohol problems later in life.

Basic human and animal research is needed in several important areas including the following: 1) to identify neurobiological and behavioral risk factors for alcohol abuse and dependence; 2) to determine the consequences of acute and chronic heavy drinking during adolescence on brain and behavioral maturation; 3) to investigate the neuropharmacological, neuroanatomical, hormonal, and behavioral mechanisms underlying the variable response to alcohol across developmental stages; and 4) to study the contribution of teenage drinking to excessive drinking and abnormal cognitive social functioning in adulthood.

Research on the neurobiological mechanisms and consequences of alcohol abuse and dependence in adolescents is in its early stages. The dearth of research in this area is due in part, to ethical and legal considerations that prohibit administering alcohol to youths. In addition, until recently, there have been few animal models available to study the effects of alcohol on the developing adolescent. Despite these challenges, we are fortunate to have as contributors to this section, four pioneers in the area of alcohol's effects on the developing adolescent brain, who have begun to address some of the key questions listed above. In the chapter, "Adolescence: Alcohol Sensitivity, Tolerance and Intake," Spear and Varlinskaya review their seminal work in rats demonstrating that adolescent animals are less sensitive to the aversive effects of alcohol (e.g., ethanol-induced motor impairment, social impairment, and withdrawal effects), but are more sensitive than adults to other alcohol effects, including alcohol-induced memory impairments and social facilitation. These developmental differences in response to alcohol appear to be related to an ontogenetic decline in acute tolerance. The authors discuss the underlying mechanisms for developmental differences in acute tolerance, as well as the implications of age-specific alcohol sensitivities on the tendency of adolescents to drink relatively high levels of alcohol.

The White and Swartzwelder chapter, "Age-related Effects of Alcohol on Memory and Memory-Related Brain Function in Adolescents and Adults," discusses the developmental effects of alcohol on memory and the neural substances that support it. These authors have shown, using in vitro as well as in behavioral studies in rats, that adolescents may be more vulnerable to hippocampal dysfunction than adult animals. Preliminary data also suggest that binge-pattern alcohol exposure during adolescence, but not adulthood, may lead to long-lasting cognitive deficits following alcohol exposure. The authors describe recent investigations of potential neural mechanisms of hippocampal vulnerability to alcohol neurotoxicity that may be responsible for the effects of repeated alcohol exposure on memory in adolescents, as well as mechanisms of neurotransmission that contribute to the decreased sensitivity of adolescents to alcohol's sedative and motor-impairing effects.

In "Adolescent Drinking and its Long-Range Consequences: Studies in Animal Models," McBride and colleagues use rodent lines selectively bred for high alcohol drinking characteristics as an animal model to study the following areas: 1) the development of alcohol drinking during adolescence, 2) the neurobiological risk factors contributing to the onset of adolescent drinking, and 3) interventions to prevent alcohol drinking during this developmental period. There is evidence in humans that heritable factors contribute to a predisposition to alcoholism, and that individuals at high risk for developing the disorder often have an early onset *of* alcohol drinking. The alcohol-preferring (P) and high alcohol drinking (HAD) lines of rats are particularly good models for studying the mechanisms of early onset drinking because they readily consume alcohol in the postnatal weaning stage and attain adult levels of intake by adolescence. These authors describe their findings that, even as soon as adolescence, innate differences are observed in the P and HAD lines in several neurobiological markers such as dopamine and serotonin receptor levels, low-dose stimulating effects of alcohol, and higher CNS functional activity, indicating a genetic susceptibility to high alcohol drinking. Research on environmental interventions during adolescence that may prevent the onset of drinking later in development are also discussed. Finally, the authors consider whether providing alcohol to adolescent animals selectively bred for high alcohol consumption results in more harmful long-term consequences because of the double jeopardy of genetic vulnerability and early onset alcohol drinking.

In "The Human Adolescent Brain and Alcohol Use Disorders," Tapert and Schweinsburg review their own research and that of others on the effects of chronic heavy drinking in human adolescents on cognition and brain functioning. Using neuropsychological testing, subtle deficits are found in learning, memory, and attention skills of youths with alcohol use disorders (AUD). New brain imaging technologies which measure structural and functional brain changes (e.g., magnetic resonance imaging, diffusion tensor imaging, and functional magnetic resonance imaging) are being applied to the important question of whether teenagers who drink heavily cause damage to their brain. Using these neuroimaging techniques, researchers have identified reduced hippocampal volumes, white matter irregularities, and functional activity abnormalities in adolescents with AUD. However, it remains unclear whether adolescent brains are more vulnerable to alcohol toxicity, or are able to recover more easily because of greater plasticity. The role of other preexisting factors such as family history of alcoholism and comorbid psychopathology are considered, as well as gender differences, which may also influence the nature and extent of alcohol's effects on the teenage brain.

As these chapters illustrate, we have made significant progress over the last decade in understanding the neurobiolpgy of adolescent drinking. However, many questions remain unanswered. Current thinking regards many types of psychopathology, including alcohol dependence, as a developmental process which is associated with multiple factors (social, environmental, genetic, biological) including brain development. With the advent of new technologies and increased knowledge of normal brain development, hopefully in the next decade, we will achieve greater understanding of the neurobiological mechanisms and consequences of adolescent alcohol abuse and dependence.

References

Johnston LD, O'Malley PM, Bachman JG: *Monitoring the Future national survey results on drug use, 1975–2002. Volume I: Secondary school students* (NIH Publication No. 03–5375). Bethesda, MD: National Institute on Drug Abuse, 2003.

Grant BF, Dawson DA: Age at onset of alcohol use and its association with DSM-IV alcohol abuse and dependence: Results from the National Longitudinal Epidemiologioc Survey. *Journal of Substance Abuse,* 9:103–110, 1997.

6

Adolescent Alcohol Drinking and Its Long-Range Consequences
Studies with Animal Models

William J. McBride, Richard L. Bell, Zachary A. Rodd, Wendy N. Strother and James M. Murphy

Abstract. This chapter reviews findings, mainly obtained from the selectively bred alcohol-preferring (P) line of rats, on (a) the development of alcohol drinking during the peri-adolescent period, (b) neurobiological factors that may contribute to adolescent drinking, (c) interventions to prevent alcohol drinking during adolescence, and (d) some long-lasting consequences of adolescent alcohol drinking. The findings indicate that P rats readily initiate alcohol drinking during the early post-weaning, adolescent and peri-adolescent periods of development. The early age-of-onset of alcohol drinking in the P compared to the NP line is associated with (a) higher densities of serotonin-1A (5-HT1A) receptors in cerebral cortical and hippocampal regions; (b) lower densities of dopamine (DA) D2 receptors in the ventral tegmental area (VTA); (c) higher functional activity in several limbic, cortical and hippocampal regions; and (d) sensitivity to the low-dose stimulating effect of ethanol. Conditioned taste aversion (CTA) training during adolescence produces long-term effects on preventing high alcohol drinking behavior of P rats. Alcohol drinking during peri-adolescence by P rats produces long-lasting effects that increase the acquisition of ethanol self-administration in adulthood, and, in addition, increase craving-like behavior and the potential for alcohol relapse. With suitable animal models, a better understanding of the mechanisms underlying adolescent alcohol drinking and its long-range consequences can be attained.

1. Introduction

Alcohol abuse among adolescents is a major health and developmental problem. The prevalence of alcohol usage is indicated by the findings that 75–90

William J. McBride, Richard L. Bell, Zachary A. Rodd, Wendy N. Strother, and James M. Murphy • Indiana University School of Medicine, Institute of Psychiatric Research, Indianapolis, Indiana 46202-4887.

% of high school students reported that they have used alcohol (Fournet, Estes & Martin, 1990; Windle, 1990; Zucker & Harford, 1983). Excessive drinking, greater than 5 or more drinks per occasion, has been reported in approximately 30 % of high school seniors (Johnston, O'Malley & Bachman, 1991, 1993; Rose, Dick, Viken & Kaprio, 2001), and there is evidence of alcohol use in pre-adolescent children (Quine & Stephenson, 1990) and eighth graders (Windle, 1990). Adolescent alcohol drinking may have enduring consequences, as indicated by an association between early onset of alcohol use and increased risk for later drug-related problems (Anthony & Petronis, 1995; Chou & Pickering, 1992), as well as more general effects on brain development and behavioral consequences.

The reviews of Witt (1994) and Spear (2000) stressed the need for developing animal models to study neurobiological mechanisms underlying adolescent alcohol drinking and the long-range consequences of adolescent alcohol drinking. Relatively few studies have been conducted using rodents to examine the effects of adolescent alcohol drinking. One study examined the influence of early post-weaning ethanol exposure on subsequent operant ethanol self-administration using Long-Evans rats (Tolliver & Samson, 1991). In this study, rats were given 10 % ethanol as the sole drinking fluid for 3 or 10 days, starting at 31 or 25 days of age, respectively. Although this schedule produced ethanol intakes of 11 g/kg/day, there was little effect of this treatment on subsequent operant performance (Tolliver & Samson, 1991). A possible concern with this study is that Long-Evans rats generally have low intakes of alcohol, thus water deprivation paradigms were needed to produce early post-weaning ethanol drinking and subsequent operant responding for ethanol. In another study (Slawecki & Betancourt, 2002), male Sprague-Dawley rats were exposed to ethanol vapor for 12 hr/day for 10 consecutive days between postnatal day (PND) 30 and 40. This treatment did not alter ethanol self-administration when measured later in life. However, this study had several weaknesses, i.e., using rats that have low alcohol intakes, did not have an ethanol drinking history during adolescence (only ethanol-vapor chamber exposure), and will not readily self-administer ethanol under operant conditions. In general, studies conducted thus far with rats and mice indicate that early exposure in life to ethanol fails to increase ethanol preference later in life (Hayashi & Tadokoro, 1985; Ho, Chin & Dole, 1989; Yashimoto, 1988). However, these studies did not employ animal models that are representative of adolescent alcohol drinking in humans.

A major problem with developing a rodent model of adolescent drinking is that most rodents do not readily and voluntarily consume ethanol without experimental manipulations. In addition, because of the relatively narrow developmental window in rodents, it is very difficult to study mechanisms underlying adolescent alcohol drinking or its long-range consequences. For the rat, an adolescent developmental window from PNDs 28–42 has been suggested (Spear 2000; Spear & Brake, 1983), with an extension to PND 60, when assessing the effects of pharmacological pretreatment for the entire adolescent period in male and female rats (Spear 2000).

One experimental approach for studying adolescent alcohol drinking in rodents would be to use rodent lines selectively bred for high alcohol drinking characteristics (McBride and Li, 1998; Murphy, Stewart, Bell, Badia-Elder, Carr, McBride, Lumeng & Li, 2002). There is convincing evidence in a large segment of the alcoholic population for hereditable factors contributing to a predisposition toward high alcohol drinking (Cloninger, 1987). Moreover, these individuals are often characterized by an early age of onset of alcohol drinking (Cloninger, Bohman, Sigvardsson, Von-Knorring, 1985; Litt, Babor, Del Boca, Kadden & Cooney, 1992).

The selectively bred alcohol-preferring (P) line of rats satisfies the criteria proposed by Cicero (1979) for an animal model of alcoholism (Table 1). The P rat will voluntarily consume 5–8 g/kg body wt/day of ethanol and attain blood alcohol concentrations of 50–200 mg % (Murphy, Gatto, Waller, McBride, Lumeng & Li, 1986). They will work to obtain ethanol when food and water are freely available (Murphy, Gatto, McBride, Lumeng & Li, 1989) and consume alcohol for its post ingestional pharmacological effects, and not solely because of taste, smell or caloric properties (Waller, McBride, Gatto, Lumeng & Li, 1984; Gatto, McBride, Murphy, Lumeng & Li, 1994; Lankford, Roscoe, Pennington & Myers, 1991). Under chronic free-choice alcohol drinking conditions, the P rat will develop metabolic (Lumeng & Li, 1986) and functional (Gatto, Murphy, Waller, McBride, Lumeng & Li, 1987) tolerance will show signs of physical de-

Table 1. Selectively Bred P Rats Satisfy Basic Criteria For an Animal Model of Alcoholism

Criteria	Experimental evidence for P rats
EtOH must be orally self-administered under free-choice conditions	P rats voluntarily drink at least 5 g EtOH/kg body weight/day (see Murphy et al., 1986, 2002)
Pharmacologically relevant BACs should be achieved as a consequence of self-administration	P rats achieve BACs of 50–200 mg % (Murphy et al., 1986, 2002)
EtOH should be positively reinforcing, e.g., as demonstrated by operant responding for EtOH	P rats operantly respond to gain access to EtOH solutions (Murphy et al., 1989)
EtOH should be consumed for its post-ingestive, pharmacological effects and not solely for its taste or calories	P rats work to self-administer EtOH intra-gastrically or directly to the VTA (Waller et al., 1984; Gatto et al., 1994)
Chronic EtOH consumption should lead to metabolic and functional EtOH tolerance	P rats develop metabolic and functional tolerance (Lumeng & Li, 1986; Gatto et al., 1987)
Chronic EtOH drinking should lead to signs of physical dependence	P rats show signs of dependence after chronic EtOH consumption (Waller et al., 1982)

pendence upon withdrawal of alcohol (Waller, McBride, Lumeng & Li, 1982). Finally, P rats demonstrate very robust alcohol relapse behavior following long-term abstinence (Sinclair & Li, 1989; McKinzie, Nowak, Yoger, McBride, Murphy, Lumeng & Li, 1998b; Rodd-Henricks, McKinzie, Shaikh, Murphy, McBride, Lumeng & Li, 2000; Rodd-Henricks, Bell, Kuc, Murphy, McBride, Lumeng & Li, 2001). Therefore, the P line of rats may be a good animal model for studying mechanisms underlying the onset of alcohol drinking during the peri-adolescent period, as well as for examining the long-range consequences of alcohol drinking during this developmental period.

This chapter will summarize data, mainly obtained with the P line of rats, on (a) the development of alcohol drinking during the peri-adolescent period, (b) neurobiological factors that may contribute to adolescent alcohol drinking, (c) interventions to prevent alcohol drinking during adolescence, and (d) some long-range consequences of adolescent alcohol drinking.

2. Development of Alcohol Drinking by High Alcohol Consuming Lines of Rats

McKinzie, Nowak, Murphy, Li, Lumeng & McBride (1998a) examined the development of alcohol drinking in male and female P rats beginning as early as PND 26. These investigators reported that both male and female P rats readily initiated free-choice intake of 10 % ethanol as early as PNDs 22–25, with intakes reaching 3–4 g/kg/day between PNDs 26–29 and attaining adult levels (5 g/kg/day or higher) by PNDs 34–37. In addition, the selectively bred high-alcohol-drinking (HAD) rats from both replicate lines also readily initiated ethanol drinking during adolescence and attained adult levels of intake (McKinzie, Eha, Murphy, McBride, Lumeng & Li, 1996; McKinzie et al., 1998a).

Bell, Rodd-Henricks, Kuc, Lumeng, Li, Murphy, & McBride (2003a) examined the development of alcohol drinking during peri-adolescence in male and female P rats, when multiple concentrations of ethanol (10, 20 and 30 %) along with water were offered. Previous studies indicated that the availability of multiple concentrations of ethanol increases alcohol intake in adult outbred (Holter, Engelmann, Kirschke, Liebsch, Landgraf & Spanagel, 1998; Wolffgramm & Heyne, 1995) and selectively bred (Rodd-Henricks et al., 2001) rats. The ethanol solutions were first given on PND 30. Over the first 10 days of free-choice access, male and female P rats given concurrent access to multiple concentrations of ethanol consumed significantly more alcohol than the group given 15 % ethanol (Fig. 1), although this difference was less evident by PND 60. The studies of Bell et al. (2003a) indicated that the amount of alcohol consumed during the peri-adolescent period was increased further by offering multiple ethanol concentrations instead of a single concentration.

The results of the above studies support the idea that the selectively bred rat lines may be good animal models for studying adolescent alcohol drinking

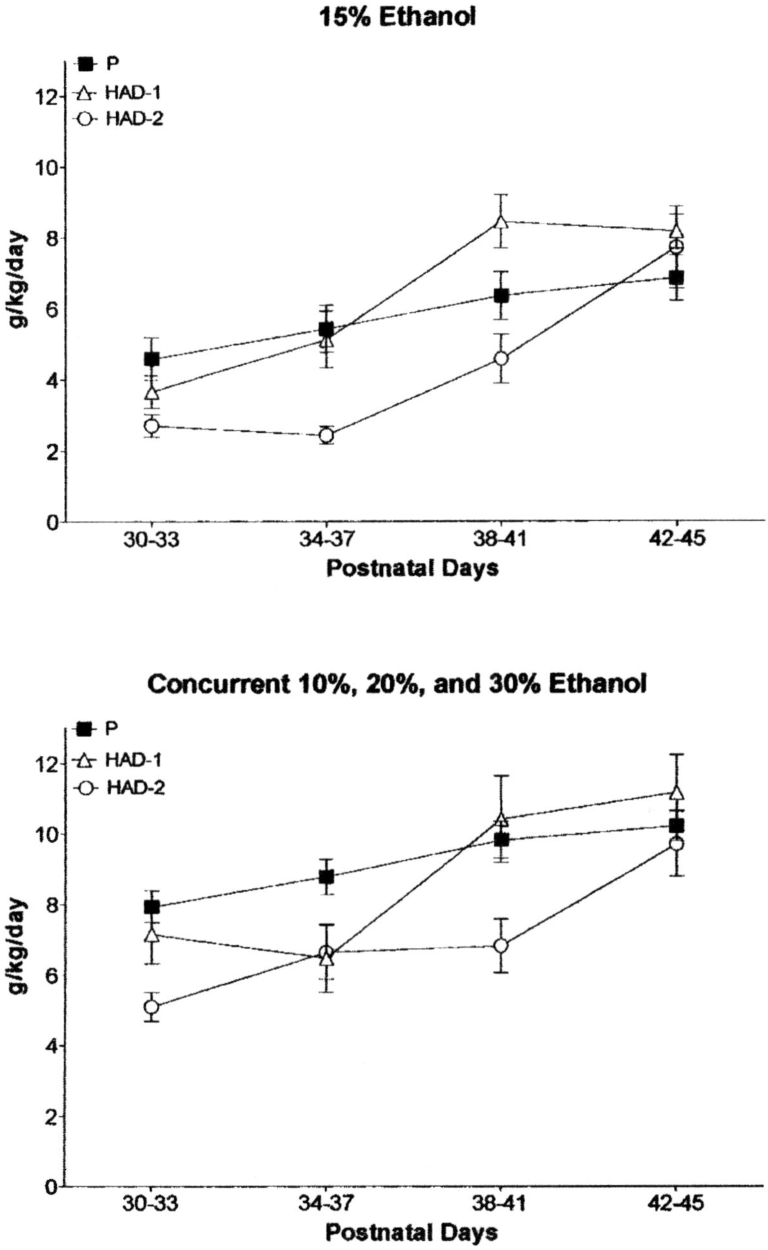

Figure 1. Development of alcohol drinking (in g ethanol/kg body wt/day) by peri-adolescent female P, HAD-1 and HAD-2 rats, beginning at postnatal day 30, given 24-hr free-choice access to either 15 % ethanol and water (top panel) or concurrent access to 10, 20 and 30 % ethanol and water (bottom panel). Data are the means ± SEM (n = 10–13 rats/group). Values for P rats are from Bell et al. (2003a).

in rodents. Moreover, by making multiple concentrations of ethanol available, significantly higher intakes can be attained (Fig. 1). Such animal models can be used to study potential interventions, and the long-range consequences of high alcohol drinking during adolescence.

3. Neurobiological Factors Contributing to Adolescent Alcohol Drinking

Numerous differences in neurotransmitter systems (e.g., DA, serotonin, opioid, etc.) and receptors (e.g., D2, 5-HT1A, 5-HT2, GABAA, mu- and delta-opioid, etc.) have been reported for the adult alcohol-preferring P line compared to the adult alcohol-non-preferring NP line (reviewed in McBride & Li, 1998; Murphy et al., 2002). Major differences were found in the mesolimbic DA system and D2 receptors, as well as in the 5-HT system and the 5-HT1A receptor. Lower contents (Murphy, McBride, Lumeng & Li, 1982, 1987) and immunoreactive fibers (Zhou, Bledoe, Lumeng & Li, 1991, 1994) were found for the 5-HT system in several CNS areas, and reduced contents of DA (Murphy et al., 1987) and tyrosine hydroxylase immunoreactive fibers projecting from the VTA (Zhou, Zhang, Lumeng & Li, 1995) to the nucleus accumbens have also been reported. Concomitant with these changes, higher densities of 5-HT1A receptors were found in the cerebral cortex (Wong, Reid, Lumeng & Li, 1993; McBride, Guan, Chernet, Lumeng & Li, 1994) and hippocampus (McBride et al., 1994) of the P than NP line. On the other hand, lower densities of D2 receptors were reported in the nucleus accumbens and VTA of the P than NP rat (McBride, Chernet, Dyr, Lumeng & Li, 1993). If any of the major differences observed are associated with the disparate alcohol drinking behaviors of the P and NP rats, then such differences might be expected to be observed at the age of onset of alcohol drinking.

Strother, Lumeng, Li, & McBride (2003a) determined the densities of 5-HT1A and D2 receptors in the CNS of P and NP pups at PND 25 using quantitative autoradiography. Approximately 20–40 % higher densities of 5-HT1A binding sites were found in cerebral cortical regions of the P than NP line. In addition, 10–20 % higher densities of 5-HT1A receptors were found in posterior hippocampal regions of the P than NP line. On the other hand, the densities of D2 binding sites were lower in the VTA of the P than NP pup (Strother et al., 2003a). These results are similar to findings observed in adult alcohol-naïve P and NP rats (McBride et al. 1993, 1994). The higher densities of postsynaptic 5-HT1A receptors may be a result of receptor up-regulation to compensate for reduced 5-HT innervation. The lower densities of D2 receptors may indicate fewer D2 autoreceptors per neuron in the VTA or fewer DA neurons. Regardless, the data suggest that the innate differences in the CNS densities of 5-HT1A and D2 are associated with the disparate alcohol drinking behaviors of the P and NP lines.

Differences in the functioning of DA systems were tested by examining the effects of amphetamine (AMPH) administration on motor activity and the acoustic startle response (ASR) in adult and peri-adolescent male and female P and NP rats. In one study, the effects of AMPH on locomotor activity (LMA) were studied in alcohol-naïve P and NP rats at PNDs 20 and 28 and in adulthood (McKinzie, McBride, Murphy, Lumeng & Li, 2002). In the 20- and 28-day old pups, AMPH dose-dependently increased LMA. However, 20-day-old female NP rats showed greater AMPH-induced increases in LMA than female P pups, whereas at 28 days of age, male NP rats showed greater activity levels than male P rats in response to AMPH. For the adult rats, the NP line also demonstrated higher AMPH-induced LMA than the P line (McKinzie et al., 2002). The results of this study suggest that the DA system mediating the effects of AMPH is functioning at a lower level in the adult P than NP line, and that this difference is evident at an early post-weaning developmental period at a time when onset of alcohol drinking is initiated. The LMA-stimulating effects of AMPH are mediated in part through its action on the mesolimbic DA system (Kelly, Seviour & Iversen, 1975; West, Boss-Williams & Weiss, 1999). It is this system that appears to have reduced DA content and immunoreactive fibers in the P than NP line (Murphy et al., 1987; Zhou et al., 1995). Therefore, the mesolimbic DA system may be functioning at a lower capacity in the adult and adolescent P rat compared to the NP line.

In the second study, the effects of AMPH on the ASR and prepulse inhibition (PPI) of adolescent (between PND 28 to 42) and adult P and NP rats were examined (Bell, Rodd, Hsu, Lumeng, Murphy & McBride, 2003b). The results of this study did not indicate that AMPH had a greater effect in the NP than P rat in either the ASR or PPI measures. Although the ASR and PPI are experimental behaviors altered by DA agonists, the neural circuits mediating these two behaviors are not the same as those mediating the LMA response to AMPH, and are likely more complex. Therefore, because of the complexity of the neurocircuitry involved in the ASR and PPI response to AMPH, it may not be possible to provide a straightforward comparison of DA function between the P and NP lines with these two behavioral measures.

The low-dose behavioral activating effect of drugs of abuse has been hypothesized to reflect their reinforcing effects and abuse liability (Wise & Bozarth, 1987). Studies with adult selectively bred rats suggest that there is an association between the low-dose motor stimulating effects of ethanol and alcohol preference. The low dose stimulating effects of ethanol have been observed in the adult P line (Waller, Murphy, McBride, Lumeng & Li, 1986), HAD rats (Krimmer & Schechter (1991), the Sardinian alcohol-preferring (sP) rats (Agabio, Carai, Lobina, Pani, Reali, Vacca & Gessa, 2001), the high alcohol consuming University of Chile (UChB) line (Quintanilla, 1999), and the ALKO alcohol (AA) rats (Paivarinta & Korpi, 1993), but this effect was not produced by ethanol in their low alcohol consuming counterparts.

If the low-dose effects of ethanol on stimulating LMA are associated with its rewarding actions and high alcohol preference, then the stimulating low-dose effects of ethanol should also be observed during adolescence around the age of onset of alcohol drinking. Rodd, Bell, McKinzie, Webster, Murphy,

Lumeng, Li & McBride (2004) examined the dose-response effects of i.p. injection of 0.25 to 1.5 g/kg ethanol on LMA of male and female adolescent P, NP, HAD and LAD rats. These investigators reported that male and female P, HAD-1 and HAD-2 adolescent rats (tested at PND 31–40) showed increased LMA following i.p. administration of 0.25–0.50 g/kg, whereas alcohol-non-preferring (NP) and low-alcohol-drinking (LAD) adolescent rats did not show stimulation (Fig. 2). These results are consistent with the findings for adult rats selectively bred for high alcohol intake. Moreover, these results are observed during the period of onset of alcohol drinking in the P and HAD lines of rats, and provide additional support for an association between the low-dose motor activity stimulating effects of ethanol and genetic vulnerability toward high alcohol drinking behavior.

The [14C]2-deoxyglucose procedure of Sokoloff, Reivich, Kennedy, Des Rosiers, Patlak, Pettigrew, Sakurada, Shinohara (1977) can be used to determine local cerebral glucose utilization (LCGU) rates, which reflect changes in functional neuronal activity. Smith, Learn, McBride, Lumeng, Li & Murphy (2001a) reported that LCGU rates were higher in several CNS regions of adult alcohol-naive P rats compared to NP and Wistar rats. Strother, Merrill, Driscoll, Lumeng, Li & McBride (2003b) examined LCGU rates in adolescent alcohol-naive P and NP rats and found that LCGU rates were also higher in the P than NP rats in several limbic regions considered to be involved in regulating the rewarding effects of ethanol and ethanol intake (Table 2). These results support the adult study and suggest that innate differences in functional activity of neuronal circuits within certain limbic structures may underlie a predisposition toward high alcohol drinking behavior.

4. Interventions to Prevent High Alcohol Drinking during Adolescence

There is evidence that early-age onset of alcohol drinking is associated with later alcohol-related problems, suggesting that childhood or adolescent exposure to the reinforcing properties of alcohol increases the probability of excessive alcohol use later in life (Cloninger 1987; Haertzen, Kocher, Miyasato, 1983). If adolescent alcohol drinking could be prevented through behavioral and/or pharmacological interventions, then this could have a positive impact on reducing alcohol-related problems later in life.

McKinzie et al. (1996) tested the hypothesis that early-in-life taste aversion training, before significant alcohol drinking experience has occurred, may be a successful treatment for preventing or delaying the initiation of alcohol drinking in subjects with a genetic predisposition for alcohol drinking, i.e., those with a family history positive (FHP) for alcoholism. Beginning at PND 26–28, alcohol-naïve P and HAD-1 rats underwent conditioned taste aversion (CTA) training, in which the aversive effects of i.p. injections of LiCl were paired with 30-min access to 10 % ethanol. There were a total of 5 training

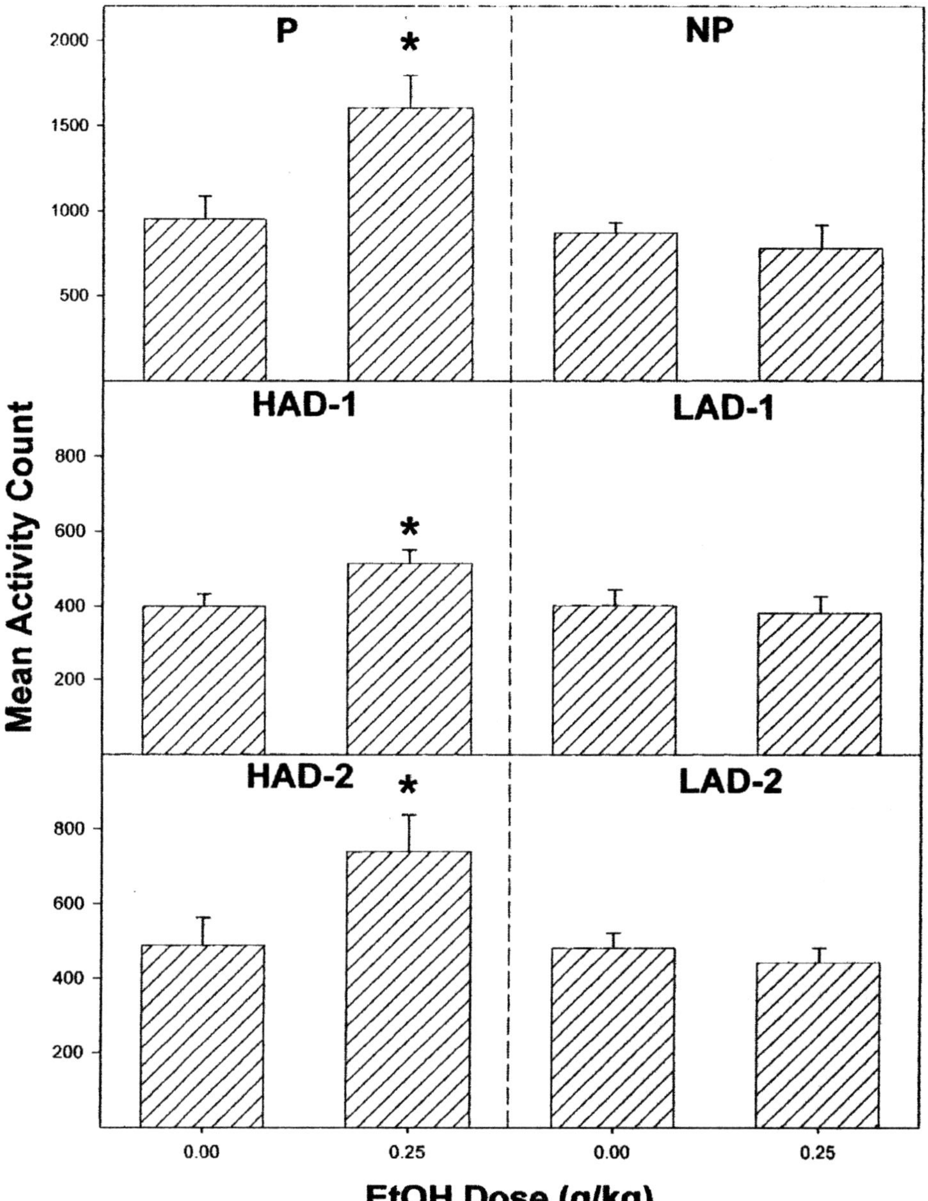

Figure 2. Total activity during the 30-min test session for male adolescent (postnatal days 33–40) P, NP, HAD-1, LAD-1, HAD-2 and LAD-2 rats following i.p. injections of saline or 0.25 g ethanol/kg body wt. Data are the means ± SEM (n = 8, 9 rats/group). *Significantly ($p < 0.05$) higher than saline. Data are from Rodd et al. (2004).

Table 2. Basal rates of local cerebral glucose utilization (mmol/100g/min) in adult and adolescent P and NP rats

Select Brain Regions:	adult P	adult NP	adol P	adol NP
Limbic Regions				
Medial Prefrontal Cortex	222 ± 12*	172 ± 8	196 ± 6*	154 ± 4
Olfactory Tubercles	224 ± 13*	177 ± 9	159 ± 7*	121 ± 5
Nucleus Accumbens				
Core	146 ± 10*	126 ± 7	142 ± 5*	114 ± 5
Shell	139 ± 11	101 ± 9	123 ± 6*	99 ± 5
Ventral Tegmental Area	125 ± 9	105 ± 9	121 ± 7*	96 ± 3
Ventral Pallidum	119 ± 9	101 ± 7	119 ± 6*	90 ± 3
Lateral Septum	107 ± 9	96 ± 9	99 ± 5*	81 ± 2
Amygdala				
Central	96 ± 9	89 ± 7	105 ± 9*	76 ± 2
Basolateral	122 ± 8	120 ± 9	134 ± 6*	108 ± 4
Hippocampus				
Anterior				
CA1	134 ± 8	103 ± 4	125 ± 7*	103 ± 4
CA3	113 ± 11	99 ± 4	115 ± 5	109 ± 4
Dentate	118 ± 8*	91 ± 5	104 ± 5	96 ± 5
Posterior				
CA1	148 ± 9*	108 ± 4	131 ± 6*	108 ± 3
CA3	122 ± 7*	104 ± 4	121 ± 6*	104 ± 3
Dentate	131 ± 10	104 ± 6	112 ± 5	104 ± 3
Cortical regions				
Cingulate	219 ± 14*	177 ± 9	196 ± 10*	154 ± 5
Frontal	176 ± 10	168 ± 11	189 ± 9*	132 ± 4
Parietal	202 ± 11	168 ± 11	158 ± 10*	129 ± 4
Temporal	228 ± 13*	172 ± 15	174 ± 9*	139 ± 5
Occipital	222 ± 12*	185 ± 7	171 ± 9*	137 ± 6
Piriform	246 ± 16*	183 ± 4	158 ± 9*	118 ± 4
Entorhinal	145 ± 11	123 ± 10	129 ± 8*	102 ± 5

Values are the means ± SEM. * Significantly different ($p < 0.05$) from corresponding NP value. Adult data from Smith et al. (2001a).

sessions, given every other day between PND 26–38; subjects were then given free-choice access to 10 % ethanol from PND 40 to 68. These results indicate that CTA training during adolescence prevented the subsequent acquisition of high alcohol drinking in male and female P and HAD rats (Fig. 3). In fact, CTA training reduced the alcohol intakes of P and HAD rats to levels observed for NP and LAD rats. These results suggest that early environmental intervention can produce long-lasting effects to prevent the onset of high alcohol drinking in FHP individuals.

Bell, Rodd, Schultz, , Lumeng, Li, Murphy & McBride (2003c) examined the effects of 9 daily treatments with naltrexone on the development of alcohol drinking in adolescent P rats. Naltrexone has received considerable attention as

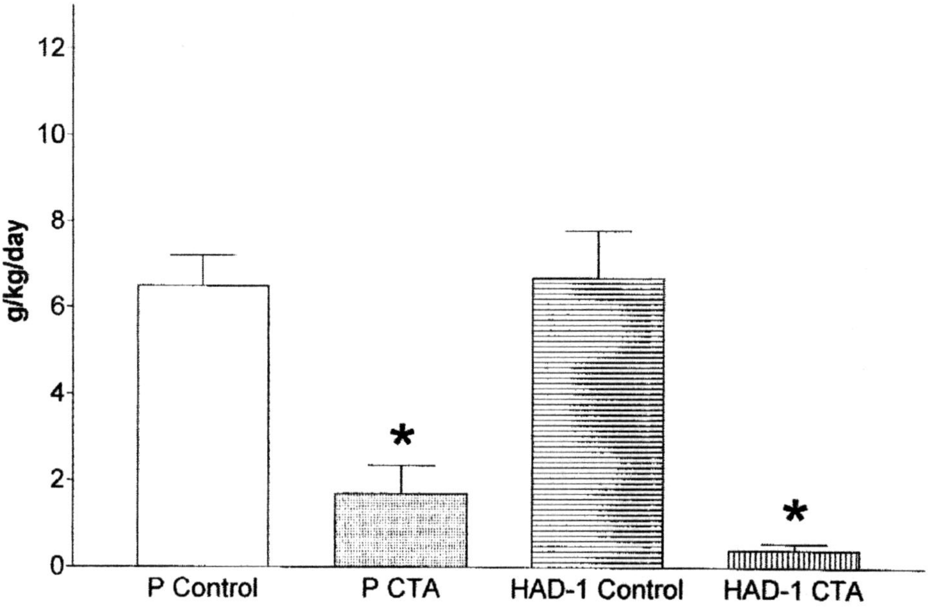

Figure 3. Effects of conditioned taste aversion (CTA) training during postnatal days 30–38 on subsequent ethanol intake of P and HAD-1 rats. Data (means ± SEM) are the average intakes at postnatal days 68–70 for the control and the CTA groups (n = 11–14 rats/group). *Significantly ($p < 0.05$) lower than control values. Data are from McKinzie et al. (1996).

a potential therapeutic agent for the treatment of alcohol abuse (O'Malley, Krishnan-Sarin, Farren, Sinha & Kreek, 2002). This treatment effectively retarded the development of adolescent alcohol drinking. Unfortunately, when the treatment was terminated, the peri-adolescent P rats readily initiated high alcohol drinking. Perhaps, a more prolonged maintenance treatment with naltrexone, or treatment of individuals without a strong genetic background for alcoholism may have produced more beneficial longer-term effects.

5. Long-Range Consequences of Alcohol Drinking during Adolescence

Adolescent alcohol drinking may have enduring consequences as suggested by the association of an early onset of alcohol and drug abuse with increased risk for later drug-related problems including alcoholism (Anthony & Petronis, 1995; Chou & Pickering, 1992). McKinzie et al. (1998b) determined the effects of free-choice alcohol drinking of 10 % ethanol beginning at PND 22 on expression of the alcohol deprivation effect (ADE) in adulthood male and female P rats. At the end of the 7 weeks of free-choice access (PND 22–71), alcohol was removed for 4 weeks. Upon restoring the 10 % ethanol, intake increased approximately 2-fold on the first day for both male and female P rats, indicating a very robust ADE. However, the expression of a robust ADE was also observed following a similar experimental paradigm in adult female P rats (Rodd-Henricks et al., 2000), although the magnitude of the ADE was smaller when ethanol drinking was initiated during adulthood.

In a more comprehensive and elegant study, Rodd-Henricks, Bell, Kuc, Murphy, McBride, Lumeng & Li (2002a) examined the long-range effects of alcohol drinking by peri-adolescent female P rats (given access to 15 % ethanol from PND 30 to 60) on subsequent acquisition and extinction of ethanol self-administration and expression of alcohol-seeking behavior in adulthood. After a 2-week alcohol-free period, ethanol-exposed and control (water only during PND 30–60) P rats were placed in two-lever operant chambers, with 15 % ethanol and water as concurrent reinforcers, to examine acquisition of ethanol self-administration using a fixed-ratio (FR) 1 schedule of reinforcement in 90-min sessions. Animals had no prior training or exposure to the operant chambers. With this self-training paradigm, the ethanol exposed group readily learned to respond on the ethanol lever and discriminate the ethanol from the water lever within the first session, whereas the control group took 4 sessions to attain lever discrimination (Fig. 4 shows the first 4 acquisition sessions). Because the rate of acquisition is considered to be correlated positively with the saliency of a reinforcer (Domjan & Burkhard, 1982; Macintosh, 1977), these results suggest that exposure to alcohol during adolescence increased the saliency of ethanol and the likelihood that alcohol drinking would be reinitiated in adulthood. In a follow-up study, Rodd-Henricks, Bell, Kuc, Murphy, McBride, Lumeng & Li (2002b) demonstrated that, using a similar paradigm, prior ethanol exposure during adulthood had no effect on the acquisition of ethanol self-administration compared to the control alcohol-naïve group. In this case, both the control and test groups learned to respond on the appropriate lever for ethanol after 4 sessions. Therefore, alcohol drinking during the peri-adolescent developmental period had a long-lasting effect that could influence initiating alcohol drinking behavior in adulthood.

Pavlovian spontaneous recovery (PSR) is a measure of the relative strength of reinforcer-seeking behavior (Domjan & Burkhard, 1982; Macintosh, 1977), possibly reflecting craving. Spontaneous recovery is defined as a recovery of responding, in the absence of the previously trained reward, which is observed after a period of rest after extinction (Domjan & Burkhard, 1982; Macintosh, 1977). Female P rats that had been exposed to ethanol during peri-adolescence showed a more robust and prolonged responding than the control group on the ethanol lever during PSR testing (Fig. 5 shows baseline values and first 4 days of PSR testing). Because ethanol is not present, the higher responding and the persistence of this responding in the ethanol exposed rats, compared to the control group, could reflect stronger alcohol-seeking behavior in the adolescent alcohol-drinking group. A difference in responding during PSR testing was not observed between ethanol exposed and control rats when

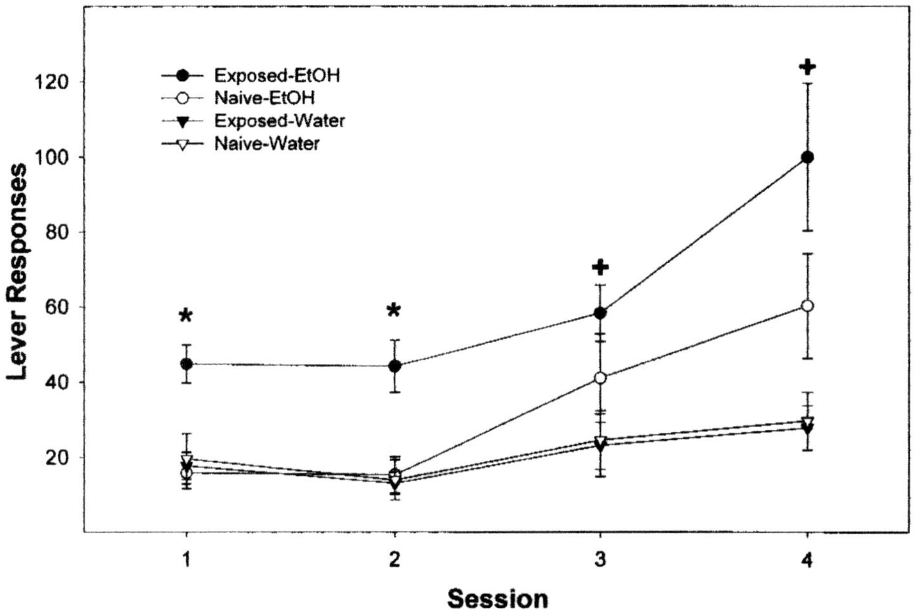

Figure 4. The mean (± SEM) responses on the ethanol (EtOH) and water levers (concurrent FR1-FR1 schedule of reinforcement for EtOH and water) during the initial four 90-min sessions (acquisition) by adult P female rats that had access to 15 % EtOH (exposed, closed symbols) or water only (naïve, open symbols) during periadolescence (postnatal days 30–60). Rats (n = 16, 17/group) were alcohol-free for 2 weeks before initiating operant sessions. Rats had no prior operant training or shaping procedures. *Indicates that responses on the EtOH lever by the group given alcohol during periadolescence (exposed group) were significantly ($p < 0.05$) higher than responses on the water lever by the exposed group, and responses on the EtOH and water levers by the naïve group. +Indicates that responses on the EtOH lever were significantly ($p < 0.05$) greater than responses on the water lever by the exposed group. Data are from Rodd-Henricks et al. (2002a).

initial exposure to ethanol was given during adulthood (Rodd-Henricks et al., 2002b). Therefore, the overall results suggest that adolescent alcohol drinking may have profound long-lasting effects into adulthood, which could increase ethanol-seeking behavior (i.e., craving), making it more difficult to stop drinking, and increasing the probability of relapse drinking in FHP individuals. These results provide experimentally controlled basic animal research that supports the conclusions from human clinical studies, suggesting that adolescent alcohol drinking can impact alcohol drinking later in life.

The findings of Rodd-Henricks et al. (2002a) suggested that adolescent alcohol drinking may produce long-lasting alterations in neuronal circuits mediating the reinforcing effects of ethanol and alcohol drinking behavior. Sable, Strother, Rodd, Lumeng, Li & McBride (2003) used the [14C] 2-DG technique to examine the effects of peri-adolescent alcohol drinking on LCGU rates

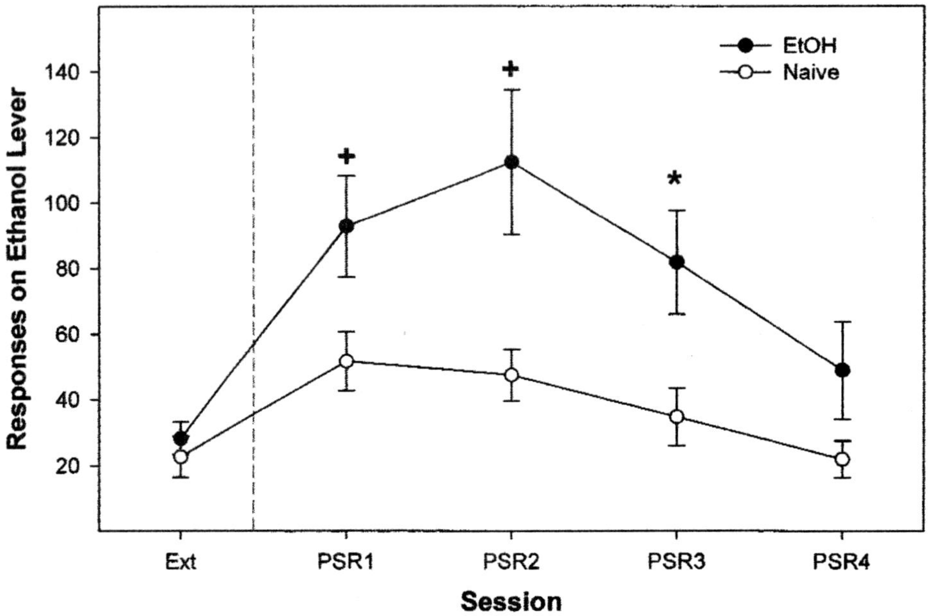

Figure 5. The mean (± SEM) responses on the ethanol (EtOH) lever by the periadolescent alcohol drinking (EtOH, closed circles) and periadolescent naïve (naïve, open circles) groups of P rats during Pavlovian spontaneous recovery (PSR) testing. The EtOH exposed group had free-choice access to 15 % EtOH and water from postnatal day 30 to 60, whereas the naïve group was given water as its sole fluid source during this period. Beginning on postnatal day 74 (after a 2-week alcohol-free period), P rats were placed in standard 2-lever operant chambers and allowed to self-train for 15 % EtOH versus water. The fixed-ratio (FR) schedule on the EtOH lever was increased from FR1 to FR5 over the 6-week acquisition-maintenance period. Both groups then underwent 9 extinction sessions. Following 2 weeks in the home cage, during which the P rats did not have access to EtOH or the operant chambers, both groups were returned to the operant chamber for PSR testing. For PSR testing, neither EtOH nor water is available. Data for responses only on the EtOH lever are shown (n = 16, 17 rats/group). Responses on the water lever during PSR testing were not significantly different than baseline extinction (Ext) levels. +Indicates that responses on the EtOH lever by both groups are significantly ($p < 0.05$) higher than Ext levels and that responses by the periadolescent EtOH exposed group are higher than responses by the periadolescent naïve group. *Indicates that responses by the periadolescent EtOH exposed group are higher than responses by the periadolescent naïve group and Ext baseline values.

in the CNS of adult P rats. No differences in LCGU rates were found in the CNS regions examined between the ethanol exposed and control groups. These results suggest that adolescent alcohol drinking is not producing overt alterations in functional activity within most CNS regions, at least none that could be detected with this technique. These results were surprising because alcohol drinking during adulthood by male P rats did produce significant changes in

LCGU rates in many limbic regions, some of which were still evident two weeks after ethanol access had ended (Smith, Learn, McBride, Lumeng, Li & Murphy, 2001b). However, it is possible that changes in functional activity are being produced but the limitations of the procedure do not permit their detection, e.g., changes in two different pathways within the same region occurring in opposite directions that cancel each other.

The results of a microdialysis study suggested small changes in the mesolimbic DA system developed as a result of periadolescent alcohol drinking (Sahr, Thielen, Lumeng, Li & McBride, 2004). These investigators used quantitative microdialysis and reported that alcohol drinking during peri-adolescence (PND 30–60) produced long-lasting effects on basal DA neurotransmission in the nucleus accumbens, and the sensitivity of this DA system to ethanol administration. Compared to control rats, male P rats exposed to alcohol during periadolescence had faster DA clearance without a change in the extracellular concentration of DA, and a more prolonged elevation in the extracellular levels of DA after a challenge dose of ethanol. These results suggest that adolescent alcohol drinking increased DA neurotransmission and increased reuptake processes (Sahr et al., 2004). The increased mesolimbic DA neurotransmission produced by adolescent alcohol drinking could contribute to the prolonged response of this DA system to a challenge dose of ethanol, and, as well, it could contribute to the enhanced saliency of ethanol and higher ethanol craving-like behavior observed in adolescent P rats exposed to ethanol (Rodd-Henricks et al., 2002a).

An earlier study (Salimov, McBride, McKinzie, Lumeng & Li, 1996) examined the consequences of adolescent alcohol drinking by P rats on subsequent behavioral performance in the cross-maze and slip-funnel tests. These tests measure a range of behaviors, e.g., anxiety when exposed to a novel environment, general motor activity, exploratory and learning, stereotypic, emotionality, behavioral despair, passive avoidance, etc. (Salimov et al., 1996). Compared to the control group, the alcohol-exposed group started exploration earlier, and made fewer defecations in the cross-maze test. In the slip-funnel test, the alcohol-exposed group spent more time immobile and less-time attempting to escape. Overall, the results of this study suggested that alcohol drinking by P rats during adolescence reduced novelty-induced anxiety and lowered response to stress induced by an inescapable situation.

6. Summary/Conclusions

Rats selectively bred for high alcohol consumption are suitable animal models for examining adolescent alcohol drinking and its long-range consequences. The P line of rats, in particular, is a good model because P rats readily consume alcohol during the early post weaning, adolescent, and peri-adolescent periods of development, and this line meets the proposed criteria for an animal model of alcoholism.

Some neurobiological factors that are found in adulthood and may contribute to the disparate alcohol drinking behaviors of P and NP rats are also observed during adolescence. The early onset of alcohol drinking in P and HAD rats is associated with the low-dose stimulating (rewarding) effect of ethanol, and higher CNS functional activity. Early environmental training can potentially prevent the onset of alcohol drinking later in life in FHP individuals.

Alcohol drinking during peri-adolescence can produce long-lasting effects in FHP subjects that increase the chance of acquiring alcohol drinking in adulthood, and increase the potential for alcohol relapse. Such profound effects of peri-adolescent alcohol drinking may be related in part to alterations in DA neurotransmission within the mesolimbic system. With suitable animal models, the potential for understanding and preventing adolescent alcohol drinking and its long-range consequences are greatly improved.

ACKNOWLEDGMENTS: The studies described in this chapter could not have been undertaken without the generous support of the National Institute on Alcohol Abuse and Alcoholism grants AA007611, AA10256, AA11261, AA10717 and AA10721.

References

Agabio, R., Carai, M. A. M., Lobina, C., Pani, M., Reali, R., Vacca, G., Gessa, G. L., & Colombo G. (2001). Alcohol stimulates motor activity in selectively bred Sardinian alcohol-preferring (sP), but not in Sardinian alcohol-nonpreferring (sNP), rats. *Alcohol, 23,* 123–126.

Anthony, J. C., & Petronis, K. R. (1995). Early onset drug use and risk of later drug problems. *Drug and Alcohol Dependence, 40,* 9–15.

Bell, R. L., Rodd-Henricks, Z. A., Kuc, K. A., Lumeng, L., Li, T-K., Murphy, J. M., & McBride, W. J. (2003a). Effects of concurrent access to a single concentration or multiple concentrations of ethanol on the intake of ethanol by male and female periadolescent alcohol-preferring (P) rats. *Alcohol, 29,* 137–148.

Bell, R. L., Rodd, Z. A., Hsu, C. C., Lumeng, L., Murphy, J. M., & McBride, W. J. (2003b). Amphetamine-modified acoustic startle responding and prepulse inhibition in adult and adolescent alcohol-preferring and—nonpreferring rats. *Pharmacology Biochemistry & Behavior, 75,* 163–171.

Bell, R. L., Rodd, Z. A., Schultz, J. A., Lumeng, L., Li, T-K., Murphy, J. M., & McBride, W. J. (2003c). Naltrexone disrupts acquisition of ethanol intake in female peri-adolescent alcohol-preferring (P) rats. *Alcoholism: Clinical and Experimental Research, 27 (suppl),* 17A.

Chou, S. P., & Pickering, R. P. (1992). Early onset of drinking as a risk factor for lifetime alcohol-related problems. *British Journal of Addiction, 87,* 1199–1204.

Cicero, T. J. (1979). A critique of animal analogues of alcoholism. In E. Majchrowicz, EP Noble (Eds.), *Biochemistry and Pharmacology of Alcohol* (Vol 2 pp 533–560). New York, Plenum Press.

Cloninger, C. R. (1987). Neurogenetic adaptive mechanisms in alcoholism. *Science, 236,* 410–416.

Cloninger, C. R., Bohman, M., Sigvardsson, S., & Von-Knorring, A. L. (1985). Psychopathology in adopted-out children of alcoholics: The Stockholm adoption study. In Galanter M (Ed): *Recent Developments in Alcoholism* (Vol 3 pp 37–51). New York, Plenum Press.

Domjam, M., & Burkhard, B. (1982). *The Principles of Learning and Behavior.* Monterey, CA: Brooks/Cole.

Fournet, G. P., Estes, R. E., & Martin, G. L. (1990). Drug and alcohol attitudes and usage among elementary and secondary students. *Journal of Alcohol and Drug Education, 35,* 81–86.

Gatto, G. J., Murphy, J. M., Waller, M. B., McBride, W. J., Lumeng, L., & Li, T-K. (1987). Chronic ethanol tolerance through free-choice drinking in the P line of alcohol-preferring rats. *Pharmacology Biochemistry & Behavior, 28,* 111–115.

Gatto, G. J., McBride, W. J., Murphy, J. M., Lumeng, L., & Li, T-K .(1994). Ethanol self-infusion into the ventral tegmental area by alcohol-preferring rats. *Alcohol, 11,* 557–564.

Haertzen, C. A., Kocher, T., & Miyasato, K. (1983). Reinforcement from the first drug experience can predict late drug habits and/or addiction: Results with coffee, cigarettes, alcohol, barbiturates, minor and major tranquilizers, stimulants, marijuana, hallucinogens, heroin, opiates and cocaine. *Drug and Alcohol Dependence, 11,* 147–165.

Hayashi, T., & Tadokoro, S. (1985). Learning retardation and enhanced ethanol preference produced by postnatal pretreatments with ethanol in adult rats. *Japanese Journal of Pharmacology, 37,* 269–276.

Ho, A., Chin, A. J., & Dole, V. P. (1989). Early experience and the consumption of alcohol by adult C57BL/6J mice. *Alcohol, 6,* 511–515.

Holter, S. M., Engelmann, M., Kirschke, C., Liebsch, G., Landgraf, R., & Spanagel, R. (1998). Long-term ethanol self-administration with repeated ethanol deprivation episodes changes ethanol drinking pattern and increases anxiety-like behavior during ethanol deprivation in rats. *Behavioral Pharmacology, 9,* 41–48.

Johnston, L. D., O'Malley, P. M., & Bachman, J. G. (1991). *Drug use Among American High School Seniors, College Students and Young Adults, 1975–1990. Volume 1: High School Seniors.* (DHHS Publication No. ADM91–1813). Superintendent of Documents, U.S. Government Printing Office, Washington, DC.

Johnston, L. D., O'Malley, P. M., & Bachman, J. G. (1993) *Drug use Among American High School Seniors, College Students and Young Adults, 1975–1990. Volume 1:Secondary Students.* (DHHS Publication No. ADM93–3597). Superintendent of Documents, U.S. Government Printing Office, Washington, DC.

Kelly, P. H., Seviour, P. W., & Iversen, S. D. (1975). Amphetamine and apomorphine responses in the rat following 6-OHDA lesions of the nucleus accumbens septi and corpus striatum. *Brain Research, 94,* 507–522.

Krimmer, E. C., & Schechter, M. D. (1991). HAD and LAD rats respond differently to stimulating effect but not discriminative effects of ethanol. *Alcohol, 9,* 71–74.

Lankford, M. F., Roscoe, A. K., Pennington, S. N., & Myers, R. D. (1991). Drinking of high concentrations of ethanol versus palatable fluids in alcohol-preferring (P) rats: Valid animal model of alcoholism. *Alcohol, 8,* 293–299.

Litt, M. D., Babor, T. F., Del Boca, F. K., Kadden, R. M., & Cooney, N. L. (1992). Types of alcoholics. II: Application of an empirically derived typology to treatment matching. *Archives of General Psychiatry, 49,* 609–614.

Lumeng, L., & Li, T-K. (1986). The development of metabolic tolerance in the alcohol-preferring P rats: Comparison of forced and free-choice drinking of ethanol. *Pharmacology Biochemistry & Behavior, 25,* 1013–1020.

Macintosh, J. J. (1977). Stimulus control: attentional factors. In W.K. Honig, J.E.R. Staddon (Eds.), *Handbook on Operant Behavior.* Englewood Cliffs NJ: Prentice-Hall.

McBride, W. J., & Li, T-K. (1998). Animal models in alcoholism: Neurobiology of high alcohol-drinking behavior in rodents. *Critical Reviews in Neurobiology, 12,* 339–369.

McBride, W. J., Chernet, E., Dyr, W., Lumeng, L., & Li, T-K. (1993). Densities of dopamine D2 receptors are reduced in CNS regions of alcohol-preferring P rats. *Alcohol, 10,* 387–390.

McBride, W. J., Guan, X-M., Chernet, E., Lumeng, L., & Li, T-K. (1994). Regional serotonin-1A receptors in the CNS of alcohol-preferring and—nonpreferring rats. *Pharmacology Biochemistry & Behavior, 49,* 7–12.

McKinzie, D. L., Eha, R., Murphy, J. M., McBride, W. J., Lumeng, L., & Li, T-K. (1996). Effects of taste aversion training on the acquisition of alcohol drinking in adolescent P and HAD rat lines. *Alcoholism: Clinical and Experimental Research, 20,* 682–687.

McKinzie, D. L., Nowak, K. L., Murphy, J. M., Li, T-K., Lumeng, L., & McBride W. J. (1998a). Development of alcohol drinking behavior in rat lines selectively bred for divergent alcohol preference. *Alcoholism: Clinical and Experimental Research, 22,* 1584–1590.

McKinzie, D. L., Nowak, K. L., Yoger, L., McBride, W. J., Murphy, J. M., Lumeng, L., & Li, T-K. (1998b). The alcohol deprivation effect in the alcohol-preferring P rat under free-drinking and operant access conditions. *Alcoholism: Clinical and Experimental Research, 22,*1170–1176.

McKinzie, D. L., McBride, W. J., Murphy, J. M., Lumeng, L., & Li, T-K. (2002) Effects of amphetamine on locomotor activity in adult and juvenile alcohol-preferring and—nonpreferring rats. *Pharmacology Biochemistry & Behavior, 71,* 29–36.

Murphy, J. M., McBride, W. J., Lumeng, L., & Li, T-K. (1982). Regional brain levels of monoamines in alcohol-preferring and—nonpreferring lines of rats. *Pharmacology Biochemistry & Behavior, 16,* 145–149.

Murphy, J. M., Gatto, G. J., Waller, M. B., McBride, W. J., Lumeng, L., & Li, T-K. (1986). Effects of schedule access on ethanol intake by the alcohol preferring P line of rats. *Alcohol, 3,* 331–336.

Murphy, J. M., McBride, W. J., Lumeng, L., & Li, T-K. (1987). Contents of monoamines in forebrain regions of alcohol-preferring (P) and—nonpreferring (NP) lines of rats. *Pharmacology Biochemistry & Behavior, 26,* 389–392.

Murphy, J. M., Gatto, G. J., McBride, W.J., Lumeng, L., & Li, T-K. (1989). Operant responding for oral ethanol in the alcohol-preferring P and alcohol-nonpreferring NP lines of rats. *Alcohol, 6,* 127–131.

Murphy, J. M., Stewart, R. B., Bell, R. L., Badia-Elder, N. E., Carr, L. G., McBride, W. J., Lumeng, L., & Li, T-K. (2002). Phenotypic and genotypic characterization of the Indiana University rat lines selectively bred for high and low alcohol preference. *Behavior Genetics, 32,* 363–388.

O'Malley, S. S., Krishnan-Sarin, S., Farren, C., Sinha, R., & Kreek, M. J. (2002). Naltrexone decreases craving and alcohol self-administration in alcohol-dependent subjects and activates the hypothalamo-pituitary-adrenocortical axis. *Psychopharmacology, 160,* 19–29.

Paivarinta, P., & Korpi, E. R. (1993). Voluntary ethanol drinking increases locomotor activity in alcohol-preferring AA rats. *Pharmacology Biochemistry & Behavior, 44,* 127–133.

Quine, S., & Stephenson, J. A. (1990). Predicting smoking and drinking intentions and behavior of pre-adolescents: the influence of parents, siblings, and peers. *Family Systems Medicine, 8,* 191–200.

Quintanilla, M. E. (1999). Effect of low doses of ethanol on spontaneous locomotor activity in UChB and UChA rats. *Addiction Biology, 4,* 443–448.

Rodd, Z. A., Bell, R. L., McKinzie, D. L., Webster, A. A., Murphy, J. M., Lumeng, L., Li, T-K., & McBride, W. J. (2004). Low-dose stimulatory effects of ethanol during adolescence in rat lines selectively-bred for high alcohol intake. *Alcoholism: Clinical and Experimental Research* 28, 535–143.

Rodd-Henricks, Z. A., McKinzie, D. L., Shaikh, S. R., Murphy, J. M., McBride, W. J., Lumeng, L., & Li, T-K. (2000). Alcohol deprivation effect is prolonged in the alcohol-preferring (P) rat after repeated deprivations. *Alcoholism: Clinical and Experimental Research, 24,* 8–16.

Rodd-Henricks, Z. A., Bell, R. L., Kuc, K. A., Murphy, J. M., McBride, W. J., Lumeng, L., & Li, T-K. (2001). Effects of concurrent access to multiple ethanol concentrations and repeated deprivations on alcohol intake of alcohol-preferring (P) rats. *Alcoholism: Clinical and Experimental Research, 25,* 140–1150.

Rodd-Henricks, Z. A., Bell, R. L., Kuc, K. A., Murphy, J. M., McBride, W. J., Lumeng, L., & Li, T-K. (2002a). Effects of ethanol exposure on subsequent acquisition and extinction of ethanol self-administration and expression of alcohol-seeking behavior in adult alcohol-preferring (P) rats. I. Periadolescent exposure. *Alcoholism: Clinical and Experimental Research, 26,* 1632–1641.

Rodd-Henricks, Z. A., Bell, R. L., Kuc, K. A., Murphy, J. M., McBride, W. J., Lumeng, L. , & Li T-K. (2002b). Effects of ethanol exposure on subsequent acquisition and extinction of ethanol self-administration and expression of alcohol-seeking behavior in adult alcohol-preferring (P) rats. II. Adult exposure. *Alcoholism: Clinical and Experimental Research, 26,* 1642–1652.

Rose, R. J., Dick, D. M., Viken, R. J., & Kaprio, J. (2001). Gene-environment interaction in patterns of adolescent drinking: regional residency moderates longitudinal influences on alcohol use. *Alcoholism: Clinical and Experimental Research, 25,* 637–643.

Sable, H. J. K. , Strother, W. N., Rodd, Z. A., Lumeng, L., Li, T-K., & McBride, W. J. (2003). Local cerebral glucose utilization (LCGU) rates in adult alcohol-preferring (P) rats are unaltered by peri-adolescent alcohol drinking. *Alcoholism: Clinical and Experimental Research, 27(suppl),* 129A.

Sahr, A. E., Thielen, R. J., Lumeng, L., Li, T-K., & McBride W. J. (2003). Long-lasting alterations of the mesolimbic dopamine system following periadolescent ethanol drinking by alcohol-preferring (P) rats. *Alcoholism: Clinical and Experimental Research* (submitted).

Salimov, R. M., McBride, W. J., McKinzie, D. L., Lumeng, L., & Li, T-K. (1996). Effects of ethanol consumption by adolescent alcohol-preferring P rats on subsequent behavioral performance in the cross-maze and slip funnel tests. *Alcohol, 13,* 297–300.

Sinclair, J. D., & Li, T-K. (1989). Long and short alcohol deprivation: effects on AA and P alcohol-preferring rats. *Alcohol, 6,* 505–509.

Slawecki, C. J., & Betancourt, M. (2002). Effects of adolescent ethanol exposure on ethanol consumption in adult rats. *Alcohol, 26,* 23–30.

Smith, D. G., Learn, J. E., McBride, W. J., Lumeng, L., Li, T-K., & Murphy, J. M. (2001a). Alcohol-naïve alcohol-preferring (P) rats exhibit higher local cerebral glucose utilization than alcohol-nonpreferring (NP) and Wistar rats. *Alcoholism: Clinical and Experimental Research, 25,* 1309–1316.

Smith, D. G., Learn, J. E., McBride, W. J., Lumeng, L., Li, T-K., & Murphy, J. M. (2001b). Long-term effects of alcohol drinking on cerebral glucose utilization in alcohol-preferring rats. *Pharmacology Biochemistry & Behavior, 69,* 543–553.

Sokoloff, L., Reivich, M., Kennedy, C., Des Rosiers, M. H., Patlak, C. S., Pettigrew, K. D., Sakurada, O., & Shinohara, M. (1977). The [14C]deoxyglucose method for the measurement of local cerebral glucose utilization: theory, procedure, and normal values in conscious and anesthetized albino rat. *Journal of Neurochemistry, 28,* 897–916.

Spear, L. P. (2000). The adolescent brain and age-related behavioral manifestations. *Neuroscience and Biobehavioral Reviews, 24,* 417–463.

Spear, L. P., & Brake, S. C. (1983). Periadolescence: age-dependent behavior and psychopharmacological responsivity in rats. *Developmental Psychobiology, 16,* 83–109.

Strother, W. N., Lumeng, L., Li, T-K., & McBride, W. J. (2003a). Regional CNS densities of serotonin-1A and dopamine D2 receptors in periadolescent alcohol-preferring P and alcohol-nonpreferring NP rat pups. *Pharmacology Biochemistry & Behavior, 74,* 335–342.

Strother, W. N., Merrill, C. C., Driscoll, C., Lumeng, L., Li, T-K., & McBride, W. J. (2003b). Effects of acute ethanol on local cerebral glucose utilization (LCGU) in adolescent alcohol-preferring P and alcohol-nonpreferring NP rats. *Society for Neuroscience Abstract* (submitted).

Tolliver, G. A., & Samson, H. H. (1991). The influence of early postweaning ethanol exposure on oral self-administration behavior in the rat. *Pharmacology Biochemistry & Behavior, 38,* 575–580.

Waller, M. B., McBride, W. J., Lumeng, L., & Li, T-K. (1982). Induction of dependence on ethanol by free-choice drinking in alcohol-preferring rats. *Pharmacology Biochemistry & Behavior, 16,* 501–507.

Waller, M. B., McBride, W. J., Gatto, G. J., Lumeng, L., & Li, T-K. (1984). Intragastric self-infusion of ethanol by the P and the NP (alcohol-preferring and—nonpreferring) lines of rats. *Science, 225,* 78–80.

Waller, M. B., Murphy, J. M., McBride, W. J., Lumeng, L., & Li, T-K. (1986). Effect of low dose ethanol on spontaneous motor activity in alcohol-preferring and—nonpreferring lines of rats. *Pharmacology Biochemistry & Behavior, 24,* 617–623.

West, C. H. K., Boss-Williams, K. A., & Weiss, J. M. (1999). Motor activation by amphetamine infusion into nucleus accumbens core and shell subregions of rats differentially sensitive to dopaminergic drugs. *Behavioral Brain Research, 98,* 155–165.

Windle, M. (1990). Alcohol use and abuse: some findings from the National Adolescent Student Health Survey. *Alcohol Health and Research World, 15,* 5–10.

Wise, R. A., & Bozarth, M. A. (1987). A psychomotor stimulant theory of addiction. *Psychological Review, 94,* 469–492.

Witt, E. D. (1994). Mechanisms of alcohol abuse and alcoholism in adolescent: a case for developing animal models. *Behavioral Neural Biology, 62,* 168–177.

Wolffgramm, J., & Heyne, A. (1995) From controlled drug intake to loss of control: the irreversible development of drug addiction in the rat. *Behavioral Brain Research, 70,* 77–94.

Wong, D. T., Reid, L. R., Li, T-K., & Lumeng, L. (1993). Greater abundance of serotonin-1A receptors in some brain areas of alcohol-preferring (P) than nonpreferring (NP) rats. *Pharmacology Biochemistry & Behavior, 46,* 173–177.

Yashimoto, K. (1988). The influence of age upon alcohol drinking behavior. *Medical Science Research, 16,* 755–756.

Zhou, F. C., Bledsoe, S., Lumeng, L., & Li, T-K. (1991). Immunostained serotonergic fibers are decreased in selected brain regions of alcohol-preferring rats. *Alcohol, 8,* 425–431.

Zhou, F. C., Bledsoe, S., Lumeng, L., & Li, T-K. (1994). Reduced serotonergic immunoreactive fibers in the forebrain of alcohol-preferring rats. *Alcoholism: Clinical and Experimental Research, 18,* 571–579.

Zhou, F. C., Zhang, J. K., Lumeng, L., & Li, T-K. (1995). Mesolimbic dopamine system in alcohol-preferring rats. *Alcohol, 12,* 403–412.

Zucker, R. A., & Hartford, T. C. (1983). National study of the demography of adolescent drinking practices in 1980. *Journal of Studies on Alcohol, 44,* 974–985.

7

Adolescence
Alcohol Sensitivity, Tolerance, and Intake

Linda Patia Spear and Elena I. Varlinskaya

Abstract. Research conducted in laboratory animals has shown adolescents to be less sensitive to numerous ethanol effects that may serve as cues to limit intake, including effects evident during intoxication (e.g., ethanol-induced motor impairment, anxiolysis, social impairment, and sedation), as well as during the post-intoxication period (e.g., "hangover"-associated anxiogenesis). Conversely, adolescents are more sensitive than adults to a few ethanol effects, including ethanol-induced social facilitation and impairments in hippocampal long-term-potentiation. These age-specific ethanol sensitivities are not simply related to developmental differences in ethanol pharmacokinetics. Instead, they appear related in part to an ontogenetic decline in expression of within session (acute) tolerance and to differential rates of development of neural systems underlying different actions of ethanol. Relatively high levels of ethanol intake often seen in adolescent rodents and their human counterparts may be related not only to an attenuated sensitivity of adolescents to negative cues that normally serve to limit drinking, but also their greater sensitivity to both the facilitation of social behavior by ethanol and the stimulation of ethanol intake by social experiences. Although data are sparse, studies in laboratory animals hint that under some circumstances chronic adolescent exposure to ethanol may influence ongoing neural maturation and later neural, cognitive, and behavioral functioning, including later sensitivity to and propensity to use ethanol. Recommendations for further research are discussed.

1. Sensitivity to Initial Ethanol Effects during Ontogeny

Work in laboratory animals has revealed that adolescent and even younger rats are surprisingly resistant to many acute effects of ethanol when compared with their adult counterparts. This relative ethanol insensitivity during adolescence has been observed for an increasingly long list of ethanol effects, including ethanol-induced motor impairment (Hollstedt et al, 1980;

Linda Patia Spear and Elena I. Varlinskaya • Binghamton University, Department of Psychology and Center for Developmental Psychobiology, Binghamton, New York 13902-6000.

Silveri & Spear, 2001; White et al, 2002a,b), suppression of locomotion (Little et al, 1996), social impairment (Varlinskaya & Spear, 2002), anxiolysis (Varlinskaya & Spear, 2002), analgesia (Hernandez & Spear, 2003), sedation (Ernst et al, 1976; Little et al, 1996; Moy et al, 1998; Silveri & Spear, 1998; although see also Keir & Deitrich, 1990), and lethality (Hollstedt & Rydberg, 1977). Sensitivity to ethanol's hypothermic effects also has been generally reported to increase ontogenetically from birth through adulthood (see Alkana et al, 1996, for review and references), although reports that adolescents are less sensitive than adults to the acute hypothermic effects of ethanol (Silveri & Spear, 2000; Ristuccia & Spear, 2003) are not ubiquitous (Swartzwelder et al, 1998; Brasser & Spear, 2002). The relative insensitivity to ethanol demonstrated by adolescent and even younger animals is often pronounced. For instance, whereas adult animals are highly sedated and do not recover their righting response for about 8 hours following challenge with 4.5 g/kg ethanol, adolescent animals recover in less than one-half the time—within about 3 hrs (Silveri & Spear, 1998).

These age-related differences in the initial response to ethanol are not simply a function of ontogenetic differences in ethanol pharmacokinetics. Indeed, the relative insensitivity to ethanol seen early in life occurs despite general ontogenetic increases in alcohol dehydrogenase activity (Raiha et al, 1967; Lad et a, 1984) and ethanol elimination rates (see Kelly et al, 1987). Although animals in the adolescent age range occasionally have been reported to show slightly elevated rates of ethanol metabolism relative to more mature animals (Hollstedt et al, 1977; Brasser & Spear, 2002), this is not a consistent finding (Kelly et al, 1987; Zorzano & Herrera, 1989; Silveri & Spear, 2000) and is insufficient to account for the attenuated sensitivity of adolescents to ethanol (e.g., see Little et al, 1996; Silveri & Spear, 2000).

Adolescents are not only less sensitive to many acute effects of ethanol, but also to certain behaviors elicited during the recovery (withdrawal) period following ethanol challenge. Symptoms of ethanol withdrawal traditionally have been characterized during the recovery period following chronic ethanol exposure, although milder signs and symptoms also may be evident following exposure to a single high dose of ethanol. These milder effects include not only physical symptoms of hangover, but also psychological symptoms such as anxiety. During the hangover phase following challenge with a high dose (4 g/kg) of ethanol, adult but not adolescent animals exhibited evidence of anxiety in the plus maze; this dramatic age difference was apparent when animals were tested either at the same post-injection time or the same time following ethanol clearance at each age (Doremus et al, 2003b). Adolescents were likewise insensitive to this hangover effect when anxiety was indexed by social suppression. Indeed, in social interaction tests adolescent rats not only failed to show as much hangover-related social suppression as adults, but also displayed instead a paradoxical increase in social interactions (play fighting) during the hangover period (Varlinskaya & Spear, 2004b). Reduced withdrawal effects in adolescent relative to adult rats also have been observed when withdrawal was indexed by "distress" ultrasonic vocalizations and rebound hyperthermia following acute ethanol challenge (Brasser & Spear, 2002), as well as by an elevation in seizure susceptibility during withdrawal from chronic ethanol (Acheson et al, 1999). Reminiscent of these findings, studies using surveys and self-reports have observed that human adolescents who abuse alcohol rarely report withdrawal symptoms upon cessation of drinking in contrast to common reports of such symptoms in adults (Martin & Winters, 1998).

Thus, adolescents appear to be considerably less sensitive than adults to many acute effects of ethanol—not only effects evident during the intoxication phase, but also those emerging during recovery following intoxication. Yet, for a few restricted effects of ethanol, younger animals through adolescence conversely are more sensitive than adults. In a well-characterized series of studies discussed elsewhere in this volume (see Swartzwelder chapter), Swartzwelder and colleagues have shown that adolescent and pre-adolescent animals are more vulnerable than adults to ethanol-induced impairments in hippocampal LTP and alterations in NMDA receptor function (Swartzwelder et al, 1995a,b; Pyapali et al, 1999; Li et al, 2002). A similar enhanced ethanol sensitivity during adolescence was also reported in terms of ethanol-related memory disruptions, findings reported in late adolescent (>21 years) college students relative to individuals several years their senior (Acheson et al, 1998), as well as in adolescent versus adult rats performing a spatial memory task in a Morris water maze (Markwiese et al, 1998). Surprisingly, when acquisition and memory of a spatial task were assessed in an appetitive situation (where animals were trained to locate hidden cereal pieces in a sandbox) rather than a presumably more stressful swim task, adults were found to be more sensitive to ethanol-induced disruption of performance than their adolescent counterparts (Pottayil & Spear, 2003). Whatever the critical distinction between the two studies that drives their opposing ontogenetic results, this difference apparently does not act purely on performance factors, given that the non-spatial versions of both tasks were resistant to ethanol disruption at the two test ages. Although considerable caution is required when comparing data across laboratories, one intriguing possibility for these opposing results is that level of stressfulness of the test situation may influence relative sensitivity of adolescents versus adults in spatial memory performance. Another hint of a possible role of stress in influencing ontogenetic patterns of ethanol sensitivity will be presented later when discussing ontogeny of acute tolerance (see also Spear, 2002).

There are a few other circumstances where adolescents display unusual sensitivities to ethanol. Adolescent rats are considerably more sensitive than their adult counterparts to ethanol-induced facilitation of social interactions, with adolescents showing increases in social interactions following challenge with low doses of ethanol in familiar (low anxiety producing) situations, social facilitation that is not evident in adults (Varlinskaya et al, 2001; Varlinskaya & Spear, 2002). There are also recent reports that adolescents may be unusually sensitive to the positive affect associated with ethanol intoxication, with low doses of ethanol sufficient to support both appetitive associative conditioning

(Fernández-Vidal et al, 2003) and conditioned place preferences (CPP) during adolescence that are not evident following the same conditioning parameters in mature animals (Philpot et al, 2003, 2004a). In the latter study, age differences in ethanol-induced CPP and place aversions were seen even within the adolescent period, findings reminiscent of other reports of ontogenetic differences in ethanol sensitivity among groups tested at different ages during adolescence (Varlinskaya & Spear, 2003, 2004a).

Taken together, the data to date from studies in laboratory animals suggest that, with some notable exceptions, adolescents are often less sensitive than their mature counterparts to many ethanol effects—both during acute exposure and the recovery ("hangover") period. While limited instances of findings reminiscent of these ontogenetic patterns of attenuated and accentuated sensitivities to ethanol in adolescence have been obtained in work with humans (Martin & Winters, 1998; Acheson et al, 1998), comparable data are limited and difficult to obtain in work with human adolescents. Even beyond ethical constraints on providing ethanol to adolescent humans, the generally longer history of ethanol use in adults, their greater exposure to intoxicated practice, and associated tolerance development seriously confound examination of patterns of acute ethanol sensitivity across age in studies conducted with humans.

2. Contributors to Ontogenetic Differences in Ethanol Sensitivity

2.1. *Neurobiology*

Ethanol exerts its effects through dose-dependent interactions with a diversity of neural systems, including GABAergic, glutaminergic, dopaminergic, serotonergic, and opiate systems (see Eckardt et al, 1998). Many of these neural systems are still maturing during adolescence. Indeed, the brain of the adolescent is a brain in transition, with the more gradual brain development seen during childhood and the relative stability of adulthood punctuated by rapid neural transformations during adolescence (see Spear, 2000, for review). This metamorphosis of adolescent brain is characterized not only by continued maturation of neural systems, but also by a loss of nearly half of the number of synaptic connections in some neural regions (Rakic et al, 1994), neural pruning that may serve to refine brain effort and increase brain efficiency during adolescence (see Chugani, 1996).

Differential rates of development of the neural systems underlying different cognitive/behavioral consequences of ethanol may contribute to the mosaic of age differences in ethanol sensitivities. For instance, as discussed elsewhere in this volume, the Swartzwelder group has convincing data that unusually potent ethanol inhibition of developmentally over-expressed NMDA receptors early in life may contribute to the greater sensitivity of adolescents to ethanol-induced disruption of neural plasticity (indexed by long-term potentiation [LTP] in the hippocampus and other brain regions) and impairment in spatial memory performance (see Swartzwelder et al, 1995a; Pyapali et al, 1999; Li et al, 2002). In contrast, we have found that developmental over-expression of NMDA receptors does not appear to be related to the notably lower sensitivity of adolescents to the sedative effects of ethanol, given that the NMDA antagonist (+)MK-801 enhances the sedative effects of ethanol similarly in young adolescents and adults (Silveri & Spear, 2002). Instead, we (Silveri & Spear, 2002) and others (Moy et al, 1998) have suggested that the attenuated sensitivity of young animals to ethanol sedation is related in part to developmental immaturity in $GABA_A$ receptor systems, a conclusion based in part on findings that young adolescents are considerably more sensitive than adults to the enhancement of ethanol sedation by the $GABA_A$ agonist muscimol (Silveri & Spear, 2002).

Together these findings illustrate how differential rates of maturation of neural substrates modulating various ethanol effects may contribute to the mosaic of increased and decreased sensitivities to ethanol during adolescence. Ontogenetic changes in expression of within session (acute) tolerance and longer-term adaptations to ethanol also may play a role in the expression of age-related differences in sensitivity to ethanol, topics considered in the sections below.

2.2. *Acute Tolerance*

The relative resistance of young organisms to many of the effects of ethanol may be attributable in part to ontogenetic differences in compensatory reactions that serve to attenuate these effects. One such sort of compensation is acute tolerance—the attenuated sensitivity to ethanol that emerges within a single ethanol exposure period. Acute tolerance can be estimated in a number of ways, many of which rely on the property that the magnitude of acute tolerance builds with time following injection. In studies of the sedative effects of ethanol, greater acute tolerance to ethanol has been reported in adolescents than adults, both when using blood ethanol concentrations (BECs) at the time of loss of the righting reflex in animals after the second of two successive ethanol challenges vs. after only one challenge (Grieve & Littleton, 1979) and when assessing BECs at recovery following higher vs. lower ethanol challenge doses (Silveri & Spear, 1998; Silveri & Spear, 2002; Silveri & Spear, 2004). Varlinskaya and Spear (2003b) estimated acute tolerance to ethanol-induced social inhibition by comparing animals tested 5 versus 30 min. following intraperitoneal (i.p.) injection of 1 g/kg ethanol. Both adolescents of various ages and adults showed equivalent ethanol-induced social inhibition at 5 min.; this social inhibition was still evident at 30 min. in adults but diminished across progressively younger ages among animals tested during adolescence. This decline in ethanol-related social impairment from 5 to 30 min. post-administration despite rising BECs is consistent with the rapid emergence of acute tolerance at the younger test ages, with such acute tolerance being particularly robust early in adolescence and declining progressively through the adolescent period and into adulthood.

Expression of this within session adaptation in young animals appears to be dependent on NMDA receptor activation (Silveri & Spear, 2004), reminiscent of other evidence for an important role of NMDA receptor systems in developmental plasticity (e.g., see McDonald & Johnston, 1990). Yet, blocking acute tolerance expression through administration of the NMDA receptor antagonist (+)MK-801 does not eliminate expression of age differences in ethanol sensitivity (Silveri & Spear, 2002; Silveri & Spear, 2004), suggesting that the greater expression of acute tolerance early in life does not solely mediate the attenuated sensitivity shown by developing animals to many ethanol effects.

The ontogenetic pattern of expression of acute tolerance can be altered by prior experiences. Studies showing robust ontogenetic differences in acute tolerance expression have typically used naïve, previously unmanipulated animals. When animals are previously exposed to ethanol or prior stressful situations, more robust evidence for acute tolerance to ethanol sedation emerges in adults, while having little further effect on the already strong acute tolerance seen in young animals (Silveri & Spear, 2004; see also Silveri & Spear, 2001). Under these circumstances, age differences in ethanol sensitivity are still maintained (Silveri & Spear, 2004), again suggesting that ontogenetic differences in expression of acute tolerance are not solely responsible for the attenuated sensitivity of young relative to mature animals to many consequences of ethanol intoxication.

2.3. *Longer-Term Adaptations and Consequences*

Ethanol tolerance not only can develop within a single ethanol episode, but also when a second exposure follows within 24–48 hr. of a previous dose (rapid tolerance) or when there is a history of many ethanol exposures (chronic tolerance)(see Kalant, 1993, for review). The relationships among these different forms of tolerance are arguable, with some researchers concluding that these different types of tolerance represent different manifestations of a common underlying process (Campanelli et al, 1988; Khanna et al, 1987), whereas others suggest that there are separable neural substrates underlying these different adaptations (e.g., Pohorecky & Roberts, 1992). Support for the latter suggestion is found in developmental data showing that, in contrast to the marked ontogenetic decline in acute tolerance to ethanol-induced sedation discussed above, rapid tolerance to ethanol-induced sedative effects does not emerge convincingly until post-adolescence (Silveri & Spear, 1999; Silveri & Spear, 2004). It may be the case that the emergence of marked within session tolerance in young animals may reduce ethanol-induced neural perturbations to such an extent as to obviate the need for longer-term adaptations expressed as rapid and chronic tolerance. To the extent that this reasoning is correct, it would be expected that chronic tolerance would likewise only emerge fairly late during ontogeny. The data are inconsistent on this point.

Evidence of the emergence of chronic tolerance to ethanol-induced motor impairment (but not hypothermia) has been reported as early as the preweaning period in rats (Hunt et al, 1993), although Lagerspetz (1972) did not find evidence for chronic tolerance to ethanol's motor impairing effects in preweanling mice. Chronic ethanol exposure during adolescence produced behavioral and electrophysiological evidence of tolerance when treated animals were tested in adulthood, although adult exposure groups were not included for comparison in this study (Slawecki, 2002). In studies comparing adolescents and adults in terms of tolerance development, chronic exposure to ethanol varyingly was reported to induce more tolerance in adolescents than adults (hypothermia: Swartzwelder et al, 1998; motor impairment: White et al, 2002b), equivalent levels of tolerance at the two ages (in a study equating initial functional motor impairment across age by dose adjustments—Silveri & Spear, 2001), or even the emergence of a later sensitized response to ethanol rather than tolerance following adolescent ethanol exposures (Lagerspetz, 1972; White et al, 2000; Washburn & Spear, unpublished data). Although the small number of available studies limits across-study comparisons, this diversity in findings does not seem to be related in any simple way to the dependent measure under examination, or to whether or not intoxicated practice was permitted during the chronic exposure period.

Reports of ethanol sensitization following adolescent exposures are particularly intriguing. In the White et al, (2000) study, adolescent rats given 3 g/kg ethanol i.p. every other day for 20 days later were found to be more sensitive to ethanol-induced disruption in a spatial working memory task than animals receiving comparable exposure beginning in adulthood as well as animals chronically exposed to saline at either age. Likewise, in recent work we observed that adolescent rats exposed to 4 g/kg intragastrically (i.g.) daily for 8 days were more sensitive to ethanol-induced disruptions in rotorod performance than their saline-exposed counterparts, whereas comparably treated adults exhibited typical tolerance on this task (Washburn & Spear, unpublished observations). In this study, animals exposed to ethanol as adolescents also tended to have more difficulty in performing the rotorod task under baseline conditions, raising the possibility that the greater sensitivity to ethanol in the chronically treated adolescents might not reflect ethanol sensitization per se, but rather an exposure-induced disruption in motor function further exacerbated by acute ethanol challenge.

The work by Lagerspetz (1972) provides some initial clues that the amount of ethanol exposure may play a role in influencing whether or not sensitization rather than tolerance is observed following adolescent exposures. In the Lagerspetz (1972) article, shorter periods of chronic ethanol exposure (i.e., 1–2 g/kg daily for 8 days) during adolescence induced ethanol tolerance, whereas a longer exposure period (i.e., 19 days) resulted in an enhanced sensitivity to ethanol relative to controls. Given that the longer exposure period also suppressed body weights, Lagerspetz (1972) concluded that "the simultaneous impairment of the physical condition of the animals may account for the relatively high alcohol sensitivity of the animals which had repeated alcohol injections" (p.506). Yet, it does not seem to be simply a matter of sensitization being associated with dosing regimens that produce reductions in weight gain. Although sensitization seen in chronically exposed adolescents in the Washburn & Spear study (unpublished observations) was accompanied by a reduction in weight gain that was not seen in adults, the ethanol exposure regimen that resulted in sensitization following adolescent exposure in White et al (2000) did not suppress body weights, whereas a higher dosing regimen used in another study by the same group (White et al, 2002b) did suppress weight gain but produced ethanol tolerance in adolescents that was greater in magnitude than in adults.

Why might ethanol exposure patterns that typically produce tolerance in adulthood sometimes produce apparent sensitization to later ethanol challenges when that exposure occurs during adolescence? One possibility is that ethanol exposure during the brain transformations of adolescence may not only trigger compensations normally expressed as tolerance, but may also perturb ongoing processes of neural development. Systems undergoing rapid ontogenetic change are often most sensitive to disruption (see Adams et al, 2000, for discussion and references), and the transformations of adolescence are a time of particularly dramatic developmental alteration. Indeed, although the available data are meager and often do not include other-aged comparison groups, a few reports have emerged showing that ethanol exposure during adolescence alters subsequent neural, hormonal, and behavioral function along a variety of dimensions.

Using a model of "binge" ethanol exposure, Crews and colleagues (2000) reported that 4 days of exposure to relatively high doses of ethanol induced more brain damage in adolescent than adult rats in a number of frontal-anterior brain regions including the olfactory-frontal cortical regions as well as anterior portions of the piriform and perirhinal cortices. Adult rats exposed as adolescents to 5- or 10-days of ethanol vapor showed a variety of electrophysiological alterations in the parietal cortex and hippocampus, findings that were interpreted as reflecting potentially more robust effects on hippocampus than reported previously in studies where the ethanol exposure was given in adulthood (Slawecki et al, 2001). Grobin et al (2001) assessed neurosteroid (3α, 21-dihydroxy-5(-pregnan-20-one: THDOC) potentiation of $GABA_A$ mediated Cl^- flux in rat cortical synaptoneurosomes at various times following chronic intermittent ethanol exposure for 1 month beginning in adolescence or adulthood, and observed greater neurosteroid potentiation in the animals that were exposed as adolescents.

These initial reports of an unusual sensitivity of adolescent brain to repeated ethanol exposures are complemented by others showing alterations in cognitive function in rats following chronic ethanol exposure during the adolescent period (Osborne & Butler, 1983; Siciliano & Smith, 2001; Lee et al, 2001). Whether similar effects would be observed following comparable dosing in mature animals is not yet known, nor is the relationship between these findings and clinical studies of adolescent alcohol abuse (see Tapert chapter in this volume for discussion of studies of adolescent brain function and alcohol use disorders in humans).

There may be other physiological and behavioral consequences of adolescent ethanol exposure. Among the acute effects of ethanol seen in adolescence are a suppression of plasma growth hormone (Tentler et al, 1997) and alterations in plasma levels of testosterone and other reproductive hormones. Developmentally-specific alterations in testosterone include an ethanol-induced increases in testosterone in adolescent male hamsters (Ferris et al, 1998) and young adolescent male rats (Little et al, 1992), with an ethanol-induced suppression of testosterone levels emerging in male rats by late adolescence (Little et al, 1992). Hormones play an important role in adolescent-associated developmental processes (e.g., see Benson & Migeon, 1975, for review), and hence it is not surprising that chronic ethanol exposure exerts greater adverse effects on reproductive endocrinology in adolescent than adult male rats (Cicero et al, 1990). These long-lasting effects may even be transmitted across generations, with a variety of similar neuroendocrine alterations in their progeny (Cicero et al, 1990). Behaviorally, ethanol-induced increases in testosterone levels during adolescence have been implicated in the increase in aggression seen in male hamsters following chronic ethanol exposure during adolescence (Ferris et al, 1998).

One final potential long-term consequence of adolescent alcohol use is the impact of this exposure on later drinking behavior. Unfortunately, the data on this issue are mixed both in studies with humans and in work using animal models (see Spear, 2002, for review), with some studies in laboratory animals reporting no increase in later ethanol consumption following periods of ethanol exposure that include adolescence (Kakihana & McClearn, 1963; Parisella & Pritham, 1964; Tolliver & Samson, 1991) contrasting with other reports that adolescent (Siciliano & Smith, 2001) or even earlier (Ho et al, 1989) ethanol exposure increases later ethanol consumption, particularly in male rats. Whether or not the ethanol exposure is voluntary and the magnitude and timing of that exposure may prove to be critical variables driving these differing results (see Smith, 2003). More basic animal and prospective human research is necessary to resolve the differing patterns of results across studies, research that is particularly critical given the importance of this issue for the prognosis for future alcohol-related problems among youth who engage in heavy alcohol use.

Taken together, the limited amount of research available to date using animal models of adolescent ethanol exposure provides disconcerting hints that the adolescent brain may respond and adapt differently to repeated episodes of ethanol exposure than the more mature brain. Whereas adolescents sometimes develop adult-typical tolerance following chronic exposure to ethanol, in other instances adolescent exposure appears to increase subsequent sensitivity to ethanol and disrupt critical ongoing processes of brain maturation, with subsequent effects on neural, cognitive, and behavioral functioning.

3. Adolescent Ethanol Intake

3.1. *Possible Relationship to Ontogenetic Differences in Ethanol Sensitivity*

What are the possible implications of these adolescent-specific sensitivities to the acute and chronic effects of ethanol for drinking behavior during adolescence and later in life? As discussed previously, adolescents are less sensitive to a number of acute effects of ethanol, such as ethanol-induced motor impairment and sedation, that presumably serve as cues to terminate intake. Adolescents are also less sensitive to the adverse effects associated with acute ethanol withdrawal/hangover, at least when indexed in terms of withdrawal-related anxiety. This attenuated sensitivity during adolescence to negative consequences of ethanol both during the intoxication and recovery (hangover) periods may serve as permissive factors to support relatively high levels of drinking. On the other hand, animal studies have shown adolescents to be more sensitive than adults to several adverse effects of ethanol that are unlikely to serve as cues to limit intake, including ethanol-induced impairment of hippocampal plasticity and spatial memory. This combination of a relative insensitivity to effects of ethanol that typically serve to moderate intake, but greater sensitivity to other adverse consequences of ethanol that are unlikely to serve as cues to limit intake—e.g., ethanol-induced disruptions of brain plasticity and memory—is an inopportune combination for the adolescent.

To the extent that human adolescents exhibit a similar pattern of attenuated sensitivity to ethanol effects serving as deterrents to excessive use, it might be expected that they would exhibit relatively high levels of ethanol drinking. Indeed, as discussed elsewhere in this volume, per episode intake levels among human adolescents are often considerable, with over 25% of all 10th and 12th grade students reporting binge drinking (i.e., 5 or more drinks in a row) during the past 2 weeks (Johnston et al, 2001), and underage college students more likely to drink to excess within a drinking episode than their older counterparts (Wechsler et al, 2002). Similar high levels of ethanol intake often are evident during adolescence in laboratory animals, with adolescent rats under some circumstances displaying at least 2–3 times higher levels of ethanol intake relative to their body weights than adults (Brunell et al, 2001; Lancaster et al, 1996; Doremus et al, 2003a). Elevated levels of ethanol intake are seen in adolescent animals when the ethanol is sweetened, with adolescent rats (like their human counterparts) initially eschewing the taste of pure ethanol. The sweetener is important, but not sufficient, with adolescents showing a considerable preference for sweetened ethanol (0.1% saccharin/10% ethanol) that is not evident in adults or in adolescents allowed comparable access to the sweetener alone (Brunell et al, 2001). Such ethanol intake by adolescents is not simply a matter of calories, with adolescent rats not showing comparable elevations in intakes relative to adults when allowed access to a calorically-equivalent solution instead of ethanol (Doremus et al, 2003a).

3.2. *Influence of Social Interactions on Ethanol Intake*

Adolescent humans drink in social situations, in part to increase ease in social situations (Beck et al, 1993; Beck & Treiman, 1996), an ethanol effect suggested to be particularly important to adolescents given the special significance of social interactions for adolescents (Smith et al, 1995). As discussed above, studies in laboratory animals have shown that alcohol facilitates social interactions more strongly in adolescents than adults—not only during the period of intoxication (Varlinskaya & Spear, 2002) but also during the post-intoxication, so-called "hangover" recovery period. To the extent that similar findings are evident in humans, ethanol-stimulated increases in peer-directed social interactions both during and following ethanol exposure could contribute to a persisting cycle of drinking in at-risk adolescents, with an increased desire for social interactions during the hangover recovery phase provoking further episodes of ethanol drinking to gain social benefits associated with drinking.

Social behavior and ethanol intake have been shown to interact in other ways as well. Among the early experiences shown in laboratory animals to alter later acceptance and preference for ethanol and ethanol-related cues (e.g., Molina et al, 1989; Chotro & Molina, 1990; Hunt et al, 1993) are social interactions with ethanol-exposed conspecifics. Early experiences with ethanol do not have to involve direct exposure of the developing organism to ethanol per se, with indirect exposure to ethanol cues via interactions with an ethanol-exposed conspecific often being sufficient to facilitate subsequent ethanol intake considerably. For instance, voluntary ethanol consumption in adolescence is elevated in rats that were exposed during the weanling period to a mother consuming ethanol relative to those without this early experience (Honey & Galef, 2003). In this experimental series, elevated consumption was not evident if the maternal exposure to ethanol occurred during gestation or the preweaning period, or if the offspring rather than their dam were allowed to consume ethanol during the weaning period, although a combination of both of these early manipulations was sufficient to enhance adolescent ethanol consumption.

Intake of ethanol during adolescence is elevated not only by earlier interactions with an ethanol-consuming mother, but also by social contact with intoxicated peers. Hunt and colleagues recently have used a demonstrator-observer paradigm developed by Galef and colleagues (Galef et al, 1985) to show that 30 min. access to an intoxicated peer was sufficient to significantly enhance intake of ethanol to levels of 8–9 g/kg over the next 24 hrs. in adolescent rats (Hunt et al, 2001). The effect was dose dependent, with a demonstrator dose of 1.5 g/kg sufficient to increase ethanol intake in experimental animals, whereas doses of 1 and 3 g/kg were ineffective. A similar effect was seen when the interaction with intoxicated peers occurred during the preweaning period, with repeated exposures sufficient to increase ethanol intake several days later (Hunt et al, 2000). Together these results illustrate the potency of interactions with an intoxicated peer for enhancing subsequent ethanol consumption, even in work using a simple animal model rather than highly social humans.

4. Summary and Conclusions

Work conducted using animal models of adolescence has revealed a number of potential contributors to the often high levels of alcohol consumption during adolescence. One potential contributor is an adolescent insensitivity to many initial effects of ethanol (such as ethanol-induced motor impairment and sedation) along with reduced hangover effects. Another is the unusual sensitivity of adolescents to ethanol/social interactions, both in terms of their greater sensitivity to ethanol-induced social facilitation as well as to the stimulation of ethanol intake by social experiences. To the extent that similar developmental differences in ethanol responsiveness are seen in humans, an attenuated sensitivity to acute effects of ethanol that normally serve to moderate drinking along with a reduced propensity of adolescents to experience ethanol withdrawal/hangover could act as permissive factors to allow relatively high consumption patterns during adolescence, consumption that may be further increased by ethanol-facilitated peer interactions. Yet, such elevated levels of ethanol consumption may exacerbate the already increased sensitivity of adolescents to ethanol-induced disruptions of hippocampal function and spatial memory.

Reminiscent of studies in laboratory animals, human adolescents report fewer "hangover" symptoms than adults (Martin & Winters, 1998), although there is a dearth of research to examine whether adolescents are less sensitive to ethanol effects normally serving as cues to moderate consumption during intoxication. Nevertheless, it is interesting that in the 2000 Monitoring the Future study, a greater percentage of 8th and 10th graders (14.1% and 26.2%, respectively) reported drinking 5 or more drinks in a row within the past 2 weeks than the percentages reporting that they had been drunk in the past month (8.3%; 23.5%)(Johnston et al, 2001). To the extent that these data are accurate and do not reflect age differences in perception of (or veracity in) reporting intoxication, these findings would be consistent with a relative insensitivity of younger adolescents to the intoxicating effects of ethanol in humans as well. Certainly, however, such survey and animal data should not be used to draw conclusions regarding the relative capacity of human adolescents to perform complex motor and decision making tasks (such as driving) during ethanol intoxication, given their considerably shorter histories of prior experience with ethanol relative to more mature drinkers.

Relative sensitivity to ethanol effects has been shown to be an important predictor of later problematic ethanol involvement. For instance, studies of individuals with a family history of alcoholism have revealed that one associated risk factor is a relative insensitivity to alcohol dysphoric (Newlin & Thomson, 1990) and perhaps euphoric (e.g, Schuckit, 1994) effects (although see Morzorati et al, 2002, for data to the contrary). A genetic-based insensitivity to undesirable dysphoric effects of ethanol, when combined with an ontogenetic insensitivity to these ethanol effects normally evident during adolescence, could potentially act as a "double whammy" to precipitate high intakes of ethanol when at-risk adolescents begin to drink, a pattern of elevated use that could place them on a trajectory for the development of alcohol-related problems.

Neural substrates underlying the notable ontogenetic differences in ethanol sensitivity remain to be elucidated, although the literature discussed in this chapter provides some initial clues. The relative resistance of adolescents to ethanol-induced sedative effects appears related in part both to the marked development of acute tolerance during the ethanol intoxication period as well as developmental immaturity in $GABA_A$ receptor systems, whereas transient over expression of NMDA receptor systems has been implicated in the unusual sensitivity of adolescents to ethanol-induced disruptions in brain plasticity and hippocampally-related memory processing. But research in this area is just beginning, with more work necessary to determine substrates underlying the mosaic of age-specific alterations in responsiveness of adolescents to ethanol.

Also remaining an important area for future study are the long-term consequences of ethanol exposure during this time of rapid neural and endocrine maturation. Although research in this area is sparse, work in laboratory animals provides initial clues that repeated ethanol use during adolescence may sometimes sensitize animals to later ethanol challenges, affect later neural, cognitive and behavioral functioning, and perhaps alter the later propensity to use and abuse ethanol. Carefully conducted ontogenetic studies in laboratory animals may serve as a valuable complement to long-term prospective studies in developing humans to determine whether there are unique long-term consequences of high levels of alcohol use during adolescence.

Acknowledgments: The writing of this of this chapter was supported by Grants R37AA12525 and R0I AA1250 to LPS and R01 AA12453 to EIV.

References

Acheson SK, Richardson R, Swartzwelder HS: Developmental changes in seizure susceptibility during ethanol withdrawal. *Alcohol* 18:23–26, 1999.

Acheson SK, Stein RM, Swartzwelder HS: Impairment of semantic and figural memory by acute ethanol: Age-dependent effects. *Alcohol Clin Exp Res* 22:1437–1442, 1998.

Adams, J., Barone, S., Jr., LaMantia, A. et al. Workshop to identify critical windows of exposure for children's health: Neurobehavioral work group summary. *Environm. Health Perspect.* 108: 535–544, 2000.

Alkana RL, Davies DL, Lê AD: Ethanol's acute effects on thermoregulation: Mechanisms and consequences, in Deitrich RA and Erwin VG (eds): *Pharmacological Effects of Ethanol on the Nervous System.* Boca Raton, CRC Press, 1996, pp 291–328.

Beck KH, Thombs DL, Summons TG: The social context of drinking scales: Construct validation and relationship to indicants of abuse in an adolescent population. *Addict Behav* 18:159–169, 1993.

Beck KH, Treiman KA: The relationship of social context of drinking, perceived social norms, and parental influence to various drinking patterns of adolescents. *Addict Behav* 21:633–644, 1996.

Benson RM, Migeon CJ: Physiological and pathological puberty, and human behavior, in Eleftheriou BE and Sprott RL (eds): *Hormonal Correlates of Behavior: A Lifespan View,* Vol. 1. New York, Plenum Press, 1975, pp 155–184.

Brasser SM, Spear NE: Physiological and behavioral effects of acute ethanol hangover in juvenile, adolescent, and adult rats. *Behav Neurosci* 116:305–320, 2002.
Brunell SC, Rajendran P, Spear LP: Ethanol intake and stress adaptation in adolescent and adult rats. Presented at the annual meeting of the Society for Neuroscience, November, 2001, San Diego, CA.
Campanelli C, Lê AD, Khanna JM, *et al:* Effect of raphe lesions on the development of acute tolerance to ethanol and pentobarbital. *Psychopharmacology (Berl)* 96:454–457, 1988.
Chotro MG, Molina JC: Acute ethanol contamination of the amniotic fluid during gestational day 21: Postnatal changes in alcohol responsiveness in rats. *Dev Psychobiol* 23:535–547, 1990.
Chugani HT: Neuroimaging of developmental nonlinearity and developmental pathologies, in Thatcher RW, Lyon GR, Rumsey J, Krasnegor N (eds): *Developmental Neuroimaging: Mapping the Development of Brain and Behavior.* San Diego, Academic Press, 1996, pp 187–195.
Cicero TJ, Adams ML, O'Connor L, *et al:* Influence of chronic alcohol administration on representative indices of puberty and sexual maturation in male rats and the development of their progeny. *J Pharmacol Exp Ther* 255:707–715, 1990.
Crews FT, Braun CJ, Hoplight B, *et al:* Binge ethanol consumption causes differential brain damage in young adolescent rats compared with adult rats. *Alcohol Clin Exp Res* 24:1712–1723, 2000.
Doremus TL, Brunell SC, Pottayil R, *et al:* Elevated ethanol consumption in adolescent relative to adult rats. Presented at the annual meeting of the Research Society on Alcoholism, June, 2003a, Fort Lauderdale, FL.
Doremus TL, Brunell SC, Varlinskaya EI, *et al:* Anxiogenic effects during withdrawal from acute ethanol in adolescent and adult rats. *Pharmacol Biochem Behav* 75:411–418, 2003b.
Eckardt MJ, File SE, Gessa GL, *et al:* Effects of moderate alcohol consumption on the central nervous system. *Alcohol Clin Exp Res* 22:998–1040, 1998.
Ernst AJ, Dempster JP, Yee R, *et al:* Alcohol toxicity, blood alcohol concentration and body water in young and adult rats. *J Stud Alcohol* 37:347–356, 1976.
Fernández-Vidal JM, Spear NE, Molina JC: Adolescent rats discriminate a mild state of ethanol intoxication likely to act as an appetitive unconditioned stimulus. *Alcohol* 30:45–60, 2003.
Ferris CF, Shtiegman K, King JA: Voluntary ethanol consumption in male adolescent hamsters increases testosterone and aggression. *Physiol Behav* 63:739–744, 1998.
Galef BG Jr, Kennett DJ, Stein M: Demonstrator influence on observer diet preference: Effects of simple exposure and the presence of a demonstrator. *Anim Learn Behav* 13:25–30, 1985.
Grieve SJ, Littleton JM: Age and strain differences in the rate of development of functional tolerance to ethanol by mice. *J Pharm Pharmacol* 31:696–700, 1979.
Grobin AC, Matthews DB, Montoya D, *et al:* Age-related differences in neurosteroid potentiation of muscimol-stimulated $36Cl^-$ flux following chronic ethanol treatment. *Neuroscience* 105:547–552, 2001.
Hernandez M, Spear LP: Ethanol-induced analgesia in adolescent and adult rats. Presented at the annual meeting of the International Society for Developmental Psychobiology, November, 2003, New Orleans, LA.
Ho A, Chin AJ, Dole VP: Early experience and the consumption of alcohol by adult C57BL/6J mice. *Alcohol* 6:511–515, 1989.
Hollstedt C, Olsson O, Rydberg U: The effect of alcohol on the developing organism: Genetical, teratological and physiological aspects. *Med Biol* 55:1–14, 1977.
Hollstedt C, Olsson O, Rydberg U: Effects of ethanol on the developing rat. II. Coordination as measured by the tilting-plane test. *Med Biol* 58:164–168, 1980.
Hollstedt C, Rydberg U: Alcohol and the developing organism: experimental and clinical aspects, in Ideström C-M (ed): *Recent Advances in the Study of Alcoholism (Proceedings of the First International Magnus Huss Symposium, Stockholm, 2–3 September 1976).* Amsterdam-Oxford, Excerpta Medica, 1977, pp. 93–100.
Honey PL, Galef BG Jr: Ethanol consumption by rat dams during gestation, lactation and weanling increases ethanol consumption by their adolescent young. *Dev Psychobiol* 42:252–260, 2003.
Hunt PS, Holloway JL, Scordalakes EM: Social interaction with an intoxicated sibling can result in increased intake of ethanol by periadolescent rats. *Dev Psychobiol* 38:101–109, 2001.

Hunt PS, Lant GM, Carroll CA: Enhanced intake of ethanol in preweanling rats following interactions with intoxicated siblings. *Dev Psychobiol* 37:90–99, 2000.

Hunt PS, Molina JC, Rajachandran L, *et al:* Chronic administration of alcohol in the developing rat: Expression of functional tolerance and alcohol olfactory aversions. *Behav Neural Biol* 59:87–99, 1993.

Johnston LD, O'Malley PM, Bachman JG: *The Monitoring the Future National Survey Results on Adolescent Drug Use: Overview of Key Findings, 2000* (NIH Publication No. 01–4923). Bethesda, National Institute on Drug Abuse, 2001, pp 1–60.

Kakihana R, McClearn GE: Development of alcohol preference in BALB/c mice. *Nature* 199:511–512, 1963.

Kalant H: Problems in the search for mechanisms of tolerance. *Alcohol Alcohol Suppl* 2:1–8, 1993.

Keir WJ, Deitrich RA: Development of central nervous system sensitivity to ethanol and pentobarbital in short- and long-sleep mice. *J Pharmacol Exp Ther* 254:831–835, 1990.

Kelly SJ, Bonthius DJ, West JR: Developmental changes in alcohol pharmacokinetics in rats. *Alcohol Clin Exp Res* 11:281–286, 1987.

Khanna JM, Campanelli C, Lê AD, *et al:* Effect of raphe lesions on the development of chronic tolerance to pentobarbital and cross-tolerance to ethanol. *Psychopharmacology (Berl)* 91:473–478, 1987.

Lad PJ, Schenk DB, Leffert HL: Inhibitory monoclonal antibodies against rat liver alcohol dehydrogenase. *Arch Biochem Biophys* 235:589–595, 1984.

Lagerspetz, KYH: Postnatal development of the effects of alcohol and of the induced tolerance to alcohol in mice. *Acta Pharmacol et Toxicol* 31:497–508, 1972.

Lancaster FE, Brown TD, Coker KL, *et al:* Sex differences in alcohol preference and drinking patterns emerge during the early postpubertal period in Sprague-Dawley rats. *Alcohol Clin Exp Res* 20:1043–1049, 1996.

Lee MH, Heaney A, Rabe A: Repeated binge exposure to alcohol of periadolescent rats produces lasting functional changes. *Abstr Soc Neurosci* 27:877.14, November, 2001, San Diego, CA.

Li Q, Wilson WA, Swartzwelder HS: Differential effect of ethanol on NMDA EPSCs in pyramidal cells in the posterior cingulate cortex of juvenile and adult rats. *J Neurophysiol* 87:705–711, 2002.

Little PJ, Adams ML, Cicero TJ: Effects of alcohol on the hypothalamic-pituitary-gonadal axis in the developing male rat. *J Pharmacol Exp Ther* 263:1056–1061, 1992.

Little PJ, Kuhn CM, Wilson WA, *et al:* Differential effects of ethanol in adolescent and adult rats. *Alcohol Clin Exp Res* 20:1346–1351, 1996.

Markwiese BJ, Acheson SK, Levin ED, *et al:* Differential effects of ethanol on memory in adolescent and adult rats. *Alcohol Clin Exp Res* 22:416–421, 1998.

Martin CS, Winters KC: Diagnosis and assessment of alcohol use disorders among adolescents. *Alcohol Res Health* 22:95–105, 1998.

McDonald JW, Johnston MV: Physiological and pathophysiological roles of excitatory amino acids during central nervous system development. *Brain Res Brain Res Rev* 15:41–70, 1990.

Molina JC, Chotro G, Spear NE: Early (preweanling) recognition of alcohol's orosensory cues resulting from acute ethanol intoxication. *Behav Neural Biol* 51:307–325, 1989.

Morzorati SL, Ramchandani VA, Flury L, *et al:* Self-reported subjective perception of intoxication reflects family history of alcoholism when breath alcohol levels are constant. *Alcohol Clin Exp Res* 26: 1299–1306, 2002.

Moy SS, Duncan GE, Knapp DJ, *et al:* Sensitivity to ethanol across development in rats: comparison to [3H]zolpidem binding. *Alcohol Clin Exp Res* 22:1485–1492, 1998.

Newlin DB, Thomson JB: Alcohol challenge with sons of alcoholics: a critical review and analysis. *Psychol Bull* 108: 383–402, 1990.

Osborne GL, Butler AC: Enduring effects of periadolescent alcohol exposure on passive avoidance performance in rats. *Physiol Psychol* 11:205–208, 1983.

Parisella RM, Pritham GH: Effect of age on alcohol preference by rats. *Q J Stud Alcohol* 25:248–252, 1964.

Philpot RM, Badanich KA, Kirstein CL: Place conditioning: Age-related changes in the rewarding and aversive effects of alcohol. *Alcohol Clin Exp Res* 27:593–599, 2003.

Pohorecky LA, Roberts P: Daily dose of ethanol and the development and decay of acute and chronic tolerance and physical dependence in rats. *Pharmacol Biochem Behav* 42:831–842, 1992.

Pottayil R, Spear LP: The effects of ethanol on spatial and non-spatial memory in adolescent and adult rats using an appetitive paradigm. Presented at a New York Academy of Sciences Conference, Adolescent Brain Development: Vulnerabilities and Opportunities, September, 2003, New York, NY.

Pyapali GK, Turner DA, Wilson WA, *et al:* Age and dose-dependent effects of ethanol on the induction of hippocampal long-term potentiation. *Alcohol* 19:107–111, 1999.

Raiha NC, Koskinen M, Pikkarainen P: Developmental changes in alcohol-dehydrogenase activity in rat and guinea-pig liver. *Biochem J* 103:623–626, 1967.

Rakic P, Bourgeois J-P, Goldman-Rakic PS: Synaptic development of the cerebral cortex: implications for learning, memory, and mental illness, in van Pelt J, Corner MA, Uylings HBM, Lopes da Silva FH (eds): *Progress in Brain Research, The Self-Organizing Brain: From Growth Cones to Functional Networks,* Vol. 102. Amsterdam, Elsevier, 1994, pp 227–243.

Ristuccia RC, Spear LP: Adolescent ethanol sensitivity: Hypothermia and acute tolerance. Presented at a New York Academy of Sciences Conference, Adolescent Brain Development: Vulnerabilities and Opportunities, September, 2003, New York, NY.

Schuckit MA: Low level of response to alcohol as a predictor of future alcoholism. *Am J Psychiatry* 151:184–189, 1994.

Siciliano D, Smith RF: Periadolescent alcohol alters adult behavioral characteristics in the rat. *Physiol Behav* 74:637–643, 2001.

Silveri MM, Spear LP: Decreased sensitivity to the hypnotic effects of ethanol early in ontogeny. *Alcohol Clin Exp Res* 22:670–676, 1998.

Silveri MM, Spear LP: Ontogeny of rapid tolerance to the hypnotic effects of ethanol. *Alcohol Clin Exp Res* 23:1180–1184, 1999.

Silveri MM, Spear LP: Ontogeny of ethanol elimination and ethanol-induced hypothermia. *Alcohol* 20:45–53, 2000.

Silveri MM, Spear LP: Acute, rapid and chronic tolerance during ontogeny: Observations when equating ethanol perturbation across age. *Alcohol Clin Exp Res* 25:1301–1308, 2001.

Silveri MM, Spear LP: The effects of NMDA and GABAA pharmacological manipulations on ethanol sensitivity in immature and mature animals. *Alcohol Clin Exp Res* 26:449–456, 2002.

Silveri MM, Spear LP: The effects of NMDA and GABAA pharmacological manipulations on acute and rapid tolerance to ethanol during ontogeny. *Alcohol Clin Exp Res,* 28:884–894, 2004.

Slawecki CJ: Altered EEG responses to ethanol in adult rats exposed to ethanol during adolescence. *Alcohol Clin Exp Res* 26:246–254, 2002.

Slawecki CJ, Betancourt M, Cole M, *et al:* Periadolescent alcohol exposure has lasting effects on adult neurophysiological function in rats. *Dev Brain Res* 128:63–72, 2001.

Smith GT, Goldman MS, Greenbaum PE, *et al:* Expectancy for social facilitation from drinking: The divergent paths of high-expectancy and low-expectancy adolescents. *J Abnorm Psychol* 104:32–40, 1995.

Smith RF: Animal models of periadolescent substance abuse: review. *Neurotoxicol Teratol* 25:291–301, 2003.

Spear LP: The adolescent brain and age-related behavioral manifestations. *Neurosci Biobehav Rev* 24:417–463, 2000.

Spear LP: The adolescent brain and the college drinker: Biological basis of propensity to use and misuse alcohol. *J Stud Alcohol Suppl* 14:71–81, 2002.

Swartzwelder HS: The adolescent brain: unique ethanol sensitivity of NMDA receptor-mediated functions *(this volume).*

Swartzwelder HS, Richardson RC, Markwiese-Foerch B, *et al:* Developmental differences in the acquisition of tolerance to ethanol. *Alcohol* 15:1–4, 1998.

Swartzwelder HS, Wilson WA, Tayyeb MI: Age-dependent inhibition of long-term potentiation by ethanol in immature versus mature hippocampus. *Alcohol Clin Exp Res* 19:1480–1485, 1995a.

Swartzwelder HS, Wilson WA, Tayyeb MI: Differential sensitivity of NMDA receptor-mediated synaptic potentials to ethanol in immature versus mature hippocampus. *Alcohol Clin Exp Res* 19:320–323, 1995b.

Tapert SF: The human adolescent brain and alcohol use disorders *(this volume).*

Tentler JJ, LaPaglia N, Steiner J, *et al:* Ethanol, growth hormone and testosterone in peripubertal rats. *J Endocrinol* 152:477–487, 1997.

Tolliver GA, Samson HH: The influence of early postweaning ethanol exposure on oral self-administration behavior in the rat. *Pharmacol Biochem Behav* 38:575–580, 1991.

Varlinskaya EI, Spear LP: Acute effects of ethanol on social behavior of adolescent and adult rats: Role of familiarity of the test situation. *Alcohol Clin Exp Res* 26:1502–1511, 2002.

Varlinskaya EI, Spear LP: Age- and time-dependent effects of ethanol on social interactions: implications for the ontogeny of acute tolerance. Presented at the annual meeting of the Research Society on Alcoholism, June, 2003, Fort Lauderdale, FL.

Varlinskaya EI, Spear LP: Changes in sensitivity to ethanol-induced social facilitation and social inhibition from early to late adolescence. *Annals of the New York Academy of Sciences,* 1021:459–461, 2004a.

Varlinskaya EI, Spear LP: Acute ethanol withdrawal (hangover) and social behavior in adolescent and adult male and female rats. *Alcohol Clin Exp Res,* 28:40–50, 2004b.

Varlinskaya EI, Spear LP, Spear NE: Acute effects of ethanol on behavior of adolescent rats: Role of social context. *Alcohol Clin Exp Res* 25:377–385, 2001.

Wechsler H, Lee JE, Nelson TF, *et al:* Underage college students' drinking behavior, access to alcohol, and the influence of deterrence policies. Findings from the Harvard School of Public Health College Alcohol Study. *J Am Coll Health* 50:223–236, 2002.

White AM, Ghia AJ, Levin ED, *et al:* Binge pattern ethanol exposure in adolescent and adult rats: Differential impact on subsequent responsiveness to ethanol. *Alcohol Clin Exp Res* 24:1251–1256, 2000.

White AM, Truesdale MC, Bae JG, *et al:* Differential effects of ethanol on motor coordination in adolescent and adult rats. *Pharmacol Biochem Behav* 73:673–677, 2002a.

White AM, Bae JG, Truesdale MC, *et al:* Chronic-intermittent ethanol exposure during adolescence prevents normal developmental changes in sensitivity to ethanol-induced motor impairments. *Alcohol Clin Exp Res* 26:960–968, 2002b.

Zorzano A, Herrera E: Decreased in vivo rate of ethanol metabolism in the suckling rat. *Alcohol Clin Exp Res* 13:527–532, 1989.

8

Age-Related Effects of Alcohol on Memory and Memory-Related Brain Function in Adolescents and Adults

Aaron M. White and H. Scott Swartzwelder

1. Overview

Adolescence, broadly defined as the second decade of life, is the period of time during which many people begin to use alcohol and other drugs, and often do so heavily. According to the 2002 Monitoring the Future survey, roughly 30% of 12th graders reported drinking five or more drinks in a row in the two weeks before being surveyed (Johnston et al, 2003). This pattern of heavy, intermittent drinking is also prevalent among college students (White et al, 2002a) and young military personnel (Bray, 1996). While levels of alcohol use among adolescents remain high, the perceived risk associated with such use appears to be declining. From 1992 to 2002, the percentage of 12th graders perceiving "great risk of harm" associated with drinking four or five drinks per day, nearly everyday, dropped from 71% to 59% (Johnston et al, 2003). It does not appear that adolescent alcohol abuse is a problem that will soon disappear.

High levels of drinking among adolescents are particularly troubling given recent evidence that, in contrast to long-held assumptions, a tremendous amount of structural and functional brain development takes place during the teenage years (Geidd et al., 1999; for review see Spear, 2000; 2002). Evidence is accruing that alcohol, and perhaps other drugs, impact brain function and behavior differently during adolescence than during adulthood. Further, preliminary data suggest that adolescents might be more vulnerable than adults to impairments following repeated alcohol exposure.

Aaron M. White and H. Scott Swartzwelder • Duke University Medical Center, Neurobiology Research Labs, Veterans Affairs Medical Center, Durham, North Carolina 27710.

In this review, we will summarize recent data regarding brain development during adolescence. We will also examine the impact of alcohol on behavior and brain function, particularly the effects of alcohol on memory and the neural substrates that support it. Finally, we will critically evaluate evidence that adolescents are more vulnerable than adults to both the short- and long-term effects of alcohol on memory formation and its neural substrates.

2. Adolescent Brain Development

Overproduction of neuronal tissue is a central theme in early brain development, from the womb to late childhood. Human infants are born with far more neurons than are present in the adult brain. The selection process that determines whether an individual cell lives or dies is based on several factors, including the transmission of neurotrophic factors from the post-synaptic cell to the pre-synaptic cell in response to excitatory synaptic activity. In this way, cells that fire together wire together, and those that do not make meaningful contacts with other cells do not survive. One key benefit of this process is that it allows a child's brain to be sculpted by his/her interactions with the outside world (Chugani, 1998).

In recent years, it has become clear that, during adolescence, as in childhood, the brain is highly plastic and shaped by experience. A substantial number of synapses are eliminated, or pruned, in the cortex during adolescence, and this process is presumably influenced, at least in part, by interactions with the outside world (Huttenlocher, 1979; Lidow et al., 1991; Seeman, 1999). It is tempting to conclude that adolescent brain development must simply be an extension of childhood brain development; that it represents a transition stage between childhood and adulthood in a manner similar to how adolescence itself has long been viewed. In actuality, it appears that many of the changes that take place during the second decade of life are novel and do not simply represent the trailing remnants of childhood plasticity.

Some of the most intriguing changes observed thus far occur in the frontal lobes, brain regions that play critical roles in memory, voluntary motor behavior, impulse control, decision-making, planning, and other higher order cognitive functions. Frontal lobe gray matter volumes, which represent dense concentrations of neuronal tissue, increase throughout childhood and do not reach their peak until roughly the age of 12, at which point they decline throughout the second decade of life. The decreased gray matter volumes appear to reflect both an elimination of synapses and an increase in myelination, a process by which glial cells surround neuronal axons and enhance the speed and distance of signal transmission. A parallel increase in overall metabolism occurs in the frontal lobes during the first decade of life and then decreases during early adolescence to reach adult levels by the age of 16–18 (Chugani, 1998). Importantly, such declines during adolescence do not reflect a diminution of frontal lobe function. Indeed, there appears to be an increased reliance on the frontal lobes in the control of behavior, a process commonly referred to as *frontalization* (Rubia et al., 2000). At the same time that gray matter volumes and metabolism decrease, neural activity during the performance of certain tasks becomes more focused and efficient (Casey, 1999; Rubia et al., 2000; Luna et al., 2001). Thus, it appears that adolescent brain development, at least in the frontal lobes, represents a very unique stage of change.

Additional research suggests that similar changes occur elsewhere in the cortex during adolescence. As in the frontal lobes, gray matter volumes in the parietal lobes, which are involved in processing sensory information and evaluating spatial relationships, peak at around age 11 and decrease throughout adolescence (Geidd et al., 1999). Gray matter volumes in the occipital lobes, which are dedicated to processing visual information, increase throughout adolescence and into the early 20s (Geidd et al., 1999). Gray matter volumes in the temporal lobes, which are critically involved in memory formation, as well as visual and auditory processing, do not reach maximum until the age of 16–17 (Geidd et al., 1999).

A variety of changes in subcortical structures have also been noted. For instance, the corpus collosum, a thick bundle of axons that allows the two cerebral hemispheres to communicate with one another, increases in size during adolescence (Geidd et al., 1999). Also, in the rat, levels of dopamine receptors in the nucleus accumbens increase dramatically between PD 25–40 (Teicher et al., 1995), an age range that falls within the window of periadolescent development (Spear, 2002). Dopamine receptor levels in the striatum also increase early in adolescence and then decrease significantly between adolescence and young adulthood (Teicher et al., 1995). Further, the numbers of GABAA receptors increase markedly in a variety of subcortical structures during early adolescence (PD 28–36), including the cerebellum and medial septal nucleus (Moy et al., 1998). As in the frontal lobes, age-related changes in brain activation during task performance have been observed in the cerebellum, superior colliculus, thalamus, striatum, parietal cortex, and hippocampus (Luna et al., 2001; Mueller et al., 1998).

It has become quite clear over recent years that alcohol impacts both behavior and brain function differently in adolescents and adults (Smith, 2003). For instance, the available evidence suggests that adolescents are more vulnerable than adults to the effects of alcohol on both memory and memory-related brain function. Following a brief overview of the impact of alcohol on memory formation, and the mechanisms underlying such effects, age-related differences in alcohol-induced memory impairments and brain dysfunction will be discussed.

3. Alcohol and Memory

Alcohol produces widespread changes in behavior and brain function. As Fleming (1935) stated nearly 70 years ago, ". . . the striking and inescapable impression one gets from a review of acute alcoholic intoxication is of the almost infinite diversity of symptoms that may ensue from the action of this single toxic agent." In addition to impairing balance, motor coordination, decision making, and a long list of other functions, alcohol impairs the ability to form new memories. Alcohol primarily disrupts the ability to form memories that are explicit in nature, including memories for facts (e.g., names, phone numbers, etc.) and events (e.g., what you did last night) (Lister et al., 1991). The impact of alcohol on the formation of new long-term explicit memories is far greater than the drug's impact on the ability to recall previously established memories or to hold new information in memory for a few seconds. When intoxicated subjects are asked to repeat new information immediately after its presentation or following short delays (e.g., a few seconds), they often do fine (see Ryback, 1971, for an early review). Similarly, subjects typically do quite well at retrieving information acquired prior to acute intoxication. In contrast, intoxicated subjects have great difficulty storing new information across delays lasting more than a few seconds, particularly if they are distracted between the stimulus presentation and testing. For instance, Acheson et al (1998) observed that intoxicated subjects could recall items on words lists immediately after the lists were presented, but had great difficulty recalling the items 20 minutes later.

Ryback characterized the impact of alcohol on memory formation as a dose-related continuum with minor impairments at one end and very large impairments at the other, with all impairments representing the same fundamental deficit in the ability store new information in memory for longer than a few seconds. Consistent with this view, research indicates that the magnitude of alcohol-induced memory impairments increases with dose but the same general pattern, greater difficulty forming new memories than recalling existing memories, remains. When doses of alcohol are small to moderate, such as those producing blood alcohol concentrations below 0.15%, memory impairments tend to be small to moderate, as well. At these levels, alcohol produces what Ryback (1971) referred to as cocktail party memory deficits, lapses in memory that one might experience after having a few drinks at a cocktail party, often manifested as "problems remembering what the other person said or where they were in conversation." Several studies have revealed difficulty forming memories for items on word lists or learning to recognize new faces at these doses. As the doses increase, the resulting memory impairments can become much more profound, sometimes culminating in blackouts, a complete inability to remember critical elements of events, or even entire events, that transpired while intoxicated (White et al., 2002a).

4. Mechanisms Underlying Alcohol-Induced Memory Impairments

Until recently, a lack of knowledge regarding the neuropharmacological effects of alcohol hampered progress toward an understanding of the mechanisms underlying alcohol-induced memory impairments. Alcohol was long assumed to affect the brain in a very general way, causing a ubiquitous depression of neural activity through non-specific mechanisms. The pervasiveness of this assumption is reflected in numerous writings during the early 20th century. For instance, Fleming (1935) wrote, "The prophetic generalization of Schmiedeberg in 1833 that the pharmacological action of alcohol on the cerebrum is purely depressant has been found, most pharmacologists will agree, to characterize its action in general on all tissues." During the 1970s, evidence led to speculation that alcohol depressed the activity of neurons by altering the movement of lipid molecules in cell membranes, leading to alterations in the activity of proteins, including ion channels, located in those membranes (e.g., Chin and Goldstein, 1977). In the 1980s, the paradigm began to shift as evidence mounted that alcohol actually has fairly selective effects on transmitter systems, altering activity at some receptor subtypes but not others (e.g., Criswell et al., 1993).

Substantial evidence now indicates that alcohol selectively alters the activity of specific receptor complexes that bind GABA, glutamate, serotonin, acetylcholine, glycine, and other transmitters (see Little, 1999 for review). In some cases, only a few amino acids appear to separate receptors that are sensitive to alcohol from those that are not (Peoples and Stewart, 2000). It remains unclear exactly how alcohol interacts with receptors to alter their activity. However, the specificity of the effects of alcohol on receptor function is difficult to reconcile with the view that alcohol produces a general effect by acting at the level of the lipid bilayer (see Peoples et al., 1996 for discussion).

5. The Role of the Hippocampus

Research conducted during the past few decades suggests that alcohol impairs memory formation, at least in part, by disrupting activity in the hippocampus (see White et al., 2000 for review). Brain damage limited to a single region of hippocampal neurons, known as CA1, dramatically disrupts the ability to form new explicit memories (Zola-Morgan et al., 1986). Such damage renders subjects incapable of forming new long-term memories for facts and events. In rodents, CA1 pyramidal cells often exhibit a striking behavioral correlate. Each cell tends to fire predominantly in a specific area of the environment. For this reason, these cells are often referred to as place-cells and the regions of the environment in which they fire are referred to as place-fields (for review see Best and White, 1998). Given the critical importance of these cells in the formation of memories for facts and events, and the clear behavioral correlates of their activity, they offer an ideal way to assess the impact of alcohol on hippocampal output in an intact, fully functional brain.

One recent project examined the impact of alcohol on hippocampal CA1 pyramidal cell activity in freely-moving rats (White and Best, 2000). Alcohol decreased the output from these cells beginning at a dose of 0.5 g/kg. Doses of 1.0 and 1.5 g/kg dramatically suppressed the firing of cells in CA1, almost shutting them off entirely in some cases.

In addition to suppressing the output from pyramidal cells, alcohol has several other effects of hippocampal function. For instance, alcohol potently disrupts the establishment of long term potentiation (LTP), an experimentally induced form of synaptic plasticity theoretically linked to memory formation (Bliss and Colinridge, 1993). It is believed that something like LTP occurs naturally in the brain during learning (see Martin and Morris, 2002 for review). Because drugs that interfere with the establishment of LTP also cause memory impairments in humans, many people believe that LTP serves as a good model for studying the neurobiology underlying the effects of drugs, like alcohol, on memory.

In a typical LTP experiment, two electrodes are lowered into a slice of hippocampal tissue kept alive by bathing it in oxygenated artificial cerebral spinal fluid (ACSF). The technique takes full advantage of the fact that, in a slice of the hippocampus, information flow progresses in a very orderly fashion from cells in the cortex, to cells in the dentate gyrus, to cells in CA3, to cells in CA1, and then back out to the cortex. The first electrode is positioned near the axons coursing from CA3 to CA1. A small amount of current is passed through the first electrode, causing the neurons in this area to send signals to cells located in CA1. The second electrode, which is located in CA1, is then used to record the response of CA1 neurons to the incoming signals. This initial response is referred to as the *baseline* response. Next, a specific pattern of stimulation intended to model the pattern of activity that might occur during an actual learning event is delivered through the first electrode. Now, when one presents the original stimulus delivered during baseline, the response detected from the cells near the second electrode is bigger (i.e., potentiated). In other words, as a result of the patterned input, cells in CA1 are now more responsive to signals sent from cells in CA3. The potentiated response often lasts for a long time, hence the label *long-term potentiation*.

Alcohol interferes with the establishment of LTP beginning at concentrations equivalent to those produced by consuming just one or two drinks (Blitzer et al., 1990). If sufficient alcohol is present in the ACSF bathing the slice of brain when the patterned stimulation is given, the response recorded later in CA1 will not be bigger than it was during baseline. Similar to the relative failure of alcohol to impair recall of previously established memories, alcohol does not disrupt the expression of LTP established prior to the application of the drug.

One of the key requirements for the establishment of LTP in the hippocampus is that the NMDA receptor, a glutamate receptor subtype, becomes activated. Activation of the NMDA receptor allows calcium (Ca2+) to enter the cell, which sets off a chain of events leading to long-lasting changes in the structure and/or function of the cell. Alcohol interferes with the activation of the NMDA receptor, thereby preventing the influx of Ca2+ and the changes that follow. This is believed to be the primary mechanism underlying the effects of alcohol on the induction of LTP, though other transmitter systems are probably also involved (Schummers and Browning, 2001).

6. Alcohol Affects Adolescents and Adults Differently

The available evidence suggests that adolescents are more vulnerable than adults to the affects of alcohol on learning and memory, though much more work needs to be done in this area. In rats, one task commonly used to assess learning and memory is called the *Morris water maze* task. This task requires rats to locate a platform submerged an inch or so beneath the surface of opaque water in a big circular tub. The ability to learn this task is very sensitive to changes in activity in the hippocampus, so it provides an easy way to assess whether drugs that disrupt hippocampal function also disrupt learning that is dependent on this structure.

Markwiese et al. (1998) discovered that adolescent rats are much more vulnerable to alcohol-induced learning impairments in the water maze than adults. Subjects were trained to locate the submerged platform over a period of five days. Subjects were administered either saline, 1.0 or 2.0 g/kg alcohol prior to each of the five days of training. Adolescents exhibited learning impairments relative to saline-treated subjects at both doses. In contrast, adults were only impaired at the highest dose.

It is difficult to determine whether adolescent humans, like adolescent rats, are more vulnerable than adults to the effects of alcohol on learning and memory. For obvious legal and ethical reasons, this research has not been carried out in young adolescent humans. However, one recent study suggests that people in their early twenties, at the trailing end of adolescence, are more vulnerable to alcohol-induced memory impairments than those in their late twenties (Acheson et al., 1998). Subjects were tested using a variety of memory tasks, including the complex figure task. In this task, subjects are shown a line drawing and are required to reproduce the drawing immediately after it is shown to them (immediate recall) and then again twenty minutes later (delayed recall). When tested under placebo, all subjects performed similarly in both the immediate and delayed components of the task. However, when tested under alcohol (the equivalent of about 2–3 drinks), subjects in their early twenties performed worse than subjects in their late twenties on both components of the task.

7. Potential Mechanisms Underlying the Age-Dependent Effects of Alcohol on Memory

As discussed above, the hippocampus plays a central role in learning and memory. Several studies have revealed that alcohol affects hippocampal function differently in adolescents and adults. For instance, it is quite clear that alcohol inhibits the induction of LTP (Swartzwelder et al., 1995a; Pyapali et al., 1999) and NMDA receptor-mediated synaptic potentials (Swartzwelder et al., 1995b) more potently in hippocampal slices from adolescent rats than in those from adults. Such findings suggest that glutamatergic neurotransmission in the hippocampus is uniquely inhibited by acute alcohol during periadolescent development.

It also appears that the unique potency of alcohol against NMDA receptor-mediated synaptic activity is not restricted to the hippocampus. Using whole-cell recording techniques in slices of the retrosplenial cortex, we found that synaptically-evoked, NMDA receptor-mediated excitatory postsynaptic currents (EPSCs) were more powerfully inhibited by alcohol in cells from juvenile rats than in those from adults (Li et al, 2002). Those findings illustrate three important points—developmental sensitivity of NMDA currents to alcohol exists outside the hippocampus, it is observable at the level of single neurons, and it is observable at alcohol concentrations as low as 5mM, roughly the equivalent of a single drink.

In contrast to the uniquely powerful effects of alcohol against excitatory glutamatergic neurotransmission and learning in adolescence, the onset of sedation following alcohol administration is slower, and the magnitude of sedation smaller, in adolescent rats than in adult rats (Little et al., 1996; Swartzwelder et al., 1998; Silveri and Spear, 1998; Moy et al., 1998). Similarly, alcohol affects motor coordination less potently in adolescents than adults (White et al., 2002b;c). In humans, the sedative and motor incoordinating effects of alcohol can limit the amount of alcohol an individual consumes. That is, the individual might find him/herself incapacitated at some point during the evening and unable to continue drinking even if they desired to do so. The existing research regarding alcohol-induced sedation and motor impairments in adolescents and adults has all involved the use of rodents. If such findings extend to humans, the decreased vulnerability of adolescents to the sedative and motor impairing effects of alcohol might allow adolescents to continue drinking for longer periods of time than adults, and perhaps achieve much higher BACs, without becoming incapacitated. As we have seen, adolescents appear to be more vulnerable than adults to some of the cognitive impairments produced by alcohol. Thus, the reduced susceptibility to alcohol-induced sedation and motor incoordination, combined with an enhanced susceptibility to alcohol-induced cognitive deficits, could be a potentially very dangerous combination of effects.

The neural mechanisms underlying the developmental differences in sensitivity to the sedative and motor impairing effects of alcohol are unclear, but are likely to involve GABA-mediated inhibition. The promotion of neuronal inhibition through enhancement of GABAA receptor activation is thought to be a primary mechanism of alcohol-induced sedation (Liljequist and Engel, 1982), and has been observed in many neural circuits and regions (Mereu and Gess, 1985). Postnatal development of GABAA receptor-mediated neurotransmission follows a linear course. In rats, after the polarity of GABAA receptor-mediated inhibition changes from depolarizing to hyperpolarizing by about postnatal day seven (Cherubini et al, 1991; Zhang et al, 1991), GABAA neurotransmission develops steadily, reaching adult functional levels by about postnatal day 60 (Behringer et al, 1996; Xia and Haddad, 1992). Accordingly, during the early adolescent period (postnatal days 28–36) levels of GABAA receptors increase markedly in a number of brain structures (Moy et al., 1998). Aguayo et al (2002) have shown a developmental sensitivity of the ability of alcohol to potentiate GABAA receptor function in tissue culture. They demonstrated that GABAA receptors in 12-day cultured hippocampal cells were not potentiated by alcohol, but if left in culture for seven more days, the cells developed alcohol sensitivity. The mechanisms underlying this are not known. These findings are consistent with other studies that have demonstrated changes in the pharmacological sensitivity of GABAA receptor-mediated currents in hippocampal neurons across postnatal development (Kapur and MacDonald, 1996; 1999). Those studies demonstrated that GABAA receptor mediated IPSCs become progressively more sensitive to the effects of both diazepam and zolpidem across juvenile and periadolescent development, reaching adult levels of sensitivity by about postnatal day 50.

These findings beg the question of whether the effects of alcohol on GABAA receptor function differ between adolescent and adult subjects. This has not as yet been definitively answered, but we have strong preliminary data suggesting that GABAA receptor-mediated inhibitory postsynaptic currents (IPSCs) in hippocampal CA1 pyramidal cells become progressively more sensitive to alcohol between two and 16 weeks of age in the rat. This would be consistent with the behavioral findings described above indicating that juvenile and adolescent animals are markedly less sensitive to the sedating effects of acute alcohol than adults.

8. Long-Lasting Consequences of Acohol Exposure: Age-Related Effects

In addition to reacting differently to the acute, or initial, effects of alcohol, it appears that adolescents are also affected differently than adults by repeated, heavy drinking. Many adolescents engage in a pattern of chronic intermittent exposure (CIE) sometimes referred to as binge drinking. Chronic intermittent exposure is a special case of chronic alcohol administration that involves discrete, repeated withdrawals. There is compelling evidence that it is the repeated withdrawals from alcohol that are responsible for many of the CNS effects of chronic alcohol exposure. For example, in laboratory animals, repeated withdrawals from alcohol result in a higher rate of seizures during withdrawal than are observed after continuous exposure of the same duration (Becker and Hale, 1993). The association of repeated withdrawals with withdrawal seizure susceptibility is also indicated in humans. In studies of alcohol detoxification, patients with a history of previous detoxifications were more likely to exhibit seizures during withdrawal (Brown et al, 1988). Although these data from human studies are correlational, the convergence of these findings with those from animal models strongly suggests that discrete, repeated withdrawals from alcohol exposure presents a unique risk for subsequent neurobehavioral impairments.

Our most recent behavioral studies have shown what we believe is a striking, long-term effect of developmental alcohol exposure (White et al, 2002c). We found that CIE treatment (5.0 g/kg IP, every 48 hrs for 20 days) during adolescence interferes with the normal increase in sensitivity to alcohol-induced motor impairments that occurs between adolescence and adulthood. As expected, under control conditions (i.e. repeated saline exposure), rats were more sensitive to the effects of alcohol on postnatal day 65 (young adulthood) then they had been on postnatal day 30 (adolescence). This is consistent with the previous reports that rats become more sensitive to the motor impairing effects of alcohol as they progress from adolescence to adulthood (White et al., 2002b). However, animals that received CIE during adolescence did not show the normal pattern of increased sensitivity to alcohol as they aged into adulthood. In these subjects, the impact of acute alcohol on motor coordination remained unchanged before, two days after, and 16 days after CIE treatment. In contrast to the effects of CIE in adolescents, CIE treatment during adulthood had little impact on the subsequent effects of alcohol on motor coordination. This suggests the possibility that the chronic exposure during adolescence may have "locked in" the adolescent insensitivity to alcohol's sedative effects, or at least significantly delayed the normal progression to greater sensitivity in adulthood.

Repeated alcohol withdrawals are also associated with subsequent cognitive deficits. For example, after repeated alcohol exposures, adult rodents exhibit impaired learning in an active avoidance paradigm (Bond, 1979). In addition, our preliminary data indicate that CIE treatment in adolescent rats results in exacerbated alcohol-induced learning deficits in adulthood (White et al, 2000). Adolescent and adult subjects with treated with CIE (5.0 g/kg, IP every 48 hrs for 20 days) and then trained on a spatial memory task. All subjects acquired the task at similar rates. However, when their memory was tested under acute alcohol (1.5 g/kg), subjects treated with CIE during adolescence performed more poorly than the other groups. Similar results have been observed in humans. Weissenborn and Duka (2003) assessed the impact of acute alcohol exposure on memory in college students. Those with a history of binge-pattern drinking performed more poorly while intoxicated than other subjects. In adult alcoholics, one of the most consistent clinical neuropsychological findings is a deficit in anterograde, declarative memory. The severity of these enduring memory deficits has been positively correlated with the number of alcohol withdrawals (Brown et al, 1988). Brown et al. (2000) observed that, among adolescents in an inpatient treatment facility, the presence of alcohol withdrawal symptoms at intake was associated with impaired cognitive functions three weeks into the program.

Cognitive impairments following repeated alcohol exposure and withdrawal may stem from neurotoxicity in the hippocampus and related structures. A study by De Bellis et al. (2000) provides preliminary evidence that, in humans, alcohol abuse during adolescence is associated with a reduction in the volume of the hippocampus. The authors utilized magnetic resonance imagine

(MRI) to assess the size of the hippocampus in subjects with adolescent-onset alcohol use disorders and in normal control subjects. Hippocampal volumes were smaller in those who abused alcohol during adolescence, and the amount of apparent hippocampal damage increased as the number of years of alcohol abuse increased (i.e., the longer one abused alcohol, the smaller the hippocampus became). Total intracranial, cortical gray and white matter, corpus callosum and amygdala volumes did not differ between groups. Such data suggest that the adolescent hippocampus is sensitive to the neurotoxic effects of alcohol, and that the earlier in adolescence one begins abusing alcohol, the greater the risk for producing hippocampal damage. However, whether adolescents are truly more vulnerable than adults to hippocampal damage following alcohol exposure remains to be seen.

Damage to the hippocampus following repeated alcohol exposure might stem from hyperactivity at NMDA receptors during alcohol withdrawal, which could allow intracellular Ca2+ levels to become neurotoxic. Repeated alcohol exposure results in an upregulation of NMDA receptors in several brain regions including the hippocampus (Grant et al, 1990; Hoffman and Tabakoff, 1994; Snell et al, 1993). Calcium channels are also upregulated after chronic alcohol exposure (Dolin and Little, 1989). Chronic exposure is also related to increased excitotoxicity of cultured neurons (Crews and Chandler, 1993) and increased NMDA-mediated Ca2+ influx (Iorio et al, 1991; 1992). Thus, repeated alcohol exposure results in neuroadaptive changes that may increase the liability for excitotoxicity during withdrawal.

As discussed above, the available evidence suggests that adolescents might be more vulnerable than adults to brain damage and, perhaps, long-lasting cognitive deficits following alcohol exposure. Given the potential role of hippocampal neurotoxicity in these effects, it is logical to speculate that adolescents might be more vulnerable than adults to hippocampal dysfunction following repeated periods of intoxication and withdrawal. However, our most recent studies have failed to show differential neuronal death or neurophysiological indices of pathology after binge-pattern alcohol exposure in adolescent rats. For example, we have done a series of experiments in which animals were exposed to doses of 5.0 g/kg of alcohol (IP) in various patterns: once per day for six days, once per 48 hours for four days, and twice per day for five days. Some of the groups were exposed during adolescent development, and some during early adulthood. The animals were perfused transcardially 1–3 days after the last alcohol treatment, and the brains were sectioned for subsequent staining with Flouro-Jade B (FJ-B), a marker for dying neurons. In no instance did we observe significant FJ-B staining, suggesting that at least with these relatively mild patterns of alcohol exposure there was no indication of frank neuronal death in rats of any of the ages tested.

As detailed above, our preliminary data suggest that binge-pattern alcohol exposure (CIE) during adolescence, but not adulthood, enhances vulnerability to alcohol-induced spatial memory impairments later in life (White et al., 2000). These behavioral findings suggested the possibility that the hippocampi of the animals that received CIE during adolescence may have been damaged in ways that would diminish the capacity for activity-induced synaptic plasticity and render these circuits more vulnerable to the acute effects of alcohol. Therefore, one week after the behavioral testing, we sacrificed the animals and prepared hippocampal slices to study the impact of alcohol on the induction of long-term potentiation (LTP) in area CA1. We found no effect of earlier intermittent alcohol treatment on LTP induction, amplitude, or maintenance in slices from animals in either age group, with or without alcohol (20 mM) added to the ACSF. While this does not fully address the question of long-term effects of intermittent alcohol exposure during adolescence on hippocampal function, it at least suggests that our current model of CIE produced no profound compromises of baseline LTP induction or the vulnerability of these circuits to acute alcohol exposure.

In similar studies we also found no effect of chronic intermittent alcohol exposure on epileptogenesis in hippocampal area CA3. Four treatment groups were prepared: CIE during adolescence, CIE during early adulthood, saline during adolescence, and saline during early adulthood. Beginning at either postnatal day 30 or 70 the animals got 5.0 g/kg of alcohol (or saline) I.P. every other day for 30 days. Twenty-four hours after the last alcohol or saline dose, the animals were sacrificed and hippocampal slices prepared. We recorded evoked, extracellular responses from area CA3 in two slices from each animal. In one slice we measured pharmacologically isolated, NMDA receptor-mediated population excitatory postsynaptic potentials (NMDA pEPSPs), and in the other we recorded spontaneous epileptiform bursts generated after bath application of 7.0 mM K+. Alcohol pretreatment did not influence the induction or amplitude of NMDA pEPSPs in area CA1 in either age group, or did it influence the time to the initial burst, the number of bursts, nor the duration of individual bursts in area CA3. Thus it does not appear that intermittent alcohol exposure during adolescence or early adulthood influences hippocampal excitatory responsiveness 24 hours after the last exposure.

The above negative findings strongly suggest that the long-term behavioral changes observed following CIE treatment in adolescence likely involve very subtle changes in neuronal circuits that do not reveal themselves through gross measures like LTP or epileptogenesis in the hippocampus. Alternatively, the changes in brain organization and function that underlie the behavioral effects might simply take place in regions that have not yet been thoroughly examined.

9. Summary

As detailed in this brief review, there is now clear evidence that adolescence represents a unique stage of brain development. Changes in brain organization and function during adolescence are widespread, and include intense rewiring in the frontal lobes and other neorcortical regions, as well as changes in a litany of subcortical structures. Recent research suggests that, because of these changes in brain function, drugs like alcohol affect adolescents and adults differently. The available evidence, much of it from research with animal models, suggests that adolescents might be more sensitive than adults to the memory impairing effects of alcohol, as well as the impact of alcohol on the brain function that underlies memory formation. For instance, when treated with alcohol, adolescent rats perform worse than adults in spatial learning tasks that are known to require the functioning of the hippocampus. Alcohol disrupts hippocampal function, and does so more potently in adolescents than adults. In contrast, adolescents appear to be far less sensitive than adults to both the sedative and motor impairing effects of alcohol. While research on this topic is still in its infancy, the findings clearly suggest that adolescence represents a unique stage of sensitivity to the impact of alcohol on behavior and brain function.

ACKNOWLEDGEMENTS: This research was supported by NIAAA grant #12478, a VA Senior Research Career Scientist award to HSS, and a grant from the Institute for Medical Research to AMW.

References

Acheson S, Stein R., Swartzwelder HS (1998) Impairment of semantic and figural memory by acute alcohol: Age-dependent effects. Alc Clin Exp Res 22:1437–1442.

Aguayo L, Peoples R, Yeh H, Yevenes G (2002) GABAA receptors as molecular sites of alcohol action: Direct or indirect actions? Current Topics in Medicinal Chemistry 2:869–885.

Becker HC, Hale RL (1993) Repeated episodes of alcohol withdrawal potentiate the severity of subsequent withdrawal seizures: An animal model of alcohol withdrawal "kindling." Alc Clin Exp Res 17:94–98.

Behringer K, Gault L, Siegel R (1996) Differential regulation of GABAA receptor subunit mRNAs in rat cerebellar granule neurons: Importance of environmental cues. J Neurochem 66:1347–1353.

Best PJ, White AM. (1998) Hippocampal cellular activity: a brief history of space. Proc Natl Acad Sci 95:2717–2719.

Bliss TVP, Collinridge GL (1993) A synaptic model of memory: Long-term potentiation in the hippocampus. Nature 361:31–39.

Blitzer RD, Gil O, Landau EM (1990) Long-term potentiation in rat hippocampus is inhibited by low concentrations of ethanol. Brain Res 537:203–208.

Bond NW (1979) Impairment of shuttlebox avoidance learning following repeated alcohol withdrawal episodes in rats. Pharmacol Biochem Behav 11:589–591.

Bray RM (1996) Department of defense survey of health related behaviors among military personnel. The Research Triangle Institute, February.

Brown AS, Tapert SF, Granholm E, Delis DC (2000) Neurocognitive functioning of adolescents: effects of protracted alcohol use. Alcohol Clin Exp Res 24:164–171.

Brown M, Anton R, Malcolm R, Ballenger J (1988) Alcohol detoxification and withdrawal seizures: Clinical support for a kindling hypothesis. Biol Psychiat 23:507–514.

Casey B (1999) Images in neuroscience. Brain development, XII: maturation in brain activation. Am J Psychiatry 156:504.

Cherubini E, Gaiarsa J, Ben-Ari Y (1991) GABA: An excitatory transmitter in early postnatal life. Trends Neurosci 14:515–519.

Chin JH, Goldstein DB (1977) Effects of low concentrations of ethanol on the fluidity of spin-labeled erythrocyte and brain membranes. Molec Pharmacol 13:435–441.

Chugani H (1998) Biological Basis of Emotions: Brain Systems and Brain Development. Pediatrics 102:1225–1229.

Crews F, Chandler L (1993) Excitotoxicity and the neuropathology of alcohol. In: *Alcohol Induced Brain Damage* (W.A. Hunt and S.J. Nixon, Eds.). NIH Publication No. 93–3549: 355–371.

Criswell HE, Simson PE, Duncan GE, McCown TJ, Herbert JS, Morrow AL, Breese GR (1993) Molecular basis for regionally specific action of ethanol on gamma-aminobutyric acidA receptors: Generalization to other ligand-gated ion channels. J Pharmacol Exp Ther 267:522–537.

De Bellis MD, Clark DB, Beers SR, Soloff PH, Boring AM, Hall J, Kersh A, Keshavan MS (2000) Hippocampal volume in adolescent-onset alcohol use disorders. Am J Psychiatry 157:737–744.

Dolin SJ, Little HJ (1989) Are changes in neuronal calcium channels involved in ethanol tolerance?. J Pharmacol Exp Ther 250:985–91.

Fleming R (1935) A psychiatric concept of acute alcoholic intoxification. Am J Psychiatry 92:89–108.

Giedd J, Blumenthal J, Jeffries N, Castllanos F, Liu H, Zijdenbos A, Paus T, Evans A, Rapoport, J (1999) Brain development during childhood and adolescence: a longitudinal MRI study. Nature Neurosci 2:861–863.

Grant K, Valverius P, Hudspith M, Tabakoff B (1990) Alcohol withdrawal seizures and the NMDA receptor complex. Eur J Pharmacol 176:289–296.

Hoffman P, Tabakoff B (1994) The role of the NMDA receptor in alcohol withdrawal. EXS 71: 61–70.

Huttenlocher P (1979) Synaptic density in human frontal cortex - developmental changes and effects of aging. Brain Res 163:195–205.

Iorio K, Reinlib L, Tabakoff B, Hoffman P (1991) NMDA-induced [Ca2+]i enhanced by chronic alcohol treatment in cultured cerebellar granule cells. Alc Clin Exp Res 15:333.

Iorio K, Reinlib L, Tabakoff B, Hoffman P (1992) Chronic exposure of cerebellar granule cells to alcohol results in increased NMDA receptor function. Mol Pharmacol 41:1142–1148.

Johnston LD, O'Malley PM, Bachman JG (2003) Monitoring the Future national survey results on drug use, 1975–2002. Volume I: Secondary school students (NIH Publication No. 03–5375). Bethesda, MD: National Institute on Drug Abuse, 520 pp.

Kapur J, MacDonald R (1996) Pharmacological properties of GABAA receptors from acutely dissociated rat dentate granule cells. Mol Pharmacol 50:458–466.

Kapur J, MacDonald R (1999) Postnatal development of hippocampal dentate granule cell GABAA receptor pharmacological properties. J Pharmacol Exp Ther 55:444–452.

Li Q, Wilson WA, Swartzwelder HS (2002) Differential effect of alcohol on NMDA receptor-mediated EPSCs in pyramidal cells in the posterior cingulate cortex of adolescent and adult rats. J Neurophysiol 87: 705–711.

Lidow M, Goldman-Rakic P, Rakic P (1991) Synchronized overproduction of neurotransmitter receptors in diverse regions of the primate cerebral cortex. Proc Nat Acad Sci 88:10218–10221.

Liljequist S, Engel J (1982) Effects of GABAergic agonists and antagonists on various alcohol-induced behavioral changes. Psychopharmacol 78:71–75.

Lister RG, Gorenstein C, Fisher-Flowers D, Weingartner HJ, Eckardt MJ (1991) Dissociation of the acute effects of alcohol on implicit and explicit memory processes. Neuropsychologia 29:1205–1212.

Little HJ (1999) The contribution of electrophysiology to knowledge of the acute and chronic effects of ethanol. Pharmacol Ther 84:333–353.

Little PJ, Kuhn CM, Wilson WA, Swartzwelder HS (1996) Differential effects of alcohol in adolescent and adult rats. Alc Clin Exp Res 20:1346–1351.

Luna B, Thulborn K, Munoz D, Merriam E, Garver K, Minshew N, Keshavan M, Genovese C, Eddy W, Sweeney J (2001) Maturation of widely distributed brain function subserves cognitive development. Neuroimage 13:786–793.

Markwiese BJ, Acheson SK, Levin ED, Wilson WA, Swartzwelder HS (1998) Differential effects of ethanol on memory in adolescent and adult rats. Alc Clin Exp Res 22:416–421.

Martin SJ, Morris RGM (2002) New life in an old idea: The synaptic plasticity and memory hypothesis revisited. Hippocampus 12:609–636.

Mereu G,Gess G (1985) Low doses of alcohol inhibit the firing of neurons in the substantia nigra, pars reticulara: a GABAergic effect? Brain Res 360:325–330.

Moy S, Duncan G, Knapp D, Breese G (1998) Sensitivity to alcohol across development in rats: comparison to [3H]zolpidem binding. Alc Clin Exp Res 22:1485–1492.

Mueller R-A, Rothermel RD, Behen ME, Muzik O, Mangner TJ, Chugani HT (1998) Developmental changes of cortical and cerebellar motor control: A clinical positron emission tomography study with children and adults. J Child Neurol 13:550–556.

Peoples RW, Li C, Weight FF (1996) Lipid vs protein theories of alcohol action in the nervous system. Annu Rev Pharmacol Toxicol 36:185–201.

Peoples RW, Stewart RR (2000) Alcohols inhibit N-methyl-D-aspartate receptors via a site exposed to the extracellular environment. Neuropharmacology 10:1681–1691.

Pyapali G, Turner D, Wilson W, Swartzwelder HS (1999) Age and dose-dependent effects of alcohol on the induction of hippocampal long-term potentiation. Alcohol 19: 107–111.

Rubia K, Overmeyer S, Taylor E, Brammer M, Williams SC, Simmons A, Andrew C, Bullmore, ET (2000) Functional frontalisation with age: mapping neurodevelopmental trajectories with fMRI. Neurosci Biobehav Rev 24:13–19.

Ryback RS (1970) Alcohol amnesia: observations in seven drinking inpatient alcoholics. Q J Stud Alcohol 31:616–632.

Ryback RS (1971) The continuum and specificity of the effects of alcohol on memory. Quart J Stud Alc 32:995–1016.

Schummers J, Browning MD (2001) Evidence for a role for GABA(A) and NMDA receptors in ethanol inhibition of long-term potentiation. Brain Research 94:9–14.

Seeman P (1999) Images in neuroscience. Brain development, X: pruning during development. Am J Psychiatry 156:168.

Silveri M, Spear L (1998) Decreased sensitivity to hypnotic effects of alcohol early in ontogeny. Alc Clin Exp Res 22:670–676.

Smith RF (2003) Animal models of periadolescent substance abuse. Neurotox Teratol 25:291–301.

Snell L, Tabakoff B, Hoffman P (1993) Radioligand binding to the NMDA receptor/ionophore complex: Alterations by alcohol in-vitro and by chronic in-vivo alcohol ingestion. Brain Res 602:91–98.

Spear L (2000) The adolescent brain and age-related behavioral manifestations. Neurosci Biobehav Rev 24:417–463.

Spear LP (2002) The adolescent brain and the college drinker: biological basis of propensity to use and misuse alcohol. J Stud Alcohol Suppl(14):71–81

Swartzwelder HS, Wilson WA, Tayyeb MI (1995a). Differential sensitivity of NMDA receptor-mediated synaptic potentials to alcohol in immature vs. mature hippocampus. Alc Clin. Exp Res 19:320–323.

Swartzwelder H S, Wilson WA, Tayyeb MI (1995b). Age-dependent inhibition of long-term potentiation by alcohol in immature vs. mature hippocampus. Alc Clin. Exp Res 19:1480–1485.

Swartzwelder HS, Richardson R, Markwiese B, Wilson W, Little P (1998) Developmental differences in the acquisition of tolerance to alcohol. Alcohol 15:311–314.

Teicher MH, Andersen SL, Hostetter JC (1995) Evidence for dopamine receptor pruning between adolescence and adulthood in striatum but not nucleus accumbens. Dev Brain Res 89:167–172.

Weissenborn R, Duka T (2003) Acute alcohol effects on cognitive function in social drinkers: Their relationship to drinking habits. Psychopharmacol 165:306–312.

White A, Bae J, Truesdale M, Ahmad S, Wilson W, Swartzwelder HS (2002c) Chronic intermittent alcohol exposure during adolescence prevents normal developmental changes in sensitivity to alcohol-induced motor impairments. Alc Clin Exp Res 26:960–968.

White AM, Best PJ (2000) Effects of ethanol on hippocampal place-cell and interneuron activity. Brain Res 876:154–165.

White, A.M., Ghia, A.J., Levin, E.D. and Swartzwelder, H.S. Binge pattern alcohol exposure: differential impact on subsequent responsiveness to alcohol. *Alcoholism: Clin. Exp. Res.* 24: 1251–1256, 2000.

White AM, Jamieson-Drake D, Swartzwelder HS (2002a) Prevalence and correlates of alcohol-induced blackouts among college students: Results of an e-mail survey. J Am College Health 51:117–131.

White AM, Matthews DB, Best PJ (2000) Ethanol, memory and hippocampal function: a review of recent findings. Hippocampus 10:88–93.

White A, Truesdale M, Bae J, Ahmad S, Wilson W, Best P, Swartzwelder HS (2002b) Differential effects of alcohol on motor coordination in adolescent and adult rats. Pharmacol Biochem Behav 73:673–677.

Xia Y, Haddad G (1992) Ontogeny and distribution of GABAA receptors in rat brainstem and rostral brain regions. Neurosci 49:973–989.

Zhang L, Spigelman I, Carlen P (1991) Development of GABA mediated, chloride dependent inhibition in CA1 pyramidal neurons of immature rat hippocampal slices. J Physiol 444: 25–49.

Zola-Morgan S, Squire LR, Amaral DG (1986). Human amnesia and the medial temporal lobe region: enduring memory impairment following a bilateral lesion limited to field CA1 of the hippocampus. J Neurosci 16:2950–2967.

9

The Human Adolescent Brain and Alcohol Use Disorders

Susan F. Tapert and Alecia D. Schweinsburg

1. Introduction

Alcohol use is common during the ages of 13 to 18, the stage commonly referred to as adolescence. An annual survey of U.S. high school students revealed that in 2002, 18% of 10th graders and 30% of 12th graders reported getting drunk in the past month (Johnston, O'Malley, & Bachman, 2003). Approximately 6% of high school students meet diagnostic criteria for alcohol abuse or dependence (Rohde, Lewinsohn, & Seeley, 1996a). The leading cause of death for teenagers is unintentional injury, primarily related to motor vehicle accidents (National Center for Health Statistics, 1999), and 20% of all traffic crashes of 16- to 20-year-olds involve alcohol (Yi, Williams, & Dufour, 2001). Drinking is associated with even greater risks of traffic accidents for youths than adults, and adolescent drivers are more likely than adults to get into accidents at lower blood alcohol concentrations (Yi et al., 2001), likely due to less driving experience (Hingson, Heeren, & Winter, 1994; Yi et al., 2001). Nonetheless, only 52% of 10th graders perceive a great risk in binge drinking each weekend (Johnston et al., 2003).

Despite the prevalence of alcohol use and related disorders in adolescence, we are just beginning to understand how protracted alcohol consumption during youth affects brain development and cognition. Central nervous system abnormalities have clearly been observed in adults with chronic heavy drinking histories (Grant, 1987; Nixon & Parsons, 1991; Nixon, Paul, & Phillips, 1998; Pfefferbaum et al., 2001; Pfefferbaum, Lim, Desmond, & Sullivan, 1996; Pfefferbaum et al., 1995; Pfefferbaum, Sullivan,

Susan F. Tapert • Department of Psychiatry, VA San Diego Healthcare System, and University of California San Diego, San Diego, California 92161.
Alecia D. Schweinsburg • University of California San Diego, Department of Psychology, La Jolla, California 92093.

Rosenbloom, Mathalon, & Lim, 1998; Pfefferbaum, Sullivan, Hegehus et al., 2000; Ryan & Butters, 1988; Sullivan, Desmond, Lim, & Pfefferbaum, 2002; Sullivan et al., 2003), but it is less clear how adolescents may be differentially affected. Understanding the neuromaturational implications of adolescent alcohol use disorders (AUD) is critical, since maladaptive patterns of use during continued development could limit educational, occupational, and social opportunities.

Substantial neuromaturation continues throughout adolescence (see Figure 1). Structural magnetic resonance imaging studies have described decreases in gray matter volume and density during adolescence, particularly in frontal and parietal brain regions (Giedd et al., 1999; Giedd et al., 1996; Jernigan, Trauner, Hesselink, & Tallal, 1991; Pfefferbaum et al., 1994; Sowell et al., 2003; Sowell, Thompson, Holmes, Batth et al., 1999; Sowell, Thompson, Holmes, Jernigan, & Toga, 1999), which may underlie cognitive maturation (Sowell, Delis, Stiles, & Jernigan, 2001). Myelination continues throughout adolescence and young adulthood (Courchesne et al., 2000; Giedd et al., 1999; Giedd et al., 1996; Pfefferbaum et al., 1994; Yakovlev & Lecours, 1967) and is thought to be related to increases in cognitive efficiency. Stages of increased cerebral blood flow support periods of rapid brain growth (Epstein, 1999). Synaptic pruning occurs until mid-adolescence, based in part on environmental stimulation (Huttenlocher, 1990; Huttenlocher & Dabholkar, 1997), resulting in decreased energy requirements and diminished glucose metabolism (Chugani, 1998). Changes in functional activity are indicative of regional specialization and maturation (Casey, Giedd, & Thomas, 2000; Klingberg, Forssberg, & Westerberg, 2002; Luna et al., 2001).

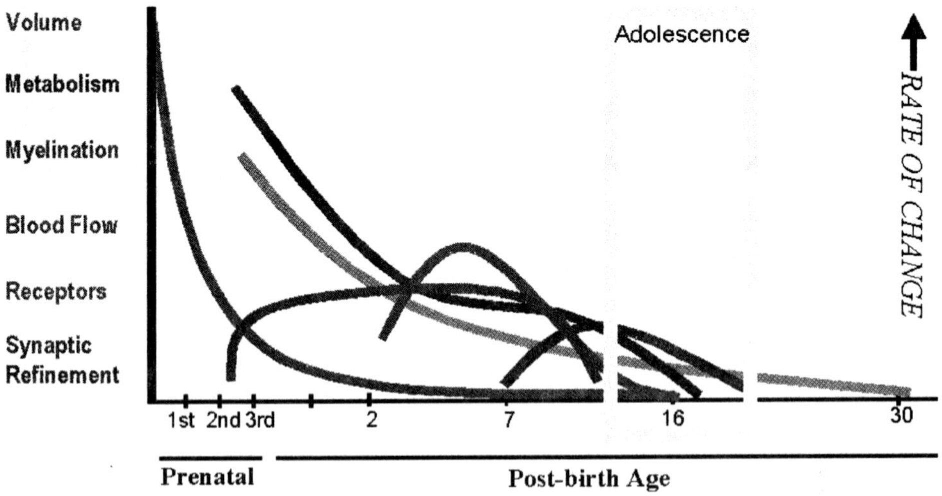

Figure 1. Neuromaturational processes during adolescence. Note that synaptic refinement and myelination continue at significant rates during the adolescent years.

2. Neurocognition in Adolescents with Alcohol Use Disorders

Neuropsychological studies of adults with AUD have consistently revealed visuospatial, executive functioning, psychomotor, and memory impairments (Grant, 1987); however, it is unclear whether teenagers might be differentially affected by protracted alcohol consumption. Few studies have examined neurocognition in adolescents with AUD, but have generally demonstrated some functional decrements. An early neuropsychological study recruited teens with AUD from treatment centers, and demonstrated subtle deficits in verbal skills among youths with AUD compared to non-abusing controls, as well as problem solving errors among girls with AUD relative to control girls (Moss, Kirisci, Gordon, & Tarter, 1994). Tarter and colleagues (Tarter, Mezzich, Hsieh, & Parks, 1995) examined cognition among 106 female youths with AUD, most of whom met criteria for other substance use disorders as well. Compared to 74 control girls, those with AUD performed poorly in several domains, including language, attention, perceptual efficiency, general intelligence, and academic achievement (Tarter et al., 1995).

In a series of studies, our group assessed AUD youths recruited from alcohol and drug treatment facilities and non-abusing control teens matched for gender, age, socioeconomic status, and family history of substance use disorders. Similar to findings with adults (Grant, 1987), youths with AUD showed a 10% deficit in the ability to retrieve verbal and nonverbal information 3 weeks after detoxification compared to control teens (Brown, Tapert, Granholm, & Delis, 2000). We followed these youths longitudinally, and tested them again 4 and 8 years after leaving treatment (Tapert & Brown, 1999b; Tapert, Granholm, Leedy, & Brown, 2002). Among those who continued substance involvement after treatment, alcohol and drug withdrawal symptoms experienced during the follow-up period predicted poorer visuospatial functioning at 4 and 8 years after treatment discharge (Tapert & Brown, 1999b; Tapert, Granholm, Leedy et al., 2002). Further, greater cumulative lifetime alcohol experiences predicted poorer attention functioning 8 years after treatment, and alcohol use following treatment was associated with poorer working memory scores at the 8-year follow-up (Tapert, Granholm, Leedy et al., 2002). These predictions remained significant even after excluding youths who had drunk heavily (≥4 drinks/occasion for females, ≥5 drinks for males) and used other substances in the 28 days prior to testing. Together, these studies suggest that heavy alcohol involvement during adolescence is associated with cognitive deficits that may worsen as heavy drinking continues.

3. Brain Structure in Adolescents with Alcohol Use Disorders

The recent advent of non-invasive neuroimaging techniques has provided unique opportunities to examine the influence of chronic alcohol use on brain structure and function in adolescents. De Bellis and colleagues used magnetic resonance imaging (MRI) to quantify volumes of several brain structures among youths ages 13 to 21 (De Bellis et al., 2000). Those with adolescent-onset AUD had reduced hippocampal volumes, but similar cortical gray and white matter, amygdala, and corpus callosum sizes compared to controls. We used diffusion tensor imaging to investigate corpus callosum microstructure integrity among 8 teenagers with AUD and 8 non-abusing controls (Tapert, Theilmann, Schweinsburg, Yafai, & Frank, 2003). All participants were free from psychiatric disorders, and had limited experience with other drugs. Preliminary results indicated that AUD youths exhibit subtle white matter abnormalities, particularly in the splenium of the corpus callosum. Thus, although adolescents with AUD show normal corpus callosum volumes (De Bellis et al., 2000), subtle abnormalities in white matter microstructure may represent the beginnings of the more profound disruption that is observed in chronic heavy drinking adults (Pfefferbaum & Sullivan, 2002; Pfefferbaum, Sullivan, Hedehus et al., 2000).

4. Brain Function in Adolescents with Alcohol Use Disorders

Functional changes have also been demonstrated among youths with AUD. Alcohol dependent young women ages 18–25 who started drinking heavily during adolescence showed significantly diminished frontal and parietal functional MRI (fMRI) response as well as less accurate performance during a spatial working memory task relative to demographically similar controls (Tapert et al., 2001). We used the same paradigm to examine brain activation among 19 teenagers with little alcohol experience and 15 teens with AUD but without histories of other psychiatric disorders or heavy drug use. In contrast to our findings with young adult women, AUD boys and girls showed increased parietal response during spatial working memory compared to control teens, despite similar task performance (Tapert et al., in press) (see Figures 2 and 3). This suggests that in the early stages of AUD, the brain may be capable of compensating for subtle alcohol-induced neuronal disturbances by recruiting additional resources, resulting in more intense and widespread activation. The fMRI findings among young adult women suggest that as heavy drinking continues, neural injury may increase (Fein et al., 1994; Schweinsburg et al., 2001), the brain may no longer be able to counteract such disruption of neuronal functioning, and behaviors may begin to show signs of impairment.

Functional neuroimaging investigations have described neural response to alcohol cue exposure among adults with AUD (George et al., 2001). We examined the neural substrates of cue reactivity in 15 teenagers with AUD and 15 demographically similar non-abusing teens (Tapert, Cheung et al., 2003). During fMRI acquisition, teens were shown pictures of alcoholic beverage advertisements and visually similar non-alcoholic beverage ads. The images presented were individualized for each teen based on drinking experiences

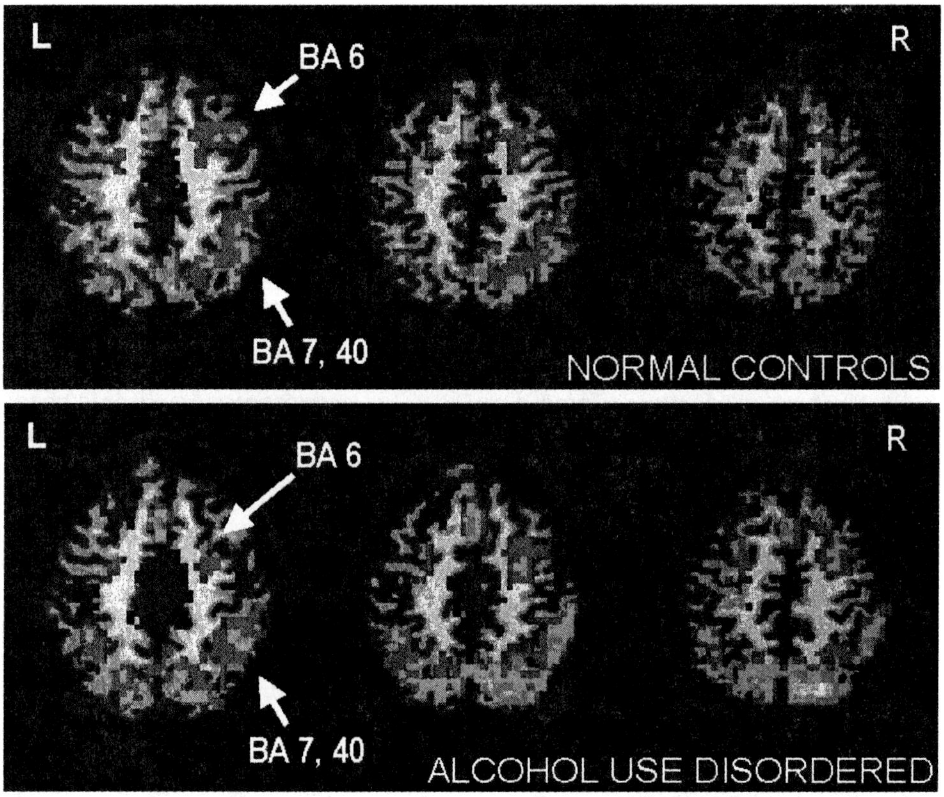

Figure 2. AUD youths showed *increased* parietal response during spatial working memory compared to control teens, despite similar task performance. These are axial slices showing significant clusters of blood oxygen level dependent response to spatial working memory relative to vigilance in control teens (n=19; top row) and AUD teens (n=15; bottom row). White clusters indicate regions of greater spatial working memory response; black clusters represent areas of greater baseline (simple vigilance) response; cluster $p<.05$, volume >943 microliters.

and preference in order to ensure familiarity with cues. Compared to control youths, teens with AUD demonstrated increased brain response to alcohol pictures in many brain regions, especially areas associated with emotion, visual processing, and reward circuitry. Although family history of AUD was also influential in both groups, personal alcohol use was a stronger predictor of brain response to alcohol cues. Moreover, AUD teens reporting greater monthly alcohol consumption and more intense desires to drink showed the greatest extent of neural response to the alcohol advertisements. Given the strong neural response to alcohol beverage advertisements among teens with AUD, it is possible that these media images may influence continued drinking among teens with alcohol problems, and may interfere with effective coping strategies in youths attempting to stop using.

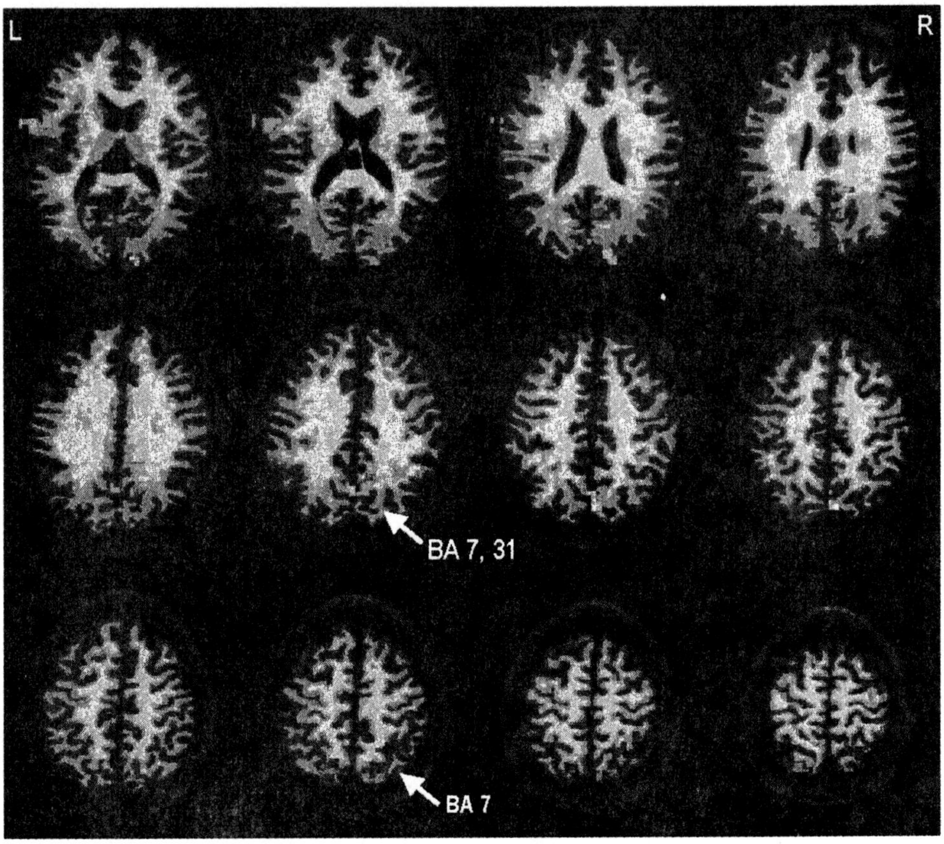

Figure 3. These are axial slices showing the statistical comparison between AUD and control teens in spatial working memory brain response. White clusters represent regions where AUD teens had *less* spatial working memory response than controls; black clusters indicate where AUD teens had *greater* spatial working memory response than controls; cluster $p<.05$, volume >943 microliters.

5. Developmental Considerations

5.1. *Age of Onset of Alcohol Use Disorder*

It remains unclear whether adolescent brains are more vulnerable to toxins, or if they are more plastic and able to recover from insult. Adults with adolescent-onset AUD show similar regional cerebral blood flow abnormalities as those with adult-onset AUD, suggesting that age of onset may not be an important predictor of neural dysfunction (Demir, Ulug, Lay Ergun, & Erbas, 2002). However, others have found that adults with early onset AUD show more pronounced cognitive deficits than those with late onset AUD, despite younger age at the time of assessment (Pishkin, Lovallo, & Bourne, 1985). Further research, including longitudinal studies, will be needed to definitively answer this important question.

5.2. *Gender Differences in Adolescents with Alcohol Use Disorders*

Studies in adults have suggested that females may be more susceptible to alcohol-related brain injury than males (Hommer, Momenan, Kaiser, & Rawlings, 2001; Schweinsburg et al., 2003), which could be due to hormonal fluctuations, differences in alcohol metabolism, or gender-specific drinking patterns. Some evidence has mounted suggesting that adolescent girls suffer greater alcohol-related neurocognitive deficits than adolescent boys. Girls with AUD show more perseveration errors than non-abusing girls, while boys with AUD show *fewer* perseverative errors than control boys, suggesting that this component of frontal lobe functioning may be more adversely affected by heavy alcohol use in girls (Moss et al., 1994). A longitudinal study evaluated the influence of gender on the extent to which substance use affects neuropsychological performance in 70 adolescents followed 8 years into young adulthood. Young women demonstrated more adverse cognitive effects related to alcohol and other drug use, especially in working memory and visuospatial functioning, whereas young men showed a greater relationship between verbal learning and substance involvement. Heavy marijuana use was associated with poorer cognitive functioning in males during mid-adolescence, while protracted marijuana use was associated with significant neurocognitive decrements in females by young adulthood (Tapert & Brown, 1999a). Overall, significant cumulative effects were observed, and more alcohol withdrawal and hangover experiences were associated with poorer performance in both young males and females (Tapert, Granholm, Leedy, & Brown, 2002), but this effect was stronger in females (Tapert & S. A. Brown, 1999a).

Our recent fMRI investigations have observed increased brain response during a spatial working memory task among both adolescent boys and girls with AUD compared to gender-matched control teens. However, the magnitude of response change was larger in females, possibly indicating that girls with AUD may be more vulnerable to alcohol-related neural dysfunction than boys on a memory for locations task (Caldwell, Schweinsburg, Nagel, Barlett, Brown, & Tapert, in preparation). Girls with AUD in this study typically attained higher blood alcohol concentrations than boys with AUD, which could explain the apparent greater functional abnormalities among alcohol-involved girls. Gender differences in fMRI response may also reflect disrupted brain development. Sexually dimorphic adolescent neuromaturation may be related in part to hormonal changes beginning in puberty (De Bellis et al., 2001; Giedd et al., 1999). Heavy alcohol consumption during this time may lead to hormonal dysregulation, which could ultimately influence neural development and functioning. Gender-specific alcohol-induced hormonal alterations may influence neurocognitive insult among teens with AUD, but further research will be needed to confirm these initial findings.

6. Neural Risk Factors

When studying alcohol-related neural sequelae, it is important to consider other sources of abnormalities that predate the onset of heavy drinking. Two such factors are familial alcoholism and personal comorbid psychopathology, both which are risk factors for developing AUD and have been associated with unique neurocognitive features.

6.1. Family History of Alcohol Use Disorders

Youths with family histories of AUD have shown neuropsychological differences compared to youths without such family histories in numerous studies, regardless of personal substance intake and controlling for maternal drinking during pregnancy. Adolescent males with family histories of AUD who do not personally abuse alcohol or other drugs commonly perform worse on tests of language functioning and academic achievement (Hegedus, Alterman, & Tarter, 1984; Najam, Tarter, & Kirisci, 1997; Peterson, Finn, & Pihl, 1992; Poon, Ellis, Fitzgerald, & Zucker, 2000; Sher, Bartholow, & Wood, 2000; Tapert & Brown, 2000; Tarter, Hegedus, Winsten, & Alterman, 1984), organization of new information (Peterson et al., 1992), executive cognitive functioning (Giancola, Martin, Tarter, Pelham, & Moss, 1996; Harden & Pihl, 1995), perseveration (Giancola, Peterson, & Pihl, 1993), working memory (Corral, Holguín, & Cadaveira, 1999; Harden & Pihl, 1995; Ozkaragoz, Satz, & Noble, 1997), nonverbal memory (Sher, Walitzer, Wood, & Brent, 1991), visuospatial skills (Aytaclar, Tarter, Kirisci, & Lu, 1999; Berman & Noble, 1995; Corral et al., 1999; Ozkaragoz et al., 1997; Ozkaragoz & Noble, 1995; Sher et al., 1991), and attention (Tapert & Brown, 2000; Tarter, Jacob, & Bremer, 1989). However, other studies have not found neurocognitive differences between individuals with and without family histories of AUD (Finn & Justus, 1999; Schuckit, Butters, Lyn, & Irwin, 1987).

Multigenerational transmission of alcohol dependence (Conrod, Pihl, & Ditto, 1995; LeMarquand, Benkelfat, Pihl, Palmour, & Young, 1999; Peterson et al., 1996; Pihl & Bruce, 1995), high familial density (Hill, Shen, Lowers, & Locke, 2000), paternal comorbid antisocial personality disorder (Poon et al., 2000), early age of alcoholism onset in the father (Tarter et al., 1989), active paternal alcoholism (Ozkaragoz et al., 1997), and certain genotypic features (Berman & Noble, 1995) have each increased the strength of the relationship between family history of AUD and neuropsychological functioning. For example, Poon and colleagues subtyped sons of alcohol dependent men according to the presence of antisocial personality disorder in the father, and found modest differences in full scale IQ and attention measures compared to sons of alcoholic but non-antisocial personality disordered men (Poon et al., 2000). In contrast, Schuckit and colleagues found no differences on neuropsychological testing or body sway indices between sons of alcoholics and sons of nonalcoholics after excluding families of fathers with antisocial personality disorder (Schuckit et al., 1987). D2 dopamine receptor alleles were considered in an examination of visuospatial performance in youths with family histories of alcoholism (Berman & Noble, 1995). Sons of active alcoholics were likely to have polymorphisms and to perform poorly on a visuoperceptual task with minimal motor and verbal demands. The authors raised the possibility that visuospatial deficits previously reported in alcoholics may predate the onset of heavy drinking (Berman & Noble, 1995).

We compared the neuropsychological functioning of non-abusing (n=50) and alcohol and drug dependent adolescents (n=101) with and without family histories of alcohol dependence. Substance dependent adolescents were tested in inpatient alcohol and drug abuse treatment programs after 3 weeks of abstinence. Participants were 44% female, ages 13 through 18, and had no histories of serious head injury or neurological disorder. Results suggested that substance involvement interacted with family history of alcohol dependence to predict language and attention functioning. Adolescents without personal or family histories of substance use disorders performed better than all other adolescents, and the pattern of results suggested that family history of alcohol dependence and adolescent substance use are separate risk factors for poorer neuropsychological performance in youth (Tapert & Brown, 2000).

In addition to neuropsychological deficits, neurophysiological abnormalities have been found in youths with family histories of AUD (Begleiter, Porjesz, & Bihiari, 1987; Pihl & Bruce, 1995; Pihl, Peterson, & Finn, 1990; Tarter, Hegedus, Goldstein, Shelly, & Alterman, 1984). The P3 component of the event-related potential is an indicator of rapid shifts in allocation of cognitive resources, and P3 amplitude and latency in response to visual and auditory stimuli appear highly heritable (Almasy et al., 1999). Children and adults with familial alcoholism commonly show a reduced P3 amplitude (Begleiter, Porjesz, Bihari, & Kissin, 1984; Porjesz et al., 1998). This feature is most consistently displayed in individuals with family histories of alcoholism who are under age 18, and after this age, family history effects diminish, suggesting an inherited developmental lag (Polich, Pollock, & Bloom, 1994). Girls with multigenerational family histories of alcohol dependence have shown greater delays than girls with only an alcohol dependent father (Holguin, Corral, & Cadaveira, 1998), and adolescent females with a family history of alcoholism show increased fast beta power and decreased theta power in left frontal regions (Bauer & Hesselbrock, 2002). Because electroencephalogram patterns are highly heritable and related to extraverted personalities, these studies may point to mechanisms whereby innate characteristics contribute to drinking practices (Wall, Schuckit, Mungas, & Ehlers, 1990).

Abnormalities in the cerebellum and basal ganglia have been implicated in youths with familial alcoholism, evidenced by delayed maturation of postural sway (Hill, Shen, Locke et al., 2000; Hill, Shen, Lowers et al., 2000). Brain volumes were compared between 17 youths with dense family histories of alcoholism and 17 age-, gender-, and IQ-matched controls. Those with positive family histories evidenced smaller right amygdala volumes than low-risk controls, which correlated with P3 amplitudes. As amygdala volumes generally increase during adolescence, the authors suggest that this indicates a developmental delay in youths with familial alcoholism (Hill et al., 2001). In contrast, family history of AUD does not appear to moderate the relationship between personal drinking and cerebral metabolic abnormalities in older adults (Adams et al., 1998). Taken together, these studies indicate that subtle neural abnormalities may underlie the heritable aspects of AUD (Begleiter & Porjesz, 1999; Pihl & Peterson, 1996). However, some studies suggest that family history of AUD primarily affects brain functioning in individuals with conduct disorder, antisocial personality disorder, sensation seeking, behavioral undercontrol, difficult temperament, or poor impulse control (Bauer & Hesselbrock, 1999a, 1999b; Schuckit, 1998; Schuckit & Smith, 1997; Tarter, Alterman, & Edwards, 1985). Understanding these brain characteristics helps us to appreciate the brain abnormalities that may be produced by personal alcohol involvement as opposed to features that are attributable to pre-drinking risk factors.

6.2. *Comorbid Disorders*

Conduct disorder refers to a "repetitive and persistent pattern of behavior in which basic rights of others, age-appropriate societal norms, or rules are violated" (American Psychiatric Association, 1994), and it occurs in 2–16% of the population (Cohen et al., 1993; Lahey et al., 1998; Rohde, Lewinsohn, & Seeley, 1996b; Zoccolillo, 1993). Conduct disorder and related circumstances (e.g., juvenile delinquency, antisocial personality disorder, disruptive behavior disorders, neurobehavioral disinhibition) have been associated with an increased risk of alcohol and other drug use disorders (Tarter et al., 2003), as well as neurocognitive disadvantages. These youths tend to perform poorly on academic achievement (Fuerst & Rourke, 1993) and IQ (Moffitt & Silva, 1988a) tests, and are more likely to demonstrate higher Performance IQ than Verbal IQ (Déry, Toupin, Pauze, Mercier, & Fortin, 1999; Haynes & Bensch, 1981; Lynam, Moffitt, & Stouthamer-Loeber, 1993; Moffitt, 1993; Prentice & Kelly, 1963; West & Farrington, 1973). Recent studies have shown poor performances on nonverbal tests as well (Toupin, Déry, Pauze, Mercier, & Fortin, 2000). Executive cognitive functioning robustly discriminates adolescents with and without conduct disorder (Deckel, Bauer, & Hesselbrock, 1995; Giancola, Mezzich, & Tarter, 1998a, 1998b; Skoff & Libon, 1987; Wolff, Waber, Bauermeister, Cohen, & Ferber, 1982). In particular, impaired functioning was noted on tests requiring sequencing, cognitive flexibility, selective attention, and initiating planned strategies, including nonverbal tests (Brickman, McManus, Grapentine, & Alessi, 1984; Moffitt & Henry, 1989; Moffitt & Silva, 1988b; White et al., 1994).

Conduct disorder and related conditions have been related to neurochemical and autonomic anomalies, such as lower resting heart rates (Delamater & Lahey, 1983; Raine & Jones, 1987), abnormal P3 amplitudes (Raine & Venables, 1987), and diminished skin conductance response (Delamater & Lahey, 1983; Garralda, Connell, & Taylor, 1991; Raine, Venables, & Williams,

1990a, 1990b). Aggressive delinquents tend to exhibit lower levels of serotonin (Kruesi et al., 1992; Kruesi et al., 1990; Virkkunen, De Jong, Bartko, Goodwin, & Linnoila, 1989) and cortisol (McBurnett, Lahey, Rathouz, & Loeber, 2000), suggesting a reduced arousal level. Overall, youths with neurobehavioral disinhibition are not only at risk for developing AUD, but are also likely to exhibit neurocognitive and other CNS functioning weaknesses. Recent event-related potential studies have suggested that P3 abnormalities previously associated with family history of AUD may be accounted for by conduct disorder (Bauer & Hesselbrock, 1999a, 1999b; Bauer, 1997). In particular, boys with histories of rule violations show a delay in maturation of frontal P3 amplitude (Bauer & Hesselbrock, 2003). These findings are supported by demonstrations of abnormal serotonin and cortisol levels that relate more to conduct disorder, aggression, or behavioral disinhibition than to familial alcohol dependence (Soloff, Lynch, & Moss, 2000; Twitchell, Hanna, Cook, Fitzgerald, & Zucker, 2000; Virkkunen & Linnoila, 1997). In summary, conduct disorder is associated with several neurocognitive abnormalities as well as increased risk of AUD, and, as many youths with AUD have conduct disorder, it is important to consider the neural features unique to conduct disorder.

Internalizing disorders have also been associated with alterations in cognitive performance and brain functioning in adolescents. In an electroencephalogram study of adolescent females, depression was associated with increased alpha power in right frontal brain regions (Bauer & Hesselbrock, 2002). Youths with familial alcoholism often show a low amplitude P3b component of the event-related potential, which has a slow rate of change during adolescence. However, in girls, this neurophysiological developmental pattern is also associated with childhood internalizing and externalizing psychopathology as well as psychiatric diagnoses in young adulthood (Hill & Shen, 2002).

7. Potential Confounds

In investigating the effects of alcohol use on brain functioning in adolescent humans, several potentially confounding factors must be considered. As described previously, some of the major risk factors for developing AUD, such as familial alcoholism and conduct disorder, are associated with some neural abnormalities. Other conditions related to these risk factors or to indirect consequences of drinking that carry neurocognitive implications will be briefly discussed. Youths with genetic vulnerabilities for AUD may have been exposed to alcohol prenatally, and fetal alcohol exposure has been linked to a range of neurocognitive deficits and brain abnormalities that persist throughout adolescence and beyond (Mattson, Schoenfeld, & Riley, 2001; Sowell et al., 2002). Traumatic brain injury, which intoxicated youths incur at elevated rates, produces significant neurocognitive problems (Verger et al., 2001).

As reviewed above, youths with AUD are more likely to have other psychiatric disorders, which may predate the onset of problem drinking or occur later, sometimes induced by substance use. Adolescents with alcohol or other drug use diagnoses are more likely to report psychiatric symptoms, especially depression and eating disorders for girls, and conduct disorder for boys. Furthermore, boys and girls with substance use disorders are more likely to report psychotic symptoms such as hallucinations and delusions than youths without substance use disorders (Shrier, Harris, Kurland, & Knight, 2003). Mood, disruptive behavior, and psychotic disorders whether primary or secondary to substance use disorders, are all associated with neurocognitive impairments.

A particularly tricky complication in studying the effects of alcohol on brain functioning is that teenagers who drink tend to use other drugs and nicotine, making it difficult to disentangle the unique effects of alcohol. Use of marijuana, stimulants (e.g., methamphetamine, methylenedioxymethamphetamine (MDMA or ecstasy)), inhalants, and dissociative drugs (e.g., phencyclidine (PCP)) have all been associated with neurocognitive decrements in adolescents (Kucuk et al., 2000; Tapert & Brown, 1999), although most studies have been small, or participants were polysubstance users and relationships between performance and drug use were inferred statistically. Nicotine has also been associated with subtle abnormalities in youth, and may possibly potentiate adverse cognitive effects of alcohol (Santerre et al., 2002; S. Tapert, Myers, Tomlinson, & Brown, 1999).

8. Recovery

In summary, we have reviewed that chronic heavy alcohol use during adolescence is associated with poorer performance on tasks requiring verbal and nonverbal learning and retrieval, attention, visuospatial functioning, and executive functioning. Additionally, subtle abnormalities have been detected by volumetric, diffusion, and functional brain imaging techniques in abstinent adolescents with histories of heavy alcohol involvement. However, it remains uncertain if these difficulties will repair with sustained abstinence, and, if so, how much sobriety is required until performance and brain integrity measures resume pre-drinking levels. Adults with histories of chronic heavy drinking have been shown to improve after extended abstinence on neuropsychological testing (Brandt, Butters, Ryan, & Bayog, 1983), magnetic resonance spectroscopy (Schweinsburg et al., 2000), and brain volume indices (Pfefferbaum et al., 1995). However, it remains to be seen if recoverability of brain integrity and cognitive function might be easier in youth, whose brains are more plastic, or if recovery is less likely because neurotoxic insult may have adversely affected the neuromaturational course.

The relationship between neurocognition and treatment outcome is complex, as thinking abilities appear to influence subsequent substance involvement. In adolescents treated for substance use disorders, a broader coping skills repertoire significantly predicted less alcohol and other drug use after treatment for those with lower levels of cognitive functioning, while coping skills did not predict outcomes for youths with higher levels of cognitive functioning (Tapert, Brown, Myers, & Granholm, 1999). In contrast, for youths with above average language skills, having more favorable alcohol expectancies predicted more substance use and dependence symptoms after treatment, while expectancies played a smaller role for young people with lower levels of language ability (Tapert, McCarthy, Aarons, Schweinsburg, & Brown, 2003). For adolescents who have not yet developed alcohol or other drug use problems, poorer functioning on neuropsychological tests of attention predicted greater alcohol and other drug use and dependence symptoms 8 years after assessment, above and beyond effects accounted for by baseline substance involvement, family history of AUD, conduct disorder, gender, education, and learning disabilities (Tapert, Baratta, Abrantes, & Brown, 2002). This series of studies suggests that youths' cognitive functioning level is important to assess during alcohol and other drug treatment, and that those with poorer scores on neurocognitive tests may be more likely to succeed if relatively concrete and practical coping responses are thoroughly imparted. Young people with strong language skills are also at risk for relapse, particularly if expectations for positive effects of drinking are strong, and they may benefit from alcohol expectancy challenge programming (Wiers et al., 2003). As youths with poor attention skills appear at risk for initiating problematic alcohol and other drug involvement, prevention programs may be more influential if designed to be effective for those with compromised concentration and processing abilities.

9. Conclusions

In summary, emerging research suggests subtle but important neurocognitive disadvantages among adolescents with alcohol use disorders (AUD) as compared to teens without AUD. Neuropsychological testing suggests that adolescents with AUD demonstrate diminished retrieval of verbal and nonverbal material, even after detoxification, and poorer performance on tests requiring attention skills. Additionally, youths who have consumed sufficient amounts of alcohol so as to experience withdrawal or hangover effects are likely to show persisting problems on visuospatial tasks. Brain imaging studies suggest reduced hippocampal volumes, white matter microstructure irregularities, and blood oxygen level dependent response abnormalities while performing challenging cognitive tasks. FMRI studies have also shown that adolescents with AUD have enhanced brain response when viewing alcohol cues (i.e., alcohol advertisements).

It is important to note the range of methodological considerations in conducting and interpreting these studies, including the patterns of neural abnormalities associated with some of the most prominent risk factors for developing AUD. Family history of alcoholism and adolescent psychopathology must be carefully considered when investigating the influence of teenage drinking on neurocognition. Other substance use, head injury, and prenatal alcohol exposure are also more likely to occur in youths with AUD, and carry unique neurocognitive effects. Thus, research into the long-term effects of alcohol use on brain functioning in adolescents must vigilantly screen for histories of these factors or appropriately manage them statistically.

Despite these recent advances, research is needed to understand how age of drinking onset and duration of abstinence at the time of assessment affect cognitive findings. To precisely determine whether heavy drinking *causes* neurocognitive insult and if damage can recover with extended sobriety, longitudinal studies of adolescents are needed. Although the magnitude of alcohol related effects observed in adolescents' neurocognition is relatively modest, the implications are major, given the prevalence of alcohol use and related disorders in our society, and the important educational, occupational, and social transitions that occur during adolescence.

References

Adams, K. M., Gilman, S., Johnson-Greene, D., Koeppe, R. A., Junck, L., Kluin, K. J., et al. (1998). The significance of family history status in relation to neuropsychological test performance and cerebral glucose metabolism studied with positron emission tomography in older alcoholic patients. *Alcoholism, Clinical and Experimental Research, 22*(1), 105–110.

Almasy, L., Porjesz, B., Blangero, J., Chorlian, D. B., O'Connor, S. J., Kuperman, S., et al. (1999). Heritability of event-related brain potentials in families with a history of alcoholism. *American Journal of Medical Genetics, 88*(4), 383–390.

American Psychiatric Association. (1994). *Diagnostic and statistical manual of mental disorders* (4th ed.). Washington, DC: American Psychiatric Association.

Aytaclar, S., Tarter, R. E., Kirisci, L., & Lu, S. (1999). Association between hyperactivity and executive cognitive functioning in childhood and substance use in early adolescence. *Journal of the American Academy of Child & Adolescent Psychiatry, 38,* 172–178.

Bauer, L., & Hesselbrock, V. (1999a). P300 decrements in teenagers with conduct problems: implications for substance abuse risk and brain development. *Biological Psychiatry, 46,* 263–272.

Bauer, L., & Hesselbrock, V. (1999b). Subtypes of family history and conduct disorder: effects on P300 during the Stroop Test. *Neuropsychopharmacology, 21,* 51–62.

Bauer, L. O. (1997). Frontal P300 decrements, childhood conduct disorder, family history and the prediction of relapse among abstinent cocaine abusers. *Drug & Alcohol Dependence, 44,* 1–10.

Bauer, L. O., & Hesselbrock, V. M. (2002). Lateral asymmetries in the frontal brain: effects of depression and a family history of alcoholism in female adolescents. *Alcohol Clin Exp Res, 26*(11), 1662–1668.

Bauer, L. O., & Hesselbrock, V. M. (2003). Brain maturation and subtypes of conduct disorder: interactive effects on p300 amplitude and topography in male adolescents. *J Am Acad Child Adolesc Psychiatry, 42*(1), 106–115.

Begleiter, H., & Porjesz, B. (1999). What is inherited in the predisposition toward alcoholism? A proposed model. *Alcoholism: Clinical and Experimental Research, 23,* 1125–1135.

Begleiter, H., Porjesz, B., Bihari, B., & Kissin, B. (1984). Event-related brain potentials in boys at risk for alcoholism. *Science, 225,* 1493–1496.

Begleiter, H., Porjesz, B., & Bihiari, B. (1987). Auditory brainstem potentials in sons of alcoholic fathers. *Alcohol Clin Exp Res, 11,* 477–480.

Berman, S. M., & Noble, E. P. (1995). Reduced visuospatial performance in children with the D2 dopamine receptor A1 allele. *Behavior Genetics, 25*(1), 45–58.

Brandt, J., Butters, N., Ryan, C., & Bayog, R. (1983). Cognitive loss and recovery in long-term alcohol abusers. *Archives of General Psychiatry, 40*, 435–442.

Brickman, A. S., McManus, M. M., Grapentine, W. L., & Alessi, N. (1984). Neuropsychological assessment of seriously delinquent adolescents. *Journal of the American Academy of Child Psychiatry, 23*, 453–457.

Brown, S. A., Tapert, S. F., Granholm, E., & Delis, D. C. (2000). Neurocognitive functioning of adolescents: effects of protracted alcohol use. *Alcoholism: Clinical and Experimental Research, 24*(2), 164–171.

Caldwell, L. C., Schweinsburg, A. D., Nagel, B. J. Barlett, V. C., Brown, S. A., & Tapert, S. F. (in preparation). Gender and adolescent alcohol use disorders on BOLD response to spatial working memory.

Casey, B. J., Giedd, J. N., & Thomas, K. M. (2000). Structural and functional brain development and its relation to cognitive development. *Biological Psychology, 54*(1–3), 241–257.

Chugani, H. T. (1998). A critical period of brain development: studies of cerebral glucose utilization with PET. *Preventative Medicine, 27*(2), 184–188.

Cohen, P., Cohen, J., Kasen, S., Velez, C. N., Hartmark, C., Johnson, J., et al. (1993). An epidemiological study of disorders in late childhood and adolescence—I. Age- and gender-specific prevalence. *Journal of Child Psychology and Psychiatry and Allied Disciplines, 34*(6), 851–867.

Conrod, P. J., Pihl, R. O., & Ditto, B. (1995). Autonomic reactivity and alcohol-induced dampening in men at risk for alcoholism and men at risk for hypertension. *Alcoholism, Clinical and Experimental Research, 19*(2), 482–489.

Corral, M. M., Holguín, S. R., & Cadaveira, F. (1999). Neuropsychological characteristics in children of alcoholics: familial density. *Journal of Studies on Alcohol, 60*, 509–513.

Courchesne, E., Chisum, H. J., Townsend, J., Cowles, A., Covington, J., Egaas, B., et al. (2000). Normal brain development and aging: quantitative analysis at in vivo MR imaging in healthy volunteers. *Radiology, 216*(3), 672–682.

De Bellis, M. D., Clark, D. B., Beers, S. R., Soloff, P. H., Boring, A. M., Hall, J., et al. (2000). Hippocampal volume in adolescent-onset alcohol use disorders. *American Journal of Psychiatry, 157*(5), 737–744.

De Bellis, M. D., Keshavan, M. S., Beers, S. R., Hall, J., Frustaci, K., Masalehdan, A., et al. (2001). Sex differences in brain maturation during childhood and adolescence. *Cereb Cortex, 11*(6), 552–557.

Deckel, A. W., Bauer, L., & Hesselbrock, V. (1995). Anterior brain dysfunctioning as a risk factor in alcoholic behaviors. *Addiction, 90*, 1323–1334.

Delamater, A. M., & Lahey, B. B. (1983). Physiological correlates of conduct problems in hyperactive and learning disabled children. *Journal of Abnormal Child Psychology, 11*, 85–100.

Demir, B., Ulug, B., Lay Ergun, E., & Erbas, B. (2002). Regional cerebral blood flow and neuropsychological functioning in early and late onset alcoholism. *Psychiatry Research, 115*(3), 115–125.

Déry, M., Toupin, J., Pauze, R., Mercier, H., & Fortin, L. (1999). Neuropsychological characteristics of adolescents with conduct disorder: Association with attention-deficit-hyperactivity and aggression. *Journal of Abnormal Child Psychology, 27*, 225–236.

Epstein, H. T. (1999). Stages of increased cerebral blood flow accompany stages of rapid brain growth. *Brain and Development, 21*(8), 535–539.

Fein, G., Meyerhoff, D. J., Discalfani, V., Ezekiel, F., Poole, N., MacKay, S., et al. (1994). 1H magnetic resonance spectroscopic imaging separates neuronal from glial changes in alcohol-related brain atrophy. In F. E. Lancaster (Ed.), *Alcohol and Glial Cells* (Vol. 27, pp. 227–241). Bethesda, MD: National Institutes of Health.

Finn, P., & Justus, A. (1999). Reduced EEG alpha power in the male and female offspring of alcoholics. *Alcohol Clin Exp Res, 23*(2), 256–262.

Fuerst, D. R., & Rourke, B. P. (1993). Psychosocial functioning of children: Relations between personality subtypes and academic achievement. *Journal of Abnormal Child Psychology, 21*, 597–607.

Garralda, M. E., Connell, J., & Taylor, D. C. (1991). Psychophysiological anomalies in children with emotional and conduct disorders. *Psychological Medicine, 21,* 947–957.

George, M. S., Anton, R. F., Bloomer, C., Teneback, C., Drobes, D. J., Lorberbaum, J. P., et al. (2001). Activation of prefrontal cortex and anterior thalamus in alcoholic subjects on exposure to alcohol-specific cues. *Archives of General Psychiatry, 58*(4), 345–352.

Giancola, P. R., Martin, C. S., Tarter, R. E., Pelham, W. E., & Moss, H. B. (1996). Executive cognitive functioning and aggressive behavior in preadolescent boys at high risk for substance abuse/dependence. *Journal of Studies on Alcohol, 57*(4), 352–359.

Giancola, P. R., Mezzich, A. C., & Tarter, R. E. (1998a). Disruptive, delinquent and aggressive behavior in female adolescents with a psychoactive substance use disorder: Relation to executive cognitive functioning. *Journal of Studies on Alcohol, 59,* 560–567.

Giancola, P. R., Mezzich, A. C., & Tarter, R. E. (1998b). Executive cognitive functioning, temperament, and antisocial behavior in conduct-disordered adolescent females. *Journal of Abnormal Psychology, 107,* 629–641.

Giancola, P. R., Peterson, J. B., & Pihl, R. O. (1993). Risk for alcoholism, antisocial behavior, and response perseveration. *Journal of Clinical Psychology, 49,* 423–428.

Giedd, J. N., Blumenthal, J., Jeffries, N. O., Castellanos, F. X., Liu, H., Zijdenbos, A., et al. (1999). Brain development during childhood and adolescence: A longitudinal MRI study. *Nature Neuroscience,* 2(10), 861–863.

Giedd, J. N., Snell, J. W., Lange, N., Rajapakse, J. C., Casey, B. J., Kozuch, P. L., et al. (1996). Quantitative magnetic resonance imaging of human brain development: Ages 4–18. *Cerebral Cortex,* 6(4), 551–560.

Grant, I. (1987). Alcohol and the brain: neuropsychological correlates. *Journal of Consulting and Clinical Psychology, 55*(3), 310–324.

Harden, P. W., & Pihl, R. O. (1995). Cognitive function, cardiovascular reactivity, and behavior in boys at high risk for alcoholism. *Journal of Abnormal Psychology, 104,* 94–103.

Haynes, J. P., & Bensch, M. (1981). The P > V sign of the WISC-R and recidivism in delinquents. *Journal of Consulting and Clinical Psychology, 49,* 480–481.

Hegedus, A. M., Alterman, A. I., & Tarter, R. E. (1984). Learning achievement in sons of alcoholics. *Alcoholism: Clinical and Experimental Research, 8,* 330–333.

Hill, S. Y., De Bellis, M. D., Keshavan, M. S., Lowers, L., Shen, S., Hall, J., et al. (2001). Right amygdala volume in adolescent and young adult offspring from families at high risk for developing alcoholism. *Biol Psychiatry, 49*(11), 894–905.

Hill, S. Y., & Shen, S. (2002). Neurodevelopmental patterns of visual P3b in association with familial risk for alcohol dependence and childhood diagnosis. *Biol Psychiatry, 51*(8), 621–631.

Hill, S. Y., Shen, S., Locke, J., Lowers, L., Steinhauer, S., & Konicky, C. (2000). Developmental changes in postural sway in children at high and low risk for developing alcohol-related disorders. *Biological Psychiatry, 47*(6), 501–511.

Hill, S. Y., Shen, S., Lowers, L., & Locke, J. (2000). Factors predicting the onset of adolescent drinking in families at high risk for developing alcoholism. *Biological Psychiatry, 48*(4), 265–275.

Hingson, R., Heeren, T., & Winter, M. (1994). Lower legal blood alcohol limit for young drivers. *Public Health Rep, 109,* 738–744.

Holguin, S., Corral, M., & Cadaveira, F. (1998). Visual and auditory event-related potentials in young children of alcoholics from high- and low-density families. *Alcohol Clin Exp Res, 22,* 87–96.

Hommer, D., Momenan, R., Kaiser, E., & Rawlings, R. (2001). Evidence for a gender-related effect of alcoholism on brain volumes. *American Journal of Psychiatry, 158*(2), 198–204.

Huttenlocher, P. R. (1990). Morphometric study of human cerebral cortex development. *Neuropsychologia, 28*(6), 517–527.

Huttenlocher, P. R., & Dabholkar, A. S. (1997). Regional differences in synaptogenesis in human cerebral cortex. *J Comp Neurol, 387*(2), 167–178.

Jernigan, T. L., Trauner, D. A., Hesselink, J. R., & Tallal, P. A. (1991). Maturation of human cerebrum observed in vivo during adolescence. *Brain, 114*(Pt 5), 2037–2049.

Johnston, L. D., O'Malley, P. M., & Bachman, J. G. (2003). *The Monitoring the Future national survey results on adolescent drug use: Overview of key findings, 2002* (No. NIH Publication No. 03-5374). Bethesda, MD: National Institute on Drug Abuse.

Klingberg, T., Forssberg, H., & Westerberg, H. (2002). Increased brain activity in frontal and parietal cortex underlies the development of visuospatial working memory capacity during childhood. *Journal of Cognitive Neuroscience, 14*(1), 1–10.

Kruesi, M. J. P., Hibbs, E. D., Zahn, T. P., Keysor, C. S., Hamburger, S. D., Bartko, J., et al. (1992). A 2-year prospective follow-up study of children and adolescents with disruptive behavior disorders. *Archives of General Psychiatry, 49,* 429–435.

Kruesi, M. J. P., Rapoport, J. L., Hamburger, S., Hibbs, E., Potter, W. Z., Lenane, M., et al. (1990). Cerebrospinal fluid monoamine metabolites, aggression, and impulsivity in disruptive behavior disorders of children and adolescents. *Archives of General Psychiatry, 47,* 419–426.

Kucuk, N. O., Kilic, E. O., Ibis, E., Aysev, A., Gencoglu, E. A., Aras, G., et al. (2000). Brain SPECT findings in long term inhalant abuse. *Nucl Med Commun, 21*(8), 769–773.

Lahey, B. B., Loeber, R., Quay, H. C., Applegate, B., Shaffer, D., Waldman, I., et al. (1998). Validity of DSM-IV subtypes of conduct disorder based on age of onset. *Journal of the American Academy of Child and Adolescent Psychiatry, 37*(4), 435–442.

LeMarquand, D. G., Benkelfat, C., Pihl, R. O., Palmour, R. M., & Young, S. N. (1999). Behavioral disinhibition induced by tryptophan depletion in nonalcoholic young men with multigenerational family histories of paternal alcoholism. *American Journal of Psychiatry, 156*(11), 1771–1779.

Luna, B., Thulborn, K. R., Munoz, D. P., Merriam, E. P., Garver, K. E., Minshew, N. J., et al. (2001). Maturation of widely distributed brain function subserves cognitive development. *Neuroimage, 13*(5), 786–793.

Lynam, D., Moffitt, T. E., & Stouthamer-Loeber, M. (1993). Explaining the relation between IQ and delinquency. *Journal of Abnormal Psychology, 102,* 187–196.

Mattson, S. N., Schoenfeld, A. M., & Riley, E. P. (2001). Teratogenic effects of alcohol on brain and behavior. *Alcohol Res Health, 25*(3), 185–191.

McBurnett, K., Lahey, B. B., Rathouz, P. J., & Loeber, R. (2000). Low salivary cortisol and persistent aggression in boys referred for disruptive behavior. *Archives of General Psychiatry, 57*(1), 38–43.

Moffitt, T. E. (1993). The neuropsychology of conduct disorder. *Development & Psychopathology, 5,* 135–151.

Moffitt, T. E., & Henry, B. (1989). Neuropsychological assessment of executive functions in self-reported delinquents. *Development and Psychopathology, 1,* 105–118.

Moffitt, T. E., & Silva, P. A. (1988a). IQ and delinquency: A direct test of the differential detection hypothesis. *Journal of Abnormal Psychology, 97,* 330–333.

Moffitt, T. E., & Silva, P. A. (1988b). Self-reported delinquency, neuropsychological deficit, and history of attention deficit disorder. *Journal of Abnormal Child Psychology, 16,* 553–569.

Moss, H. B., Kirisci, L., Gordon, H. W., & Tarter, R. E. (1994). A neuropsychologic profile of adolescent alcoholics. *Alcoholism: Clinical and Experimental Research, 18*(1), 159–163.

Najam, N., Tarter, R. E., & Kirisci, L. (1997). Language deficits in children at high risk for drug abuse. *Journal of Child & Adolescent Substance Abuse, 6,* 69–80.

National Center for Health Statistics. (1999). *10 leading causes of death, United States.* Atlanta, GA: Office of Statistics and Programming, National Center for Injury Prevention and Control, Center for Disease Control.

Nixon, S. J., & Parsons, O. A. (1991). Alcohol related efficiency deficits using an ecologically valid test. *Alcohol Clin Exp Res, 15*(4), 601–606.

Nixon, S. J., Paul, R., & Phillips, M. (1998). Cognitive efficiency in alcoholics and polysubstance abusers. *Alcoholism: Clinical and Experimental Research, 22*(7), 1414–1420.

Ozkaragoz, T., Satz, P., & Noble, E. P. (1997). Neuropsychological functioning in sons of active alcoholic, recovering alcoholic, and social drinking fathers. *Alcohol, 14,* 31–37.

Ozkaragoz, T. Z., & Noble, E. P. (1995). Neuropsychological differences between sons of active alcoholic and non-alcoholic fathers. *Alcohol and Alcoholism, 30*(1), 115–123.

Peterson, J., Finn, P., & Pihl, R. (1992). Cognitive dysfunction and the inherited predisposition to alcoholism. *J Stud Alcohol, 53*, 154–160.

Peterson, J. B., Pihl, R. O., Gianoulakis, C., Conrod, P., Finn, P. R., Stewart, S. H., et al. (1996). Ethanol-induced change in cardiac and endogenous opiate function and risk for alcoholism. *Alcoholism, Clinical and Experimental Research, 20*(9), 1542–1552.

Peterson, J. L., Coates, T. J., Catania, J. A., Middleton, B. A., Hilliard, B., & Hearst, N. (1992). High-risk sexual behavior and condom use among gay and bisexual African-American men. *American Journal of Public Health, 82*, 1490–1494.

Pfefferbaum, A., Desmond, J., Galloway, C., Menon, V., Glover, G., & Sullivan, E. (2001). Reorganization of frontal systems used by alcoholics for spatial working memory: an fMRI study. *NeuroImage, 14*, 7–20.

Pfefferbaum, A., Lim, K., Desmond, J., & Sullivan, E. (1996). Thinning of the corpus callosum in older alcoholic men: A magnetic resonance imaging study. *Alcohol Clin Exp Res, 20*, 752–757.

Pfefferbaum, A., Mathalon, D. H., Sullivan, E. V., Rawles, J. M., Zipursky, R. B., & Lim, K. O. (1994). A quantitative magnetic resonance imaging study of changes in brain morphology from infancy to late adulthood. *Archives of Neurology, 51*(9), 874–887.

Pfefferbaum, A., Sullivan, E., Mathalon, D., Shear, P., Rosenbloom, M., & Lim, K. (1995). Longitudinal changes in magnetic resonance imaging brain volumes in abstinent and relapsed alcoholics. *Alcoholism: Clinical and Experimental Research, 19*, 1177–1191.

Pfefferbaum, A., Sullivan, E., Rosenbloom, M., Mathalon, D., & Lim, K. (1998). A controlled study of cortical gray matter and ventricular changes in alcoholic men over a 5-year interval. *Arch Gen Psychiatry, 55*, 905–912.

Pfefferbaum, A., & Sullivan, E. V. (2002). Microstructural but not macrostructural disruption of white matter in women with chronic alcoholism. *Neuroimage, 15*(3), 708–718.

Pfefferbaum, A., Sullivan, E. V., Hedehus, M., Adalsteinsson, E., Lim, K. O., & Moseley, M. (2000). In vivo detection and functional correlates of white matter microstructural disruption in chronic alcoholism. *Alcoholism: Clinical and Experimental Research, 24*(8), 1214–1221.

Pfefferbaum, A., Sullivan, E. V., Hegehus, M., Adalsteinsson, E., Lim, K. L., & Moseley, M. (2000). In vivo detection and functional correlates of white matter microstructural disruption in chronic alcoholism. *Alcoholism: Clinical and Experimental Research, 24*, 1214–1221.

Pihl, R., & Bruce, K. (1995). Cognitive impairment in children of alcoholics. *Alcohol Health & Research World, 19*, 142–147.

Pihl, R. O., & Peterson, J. (1996). Characteristics and putative mechanisms in boys at risk for drug abuse and aggression. In T. G. Craig F. Ferris (Ed.), *Understanding aggressive behavior in children. Annals of the New York Academy of Sciences, Vol. 794.* (pp. 238–252): New York Academy of Sciences, New York, NY, US.

Pihl, R. O., Peterson, J., & Finn, P. R. (1990). Inherited predisposition to alcoholism: Characteristics of sons of male alcoholics. *Journal of Abnormal Psychology, 99*, 291–301.

Pishkin, V., Lovallo, W. R., & Bourne, L. E., Jr. (1985). Chronic alcoholism in males: cognitive deficit as a function of age of onset, age, and duration. *Alcoholism: Clinical and Experimental Research, 9*(5), 400–406.

Polich, J., Pollock, V. E., & Bloom, F. E. (1994). Meta-analysis of P300 amplitude from males at risk for alcoholism. *Psychological Bulletin, 115*, 55–73.

Poon, E., Ellis, D. A., Fitzgerald, H. E., & Zucker, R. A. (2000). Intellectual, cognitive, and academic performance among sons of alcoholics during the early school years: Differences related to subtypes of familial alcoholism. *Alcoholism: Clinical & Experimental Research, 24*, 1020–1027.

Porjesz, B., Begleiter, H., Reich, T., Van Eerdewegh, P., Edenberg, H., Foroud, T., et al. (1998). Amplitude of visual P3 event-related potential as a phenotypic marker for a predisposition to alcoholism: Preliminary results from the COGA project. *Alcohol Clin Exp Res, 22*(6), 1317–1323.

Prentice, N. M., & Kelly, F. J. (1963). Intelligence and delinquency: A reconsideration. *Journal of Social Psychology, 60*, 327–337.

Raine, A., & Jones, F. (1987). Attention, autonomic arousal, and personality in behaviorally disordered children. *Journal of Abnormal Child Psychology, 15*, 583–599.

Raine, A., & Venables, P. H. (1987). Contingent negative variation, P3 evoked potentials, and antisocial behavior. *Psychophysiology, 24*, 191–199.

Raine, A., Venables, P. H., & Williams, M. (1990a). Autonomic orienting responses in 15 year-old male subjects and criminal behavior at age 24. *American Journal of Psychiatry, 147*, 933–937.

Raine, A., Venables, P. H., & Williams, M. (1990b). Relationships between central and autonomic measures of arousal at age 15 and criminality at age 24 years. *Archives of General Psychiatry, 47*, 1003–1007.

Rohde, P., Lewinsohn, P. M., & Seeley, J. R. (1996a). Psychiatric comorbidity with problematic alcohol use in high school students. *Journal of the American Academy of Child and Adolescent Psychiatry, 35*(1), 101–109.

Rohde, P., Lewinsohn, P. M., & Seeley, J. R. (1996b). Psychiatric comorbidity with problematic alcohol use in high school students. *Journal of the American Academy of Child & Adolescent Psychiatry, 35*, 101–109.

Ryan, C., & Butters, N. (1988). Neuropsychology of alcoholism. In D. Wedding & H. MacNeil, Jr. (Eds.), *The Neuropsychology Handbook: Behavioral and Clinical Perspectives* (pp. in press).

Santerre, L., Dager, A., Cheung, E., Meloy, M., Paulus, M., Brown, G., et al. (2002). Chronic smoking and fMRI response in alcohol use disordered adolescents. *Alcoholism: Clinical and Experimental Research, 26*, 711.

Schuckit, M. A. (1998). Biological, psychological and environmental predictors of the alcoholism risk: A longitudinal study. *Journal of Studies on Alcohol, 59*(5), 485–494.

Schuckit, M. A., Butters, N., Lyn, L., & Irwin, M. (1987). Neuropsychologic deficits and the risk for alcoholism. *Neuropsychopharmacology, 1*(1), 45–53.

Schuckit, M. A., & Smith, T. L. (1997). Assessing the risk for alcoholism among sons of alcoholics. *Journal of Studies on Alcohol, 58*(2), 141–145.

Schweinsburg, B. C., Alhassoon, O. M., Taylor, M. J., Gonzalez, R., Videen, J. S., Brown, G. G., et al. (2003). Effects of alcoholism and gender on brain metabolism. *American Journal of Psychiatry, 160*(6), 1180–1183.

Schweinsburg, B. C., Taylor, M. J., Alhassoon, O. M., Videen, J. S., Brown, G. G., Patterson, T. L., et al. (2001). Chemical pathology in brain white matter of recently detoxified alcoholics: a 1H magnetic resonance spectroscopy investigation of alcohol-associated frontal lobe injury. *Alcoholism: Clinical and Experimental Research, 25*(6), 924–934.

Schweinsburg, B. C., Taylor, M. J., Videen, J. S., Alhassoon, O. M., Patterson, T. L., & Grant, I. (2000). Elevated myo inositol in gray matter of recently detoxified but not long term abstinent alcoholics: a preliminary MR spectroscopy study. *Alcohol Clin Exp Res, 24*(5), 699–705.

Sher, K. J., Bartholow, B. D., & Wood, M. D. (2000). Personality and substance use disorders: A prospective study. *Journal of Consulting & Clinical Psychology, 68*(5), 818–829.

Sher, K. J., Walitzer, K. S., Wood, P. K., & Brent, E. E. (1991). Characteristics of children of alcoholics: Putative risk factors, alcohol and other drug use and abuse, and psychopathology. *Journal of Abnormal Psychology, 100*, 427–448.

Shrier, L. A., Harris, S. K., Kurland, M., & Knight, J. R. (2003). Substance use problems and associated psychiatric symptoms among adolescents in primary care. *Pediatrics, 111*(6 Pt 1), MID-12777342.

Skoff, B. F., & Libon, J. (1987). Impaired executive functions in a sample of male juvenile delinquents. *Journal of Clinical and Experimental Neuropsychology, 9*, 60.

Soloff, P. H., Lynch, K. G., & Moss, H. B. (2000). Serotonin, impulsivity, and alcohol use disorders in the older adolescent: A psychobiological study. *Alcoholism: Clinical & Experimental Research, 24*, 1609–1619.

Sowell, E. R., Delis, D., Stiles, J., & Jernigan, T. L. (2001). Improved memory functioning and frontal lobe maturation between childhood and adolescence: a structural MRI study. *J Int Neuropsychol Soc, 7*(3), 312–322.

Sowell, E. R., Peterson, B. S., Thompson, P. M., Welcome, S. E., Henkenius, A. L., & Toga, A. W. (2003). Mapping cortical change across the human life span. *Nature Neuroscience, 6*(3), 309–315.

Sowell, E. R., Thompson, P. M., Holmes, C. J., Batth, R., Jernigan, T. L., & Toga, A. W. (1999). Localizing age-related changes in brain structure between childhood and adolescence using statistical parametric mapping. *Neuroimage, 9*(6 Pt 1), 587–597.

Sowell, E. R., Thompson, P. M., Holmes, C. J., Jernigan, T. L., & Toga, A. W. (1999). In vivo evidence for post-adolescent brain maturation in frontal and striatal regions. *Nature Neuroscience, 2*(10), 859–861.

Sowell, E. R., Thompson, P. M., Mattson, S. N., Tessner, K. D., Jernigan, T. L., Riley, E. P., et al. (2002). Regional brain shape abnormalities persist into adolescence after heavy prenatal alcohol exposure. *Cereb Cortex, 12*(8), 856–865.

Sullivan, E. V., Desmond, J. E., Lim, K. O., & Pfefferbaum, A. (2002). Speed and efficiency but not accuracy or timing deficits of limb movements in alcoholic men and women. *Alcohol Clin Exp Res, 26*(5), 705–713.

Sullivan, E. V., Harding, A. J., Pentney, R., Dlugos, C., Martin, P. R., Parks, M. H., et al. (2003). Disruption of frontocerebellar circuitry and function in alcoholism. *Alcohol Clin Exp Res, 27*(2), 301–309.

Tapert, S. F., Baratta, M., Abrantes, A., & Brown, S. (2002). Attention dysfunction predicts substance involvement in community youth. *Journal of the American Academy of Child and Adolescent Psychiatry, 41*, 680–686.

Tapert, S. F., Schweinsburg, A. D., Barlett, V. C., Brown, S. A., Frank, L. R., Brown, G. G., & Meloy, M. J. (in press). BOLD response and spatial working memory in adolescents with alcohol use disorders. *Alcoholism: Clinical and Experimental Research.*

Tapert, S. F., Myers, M., Tomlinson, K., & Brown, S. (1999). Influence of smoking and substance withdrawal on cognitive efficiency among young adults. *Annals of Behavioral Medicine, 21*, S190.

Tapert, S. F., Brown, G. G., Kindermann, S. S., Cheung, E. H., Frank, L. R., & Brown, S. A. (2001). fMRI measurement of brain dysfunction in alcohol-dependent young women. *Alcoholism: Clinical and Experimental Research, 25*(2), 236–245.

Tapert, S. F., & Brown, S. A. (1999a, 1999, August). *Gender differences in neuropsychological functioning of young adult substance abusers.* Paper presented at the Annual Meeting of the American Psychological Association, Boston, MA.

Tapert, S. F., & Brown, S. A. (1999b). Neuropsychological correlates of adolescent substance abuse: Four-year outcomes. *Journal of the International Neuropsychological Society, 5*(6), 481–493.

Tapert, S. F., & Brown, S. A. (1999). Neuropsychological correlates of adolescent substance abuse: Four-year outcomes. *Journal of the International Neuropsychological Society, 5*, 481–493.

Tapert, S. F., & Brown, S. A. (2000). Substance dependence, family history of alcohol dependence, and neuropsychological functioning in adolescence. *Addiction, 95*, 1043–1053.

Tapert, S. F., Brown, S. A., Myers, M. G., & Granholm, E. (1999). The role of neurocognitive abilities in coping with adolescent relapse to alcohol and drug use. *Journal of Studies on Alcohol., 60*, 500–508.

Tapert, S. F., Cheung, E. H., Brown, G. G., Frank, L. R., Paulus, M. P., Schweinsburg, A. D., et al. (2003). Neural response to alcohol stimuli in adolescents with alcohol use disorder. *Archives of General Psychiatry, 60*(7), 727–735.

Tapert, S. F., Granholm, E., Leedy, N., & Brown, S. A. (2002). Substance use and withdrawal: Neuropsychological functioning over 8 years in youth. *Journal of the International Neuropsychological Society, 8*, 873–883.

Tapert, S. F., Granholm, E., Leedy, N. G., & Brown, S. A. (2002). Substance use and withdrawal: neuropsychological functioning over 8 years in youth. *Journal of the International Neuropsychological Society, 8*(7), 873–883.

Tapert, S. F., McCarthy, D. M., Aarons, G. A., Schweinsburg, A. D., & Brown, S. A. (2003). Influence of language abilities and alcohol expectancies on the persistence of heavy drinking in youth. *J Stud Alcohol, 64*, 313–321.

Tapert, S. F., Theilmann, R. J., Schweinsburg, A. D., Yafai, S., & Frank, L. R. (2003). Reduced fractional anisotropy in the splenium of adolescents with alcohol use disorder.

Tarter, R., Jacob, T., & Bremer, D. (1989). Specific cognitive impairment in sons of early onset alcoholics. *Alcohol Clin Exp Res, 13,* 786–789.

Tarter, R. E., Alterman, A. I., & Edwards, K. L. (1985). Vulnerability to alcoholism in men: A behavior-genetic perspective. *Journal of Studies on Alcohol, 46,* 329–356.

Tarter, R. E., Hegedus, A. M., Goldstein, G., Shelly, C., & Alterman, A. I. (1984). Adolescent sons of alcoholics: Neuropsychological and personality characteristics. *Alcoholism: Clinical and Experimental Research, 8,* 216–222.

Tarter, R. E., Hegedus, A. M., Winsten, N. E., & Alterman, A. L. (1984). Neuropsychological, personality, and familial characteristics of physically abused delinquents. *Journal of the American Academy of Child Psychiatry, 23,* 668–674.

Tarter, R. E., Kirisci, L., Mezzich, A., Cornelius, J. R., Pajer, K., Vanyukov, M., et al. (2003). Neurobehavioral disinhibition in childhood predicts early age at onset of substance use disorder. *Am J Psychiatry, 160*(6), 1078–1085.

Tarter, R. E., Mezzich, A. C., Hsieh, Y. C., & Parks, S. M. (1995). Cognitive capacity in female adolescent substance abusers. *Drug and Alcohol Dependence, 39*(1), 15–21.

Toupin, J., Déry, M., Pauze, R., Mercier, H., & Fortin, L. (2000). Cognitive and familial contributions to conduct disorder in children. *Journal of Child Psychology and Psychiatry and Allied Disciplines, 41*(3), 333–344.

Twitchell, G. R., Hanna, G. L., Cook, E. H., Fitzgerald, H. E., & Zucker, R. A. (2000). Serotonergic function, behavioral disinhibition, and negative affect in children of alcoholics: The moderating effects of puberty. *Alcoholism: Clinical & Experimental Research, 24,* 972–979.

Verger, K., Junque, C., Levin, H. S., Jurado, M. A., Perez Gomez, M., Bartres Faz, D., et al. (2001). Correlation of atrophy measures on MRI with neuropsychological sequelae in children and adolescents with traumatic brain injury. *Brain Inj, 15*(3), 211–221.

Virkkunen, M., De Jong, J., Bartko, J., Goodwin, F. K., & Linnoila, M. (1989). Relationship of psychobiological variables to recidivism in violent offenders and impulsive firesetters: A follow-up study. *Archives of General Psychiatry, 46,* 600–603.

Virkkunen, M., & Linnoila, M. (1997). Serotonin in early-onset alcoholism. In E. Marc Galanter & et al. (Eds.), *Recent developments in alcoholism, Vol. 13: Alcohol and violence: Epidemiology, neurobiology, psychology, family issues.* (pp. 173–189). New York: Plenum Press.

Wall, T. L., Schuckit, M. A., Mungas, D., & Ehlers, C. L. (1990). EEG alpha activity and personality traits. *Alcohol, 7,* 461–464.

West, D. J., & Farrington, D. P. (1973). *Who becomes delinquent?* : London: Heinemann Educational Books.

White, J. L., Moffitt, T. E., Caspi, A., Bartusch, D. J., Needles, D. J., & Stouthamer-Loeber, M. (1994). Measuring impulsivity and examining its relationship to delinquency. *Journal of Abnormal Psychology, 103,* 192–205.

Wiers, R. W., Wood, M. D., Darkes, J., Corbin, W. R., Jones And, B. T., & Sher, K. J. (2003). Changing expectancies: cognitive mechanisms and context effects. *Alcohol Clin Exp Res, 27*(2), 186–197.

Wolff, P. H., Waber, D., Bauermeister, M., Cohen, C., & Ferber, F. (1982). The neuropsychological status of adolescent delinquent boys. *Journal of Child Psychology and Psychiatry, 23,* 267–279.

Yakovlev, P. I., & Lecours, A. R. (1967). The myelogenetic cycles of regional maturation of the brain. In A. Mikowski (Ed.), *Regional Development of the Brain in Early Life* (pp. 3–70). Oxford, England: Blackwell Scientific.

Yi, H.-y., Williams, G. D., & Dufour, M. C. (2001). *Surveillance report #56: Trends in alcohol-related fatal traffic crashes, United States, 1977–99.* Bethesda, MD: National Institute on Alcohol Abuse and Alcoholism.

Zoccolillo, M. (1993). Gender and the development of conduct disorder. *Development & Psychopathology, 5,* 65–78.

III

Prevention

Gayle M. Boyd, *Section Editor*

The chapters in this section provide a survey of issues, models and intervention approaches for the prevention of alcohol-related problems in adolescents. Collectively, they address the breadth of prevention strategies (e.g., school-family- and community-based and comprehensive interventions) and discuss issues relevant to specific populations defined by race/ethnicity or presumed level of risk. The final chapter presents an integrated set of strategies developed by a Task Force of the National Advisory Council on Alcohol Abuse and Alcoholism[1] to reduce alcohol-problems among college students.

Prevention may be viewed as falling along one end of a continuum that also includes treatment and maintenance. Older descriptors for classifying medical preventive interventions—primary, secondary and tertiary—have been replaced by a system that is better adapted for prevention of mental health and behavioral disorders.[2] Interventions are classified according to the risk level of the populations for which they are intended: *universal* preventive interventions are directed toward the general population regardless of risk; *selective* interventions are directed toward populations or individuals presumed to be at higher than average risk; and *indicated* interventions are directed toward individuals who are manifesting early signs or symptoms of a disorder or who have biological markers indicating increased risk.

This system of classification can be useful for program planning. Selection and deployment of strategies cannot be divorced from practical considerations of cost and anticipated benefit. Usually, there is a gradient of intervention intensity and cost per individual from universal through selective and indicated approaches. A tiered or stepped approach in which more intensive programs are delivered to groups at higher risk or individuals who have not responded to universal approaches has been recommended by a number of writers as an efficient way to utilize resources.[3,4,5] The majority of

Gayle M. Boyd • Health Scientist Administrator, Prevention Research Branch, NIAAA Division of Clinical and Prevention Research, Bethesda, Maryland 20892-7003.

existing prevention interventions are universal, and there are relatively few well-tested programs for higher risk youth.

Interventions can be loosely described as operating at the level of the environment, the individual, or both. Environmental interventions seek to reduce opportunities (availability) for underage drinking, increase penalties or the probability of incurring penalties for violation of the minimum legal drinking age (MLDA) or other laws and policies related to alcohol use, and reduce community tolerance for alcohol use and misuse by youth. Environmental interventions are among the recommendations included in the recent National Research Council and Institute of Medicine report,[6] "Reducing Underage Drinking: A Collective Responsibility." Individual-level interventions seek to change knowledge, expectancies, attitudes, intentions, motivation and skills so that youth are better able to resist the pro-drinking influences and opportunities that surround them. School prevention curricula are a prime example.

Policy change is the keystone of preventive environmental interventions. The chapter by Wagenaar, Lenk and Toomey reviews the research literature on relationships between alcohol policies and underage drinking. They structured their chapter by policy categories and ordered them according to the number and methodological strength of available research studies. It begins with studies on the MLDA and price effects, for which the evidence is strongest, and proceeds through policies for which only moderate (e.g., server training) or minimal (e.g., compliance checks) support is available. They conclude with a section on policies that have not been researched but that have considerable face value, such as home-delivery restrictions and shoulder-tap enforcement, which provides clear direction for future research.

Policies do not exert effects in a vacuum. As Wagenaar et al., point out, enforcement is key to policy effectiveness. They note that, had it been vigorously enforced, the positive effects associated with raising the MLDA to 21 would probably have been even greater than those observed. And they warn against discounting the potential utility of policies that appear ineffective if their evaluation was based on instances that lacked robust enforcement. Additionally, the target population must be aware of both the policy and its enforcement. Communities that undertake new policies or changes in enforcement are urged to include publicity as part of their overall strategy.

It should be noted that alcohol policies are usually considered an universal prevention approach because they apply equally to the entire population. Evaluations have conformed to this model and are generally based on population outcomes. However, there is no reason to assume that effects are uniform across population subgroups; and some groups may respond differentially. For instance, how are policies perceived by different racial/ethnic groups; are they enforced differently in some groups than others; are some groups more or less responsive to specific policies? (Sussman, this volume) An especially intriguing question is how individuals at higher levels of risk (e.g., children of alcoholics, youth who are already drinking heavily, youth with co-morbid conditions) are affected by their policy environment. If environmental strategies are effective for higher risk groups and groups that are hard to reach (e.g., school dropouts), then there is even greater support for their use.

Comprehensive prevention interventions are reviewed by Komro, Stigler and Perry. Ideally these approaches include a mix of environmental and individual-level strategies. Unfortunately, the environmental aspect is often confined to school and family environments; and to date there has only been one comprehensive intervention trial focused specifically on alcohol that incorporated community-level action. Findings from this successful randomized multi-site trial, Project Northland, are reported in the chapter by Komro et al. It should be noted that this trial took place in racially homogeneous small rural communities, and therefore it is now being replicated in multi-ethnic urban neighborhoods.

Komro et al. describe the logic process that underlies sound intervention design, and this can be applied to single component as well as comprehensive programs. The factors or influences that are targeted for change should be selected on the basis of theoretical models that incorporate existing knowledge about the etiology of drinking or other problem behaviors. Comprehensive models, such as the Theory of Triadic Influences,[7] synthesize findings across multiple domains (e.g., individual; family; community) and can be used to identify targets for change with the greatest potential for improving youth outcomes. Other sections in this volume review epidemiological and neurobiological research that inform these models. A second level of theory, action models, are needed to link specific change targets to intervention strategies.

Prevention programs for adolescents must specify exactly what is to be prevented to insure that appropriate interventions are being selected, that there is a correspondence between program goals and evaluation measures, and that programs meet the needs and expectations of communities. The formal goal is usually prevention of all underage drinking, and there is strong support for the importance of this goal. As discussed in other sections of this volume, there is a robust correlation between early initiation of drinking and experiencing subsequent alcohol-related problems during adolescence, adult alcohol abuse and/or dependence, lifetime experience of alcohol-related injury, being in a fight after drinking, and psychopathology.[8 9 10 11 12 13 14] Although it is not clear whether early initiation is causally related to these problems, it is at the very least a marker for risk.

However, youth who drink early are not only at risk for escalating alcohol involvement and future problems; they experience risk for immediate adverse consequences, injury and alcohol poisoning. These potential outcomes are also described elsewhere in this volume. It is clear that reducing risk for immediate harm is another important possible program goal, which can be accomplished by reducing high-quantity ("binge") drinking and drinking in risky situations (e.g., driving). With increasing age, alcohol use becomes increasingly normative and high-risk drinking practices become increasingly prevalent. Tension may result between goals of promoting alcohol abstinence, the only legal option for youth, and reducing high-risk drinking. Balancing goals so that public health needs are met, messages do not undermine each other, and community values are not offended is a major challenge for program planners. Attention to the developmental appropriateness of interventions and audience risk level should help in meeting this practical challenge.

The chapter by Saltz summarizes the findings and recommendations of the Task Force on College Drinking of the National Advisory Council on Alcohol Abuse and Alcoholism.[1] This Task Force was formed in response to increasing concern about the prevalence of serious alcohol-related problems on and around college campuses, including an estimated 1,400 deaths each year. They reviewed the available literature and provided recommended intervention strategies according to the strength of evidence supporting them. There has been more research on individual-focused interventions for this population, especially cognitive-behavioral skills training and brief motivational enhancement, than on environmental strategies. However, based on extrapolation from the general population, environmental interventions such as increased enforcement of MLDA and drunk driving laws were recommended as useful strategies. On many campuses heavy drinking has become a part of the culture of college life, and this culture is not likely to be affected by single short-lived interventions. Colleges are urged to join with surrounding communities to develop and implement comprehensive strategies that address environmental conditions that facilitate high risk and underage drinking, as well as promoting abstinence or moderation by influencing individual student attitudes, motivation and skills . The overall approach and need for underlying logic models are similar to that described by Komro et al.

The prevalence of periodic heavy or high-risk drinking, as indicated by self-reports of consuming five or more drinks on a single occasion, is greatest among young adults compared to older adults; and among young adults, college students have the highest prevalence of high-risk drinking.[15] Longitudinal studies indicate that drinking increases with entrance into college, but drinking during high school sets the stage. Many students arrive on campus with preexisting patterns of high-risk drinking, and the need for intervention among younger adolescents is clear.

Most prevention strategies for young adolescents have been school-based. School curricula to prevent alcohol and other substance use have a long history, but the use of empirical findings to guide content development and systematic evaluation to inform improvements is a more recent development [16] [17]. Initial efforts were primarily informational and often used scare tactics. It was assumed that if youth understood the dangers inherent in alcohol misuse they would choose to abstain. These programs were ineffective. There has been steady progress in both underlying theory for school prevention curricula and in research methodology; and superior programs are now available, although they are not necessarily selected for use[18] or implemented as designed.[19] Methodological issues remain a critical barrier to interpreting the large number of published studies. Variations in design and methodology make comparisons across studies difficult, and the vast majority do not meet even minimum standards of rigor.[20,21]

These methodological problems pertain equally to interventions for special populations, reviewed by Sussman (this volume). He provides a comprehensive inventory of prevention programs for various subpopulations defined by race/ethnicity, region or socio-economic status. Although instances of successful programs are identified, it is difficult to make comparisons across studies to address broader questions. For example, Sussman asks whether interventions developed for the general population can be adapted with only minimal (surface structure) modifications or must cultural values and traditions inform all phases of intervention development (deep structure). The answer to this question has clear implications for program costs, as well as for the feasibility of developing interventions for multi-cultural communities.

Sussman, Zucker and Wong, and Komro et al. all identify family-based interventions as having utility for preventing alcohol onset. These interventions operate dually at the individual and environmental level. Typically they encourage parents to be aware of risks from underage drinking, to communicate with children, to clarify expectations regarding alcohol use, to set rules and consequences for violations, to monitor children's activities, and to reduce the availability of alcohol in the home. By changing parent practices they affect a primary social environment for the child and can both reduce alcohol availability and increase "costs" associated with drinking.

Parent-directed programs have been included with school-based interventions, some of which have evidence of success; but these components are rarely evaluated separately.[22] Sussman cites one study in which previously tested family skills training and school-based programs were combined, and the addition of the family component was found to greatly increase the effectiveness of the school program to delay drinking onset.[23] Stand-alone family interventions have also been successful in reducing alcohol use and other risk behaviors[24] (Komro et al. this volume). The Iowa Strengthening Families Program (ISFP), delivered when students were in grade six in rural communities, has shown long-lasting preventive effects on alcohol use, even when evaluated on the basis of intent-to-treat;[25] and a recent Cochrane review identified the ISFP as one of two potentially effective interventions for the primary prevention of alcohol misuse by youth.[20]

Zucker and Wong review what is known about markers of risk for future alcohol problems that can be observed in young children, and they discuss the implications of these studies for prevention programming. Markers include a family history of alcoholism, internalizing behaviors (e.g., shyness/social inhibition), and externalizing behaviors (e.g., behavioral undercontrol, aggression, high novelty seeking, low harm avoidance). The authors describe their own research on developmental trajectories of risk in which they track child problem behaviors over time in families with and without alcohol problems. Their measure of family alcohol problems incorporates both the presence and the severity of alcohol use disorders in parents, which enables a more refined consideration of the family context in which these children live. Both internalizing and externalizing problems at ages 12–14 could be predicted by family environment and child characteristics at age 3–5, although they followed different trajectories. As the authors point out, it is not clear whether it is optimal to intervene in early or middle childhood; but their findings clearly support the need for intervention prior to adolescence. It is striking that so few selective and indicated interventions for children at risk have been tested. This population is large—approximately 15% of youth under age 17 live in households with one or more adults who abuse or are dependent on alcohol.[26] The authors suggest that stigma associated with labeling children or families as at risk is one barrier. Stigma is also a barrier for seeking treatment for dependence, and the reduction of stigma is part of the National Institute on Alcohol Abuse and Alcoholism vision statement.[27]

Collectively, these chapters provide strong support for the need for comprehensive prevention strategies that combine universal, selected and indicated interventions, address youth environments (family, school, neighborhood, community) in ways that reduce alcohol availability and increase real and perceived costs associated with underage or high risk drinking, have both theoretical and empirical support, and are acceptable and appropriate for the populations and communities for which they are designed. The importance of cost-effectiveness analyses to guide program decisions is consistently evident. Each of the papers poses important research questions that should provide direction for the next generation of research.

References

Task Force of the National Advisory Council on Alcohol Abuse and Alcoholism. (2002) *A Call To Action: Changing The Culture Of Drinking At U.S. Colleges.* NIAAA, NIH, U.S. Department of Health and Human Services, NIH Publication No. 02–5010, 2000.

Institute of Medicine. (Mrazek, P.J. and Haggerty, R.J., Eds.) (1994) *Reducing Risks for Mental Disorders: Frontiers for Preventive Intrvention Research.* Committee on Prevention of Mental Disorders, Division of Biobehavioral Sciences and Mental Disorders, Institute of Medicine, Washington, D.C.: National Academy Press, pp 19–29.

Dishion, T.J. and Kavanagh, K. (2000) A multilevel approach to family-centered prevention in schools: Process and outcome. *Addictive Behaviors,* 25(6), 899–911.

Larimer, M. E. and Cronce, J.M. (2002) Identification, prevention and treatment: A review of individual-focused strategies to reduce problematic alcohol consumption by college students. *JSA,* Supplement No. 14, 148–163.

Sanders, M.R. (2000) Community-based parenting and family support interventions and the prevention of drug abuse. *Addictive Behaviors,* 25(6), 929–942.

National Research Council and Institute of Medicine (2004). *Reducing Underage Drinking: A Collective Responsibility.* Committee on Developing a Strategy to Reduce and Prevent Underage Drinking, Richard J. Bonnie and Mary Ellen O-Connell, Eds. Board on Children, Youth, and Families, Division of Behavioral and Social Sciences and Education. Washington, DC: National Academies Press.

Flay, B.R., & Petraitis, J. (1994) The theory of triadic influence: A new theory of health behavior with implications for preventive interventions. *Advances in Medial Sociology,* Vol 4, 19–44.

Ellickson, P.L., Tucker, J.S. and Klein, D.J. (2003) Ten-year prospective study of public health problems associated with early drinking. *Pediatrics,* 111 (5), 949–955, .

Grant, B.F. & Dawson, D.A. (1997) Age at onset of alcohol use and its association with DSM-IV alcohol abuse and dependence: Results from the National Longitudinal Alcohol Epidemiologic Survey. *Journal of Substance Abuse*, vol. 9, 103–110.

Grant, B.F., Stoinson, F.S. & Harford, T.C. (2001) Age at onset of alcohol use and DSM-IV alcohol abuse and dependence: A 12-year follow-up. *Journal of Substance Abuse*, Vol 13, 493–504.

Hawkins, J.D., Graham, J.W., Maguin, E., Abbott, R., Hill, K.G. & Catalano, R.F. (1997) Exploring the effects of age of alcohol use initiation and psychosocial risk factors on subsequent alcohol misuse. *Journal of Studies on Alcohol*, vol. 58, 280–290.

Hingson, R.W., Heeren, T., Jamanka, A. & Howland, J. (2000) Age of drinking onset and unintentional injury involvement after drinking. *JAMA*, Vol 284, No.12, 1527–1533.

Hingson, R.W., Heeren, T. & Zakocs, R. (2001) Age of drinking onset and involvement in physical fights after drinking. *Pediatrics*, Vol. 108 No. 4, 872–877.

McGue, M., Iacono, W.G., Legrand, L.N. Malone, S. & Elkins, I. (2001) Origins and consequences of age at first drink. I. Associations with substance-use disorders, disinhibitory behavior and psychopathology, and P3 amplitude. *Alcohol Clin Exp Res*, Vol. 25, No. 8, 1156–1165

Johnston, L.D., O'Malley, P.M., & Bachman, J.G. (2003). *Monitoring the Future national survey results on drug use, 1975–2002. Volume II: College students and adults ages 19–40* (NIH Publication No. 03-5376). Bethesda, MD: National Institute on Drug

Bangert-Drowns, R.L. (1988) The effects of school-based substance abuse education—a meta-analysis. *J of Drug Ed., 18* (3), 243–264.

Dielman, T.E. (1995) School-Based research on the prevention of adolescent alcohol use and misuse: Methodological issues and advances. In (Boyd, G.M., Howard, J. and Zucker, R.A. (Eds.) *Alcoholl problems among adolescents: Current directions in prevention research.* Hillsdale, N.J: Lawrence Erlbaum Associates, Publishers pp.125–146.

Silvia, E.S., Thorne, J. and Tashjian, C.A. (1997) School-based drug prevention programs: A longitudinal study in selected school districts. Final report. Washington, DC: U.S. Department of Education.

Dusenbury, L., Brannigan, R., Falco, M. and Hansen, W. (2003) A review of research on fidelity of implementation: Implications for drug abuse prevention in school settings. *Health Education Research, 18* (2), 237–256.

Foxcroft, D.R., Ireland, D, Lister-Sharp, D.J., Lowe, G. and Breen, R. (2003) Longer-term primary prevention for alcohol misuse in young people: a systematic review. *Addicition, 98*, 397–411.

Tobler, N.S., Roona, M.R., Ochshorn, P., Marshall, D.G., Streke, A.V. and Stackpole, K.M. (2000) School-based adolescent drug prevention programs: 1998 meta-analysis. *Journal of Primary Prevention*, Vol. 20, No. 4, 275–336.

Flay, B.R. (2000) Approaches to substance use prevention utilizing school curriculum plus social environment change. *Addictive Behaviors, 25* (6), 861–885.

Spoth R.L., Redmaond, C., Trudeau, L., and Shin, C. (2002) Longitudinal substance initiation oucomes for a universal preventive intervention combining family and school programs. *Psychology of Addictive Behaviors*, Vol. 16, 129–134.

Komro, K.A. and Toomey T.L. (2002) Strategies to prevent underage drinking. *Alcohol Research & Health, 26* (1), 5–14.

Spoth, R.L., Redmond, & Shin, C. (2001) Randomized trial of brief family interventions for general populations: Adolescent substance use outcomes 4 years following baseline. Journal of Consulting and Clinical Psychology, 69(4), 627–642.

Grant, B.F. (2000) Estimates of U.S. children exposed to alcohol abuse and dependence in the family. *AJPH*, Vol. 90, No. 1, 112–115.

NIAAA web site: www.niaaa.nih.gov.

10

Comprehensive Approaches to Prevent Adoloscent Drinking and Related Problems

Kelli A. Komro, Melissa H. Stigler, and Cheryl L. Perry

A number of single component strategies have proven effective at reducing underage drinking (Komro & Toomey, 2002). Some of these strategies include interactive classroom curricula driven by the social influences model [e.g., Life Skills Training (Botvin, Baker, Dusenbury, Botvin, & Diaz, 1995)], parenting programs that emphasize skill development [e.g., Strengthening Families Program: For Parents and Youth 10–14 (Spoth, Redmond, & Lepper, 1999)], and public policies that reduce the availability of alcohol [e.g., minimum legal drinking age (Wagenaar & Toomey, 2000)]. The effects of these strategies alone, however, are often limited in duration and scope. Few classroom curricula, for example, have been able to achieve long-term reductions in alcohol use (Komro & Toomey, 2002), and the success of alcohol-related policies appears to be constrained by modest enforcement levels (Wagenaar & Wolfson, 1994).

Therefore, in order to achieve a more substantial and sustained intervention effect, an increasingly adopted approach to prevention over the last decade has been the use of more comprehensive strategies that combine two or more of these single components into a multiple component intervention. To date, most multiple component alcohol prevention interventions have combined a classroom curriculum with other strategies that better address the social environment of youth, like school-wide climate change programs, mass media, parent programs, and/or community organizing (Flay, 2000). The pur-

Kelli A. Komro, Melissa H. Stigler, and Cheryl L. Perry • University of Minnesota, School of Public Health-Division of Epidemiology, Minneapolis, Minnesota 55454.

pose of this chapter is to review multiple component interventions that have been rigorously evaluated in regards to their effect on underage drinking. The chapter starts with a discussion of the theory and rationale underlying this approach to prevention and then ends with potential limitations of current research and recommendations for future research.

1. Theory and Rationale

The most effective preventive interventions are those guided by a theoretical framework (Pentz, 2003). Theories serve as an important frame of reference and are relevant to the design, implementation, and evaluation of any kind of intervention (Chen, 1990). In prevention science, there are two types of theory that are particularly critical: conceptual theory and action theory. *Conceptual theory* provides the basis for the design of an intervention—it is the theory, driven in large part by etiologic research, that connects intervening (or mediating) variables like personal, social, and/or environmental factors (e.g., life skills, social norms) to the behavioral outcome of interest (e.g., alcohol use) (Chen, 1990). *Action theory,* in turn, identifies the strategies an intervention utilizes to achieve its program effects—it is the theory that links and drives the development of program components (e.g., skills training, policy change) in order to change the intervening (or mediating) variables that have been identified by conceptual theory (e.g., life skills, social norms) (Chen, 1990). Figure 1 illustrates how these two types of theories are related. Action theories are most relevant to program planners, administrators, and other individuals interested in how best to devise and implement an intervention, while conceptual theories are most germane to basic (i.e., etiologic) research scientists. Conceptual theories regarding health behavior are historically well developed and have been investigated extensively over time (e.g., Glanz, Rimer, & Lewis, 2002). Action theories, in contrast, have neither been described nor explored as much. The rationale for using a multiple component intervention to address youth drinking is outlined below from the perspective of both conceptual and action theories.

1.1. *Conceptual Theory*

A wide range of risk and protective factors influence the onset and escalation of adolescent drinking (Derzon, 2000; Hawkins, Catalano, & Miller, 1992; NIAAA, 1997). Notably, these factors occur across all of the different spheres of an adolescent's social environment. That is to say, they include peer- (e.g., friends with attitudes favorable towards alcohol use), parent- (e.g., poor family management practices), school- (e.g., academic failure), and community-level

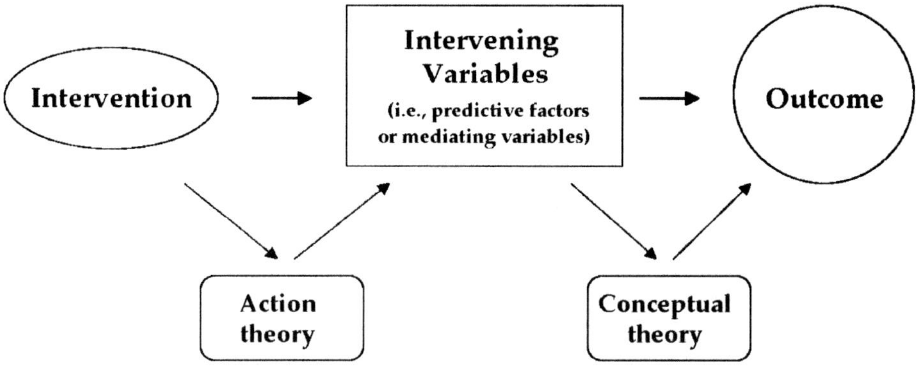

Figure 1. The relationship between action theory and conceptual theory. (Adapted from Chen, 1990.)

(e.g., availability of alcohol) factors, as well as individual-level influences (e.g., genetic susceptibility to alcohol and personality characteristics) (Windle, Shope, & Bukstein, 1996). The development of drinking behavior throughout adolescence is certainly a dynamic process. These different influences do not occur independently but, instead, frequently cluster together and interact with one another in developmentally dependent ways (Flay & Petraitis, 1994; Windle, Shope, & Bukstein, 1996; Windle & Windle, 1999).

Conceptual theories that typically underlie multiple component approaches to alcohol prevention recognize the complexities inherent in the etiology of underage drinking. Examples of conceptual theories used in multiple component interventions include an integrated meta-theory of drinking behavior (Wagenaar & Perry, 1994), Social Cognitive Theory (Bandura, 1977), and the theory of triadic influence (Flay & Petraitis, 1994). The theory of triadic influence (TTI) offers a comprehensive look at the influences on health behavior, including the early onset and use of drugs and alcohol among adolescents (Petraitis, Flay & Miller, 1995). The TTI (Flay & Petraitis, 1994) integrates factors from several social behavioral theories. In this macro-level theory, behaviors are seen as resulting from a person's current social situation, general environment, and personal characteristics. Factors within these domains can further be arranged on a proximal (e.g., cognitions) to distal (e.g., cultural influences) dimension. Interventions appear to be most successful when they are able to make changes in all three of these domains and along both proximal and distal dimensions (Flay & Petraitis, 1994). Addressing distal factors seems to be particularly critical for the maintenance of behavior change (Komro, Hu & Flay, 1997).

Figure 2 provides a diagram using the framework of the TTI of important intervening variables to be targeted in multiple component interventions to prevent alcohol use and alcohol-related problems among adolescents. According to the TTI, behaviors, such as early onset of alcohol use among adolescents, are most immediately controlled by decisions or intentions to use or avoid alcohol, and decisions are a function of social normative beliefs about alcohol use, attitudes toward alcohol use, and self-efficacy to use or avoid alcohol use.

Social normative beliefs about alcohol use are thought to originate in the current social context, including the behaviors and attitudes of others in the adolescent's social world as well as how bonded the adolescent is with those individuals. Others' behaviors and attitudes related to alcohol use and level of bonding are thought to influence perceived norms about alcohol use and motivation to comply with those in one's social world, which, in turn influence an adolescent's social normative beliefs about alcohol use. Derzon (2000) conducted a thorough meta-analysis using longitudinal data sets of risk factors for alcohol use among adolescents. The meta-analysis provides empirical support for the influence of the social context on adolescent alcohol use, with specific support for ties with delinquent peers (others' behaviors in one's social world), opportunities for positive family involvement, low attachment, and social norms that condone substance use (Derzon, 2000).

Attitudes toward alcohol use are thought to originate in the cultural environment, including such things as alcohol availability, media portrayals of alcohol use, and cultural values around alcohol use. The cultural environment influences the adolescent's own knowledge about alcohol use and consequences/benefits of use and values related to alcohol use, which influence adolescents' expectations related to consequences/benefits of alcohol use and evaluations of the importance of consequences/benefits of drinking alcohol. Expectations and evaluations, in turn, influence alcohol-related attitudes. There is also empirical support for the importance of cultural environmental influences on adolescent alcohol use, including the availability of alcohol, community disorganization, opportunities for conventional involvement, low perceived risks of drug use, and positive attitudes towards substance use (Derzon, 2002).

Self-efficacy to use or avoid alcohol use is thought to originate from an adolescent's personality, social competence, and sense of self. General social competence and sense of self are thought to influence an adolescent's social skills and self determination about their ability to use or avoid alcohol, which, in turn influence an adolescent's level of self-efficacy to use or avoid. Empirically there is support for the more distal intrapersonal influence on adolescent alcohol use, including sensation seeking, impulsiveness, rebelliousness, and academic failure (Derzon, 2000).

There is still a need for continued research into the predictors of alcohol use among adolescent. Research is especially needed regarding the various levels of influence, including both distal and proximal variables, and testing both direct and indirect effects using complicated path analytical approaches. Understanding the many influences on adolescent alcohol use is complicated, but a more in-depth understanding is critical in order to develop comprehensive prevention strategies that target predictors of alcohol use at multiple levels.

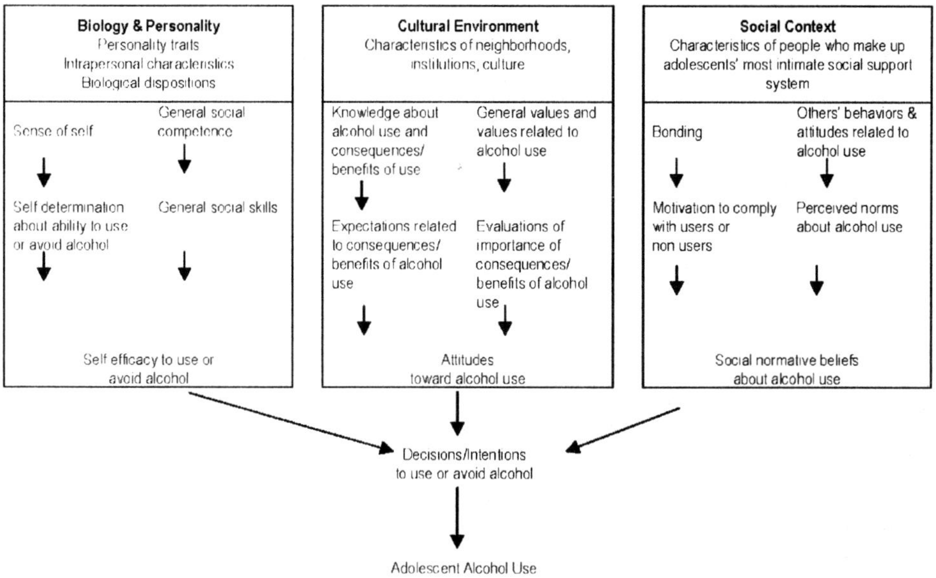

Figure 2. The theory of triadic influence and adolescent alcohol use. (Adapted from Flay, B.R., & Petraitis, J, 1994; Petraitis, Flay & Miller, 1995.)

Driven by more comprehensive theories, such as the TTI, multiple component interventions usually target multiple intervening variables at multiple levels of a young person's personal, social and environmental context, in order to prevent and/or reduce alcohol use and its related problems. Although many single component interventions also address several intervening variables within the same program (e.g., Hansen, 1992), the scope of these factors is usually broader in a multiple component intervention. The latter recognizes that effective intervention efforts require changes in both proximal (e.g., individual-level) and distal (e.g., cultural-environmental level) spheres of a young person's life in order to maximize short-term effects and maintain them in the long-term (Flay & Petraitis, 1994; Wagenaar & Perry, 1994).

1.2. *Action Theory*

While conceptual theory and empirical research directs us to different personal, social and environmental factors that should be changed to reduce underage drinking, action theory explains *how* an intervention strategy endeavors to modify these factors. This kind of theory has also been referred to elsewhere as theory related to prevention process (e.g., theories of community organizing) and/or prevention structure (e.g., theories related to organizational development) (Pentz, 2003). Some important elements of a theory of action, or change, to consider include intervention characteristics related to program component, content, and setting. These features are described below in regards to multiple component interventions that have been used to address underage drinking. Combining and synthesizing program components is thought to contribute to a more potent and pervasive influence on important mediators of adolescent alcohol use than are single component approaches able to do alone.

Multiple component interventions usually target multiple intervening variables in multiple ways, at the same time. In doing so, different components may address the same (set of) intervening variable(s) (e.g., school curriculum and community organizing may both target changes in social norms), and/or they may address different (sets of) intervening variables (e.g., school curriculum may be used to enhance general social skills, while community organizing may be used to decrease the availability of alcohol). The development of program content specific to the different components is driven by conceptual theory, as noted previously. Different components of a multiple component intervention, in turn, typically represent different delivery mechanisms, or vehicles of change. Parent involvement programs [e.g., family skills training programs (Spoth, Redmond, Trudeau, & Shin, 1999)] may be used to address intervening variables at the family-level, while environmental change strategies [e.g., community organizing (Perry et al., 2000)] may be used to address relevant community-level variables (Perry, 1999).

Table 1 links program components that were used in a multiple component alcohol use prevention program, Project Northland, with the intervening variables they were designed to address (Perry et al., 1993; Perry et al., 2000). Project Northland's intervention included classroom curricula, parent education and family involvement, youth development, community organizing, and policy development. TTI (see Figure 2) is used to organize the intervening variables outlined in this table. As can be seen in Table 1, intervening variables within the three domains of the TTI, personal social, and environmental, were targeted by various components of the Project Northland intervention. In addition, many intervening variables were targeted by more than one intervention component. The intervention was intentionally designed in this way so as to provide consistent and repetitive messages and influences in the adolescents' social worlds.

Importantly, multiple component interventions recognize the need for consistent and simultaneous messages and actions at multiple levels of youths' social environment, so they often employ both demand and supply reduction strategies simultaneously (Wagenaar & Perry, 1994). Moreover, this kind of intervention typically targets not only young people, but also their parents and members of their community (e.g., alcohol merchants). As a result, these interventions are usually implemented in several different settings (e.g., school, home, community). In doing so, they strive to identify ways in which members of the target audience, including the young people themselves, as well as their parents and neighbors, can become active participants in creating and subsequently reinforcing a positive social and physical environment that supports youth abstinence from drinking (Wagenaar & Perry, 1994).

Table 1. Hypothesized direct effects (X) of program components on intervening (or mediating) variables in Project Northland, a multiple component intervention.

Level	Intervening Variables within the Framework of the TTI	Project Northland Program Components				
		Classroom Curricula	Parent Education & Family Involvement	Youth Development	Community Organizing	Policy Development
Ultimate	1. Biology & Personality					
	a. Personality Characteristics					
	b. Intrapersonal Characteristics					
	c. Biological Disposition					
	2. Sense of Self			X		
	Social Competence	X		X		
	3. Self Determination	X		X		
↓	Social Skills	X	X	X		
Proximal	4. Self-efficacy	X	X	X		
Ultimate	1. Social Context					
	a. Proactive Family Management		X			
	b. Parenting Skills		X			
	c. Parent Values		X		X	
	d. Peer Values	X		X		
	2. Social Learning	X	X	X	X	X
	Social Bonding					
	a. Family Bonding		X			
	b. Family Involvement		X			
	c. School Bonding					
	3. Motivation to Comply	X	X	X		
↓	Perceived Norms	X	X	X	X	
Proximal	4. Social Normative Beliefs	X	X	X	X	
Ultimate	1. Cultural Environment					
	a. Availability		X		X	X
	b. Media Exposure		X		X	X
	c. Public Policies				X	X
	d. Cultural Values				X	
	e. Neighborhood Characteristics				X	
	2. Knowledge	X	X	X	X	
	Values	X	X	X	X	
	3. Expectations from Behavior	X	X	X	X	X
↓	Evaluations of Consequences	X	X	X	X	
Proximal	4. Attitudes	X	X	X		

The extant research literature supports the theoretical basis for use of more comprehensive, multiple component strategies to prevent adolescent alcohol use. A meta-analysis of drug and alcohol prevention programs found that "system-wide change" programs were the more effective in preventing overall drug use, including alcohol use, than were classroom-based social influences and comprehensive life approaches (Tobler et al., 2000). Most studies of system-wide change have included a more comprehensive approach, including family and community components (Flay, 2000). The following section summarizes research studies that have used more than one component (e.g., school, family and community strategies) to prevent or reduce alcohol use among adolescents. Where available, results of mediation analyses of these programs are also presented. Mediation analysis explicitly tests the relationship between an intervention's action theory and the conceptual theory upon which it was based (see Figure 1). In the absence of mediation analysis, intervention effects on intervening variables targeted by the program are noted.

2. Comprehensive Preventive Interventions

2.1. *Life Skills Training and the Strengthening Families Program: For Parents and Children 10–14*

The sole curricula-only prevention program that has reported long-term effects on alcohol use is Life Skills Training (Botvin et al. 1990; 1995). This program consists of 3 years of prevention curricula for middle or junior-high school students and includes 15 sessions during the first year, 10 sessions during the second year, and 5 sessions during the third year. The curricula cover drug information, drug-resistance skills, self-management skills, and general social skills. A long-term follow-up study indicated that this program had long-term effects on tobacco, alcohol, and marijuana use through grade 12 (Botvin et al. 1995); however, no alcohol results were reported on in the paper presenting results from 1 year past high school (Botvin et al. 2000). No mediation analyses of this curriculum in regards to its effects on alcohol use have been published, either. The Life Skills Training curricula focus on changes only at the individual level. A recent etiological analysis conducted by the authors of Like Skills Training, however, indicates that individual-level variables only account for a small percent of the variance in alcohol use among adolescents (Griffin et al. 2000). Accordingly, Griffin and colleagues (2000) concluded that classroom-based prevention efforts should be complemented with family, community, and policy initiatives that facilitate change in the larger social environment.

Recently a study was completed that implemented the Life Skills Training (LST) curriculum (Botvin et al., 1995) with a well-researched and successful family program, entitled Strengthening Families Program: For Parents and

Children 10–14 (SFP 10–14) (Spoth, Reyes, Redmond & Shin, 1999; Spoth, Redmond & Lepper, 1999; Spoth, Redmond, Trudeau & Shin, 2002). The first year of the LST curriculum was implemented with seventh grade students. It included 15 sessions and included skill development and knowledge acquisition related to the avoidance of drug use. The curriculum is interactive and includes coaching, facilitating, role modeling, and feedback and reinforcement. The goals of the SFP 10–14 are to enhance parental skills in nurturing, limit setting, and communication, as well as youth pro-social and peer resistance skills. Seven sessions were conducted in the evenings once each week for seven consecutive weeks when youth were in the second semester of seventh grade. The sessions were two hours, the first hour was a separate training for parents and children, and the second hour was a family training session. Ninety-four percent of students participated in the classroom-based LST program, and 38% of eligible families participated in the SFP 10–14 program.

The program was evaluated with a randomized controlled trial (Spoth et al., 2002). Thirty-six randomly selected rural schools were randomly assigned to one of three conditions: 1) LST with the SFP 10–14 program, 2) LST only, and 3) control. The mean Substance Initiation Index score was lowest for the LST + SFP 10–14 condition, next highest score was in the LST condition, and the highest score was in the control condition. For alcohol use initiation specifically, the same pattern was apparent, with the lowest prevalence of new users of alcohol among the LST + SFP 10–14 condition, next highest was in the LST condition, and the highest was in the control condition. However, only the combined condition was significantly different from the other two conditions. These results suggest that adding a family program to a successful classroom program significantly enhances the positive results. The outcome paper for this trial only presented results for the main behavioral outcomes, without any information on intervening variables.

2.2. *Midwestern Prevention Project (Project STAR)*

The Midwestern Prevention Project or Project STAR was not specific to alcohol use but addressed all types of drug use. The intervention consisted of the following five components: 1) a 10-session school program emphasizing drug use resistance skills training, delivered in grade 6 or 7; 2) the school component also included homework sessions involving active interviews and role plays with parents and family members; 3) a parent organization program for reviewing school prevention policy and training parents in positive parent-child communication skills; 4) initial training of community leaders in the organization of a drug abuse prevention task force; and 5) mass media coverage of the program.

The study included eight representative Kansas City communities that were assigned to the full program including all four components or to a comparison program including only the community organization and mass media components. Assignment to full program was not by randomization, but rather based on school administrator's scheduling flexibility. After the first year of implementation, the students who received the full program had significantly lower rates of tobacco, marijuana and alcohol use. The net increase in drug use prevalence among the full program schools was half that of the comparison schools (Pentz et al., 1989). Besides the alcohol and other drug use outcomes, the intervention had a significant effect on intentions, communication skills, friends' reactions to use (perceived norms), and beliefs about positive consequences (expectations from behavior) (MacKinnon et al., 1991). Mediation analyses conducted on the first year outcomes revealed that friends' reactions to use was the most substantial mediator of program effects on alcohol use (MacKinnon et al., 1991). Intentions to use was a marginally significant mediator of program effects on alcohol use. Despite the positive outcomes after the first year, after 3 years, students in the communities implementing the full program had lower rates of tobacco and marijuana use, but not alcohol use (Johnson et al., 1990). The results of the second phase of the study, a replication with a randomized design in Indianapolis, have not been reported (Flay, 2000).

2.3. *Project Northland*

Project Northland was designed to prevent or reduce alcohol use among young adolescents using a comprehensive, multiple component intervention that targeted both the supply of and demand for alcohol. Project Northland was evaluated using 20 school districts from northeastern Minnesota that were randomly assigned to the treatment or control condition. The students participating in the study were surveyed from grades 6 through 12. The intervention was conducted in three stages: a first intervention phase, an interim phase, and a second intervention phase. The first intervention phase, which was conducted when the students were in grades 6 through 8, included: (1) social behavioral curricula, (2) peer leadership and extracurricular social opportunities, (3) parental involvement and education, and (4) community-wide task forces (Perry et al. 1993). At the end of 3 years, a smaller percentage of students in the intervention communities reported drinking or beginning to drink compared with students in the control communities. Furthermore, among students in all districts who at the beginning of sixth grade reported never having consumed alcohol, those in the intervention communities were not only less likely to drink 3 years later but also had lower rates of cigarette and marijuana use (Perry et al. 1996). Besides the behavioral effects, the intervention has significant effects on self-efficacy to resist alcohol use among baseline nondrinkers, family management around alcohol use issues, peer influence (social learning and perceived norms), social normative beliefs, and evaluations of consequences (Perry et al., 1996). Mediation analysis conducted after the first phase of the intervention indicated that the following were important and significant mediators: 1) peer influence to use (social learning and perceived norms), 2) evaluations of consequences, 3) attitudes and behaviors associated with alcohol and drug problems like stimulus seeking, rule violations and bad judgment, and 4) parent-child alcohol-related communications (Komro et al., 2001). In addition, among those students who were non-drinkers at baseline, self-efficacy to refuse offers of alcohol use was a significant mediator.

The interim phase of the study occurred when the students were in grades 9 and 10. During those years, only minimal intervention (i.e., a five-session classroom program) took place, and drinking rates between the treatment and control groups began to converge. In fact, by the end of grade 10, no significant differences existed between the two groups (Williams & Perry, 1998).

In the second intervention phase, when the students were in grades 11 and 12, they were exposed to various interventions, including an 11th grade classroom curriculum, parent postcards, mass media involvement, youth development activities, community organizing and policy development (Perry et al. 2000). As a result of the intensified intervention, the alcohol use patterns of the treatment and control groups began to diverge again by the end of the 11th grade, and the differences between groups were marginally significant for those students who had not used alcohol at the beginning of 6th grade (Williams et al. 1999).

An analysis comparing the trajectories of alcohol use between the treatment and control groups (i.e., a growth curve analysis) was conducted for all three phases of Project Northland. During the first intervention phase, the increase in alcohol use was significantly greater in the control group than in the intervention group. Conversely, the increase in alcohol use was significantly greater in the intervention group than in the control group during the interim phase, when there were minimal program efforts. The students seemed to return to the level of drinking that was normative in their communities. Fortunately, that trend was reversed again during the second intervention phase. During that period, the increase in alcohol use was again greater in the control group than in the intervention group ($p<0.02$), demonstrating the positive and significant impact of the second intervention phase (Perry et al. 2003). In addition, the community-organizing intervention component during the second intervention phase, which focused on community action team-initiated compliance checks of alcohol outlets, successfully reduced the ability of youthful-appearing 21-year-olds to purchase alcohol without age identification ($p=.05$) (Perry et al. 2003).

Because of the positive and significant outcomes of Project Northland, it is now being updated and adapted for a multi-ethnic urban population in Chicago (Komro et al., 2004). There are 61 Chicago public schools participating in a randomized controlled trial to test the effectiveness of the revised Project Northland. The first phase of Project Northland interventions are being updated, adapted and implemented with 6th, 7th, and 8th grade students during 2002–2005. Outcomes of the trial will then be available.

2.4. *D.A.R.E. Plus*

D.A.R.E. Plus was designed to prevent or reduce alcohol, tobacco and marijuana use, as well as violence among young adolescents. The intervention design for the "Plus" components were based on Project Northland and meant to enhance the effectiveness of the D.A.R.E. middle school curriculum (Perry et al., 2000). The D.A.R.E. middle school curriculum provides 10 sessions of skills in recognizing and resisting influences to use drugs and to handle violent situations. It also focuses on character-building and becoming a citizen in our communities. The first and second component of D.A.R.E. Plus is a classroom-based and parental involvement program, entitled "On the VERGE" or "VERGE." VERGE is a four-session classroom program implemented by trained teachers once a week for four weeks. The activities are imbedded in four teen magazines. The classroom activities were primarily led by elected and trained peer leaders, with 5–6 peer leaders for each classroom. The last part of the magazine includes activities for the students to complete with their parents around specific themes. As a follow-up for students, a theater performance was conducted and postcards were sent to 8th grade students that complemented a state-wide tobacco use prevention campaign. As a follow-up for parents, postcards were sent about every eight weeks with short and relevant behavioral messages and with attractive. The third component of D.A.R.E. Plus involved after-school activities for students. Student groups, called youth action teams, were organized at each of the eight D.A.R.E. Plus schools. Students were recruited to participate in these groups to help create widespread normative changes at the school level. Activities were held after school and on weekends. The final component of D.A.R.E. Plus involved neighborhood action teams, which were formed at each D.A.R.E. Plus school to address neighborhood and school-wide issues related to drug use and violent behavior. Eight community organizers were hired to create and facilitate the teams and extracurricular programs in the D.A.R.E. Plus schools.

The study design involved 24 middle schools in Minnesota which were matched on socio-economic measures, drug use, and size, and randomly assigned to one of three conditions: 1) D.A.R.E. Plus, 2) D.A.R.E. junior high curriculum only, or 3) delayed-program control condition (Perry et al., 2003). One group of students formed the study cohort and was followed from the seventh through eighth grade. The behavioral effects of the D.A.R.E. curriculum and D.A.R.E. Plus intervention were evaluated using three student surveys, one baseline and two follow-ups. There were no significant differences between the D.A.R.E. curriculum only compared with the control group. Boys in the D.A.R.E. Plus schools were significantly less likely than boys in the control schools to report current smoking or drinking, and lower levels of violence. Girls in the D.A.R.E. Plus schools were significantly less likely than girls in the D.A.R.E. only schools to report ever being drunk. There were also significant differences between conditions in psychosocial variables with positive and significant effects among the D.A.R.E. Plus group boys compared to the control group boys on: 1) drug-related perceived norms, 2) violence-related normative expectations, 3) access and offers to drugs, 4) tobacco-related outcome expectations, and 5) violence-related outcome expectations. Parent rules around drugs and violence were marginally significant.

2.5. *Seattle Social Development Project*

Unique among the comprehensive programs reviewed so far, the Seattle Social Development Project begins interventions during the early elementary school years and continues through grade six. The purpose of the intervention is to prevent a multitude of problem behaviors, including alcohol use. The intervention spans six years and combines classroom social competence training (in grades 1 and 6), classroom management in-service training for teachers (for grades 1 through 6), and developmentally appropriate parent training programs (in grades 1 through 3 and 5 through 6) (Hawkins et al., 1999).

A quasi-experimental research design was employed with partial randomization to intervention or comparison conditions based on both the school and student (Hawkins et al., 1999; Flay, 2000). At the beginning of the fifth grade, students in the intervention group compared to the control group reported significantly lower prevalence of alcohol use and delinquency (Hawkins et al., 1992). In addition to these behavioral outcomes there were positive and significant differences between the intervention and control groups. Students in the intervention group reported significantly: 1) more proactive family management, 2) greater family communication, 3) greater family involvement, 4) greater bonding to family, 5) higher perceptions of school as rewarding, 6) more attachment to school and 7) more commitment to school. No differences were found between the intervention and controls students on drug-related norms, belief in moral order, or getting into trouble at school.

Students were followed to the age of 18. The long-term effects of the program were positive and statistically significant, with reductions in heavy drinking, violent delinquent acts, and sexual risk taking behaviors. There were no significant effects for lifetime use of alcohol, tobacco, marijuana, or other drug use. In addition, students in the intervention compared to the control group reported more commitment and attachment to school, better academic achievement, and less school misbehavior. Students who received the program only in grades 5 and 6, and not in the early elementary grades, did not have any significant positive effect on their behaviors. These results suggest a long-term program is necessary to maintain changes through high school.

2.6. *Project SAFE (Strengthening America's Families and Environment)*

A similar program that intervened during early childhood with schools and parents is Project SAFE (Kumpfer, Alvarado, Tait & Turner, 2002). Project SAFE combined a classroom program for first grade students called I Can

Problem Solve (ICPS), with the Strengthening Families (SF) program for parents of first grade students. The ICPS program is directed as enhancing problem-solving and critical thinking skills. It includes games, stories, puppets and role playing during 83 30-minute sessions held throughout the school year. The SF program is a 14-session family skills training program, which includes parent skills training, children skills training, and family skills training.

A randomized controlled trial was conducted within 12 schools. Families of first grade students were randomly assigned to one of four conditions: 1) ICPS + SFP (Parent Only), 2) ICPS + SFP, 3) ICPS Only, and 4) Control. Parents, students and teachers were assessed pre- and post-intervention. The findings indicated that the most effective program delivery consisted of the ICPS + full SFP. Significant improvement was observed on all five constructs accepted to be associated with future risk of drug use. These constructs included school bonding, parenting skills, social competence, family relationships, and self-regulation. Actual drug or alcohol use was not assessed because of the early age of the participants. It will be important for a full assessment of this program to follow these young people into their adolescent years to evaluate whether or not the program had an effect on preventing the early onset of alcohol use.

3. Discussion

Preventing drinking among adolescents remains the most difficult drug-related behavior to intervene upon, with few studies finding sustained long-term effects (Komro & Toomey, 2002). The Midwestern Prevention Program and Project Northland are two of the most comprehensive approaches. Yet only Project Northland achieved long-term effects on alcohol use, and only with sustained interventions through high school graduation. The Social Development Project did achieve long-term effects on heavy alcohol use. The Social Development Project intervention included school and parent components and began in the early elementary school years. Similarly, the SAFE Project intervened during early elementary school years, and the short-term results are promising. The inclusion of school and family components were included in each of the effective interventions. Therefore, major themes from this review of complementary programs include the importance school and family components, sustained intervention efforts over multiple years, and intervening early and throughout high school.

These multiple component approaches have had short and some long-term success in reducing alcohol use and some associated intervening variables among adolescents. Table 2 summarizes the results of the comprehensive programs on intervening variables. As can be seen, although these programs have multiple components, there are many important intervening variables, highlighted in the TTI, that are not being targeted by the intervention and/or not being measured in the evaluation. The Midwestern Prevention Program included classroom, family, and community strategies. Yet only four (three

Table 2. Specific multiple component programs and their effects on intervening variables.

Level	Intervening Variables within the Framework of the TTI	Program				
		MPP	PN	DARE	SDP	SAFE
Ultimate	1. Biology & Personality					
↓	a. Personality Characteristics					
↓	b. Intrapersonal Characteristics					
↓	c. Biological Disposition					
↓	2. Sense of Self					
↓	Social Competence				X	X
↓	3. Self Determination					
↓	Social Skills	X				
Proximal	4. Self-efficacy		X			
Ultimate	1. Social Context					
↓	a. Proactive Family Management		X	X	X	
↓	b. Parenting Skills					X
↓	c. Parent Values					
↓	d. Peer Values					
↓	2. Social Learning		X			
↓	Social Bonding					
↓	a. Family Bonding				X	X
↓	b. Family Involvement				X	
↓	c. School Bonding				X	X
↓	3. Motivation to Comply					
↓	Perceived Norms	X	X	X	NS	
Proximal	4. Social Normative Beliefs		X			
Ultimate	1. Cultural Environment					
↓	a. Availability		X	X		
↓	b. Media Exposure					
↓	c. Public Policies					
↓	d. Cultural Values					
↓	e. Neighborhood Characteristics					
↓	2. Knowledge					
↓	Values					
↓	3. Expectations from Behavior	X				
↓	Evaluations of Consequences		X			
Proximal	4. Attitudes					

Note:
MPP = Midwestern Prevention Project included classroom curricula, parent education, family involvement, community organizing, policy development, and media (formal mediation analysis was conducted)
PN = Project Northland included classroom curricula, parent education, family involvement, youth leadership, community organizing and policy development (formal mediation analysis was conducted)
D.A.R.E. = D.A.R.E. Plus included classroom curricula, parent education, family involvement, youth leadership, and community organizing
SDP = Social Development Program included classroom curricula, teacher training in classroom management and parent education
SAFE = Project SAFE included a classroom curriculum, parent education and family involvement
NS = Intervening variable was not affected by program
X = Intervening variable was significantly affected by program
☐ = Intervening variable was not targeted by the intervention and/or not measured in the evaluation

reported in table plus intentions to use) intervening variables were reported on in their report on mediating mechanisms (MacKinnon et al., 1991). However, it seems clear that their programs targeted many more intervening variables, and in all three domains of influence. And the same was found for Project Northland and the D.A.R.E. Plus studies. As presented in Table 1, Project Northland's intervention was designed to target many intervening variables in each of the three domains. The challenge then, appears to be to design a more comprehensive evaluation that can validly measure changes in all of these domains and levels of influence. Such comprehensive evaluation plans are critical to thoroughly evaluate comprehensive programs and their effectiveness, in order to gain a better and more thorough understanding of the complexities and areas of effectiveness in preventing alcohol use among adolescents.

Implementing multiple component interventions and evaluating them requires a great deal of resources (e.g., time, money, and personnel) such that, logistically, they can be challenging to execute. Often it is difficult to determine which component(s) of a multiple component intervention actively contribute to its success (Flay, 2000; Stigler, 2002). It is often assumed that the addition of extra components simply increases the efficacy of the at least minimally effective school-based curriculum that often serves as the foundation of a multiple component intervention (Flay, 2000; Tobler, et al., 2000). Unfortunately however, the research design of most studies of these programs has not allowed for an estimation of the separate effect of each component. Future research should address this concern so that this approach to intervention can be optimized (Stigler, 2002).

From this review of conceptual and action theory related to comprehensive programs to prevent adolescent drinking the following recommendations are put forth. It is recommended that the development of comprehensive programs to prevent adolescent alcohol use include 1) coordinated and complementary intervention components, accompanied by better explanations of how action theory is used to drive these interventions and target multiple intervening variables, 2) measurement of the intervening variables that are being targeted by the intervention components, and 3) thorough analysis of intervening variables, including analyses of mediating mechanisms.

References

Bandura, A. *Social Learning Theory.* Englewood Cliffs, NJ: Prentice-Hall, 1977.

Botvin, G.J., Baker, E., Dusenbury, L., Botvin, E.M., & Diaz, T. Long-term follow-up results of a randomized drug abuse prevention trial in a white middle-class population. *Journal of the American Medical Association, 273*(14): 1106–1112, 1995.

Botvin, G.J., Baker, E., Dusenbury, L., Tortu, S., & Botvin, E.M. Preventing adolescent drug abuse through a multimodal cognitive-behavioral approach: Results of a 3-year study. *Journal of Consulting and Clinical Psychology, 58*(4): 437–466, 1990.

Botvin, G.J., Griffin, K.W., Diaz, T., Scheier, L.M., Williams, C., & Epstein, J.A. Preventing illicit drug use in adolescents: Long-term follow-up data from a randomized control trial of a school population. *Addictive Behaviors, 25*(5): 769–774, 2000.

Chen, H-T. *Theory-driven evaluations*. Newbury Park, CA: Sage Publications, 1990.

Derzon, J.H. A synthesis of research on predictors of youth alcohol, tobacco, and marijuana use. In: *Improving Prevention Effectiveness*, W.B. Hansen, S.M. Giles, & M.D. Fearnow-Kenney (Eds). Greensboro, NC: Tanglewood Research, 2000, pp. 105–114.

Flay, B.R. Approaches to substance use prevention utilizing school curriculum plus social environment change. *Addictive Behaviors, 25*(6): 861–885, 2000.

Flay, B.R., & Petraitis, J. The theory of triadic influence: A new theory of health behavior with implications for preventive interventions. *Advances in Medial Sociology, 4*:19–44, 1994.

Glanz, K., Rimer, B.K., & Lewis, F.M. *Health Behavior and Health Education: Theory, Research, and Practice*. San Francisco, CA: Josey-Bass Publishers, 2002.

Griffin, K.W., Botvin, G.J., Epstein, J.A., Doyle, M.M., Diaz, T. Psychosocial and behavioral factors in early adolescence as predictors of heavy drinking among high school seniors. *Journal of Studies on Alcohol, 61*(4):603–606, 2000.

Griffin, K.W., Scheier, L.M., Botvin, G.J., & Diaz, T. Ethnic and gender differences in psychosocial risk, protection, and adolescent alcohol use. *Prevention Science, 1*(4):199–212, 2000.

Hansen, W.B. School-based substance abuse prevention: A review of the state of the art in curriculum, 1980–1990. *Health Education Research, 7*(3):403–430, 1992.

Hawkins, J.D., Catalano, R.F., Kosterman, R., Abbott, R., & Hill, K.G. Preventing adolescent health-risk behaviors by strengthening protection during childhood. *Archives of Pediatric and Adolescent Medicine, 153*:226–234, 1999.

Hawkins, J.D., Catalano, R.F., & Miller, J.Y. Risk and protective factors for alcohol and other drug problems in adolescence and early adulthood: Implications for substance abuse prevention. *Psychological Bulletin, 112*(1):64–105, 1992.

Johnson, C.A., Pentz, M.A., Weber, M.D., Dwyer, J.H., Baer, N., MacKinnon, D.P., Hansen, W.B. Relative effectiveness of comprehensive community programming for drug abuse prevention with high-risk and low-risk adolescents. *Journal of Consulting and Clinical Psychology, 58* (4):447–456, 1990.

Komro, K.A., Hu, F.B., & Flay, B.R. A public health perspective on urban adolescents. In: *Children and Youth: Interdisciplinary Perspectives*. H.J. Walberg , O. Reyes, & R.P. Weissberg (Eds.). Thousand Oaks, CA: Sage Publications, 1997, pp. 253–298.

Komro, K.A., Perry, C.L., Veblen-Mortenson, S., Bosma, L.M., Dudovitz, B.S., Williams, C.L., Jones-Webb, R., & Toomey, T.L. Brief report: The adaptation of Project Northland for urban youth. *Journal of Pediatric Psychology*, 29(6):457–466. 1994.

Komro, K.A., Perry, C.L., Williams, C.L., Stigler, M.H., Farbakhsh, K., & Veblen-Mortenson, S. How did Project Northland reduce alcohol use among young adolescents? Analysis of mediating variables. *Health Education Research: Theory & Practice, 16*(1), 59–70, 2001.

Komro, K.A., & Toomey, T.L. Strategies to prevent underage drinking. *Alcohol Research & Health, 26*(1): 5–14, 2002.

Kumpfer, K.L., Alvarado, R., Tait, C., & Turner, C. Effectiveness of school-based family and children's skills training for substance abuse prevention among 6–8-year-old rural children. *Psychology of Addictive Behavior, 16*(4S): S65-S71, 2002.

MacKinnon, D.P., Johnson, C.A., Pentz, M.A., & Dwyer, J.H. Mediating mechanisms in a school-based drug prevention program: First-year effects of the Midwestern Prevention Project. *Health Psychology, 10*(3): 164–172, 1991.

National Institute on Alcohol Abuse and Alcoholism. Youth drinking: Risk factors and consequences. Alcohol Alert, No. 37. Washington, DC: National Institute on Alcohol Abuse and Alcoholism, 1997.

Pentz, M.A. Evidence-based prevention: Characteristics, impact, and future direction. *Journal of Psychoactive Drugs, SARC Suppl 1*:143–152, 2003.

Pentz, M.A., Dwyer, J.H., MacKinnon, D.P., Flay, B.R., Hansen, W.B., Wang, E.Y., and Johnson, C.A. A multi-community trail for primary prevention of adolescent drug abuse. *Journal of the American Medical Association, 261*:3259–3266, 1989.

Perry, C.L. *Creating health behavior change: How to develop community-wide programs for youth*. Thousand Oaks, CA: Sage Publications, 1999.

Perry, C.L., Komro, K.A., Veblen-Mortenson, S., Bosma, L.M., Farbakhsh, K., Munson, K.A., Stigler, M.H., & Lytle, L.A. A randomized controlled trial of the Middle and Junior High D.A.R.E. and D.A.R.E. Plus Programs. *Archives of Pediatrics and Adolescent Medicine,157*(2):178–184, 2003.

Perry, C.L., Williams, C.L., Forster, J.L., Wolfson, M., Wagenaar, A.C., Finnegan, J.R., McGovern, P.G., Veblen-Mortenson, S., Komro, K.A., & Anstine, P.S. Background, conceptualization and design of a community-wide research program on adolescent alcohol use: Project Northland. *Health Education Research, 8*(1):125–136, 1993.

Perry, C.L., Williams, C.L., Veblen-Mortenson, S., Toomey, T., Komro, K., Anstine, P.S., McGovern, P., Finnegan, J.R., Forster, J.L., Wagenaar, A.C.,& Wolfson, M. Outcomes of a community-wide alcohol use prevention program during early adolescence: Project Northland. *American Journal of Public Health, 86*(7):956–965, 1996.

Perry, C.L., Williams, C.L., Komro, K.A., Veblen-Mortenson, S., Forster, J.L., Lachter, R.B., Pratt, L.K., Dudovitz, B., Munson, K.A., Farbakhsh, K., Finnegan, J., & McGovern, P. Project Northland high school interventions: Community action to reduce adolescent alcohol use. *Health Education and Behavior, 27*(1):29–49, 2000.

Petraitis, J., Flay, B.R., & Miller, T.Q. Reviewing theories of adolescent substance use: Organizing pieces of the puzzle. *Psychological Bulletin, 117* (1):67–86, 1995.

Spoth, R., Redmond, C., & Lepper, H. Alcohol initiation outcomes of universal family-focused preventive interventions: One- and two-year follow-ups of a controlled study. *Journal of Studies on Alcohol, Supplement 13*:103–111, 1999b

Spoth, R.L., Redmond, C., Trudeau, L., & Shin, C. Longitudinal substance initiation outcomes for a universal preventive intervention combining family and school programs. *Psychology of Addictive Behaviors, 16*(2):129–134, 2002.

Spoth, R., Reyes, M.L., Redmond, C. & Shin, C. Assessing a public health approach to delay onset and progression of adolescent substance use: Latent transition and log-linear analyses of longitudinal family preventive intervention outcomes. *Journal of Consulting and Clinical Psychology, 67*(5):619–630, 1999a

Stigler, M. H. *Teasing apart a multi-component approach to adolescent alcohol prevention: What worked in Project Northland?* Ann Arbor, MI: University of Michigan Dissertation Services, 2002.

Tobler, N.S., Roona, M.R., Ochshorn, P., Marshall, D.G., Streke, A.V., & Stackpole, K.M. School-based adolescent drug prevention programs: 1998 meta-analysis. *The Journal of Primary Prevention, 20*(4):275–335, 2000.

Wagenaar, A, & Perry, C.L. Community strategies for the reduction of youth drinking: Theory and application. *Journal of Research on Adolescence, 4*(2):319–345, 1994.

Wagenaar, A. C., & Toomey, T. *Effects of minimum drinking age laws: Reviews and analyses of the literature.* Prepared for the Advisory Council on College Drinking, National Institute on Alcohol Abuse and Alcoholism, 2000.

Wagenaar, A.C. & Wolfson, M. Enforcement of the legal minimum drinking age in the United States. *Journal of Public Health Policy, 15*:37–53, 1994.

Williams, C.L. & Perry, C.L. Lessons from Project Northland: Preventing alcohol problems during adolescence. *Alcohol Health & Research World* 22(2):107–116, 1998.

Williams, C.L., Perry, C.L., Farbakhsh, K., Veblen-Mortenson, S. Project Northland: Comprehensive alcohol use prevention for young adolescents, their parents, schools, peers, and communities. *Journal of Studies on Alcohol, Supplement 13*:112–124, 1999.

Windle, M., Shope, J.T., & Bukstein, O. Alcohol use. In: *Handbook of Adolescent Health Risk Behavior.* R. J. DiClemente, W. B. Hansen, & L.E. Ponton (Eds.) New York: Plenum Press, 1996. pp. 115–160.

Windle, M., & Windle, R. C. Adolescent tobacco, alcohol, and drug use: Current findings. *Adolescent Medicine, 10*(1):153–163, 1999.

11

Prevention of Adolescent Alcohol Problems in Special Populations

Steve Sussman

Abstract. Research on the prevention of alcohol abuse in America has only recently begun to consider the needs of special populations. This chapter will consider alcohol prevention as a function of four major special population divisions: gender, ethnicity, region (population density), and socioeconomic status. Specific ethnic groups examined will include Hispanics, African-Americans, Asian-Americans, and Native Americans. In general, there is some support for the utility of current alcohol prevention approaches on special populations. Much population-specific work completed to date has not been rigorously designed or evaluated, though it appears likely that partnering with population gatekeepers and showing cultural respect and sensitivity to the population, and providing material that is relevant to the population's adaptation to their environment are essential.

1. Introduction

Minority youth, together with adolescents defined by other sociodemographic characteristics, require special attention from alcohol researchers. In America today, youth from special populations are under-researched, underserved, and poorly represented in alcohol prevention studies. Within the National Institutes of Health, special populations research is becoming a focal point, as illustrated by the significant investment by the National Institute on Alcohol Abuse and Alcoholism in the prevention of teenage alcohol-related problems in special populations.[1] Most often, demographics delineate special populations. Consequently, this chapter considers alcohol prevention as a function of gender, ethnicity, region (population density), and socioeconomic status.

To set the stage for this discussion, the research backdrop for special population research must be articulated. Research on special populations is

Steve Sussman • University of Southern California, Departments of Preventive Medicine and Psychology, Alhambra, California 91803.

sometimes assumed to be needed because of another assumption—that a body of knowledge has all ready been accumulated on general populations, and that this body of knowledge may not apply well or maximally to populations less often studied carefully. This latter assumption may not apply well to the field of alcohol prevention research. The limit of progress in special population work is rendered difficult by the current general status of alcohol prevention knowledge.

Prevention of alcohol abuse has been relatively difficult to effect among substances of abuse.[2] At least five major reasons exist for this quandary. First, ambiguity surrounds information about the dangers of alcohol use. Small doses of alcohol are purportedly healthy, at least among an adult population.[3] Generally, available guidelines suggest that no more than one drink a day for women and two drinks a day for men (12 oz beer, 5 oz wine, 1.5 oz 80-proof spirits) are considered a ceiling of healthy drinking.[3] Arguably any drinking is dangerous for a young teen because it could set up a pattern for heavy drinking as a young adult. Among youth, it is not clear that small doses are injurious although they are illegal. Certainly, larger doses of alcohol may be dangerous particularly while one's nervous system is still in development.[4] Unfortunately, there is a widespread acceptability of alcohol use across many societies alongside a widespread denial that alcohol use is dangerous.[5] As a corollary to this large social climate attitude, relatively few treatment agents will warn youth about the dangers of alcohol use. For example, at present only about 50% of primary care physicians will warn their young patients about the risks of alcohol abuse.[6]

Second, that alcohol use is illegal among youth but not among adults may present alcohol as "forbidden fruit" among teens. Because adults can legally drink, youth may be more tempted to drink than if drinking were not appropriate for anyone. Third, many cultures through use of rituals, special events, specialty shops, or in their mass media, promote use of alcohol as a means of social lubrication, sophistication, or as rites of passage to adulthood. Many movies depict teens drinking to excess and experiencing almost transcendent pleasure.

Fourth, alcohol generally is easy to obtain by teens as well as by adults. It can even be manufactured at home with readily available products. Finally, many researchers popularly assert that different youth are differentially vulnerable to suffering chronic problems with alcohol. Possibly, up to 50% of "alcoholism" has a genetic basis[7], which may be related to relatively early onset and sensation seeking tendencies. From such assertions, some people may assume that a progression of alcohol use among vulnerable persons is intractable. That is, prevention would not be successful. (These assertions run parallel to and separate from other findings that suggest social and environmental variables are largely responsible for delayed initiation of alcohol use; see ref. 4) Even though a blanket of skepticism clouds the progress of alcohol prevention work, such work does and should continue to prevent the consequences that adolescents who drink alcohol may suffer.

2. Consequences of Teen Alcohol Use

Alcohol use results in numerous life problems. Alcohol accounts for two-thirds of substance abuse disorder treatment worldwide,[8] and incurs enormous health care costs due to alcohol use-related accidents or injuries, fetal effects, and diseases such as alcoholic liver disease.[5] Negative effects on one's productivity in society are additional dire consequences of use.

Among youth, these consequences begin with increased tolerance to alcohol and much time sacrificed to obtain and use alcohol. Then, youth who drink may suffer impairments in their social and role functioning. Eventually, youth may begin to desire to control use and find that they are having difficulty doing so, resulting in or related to new problems such as fights, poor school performance, and illegal or dangerous behavior.[9] Serious and fatal consequences can occur with very occasional use. Any high quantity drinking can result in alcohol poisoning. Traffic fatalities are the number one cause of death among adolescents and many are alcohol-related. Alcohol is associated with many other unintentional injuries including drowning, boating accidents, and fire burns.[10] Drinking is associated with violence, including rioting as well as fights and assaults; adolescents who are under the influence of alcohol are vulnerable to assaults, especially sexual assaults. Hangovers are incompatible with schoolwork. Drinking exacerbates depression and alcohol use increases the risk for suicide. Decision making is impaired and may lead to having unprotected sex (e.g., see refs. 10,11,12,13).

Perversely, youth seek out alcohol often to improve social functioning, and then later suffer social consequences related to alcohol use. Youth look to alcohol as an enjoyable distraction and then become preoccupied with its use to the exclusion of other activities. If they become accustomed to using alcohol at an early age, they are relatively likely to suffer the more severe alcohol-related problems in adulthood.[2,5] Many researchers have searched for means to delay youth from using alcohol or prevent youth from abusing alcohol, to try to curb the negative consequences that eventually would result otherwise. Any program that delays the onset or increases in alcohol use also is likely to succeed in interrupting the cascade of increasing risk.

3. Universal Prevention Program Effects

Before examining alcohol use prevention programming among special populations, this chapter first examines what is known about alcohol use prevention, in general. This knowledge sets a limit, perhaps, on what can be discerned among special populations since, by definition, there is less known and available to assist special populations. Numerous types of alcohol use prevention strategies are being attempted. One general type of programming focuses on changes in the alcohol use environment (sometimes referred to as "supply reduction"; see 14). Environmental prevention strategies include traffic safety education, policy mechanisms (e.g., raising the minimum drinking age, alcohol taxation, BAL limits and enforcement, zoning), server training, and community involvement (coalitions, point-of-sales stings, community leader and business involvement, media and family involvement; see 2, 4, 5). Some environmental manipulations, such as use of warning labels and provision of alternative youth activities outside of school may serve to reduce demand for alcohol, as well as potentially limit expose to alcohol. Results of these programs are promising; they have effected decreases in heavy drinking among youth and decreases in numbers of fatal car crashes (see review in refs 2, 15). These various prevention program components attempt to make alcohol use less accessible, less desirable socially, as well as make one's social environment more supportive to nonuse.[2,4,5] These programs are likely to be of relative importance in the prevention of youth alcohol use because alcohol is so widely available to youth, both outside and inside the home (see refs. 15,16).

Alcohol demand reduction programs also have been evaluated. Social influences and comprehensive life skills programs have been considered to be relatively effective demand reduction programs.[17] Social influences programming provides normative information and skill instruction (e.g., corrective prevalence and peer approval norms, awareness of social influences, refusal assertion skill instruction, making a public commitment not to use). The theoretical basis of social influences programming in its simplest form is that inoculation against direct or indirect social pressure to use alcohol will help prevent use when youth enter alcohol use situations. Comprehensive life skill programming subsumes social influence material, and adds life skill information (e.g., problem solving, general social skills, and coping skills). However, some recent empirical reviews and meta-analyses question the clinical significance of programming designed to reduce alcohol use prevalence among teens at a 1-year follow-up.[2,18,19,20,21,22] Even iatrogenic effects have been suggested among those youth who are drinkers prior to program implementation.[22] One suggestion made is that social skills training programs attempt to influence a very narrow range of factors that influence the development of drinking behavior. In particular, these programs are argued to focus on interpersonal factors, whereas correction of erroneous (intra-personal) alcohol-related beliefs, counteraction of widespread acceptability and tolerance of alcohol use, tailoring of delivery to different groups, or multi-faceted modalities of implementation are needed.[20,21]

Very recently, Skara & Sussman[23] examined all school-based alcohol and drug abuse prevention education programs (which may also include family and community involvement) that reported data of at least a two-year follow-up, extending at least from junior high school to high school age. A total of nine social influences or comprehensive life skill studies summarize the total pool of programming that reported longer-term quantitative data on alcohol-specific program effects in that review. Ten other alcohol prevention studies were added here to provide information on all work that provides at least a two-year follow-up. Six of these ten studies do not cross over from junior high school to high school age.[21,25,26,27,28] Four studies do cross over this transition period.[29,30,3132,33] One pioneer, brief pilot study program (3 sessions plus booster activities), that utilized a very small sample of 9th grade youth (91 social influences program participants and 30 controls from one high school), is not reported among this total set of 19 programs (i.e., ref. 34). While a 3-year behavioral follow-up in 11th grade was reported, the sample is too small and limited to include other than as a historical note. (No effects were found at the 3-year follow-up.)

These programs are presented in Table 1. Some of these programs had initial effects that later decayed. At 1-year follow-up, the MMCSHE project found no difference in frequency of drinking but did find a difference in numbers of drinks per sitting (mean difference=.52 drinks). This number-of-drinks effect vanished by the 6-year follow-up. AMPS found an effect at 27-months follow-up only on the baseline "unsupervised use" subgroup (8% of the sample) for which the rate of alcohol misuse was halved compared to the control sample. This subgroup effect disappeared by the last, 4-year follow-up time-point[19,33,35]. Project Northland found effects on weekly use that vanished by the 5-year follow-up, although effects on binge drinking remained. Project ALERT found only a temporary effect on baseline non-drinkers. Finally, Project TND found a 10% relative reduction effect among baseline drinkers on 30-day alcohol use at a 1-year follow-up that vanished by the 2-year follow-up.

A brief summary of these 19 long-term follow-up studies is enlightening. These studies primarily were implemented with young teens at baseline that received a mean of 14.9 sessions of program material. Primarily white youth were targeted in 11 of the studies (ethnicity was not reported in two studies). A total of 13 studies used an experimental design, and 6 were quasi-experimental. A total of 10 studies were social influence-oriented, and 8 studies were comprehensive life skills oriented (i.e., social influences programming plus material on coping skills and communication skills). One other study also included motivation enhancement material along with comprehensive life skill material (Project TND). These 19 long-term follow-up studies involved an average of 3.8 years follow-up. Interestingly, 11 studies demonstrated program effects at final follow-ups. Albeit effect sizes were small, eight studies achieved effects on problematic use, over varying geographic regions.

Though a majority of the studies targeted mostly white subjects, ethnic minorities were represented in several studies. Of the 17 studies that reported ethnicity, 14 included whites, eight included Hispanics, eight included African-Americans, four included Asians, and two included Native Americans, as composing at least 5% of the sample in the study. In addition, 10 of the studies were conducted at least in part in rural areas, and four took a focus on poor youth. Alcohol abuse prevention shows some promise long-term among general and special populations.

4. Special Populations and Alcohol Prevention

Special populations are those which require specially focused attention by virtue of social and historical circumstance, process or elements of culture, or having been significantly neglected in past studies or programs.[1] This section will discuss what is known about alcohol prevention as a function of four special population divisions: gender, ethnicity, region, and socioeconomic status.

4.1. *Gender*

Males are more likely than females to have ever been drunk by 12th grade (65.1% versus 62.2%) and are more likely to report having been drunk in the last 30 days (37.0% versus 28.4%). They are also more likely to consume large quantities in a single sitting.[7] Males also are at greater risk for poor refusal skills, which is associated with greater risk for alcohol use.[36] Conversely, girls may be pressured into drinking by their peers more so than are boys[37] Gender differences have failed to be found regarding alcohol abuse and dependence among teen drug abusers attending drug clinics.[38] Also prevention program findings on alcohol use apply across gender. Many prevention studies did not examine alcohol use results by gender. Rather, gender was not discussed or it was entered as a covariate (adjustment variable). But among those studies that directly examined gender effects, no differences were revealed (see refs. 17, 23, 28, 39, 40). Even so, some specialized prevention studies focus only on delivery to females (e.g., ref. 41), and there may be gender-specific issues that youth would not want to share only with the other gender (e.g., physical maturation).

4.2. *Ethnicity*

Whites are relatively likely to have been ever drunk by 12th grade compared to African-Americans and Hispanics (67.9 versus 40.5% and 63.8%) and are relatively likely to report having been drunk in the last 30 days (37.7% versus 25.5% and 12.0%; ref. 42). Generally, Asian-Americans show the lowest level of drinking among ethnic groups, though notable differences exist between different Asian groups.[1] With great variation across tribes, Native Americans show the highest rate of alcoholism-related consequences among any ethnic group.[43,44] While whites report greater prevalence of alcohol use, alcohol use is understudied among other ethnic groups, and these groups do suffer alcohol-related consequences. Arguably, one may have more confidence in prevalence data on alcohol use among white persons because there is more data about them. The following subsections present the information on alcohol prevention as applied to Hispanics, African-Americans, Asian-Americans, and Native-Americans ethnic groups.

4.2.1. Hispanics. Ethnic minorities are underrepresented in alcohol research, and studies that are completed generally do not consider within (molar) group label variability.[45] For example, in the few prevalence comparison studies completed with Hispanics, Mexican-Americans generally have been found to report higher drinking rates and alcohol-related problems than Puerto Rican or Cuban-Americans.[45] One reason for this disparity in reporting among Hispanic ethnic groups could include differential cross-cultural influences. In particular, Mexican Americans experience easy and proximal travel between Mexico and the U.S., leading to a relatively greater number of communications across cultures. These frequent communications might lead some Mexican-Americans to search for ways to maintain their cultural uniqueness and pride while traveling to and from the wealthier, dominant culture. Inadequate preparation and flexibility in adapting to experiences in both cultures may lead to alcohol use as an escapist means of coping. Interestingly, Cinco de Mayo is a Mexican holiday that celebrates Mexican determination to retain hard-fought independence from invaders. This holiday has achieved greater importance among Mexican-Americans than Mexicans, perhaps because Mexican-Americans may have a relatively greater desire to instill or maintain ethnic pride amidst the presence of the dominant culture. The alcohol industry has responded to this holiday by a promotion that has linked the holiday and "being Mexican" to drinking beer,[46] anecdotally resulting in much drinking occurring on this day among Mexican Americans, particularly males. Not so surprisingly, perhaps, Mexican-American males are at relatively high risk for alcohol-related problems (e.g., Alcoholic Liver Disease), when compared to whites.[47]

Among Mexican-American youth, there appears to be a relation between using the language of the dominant culture (English) and alcohol use. Language-based acculturation measures predict 30-day drinking among Mexican-American youth, including those who are migrant farm children.[32,48] Possibly, these youth that learn English find themselves at a greater emotional distance from their Spanish-only speaking parents. Certainly, acculturation processes are complicated and need continued research.

Some prevention programming developed for Latinos has been delivered to multiple ethnic groups, among which Latinos are a large minority or a majority. For example, Botvin, Schinke and colleagues[29,49] developed a culturally tailored intervention for Latinos and African American youth. This program made use of a professional "story teller" who told mythic stories drawn from African, Spanish, and Greek cultures to relay important social or life skills. Also used were biographies of minority heroes who used their skills to overcome adversity; a rap video that instructs how skills are used in different situations; and peer leaders who assisted adult leaders. This program was compared to standard Life Skills Training (both were 23 sessions long) and an 8-session information-only control condition (IC) at six inner city schools (mean age=12.7 years; n=757 at pretest; two schools per condition), in which 49% were African American and 37% were Latino. Results at 2-year follow-up indicated that youth in the culturally sensitive program (Culturally Focused Intervention; CFI) reported less drinking than those in the Life Skills Training condition, although both conditions reported less drinking and drunkenness than youths in the control condition. Use in the last 30 days was 13% for IC, 10% for LST, and 6% for CFI. This study appeared promising, but the number of schools per condition was small (see Table 1).

Table 1. Long-term Evaluations of Youth Alcohol Prevention Programs

Name of Program Developers	Name of Program	Grade of Subjects at Baseline	Length of Follow-up (years)	Number of Program Sessions	Method-ological Design	Outcomes*	Subject Ethnicity	Region	Type of Program
Botvin et al.	Life Skills Training (LST)	7th	6	30	Exp.	7% monthly drunkenness	91% White	Suburban/ rural NY	CLS; S
Pentz et al.	Midwest Prevention Project (MPP)	6th and 7th	6	15 and comm. support	Quasi-Exp. KS Exp. Ind.	2% last week use; 17% KC, 1% Ind. monthly drunk	77% White, 19% Afr. Am., 2% Hisp.	Urban/ suburban/ rural KS and IN	CSI; S,F,M,SR
Hansen et al.	Adolescent Alcohol Prevention Trial (AAPT)	5th and 7th	5	10	Exp.	Small effect on light drinkers	47% White, 28% Hisp., 16% Asian Am., 2.5% Afr. Am.	Urban/ suburban CA	CSI; S
Flynn et al.	Mass Media and School Intervention (MMSI)	4th, 5th, and 6th	5	22 and media support	Quasi-Exp.	6% drinking beer more than once	96% White	Suburban MT, NY, and VT	SI; S
Shope et al.	Michigan Model for Comprehensive School Health Education (MMCSHE)	6th	6	23	Quasi-Exp.	No effect	94% White	Suburban/ rural Midwest	SI; S
Perry et al.	Project Northland	6th	5	20 and comm. support	Exp.	.09 growth of binge drinking (5+/ 3 weeks)	94.5% White, 5.5% Nat. Am.	Rural Midwest, poor	CSI; S,F,SR
Ellickson et al.	Adolescent Learning Experiences in Resistance Training (ALERT)	7th	5	11	Exp.	No effect	67% White, 10% Hisp., 10% Afr. Am., 8% Asian Am.	Urban/ Suburban/ Rural CA and OR	CSI; S

Loveland-Cherry et al.	Child and Parent Relations Project (CPRP)	4th	4	3 (to family)	Exp.	No overall effect**	86% White	Suburban/ rural Midwest	CLS; S,F
Wynn et al. (Dielman)	Alcohol Misuse Prevention Study (AMPS)	6th	4	17	Exp.	No overall effect	77% White, 13% Afr. Am.	Suburban/ rural Midwest	SI; S
Schinke et al., 2000	Bicultural Life Skills Program (BLSP)	3rd, 4th, and 5th	3.5	15 plus comm. support	Exp.	20% 4+ drinks per week (6% difference)	100% Nat. Am.	Rural ID OK, MT, ND, SD	CLS with cultural material; S,F, SR
Hawkins et al.	Preparing for The Drug Free Years (PDFY)	7th	3.5	5 (multi-media, to parents)	Exp.	16% monthly use; 10% been drunk	100% White	Rural Midwest, poor	CLS; F
Cuijpers et al.	Healthy School and Drugs Project (HSDP)	7th	3	9	Quasi-Exp.	12.7% weekly use; 1 less drink per occasion	?	Holland	CSI; S
Hansen et al.	Tobacco and Alcohol Prevention Program (TAPP)	6th and 7th	3	15	Quasi-Exp.	No effect	60% White, 15% Asian Am., 10% Hisp., 5% Afr. Am.	Urban CA	CSI; S
Sussman et al.	Project Towards No Drug Abuse (TND)	9th, 10th, 11th, 12th; mean of 17 years	2	12	Exp.	No effect	45% White, 42% Hisp, 10% Afr. Am.	Urban/ suburban CA	MSD; S
Botvin et al., 1995	Culturally Focused Life Skills Training (CFI)	7th	2	23	Exp., but 2 schools per condition	CFI=6%, LST=10%, 5% White, 37% Hisp, 49% Afr. Am.	IC=13% alcohol use last 30 days	Urban NYC	CLS with cultural material; S
Botvin et al., 2001	Culturally Focused Life Skills Training-2 (CFI-2)	7th	2	25	Exp., 16 program, 13 control schools	CFI-2=2.2%, Control=5.2% binge drinking, typically	3% White, 8% Asian Am., 24% Hisp, 57% Afr. Am.	Urban NYC	CLS with cultural material; S

Table 1. Long-term Evaluations of Youth Alcohol Prevention Programs

Name of Program Developers	Name of Program	Grade of Subjects at Baseline	Length of Follow-up (years)	Number of Program Sessions	Method-ological Design	Outcomes*	Subject Ethnicity	Region	Type of Program
Elder et al.,	Sembrando Salud	5th to 10th grade	2	8	Exp.	No effect; 5.3% in attention control, 6.8% in program group	100% Hisp.	Urban/ Suburban/ Rural CA, poor	CLS with cultural material; S, F
Schinke et al., in press	Thinking Not Drinking: A SODAS City Adventure (T:S)	8 to 10 years old	2	10	Exp.	46% less likely to be drunk in last month, two program groups; no other alcohol effects (lifetime, 30-day use)	11% White, 30% Hisp, 54% Afr. Am.	Urban NYC, poor	CLS; M (CD-ROM computer-based, urban landscape), F
Telch et al.	Counseling Leadership about Smoking Prevention (CLASP)	9th, 10th, 11th, 12th; mean of 17 years	2	12	Exp.	No effect	45% White, 42% Hisp, 10% Afr. Am.	Urban/ Suburban CA	

Notes. comm. support = community support; Quasi-exp. = quasi-experimental; Exp. = experimental; K.S. = Kansas City' Ind. = Indianapolis; * Outcomes refers to a comparison of relative effects of a program condition with a control condition, generally a difference score; ** refers to a small (0.3) difference in drinks per week over the last year favoring the program condition, for baseline non-drinkers–whereas for baseline drinkers the program appears to exert an iatrogenic effect (1.6 difference in drinks per week over last year); Hisp. = Hispanic; Asian Am. = Asian American; Afr. Am. = African American; Nat. Am. = Native American; initials in Region category refer to the States the study was conducted in; SI = traditional social influences program (refusal assertion focused) and decision making); CSI = comprehensive social influences program (includes public commitment, normative education components); CSL = comprehensive life skills (also includes communication and self-control skill material); ? = information not provided; S, F, M, and SR =school, family, media, and supply components, respectively.

Schinke, Botvin and their colleagues followed this study with the development of an adapted Life Skills Training Program that was much less drastically altered than the prior study version. This newer program subsequently was shown to prevent binge drinking at a 2-year follow-up, targeting African-American and Latinos (as described in the next subsection on African Americans; see refs. 30, 31).

Sussman and colleagues' drug abuse prevention programming with alternative and regular high school youth (Project TND) showed a 10% relative reduction in alcohol use across three randomized trials at a one-year follow-up among baseline drinkers in a sample that is 40% Latino.[40] This project involves only a little cultural tailoring (e.g., names used in activities). However, effects on alcohol use were found to dissipate by 2-year follow-up in one of those trials.[28]

Eisen, Zellman, & Murray[50] provided a 1-year post-program evaluation of the Lions-Quest Skills for Adolescence drug education program. The program was delivered at four program sites [Los Angeles, Detroit (city and suburb), and Washington-Baltimore] to 7,400 6th grade youth in a randomized design. Of these youth, 34% were Latino, 26% were White, 18% were African American, and 7% were Asian. Youth received 40 program sessions over a full school year, which involved building self-competence while becoming a teen, communication skills, mood management, refusal assertion training and managing friendships, and healthy living and being drug-free (e.g., instruction on harm of drug use). No main effects were found on alcohol use compared to a standard care control condition. There was one significant treatment by pretest use interaction. Baseline binge drinkers (drinking 3 or more times in last 30 days) in the program condition were less likely to binge drink at follow-up (27% versus 37%).

Valentine et al.[51] provided a 6-month evaluation of an approximately 10-session student-counseling program among 439 middle and high school youth in Boston (Urban Youth Connection Program). Counseling sessions were provided at the schools to individuals, pairs, or larger groups by graduate student interns (in Education). Contents of the counseling were not specified. No behavioral effects were found among this sample (43% Latino, 42% African American and 12% white), in this quasi-experimental design.

Some alcohol prevention programming has emphasized a specific focus on a Latino culture. For example, La Familia is a community-based alcohol and drug use prevention program that targets Latino families with high-risk youth 6 to 11 years old.[52] The approach involves building protective environments by engaging multiple families in the process of learning healthy lifestyles and how to build "social capital" (i.e., time and energy that adults exert to support each other in reciprocal relationships). In addition apparently the Strengthening Families Program was implemented within La Familia.[53] Parent-child communication, drug education, problem solving, and instruction in community responsibility were emphasized. Approximately 30 sessions of material were delivered to each family. The authors mention that over the two years the program had been in existence, 219 Hispanic youths and 61 families had been enrolled. The program retention rate was 92%. However, over the time of the evaluation only 20 youth had tried alcohol 1–10 times, and none had used alcohol more than 10 times. The behavioral effects of this study are not interpretable given the low prevalence of use, along with lack of a comparison group.

Another Latino-specific alcohol prevention program involves the development of "novelas" (episodics) for youth and their families. Specifically, a TV, radio, and storybook episodic (La Esperanza del Valle) was implemented to improve family communications and youth attitudes about alcohol use. Subjects were relatively poor, rural Latinos in Washington State. Latino rituals (e.g., coming of age ceremony for a teenage girl), appreciating the family as a unit, and cultural values (e.g., Dignidad-self worth, Repeto-value of rituals, Caridad-assisting other Latinos in need, La unidad de familia-family alliance) were included in the novelas, with an overall theme of family bonding and protection. The TV version (telenovela) consisted of 6 22-minute episodes. Airings occurred numerous times over the different communication systems (two TV stations, radio, print). There was a small improvement in alcohol attitude scores after viewing the telenovela among approximately 800 Latino youths 11 to 19 years of age. No behavioral effects are reported.[54]

Litrownik, Elder, and colleagues[32,55] involved 660 Latino migrant families in a randomized design which involved exposure to an 8-session culturally sensitive program (Sembrando Salud) presented by bilingual/bicultural college students (see Table 1). Youth were recruited at 22 schools into 70 total groups. Parents attended three of these sessions, and assisted in helping their children complete relevant homework assignments. Students were taught about tobacco and alcohol consequences, communication skills (listening, speaking, and refusal assertion), and development of parent-child communication skills to support youth decision-making. Cultural values such as familismo and respeto (parental respect) were incorporated into the refusal assertion role plays, and other material, to increase the cultural relevance of the material. This program was compared with one involving learning first aid and home safety. Data were collected at an immediate posttest two months after the pretest, and at one and two year follow-ups. No effects on alcohol use behavior were reported at any time point, and a favorable parent-child communication effect only was reported among families with a relatively small family size.

One other pilot study program (Project HOPE) was delivered to 130 Latino 7th and 8th graders in English as a Second Language (ESL) class[56]. A-12 session drug education and career development curriculum was offered as well as team-building leadership activities and counseling by bicultural specialists. In addition, a 9-session parenting skill workshop and school advocacy for the parents of these youth was offered. A normative data comparison at an approximately 2-year follow-up showed that 11% of the project sample reported alcohol use in the last 30-days compared to 40% of a large normative comparison. However, changes in alcohol use by sample or comparability of samples were not reported. These behavioral data are difficult to interpret.

4.2.2. African-Americans. While heavy drinking is a stereotype that has proliferated about African-Americans (with Ripple or malt liquor in hand), across the life span African-Americans generally show a relatively lower level of alcohol use than whites.[45] Still, among substances of abuse, alcohol is the most abused substance among African American adolescents and adults, and its use may remain stable with increasing age (instead of decreasing as with whites; see ref. 57). Relatively low socioeconomic status, social disorganization, allostatic stresses, and relatively older age have been thought to be most descriptive of continued heavy drinking among African-Americans.

Prevention programming for African Americans has attempted to be culturally sensitive through use of materials that portray African American youth as pathfinders, provide situations that reflect African American contexts, and use language or expressions familiar to the target population[30]. Botvin et al. tested a 25 session version (15 core, 10 booster) of Life Skills Training among a sample of 3,041 baseline 7th grade inner city youth (1,713 that received the program) from 29 schools in New York City. Of these youth, 57% were African American, 24% were Latino, 8% were Asian, 3% were white, and 7% were of mixed or other backgrounds (see Table 1). This curriculum was adapted by depicting African American characters in illustration, modifying role plays to refer to familiar situations, and adapting language. A two-group blocked randomized design was used. Results at a 1-year follow-up indicated small but significant program effects on drinking frequency, drunkenness frequency, and drinking quantity. These effects were statistically mediated by reductions in intention to drink and risk taking. At the 2-year follow-up, effects were maintained on binge drinking (those who typically consume 5 or more drinks on drinking occasion). Approximately, 5.2% versus 2.2% of control versus program youth reported binge drinking.[31]

Four culture-specific substance abuse prevention programs for African-American teens were located in the published literature.[58,59,60,61] For example, Maypole & Anderson's[60] program ("Soulbeat") was developed to complement church and school-based programs and involves participation in plays that dramatizes the problems of drug abuse, peer pressure, parent-teacher relations, and institutional racism, followed by discussion among church members. The only data provided were training data (only 4 of 14 teens attended over half of the five training sessions), and anecdotal reports that church members enjoyed the play and discussion after it.

In Cherry et al.[59], the "NTU" (Bantu African culture word for "essence of life") program had involved 85 5th grade youth in a quasi-experimental design. The program included a "rites of passage," substance abuse prevention, education, and parenting components. The "rites of passage" component involved instruction in principles of Kwanzaa and other Africentric principles (e.g., Heshema-respect for others, Ujima-importance of family, Nia-purpose, and Ujamaa-cooperative economics) in a total of 42 group sessions and retreats, field trips or ceremonies. The substance abuse prevention component involved an average of 10 sessions on drug education. The parenting program involved 6–8 parent education sessions with an additional 5 in-home counseling sessions. While a great deal of programming was offered, only 25% of the youth reported ever drinking wine or beer, and most held negative attitudes toward drug use, at baseline. No significant relative changes on alcohol use were found over a 1-year period. The other two culture-specific programs were family-oriented, emphasized cultural specificity in contents and language, and one contained competency-based skills education; however, neither provided a behavioral outcomes evaluation (see ref. 58, Safe Haven; ref. 61, Project SAFE).

4.2.3. Asian-Americans. There are up to as many as 60 different groups that may be classified as Asian-Americans or Pacific Islanders. Vietnamese-Americans and Japanese-Americans report the heaviest drinking. Fillipino-Americans and Korean-Americans generally report somewhat less heavy drinking. Generally, Chinese-Americans report the lowest levels of drinking[1,45]. There is no simple explanation for these differences. Generally, though, Asian-Americans show a lower prevalence of drinking than other groups, perhaps due to cultural influences, a tendency to exhibit a flushing response, or other factors; and Asian American women show much lighter levels of drinking than the men. Those persons who are subjected to rapid economic growth and changing demands on lifestyle, social isolation, and barriers related to recent immigration are relatively likely to use alcohol to excess.

Little knowledge exists on effective alcohol prevention programming among Asian Americans.[62] Many predictors of drug use are similar across ethnic groups, including peer use and problem behavior[62]. Five prevention programs were located that provided behavioral data on Asian Americans. Project SMART utilized a quasi-experimental design in urban/suburban southern California, and compared exposure to program (there were two types, both generally social influence oriented, combined for this assessment) versus a standard care control condition. Subjects were 5,070 7th graders, of whom 6% were Asian American, 20% were African-American, 31% were Hispanic, and 43% were white. The results at a 1-year follow-up revealed program effects for alcohol use, with relatively strong effects among non-whites compared to whites. For alcohol, the program effect was strongest for Asians, with Hispanics, African-Americans, and whites successively less affected by the program[39]. The effect size on a 3-item index of lifetime and current alcohol use was small, and no numerical measure of mean effect or percentage difference was offered regarding the alcohol ethnicity by condition-type analysis. Two other programs reviewed in this chapter that intervened on multiple ethnic groups including Asian Americans showed effects on drinking (Projects AAPT and CFI-2), whereas two other studies failed to show effects on drinking (Projects ALERT and TAPP; see Table 1). No culturally tailored study was located that focused on alcohol prevention among Asian Americans.

4.2.4. Native-Americans. Great variations in attitudes toward drinking exist across the more than 500 Native American tribes living in the United States today. Some tribes show very low rates of drinking and high disapproval of drinking (e.g., many Southern tribes), whereas others do not (many Northern tribes). Still, Native Americans show the highest rate of alcoholism-related consequences among any U.S. ethnic-racial group, including driving and other accidents and fetal alcohol syndrome.[43,44] Very little empirical data exists to explain differences in drinking among these many tribes, although many theories (e.g., poverty, lack of integration, or hopelessness) continue to be presented.[45] These theories might suggest that non-use of alcohol may lead to depression among youth unless some means of upward mobility or meaningfulness is offered in its place (see ref. 63).

Generalizations about Native American youth are difficult to make. Nonetheless, prevalence of teen alcohol use among these youth may not be higher than among Anglos. However, the amount of alcohol consumed by Native youths on occasions of use is relatively high with worse consequences; and family influences may be relatively important.[1]

At least three comprehensive empirical reviews of alcohol prevention among Native Americans have been written.[64,65,66] Across these three reviews, 26 different studies were located. In 20 of these studies, all subjects were Native Americans. However, only 11 studies included comparison groups and, of them, only five used experimental designs. In addition, half of the studies included sample sizes less than 100. Effects on alcohol use were reported in 13 of these studies, eight of which included comparison groups and four of which involved experimental designs.

All three reviews suggest that including cultural objects and events into programming are means to enhance effectiveness of alcohol prevention efforts. These culturally sensitive efforts include adding traditional songs, dances, ceremonies, and crafts, and involvement of the elders and other community leaders in prevention activities or decision making (also see refs. 67, 68). These efforts can energize core learning or policy change efforts.

In terms of core learning activities, skill enhancement programs show promise.[27,44,69] For example, Carpenter and colleagues (1985) instructed a peer-managed drinking self-control program in a residential high school to 30 at risk youth. Youth were randomly assigned to three program groups, involving incremental amounts of programming (alcohol education, self-monitoring, and self-control). The investigators found decreases in drinking that were maintained over a 1-year period (with breath test validation of self-reports), but no condition differences were revealed between minimal and full program conditions, and no standard care control group was included.

Schinke and colleagues[69] found a small to moderate effect on alcohol use (use in last 14 days rating scale item; means=3.76 versus 4.92 days of use), at a 6-month follow-up, using a 10-session program that focused on bicultural competence skills. This program included 137 12-year old youth from two western Washington reservation sites, comparing program versus control conditions in a small, randomized design. The purpose was to teach youth how to cope with pressures from within the Native American community and within the majority culture. Culturally focused program material included instruction on myths and facts about Indian drinking, involvement of peer and adult tribal speakers, and inclusion of healthful concepts such as "thinking like an elder."

This program influenced development of the Schinke, Tepavac, & Cole study,[27] which studied approximately 1,400 Native American youth, and included a 3 1/2 year follow-up (also see Table 1). Schinke and colleagues used an experimental design (standard care, school-based, school plus community involvement). The skill condition included instruction in Native American legends, values, and stories (15 weekly sessions), and the community condition also involved the school-based program plus community-wide awareness efforts. Core learning activities were derived from Life Skills Training, and included problem-solving, personal coping, interpersonal communication skills, and refusal assertion, all culturally woven. No differences were found between the two intervention arms. Youths in each of the intervention arms showed less drinking at a long-term follow-up compared to the standard care condition (24% versus 30% drinking). This study involved baseline 3rd, 4th, and 5th grade Native American youth (mean age=10 years) from rural schools located in 10 reservations in North and South Dakota, Idaho, Montana, and Oklahoma.

One pilot program (the Seventh Generation—which refers to a "time of healing") developed and evaluated a culturally focused after-school alcohol prevention program for Native American 4th to 7th graders in Denver, utilizing a quasi-experimental design (257 program youth, 121 control youth; ref. 65). The program aimed to correct inaccurate stereotypes about Native American alcohol consumption, enhance values in conflict with alcohol use, provide refusal assertion training, teach decision making, and coach making a personal commitment to not use alcohol. In addition, to enhance Indian identify, Native American values of harmony, respect, generosity, courage, wisdom, humility, and honesty were instructed (e.g., as reflected in the Medicine Wheel), as part of this 18-week program. At a one-year follow-up of this program the program group reported better decision making, less positive beliefs about alcohol use effects, a more positive self-concept, and only 5.6% of the program versus 19.7% of the comparison group, reported drinking in the last 30 days. Pretest differences across groups were minimal.

Another pilot program (Family Circle Prevention Program) took a bicultural educational approach with a strong emphasis on Native American cultural enhancement within the context of family systems education (24-week program; see refs. 65,70). Eight rural schools participated, focusing on nine to 18 year old youth (N = 1,937). A culturally focused school-based substance abuse curriculum was developed and implemented, including instruction in tribal legends, cooperative learning, and building resiliency skills. Classes also included instruction in the Ojibwe Native American language. A community curriculum also was developed and implemented with a family focus. Role modeling a "good way of life" was imparted by involvement of respected community elders, who told stories and instructed youth on how to live like they did. The program emphasized a four-fold message regarding the collective physical, spiritual, emotional and intellectual selves. Instruction in self-esteem building, positive thinking, self-awareness, creation myths, and Native American family values was emphasized. Further, counteraction of a sense of communal powerless was targeted. A pretest-posttest comparison group design was employed, and a school in another community served as a comparison. The program appeared to slow the rise of alcohol use, but no difference was found in perceived likelihood of accepting alcohol from friends, and the adequacy of the comparison group was not well established.

Also, a few empowerment-centered programs have been implemented (e.g., ref. 68), which show effective action to create alternatives to alcohol use (e.g., building a teen center) but provide no data on effects on alcohol use behavior. Little policy, school based, family, or media prevention research exists that demonstrates behavioral effects on Native American youths' drinking behavior[1].

4.3. *Region*

While there have been many fluctuations over the last 10 years, in 2001, lifetime prevalence of alcohol use was higher among 8th graders in relatively low population density areas (Non-MSA=53.5% and Large MSA=49.1%). Likewise, prevalence of ever having been drunk was higher among 8th graders in relatively low population density areas (Non-MSA=26.7%; Large MSA=21.1%). Difference in lifetime prevalence was not evident by 12th grade (Non-MSA=78.9%, Large MSA=79.9%), but reporting having ever been drunk remained higher among rural youth (Non-MSA=66.3%, Large MSA=61.6%). This same pattern of reporting was observed for 30-day prevalence (i.e., in 12th grade; alcohol use in last 30 days=50.0% and 49.7%, and having been drunk in the last 30 days=36.7% and 30.6%, respectively in Non-MSA versus Large MSA areas). Differences were especially pronounced among youth living in rural areas in the North Central region of the country.[42] Thus, there is some evidence of increased risk for alcohol-related problems among rural youth.

D'Onofrio[67] provided a comprehensive review of this arena. Among the problems stated in the review regarding the alcohol prevention literature included disparities in the definition of "rural." At least three have been used: (1) Standard Metropolitan Statistical Area (SMSA) < 25,000 people; (2) non-Metropolitan Statistical Area (MSA), < 100,000 people, with no economic relation with an adjoining central city; or (3) Census Bureau, < 2,500 people outside of urbanized areas. Use of these different definitions led to variation in composition and number of rural regions. For example, 15% to 30% of the U.S. can be considered to be rural depending on which of these three definitions is used[67]. Even given definitional limitations, some generalities have been found across several studies. In particular, common risk factors for alcohol use and abuse exist between urban and rural sites (e.g., peer and family influences, sensation seeking). Relative sparseness of social support and services, combined with economic hardship, may be of relative unique importance in predicting alcohol use in rural areas.

No distinctively rural prevention strategy was uncovered by D'Onofrio[67], in her search of the literature. Four recent studies not in her review also were not tailored for rural areas. A prevention study targeting alcohol prevention among 4406 rural youth in New Hampshire[71] presented a 3-year follow-up that contrasted the Here's Looking at You 2000 school-based curriculum, a Parent Communication Course along with a community task force, and a delayed intervention control. The school-based curriculum was implemented in grades one through 12. Program contents, number of sessions, degree of exposure to the program, or success of follow-up tracking were not located. This study failed to find a program effect on alcohol use. The conclusion of the authors is that by the end of high school most students are drinking regularly, and the only predictor of multiple drunkenness is regular drinking in middle school and early high school.

Another recent outcome study that was implemented among primarily rural white youth was Project Northland. Perry et al.[26] used classroom (a total of 20 comprehensive social influence sessions), parent involvement, peer leader, print media, peer activism and activities (an average of four activities per school), and community task force components over three years of implementation. They did find effects on binge drinking (through use of growth curve analysis), and ability to obtain alcohol, but not on regular drinking. Effects were relatively strong on baseline non-drinkers (see Table 1).

A test of Life Skills Training versus Life Skills Training-plus the Strengthening Families Program (the latter, a 7-session version) recently was completed among 7th graders from 36 Midwestern rural schools (96% white). This was a 3-condition experimental study (LST+SFP, LST only, or standard care control). The study revealed at a 1-year follow-up that Life Skills training showed a 1.5% lower onset of alcohol use, and the combined condition showed an 11% lower onset of alcohol use, than the control condition.[72] Only 38% of eligible families were recruited into SFP. Thus, while the results show potential importance of family-based prevention of alcohol onset, and other meta-analytic work suggests that the SFP program is promising,[19] involvement of families in this programming remains a challenge.

One recent quasi-experimental pilot study (see ref. 72; Families in Action; 43 program participant "graduates") offered 6 2 1/2 hour family sessions to young teens and their parents, involving skill building (decision making, assertiveness, responsibility) and family systems elements. No behavioral data was presented during the one-year follow-up in this rural Michigan sample. However, Pilgrim and colleagues did report a main effect of programming on treatment seeking (talking to counselors), reporting appropriate attitudes regarding alcohol use (by boys only), and reporting improvements in school and peer attachment (for boys only). Parents reported more involvement in family counseling and school activities than did non-participants.

4.4. *Socioeconomic Status*

Lifetime or 30-day likelihood of having been drunk is inversely associated with plans to attend college, but is positively (although weakly) associated with parental education.[42] Alcohol prevention programs have been implemented among youth varying widely in economic background. Prevention program effectiveness has not been found to vary as a function of socioeconomic status in these many studies (e.g., MPP, LST, TND, and AAPT).

Only four published studies (and one in press) were located that reported placing a focus of their alcohol prevention program on economically disadvantaged youth (Werch and colleagues' work, STARS for Families, Preparing for the Drug Free Years (PDFY), Northland, Sembrando Salud, and T:S). Werch and colleagues' STARS for Families program was implemented with 211 economically disadvantaged youth at urban, suburban, and rural schools in northern Florida.[73] This program was developed for middle and junior high school youth (11 to 15 years old), and involved a nurse health care consultation (for youth who are considering being on a sports team at school), key fact postcards sent to parents, and four family take-home lessons. STARS for Families found effects on alcohol use behavior that vanished by 1-year follow-up.

PDFY involved a 5-session multi-media skills-training program for parents of 7th grade, white youth at 33 relatively poor Midwestern rural schools (see ref. 25). Project Northland focused on 20 school districts in Northeastern Minnesota, from poor, rural communities. Northland and PDFY did find effects that lasted several years (see Table 1). Sembrando Salud, presented previously in this chapter, involved Hispanic migrant families and failed to show effects on alcohol use. T:S (see ref.) was CD-ROM based and did achieve effects among poor Hispanic and African American youth on 30-day likelihood of getting drunk. However, this program did not impact 30-day use or lifetime use of alcohol. Since youth were 8–10 years old at baseline, the long-term importance of these results are not clear (see Table 1). None of these programs were developed with material that reflects the perspective or stories of poor people.

5. Summary of the Outcomes of Programs for Special Populations

This section provides a brief summary regarding the status of alcohol abuse prevention among the different populations described in this chapter (aside from socioeconomic status). A total of 16 of the 19 long-term studies (Table 1) contained at least some element relevant for special populations. Also, 18 other studies were not presented in Table 1, but were discussed within specific population sections of the text (five on Hispanics, four on African-Americans, one on Asian-Americans, five on Native Americans, and three on rural regions). Taken together, subsets of these 34 studies were used to generate an overall sense on whether previously developed programming may be impacting on each population.

Regarding Hispanic youth, of 14 studies total, there were 10 studies delivered to mixed ethnic samples (seven of the 19 long-term studies in Table 1 and 3 studies discussed only in the text). Four studies (one in Table 1 and three discussed only in the text) targeted only Hispanics. Seven of the programs that intervened on multiple ethnic groups showed at least 1-year follow-up effects on drinking (Projects AAPT, CFI, CFI-2, Quest, SMART, T:S, and TND). Three mixed-group studies failed to find effects (Projects ALERT, TAPP, and the culturally tailored Urban Youth Connection). Two of the Hispanic-only programs did not report behavior effects (La Familia, La Esperanza del Valle), a third well-designed study failed to find effects (Sembrando Salud), and a fourth program's effects were not interpretable (Project HOPE).

Regarding African-American youth, there were 11 studies delivered to mixed ethnic samples (eight of the 19 long-term studies in Table 1 and 3 studies in the text). Four studies (in the text) targeted only African-Americans. Seven programs that intervened on multiple ethnic groups showed at least 1-year follow-up effects on drinking (CFI, CFI-2, MPP, Quest, SMART, T:S, and TND). Four mixed-group studies failed to find effects (Projects ALERT, TAPP, AMPS, and the Urban Youth Connection). Four African-American only programs were located (Soulbeat, NTU, Safe Haven, and Project SAFE), but behavioral outcome data were provided in only one of them (NTU), failing to find effects on alcohol use.

Regarding Asian-American youth, there were 5 studies that were delivered to mixed ethnic samples (four of the 17 long-term studies in Table 1 and one study in the text), and no studies that targeted only Asian-Americans. Three programs that intervened on multiple ethnic groups showed effects on drinking at a 1-year follow-up (Projects AAPT, CFI-2, and SMART). Two mixed-group studies failed to find effects (Projects ALERT and TAPP).

Regarding Native American youth, among the studies discussed specifically in the chapter, one study involved a mixed ethnic sample (one of the 19 long-term studies in Table 1), and 6 studies that targeted only Native-Americans (one of which is also in Table 1). One program that intervened on multiple ethnic groups may have exerted effects on drinking among Native Americans (Project Northland, although the Native American sample was too small to analyze program effects as a function of white versus Native American ethnicity; refs. 4,26). Two small-sampled culturally tailored Native American focused pilot studies reported finding effects (see refs. 69,76), and two did not report data on behavioral effects.[68,70] One quasi-experimental trial of culturally-focused programming (Seventh Generation) found strong effects at a 1-year follow-up on 30-day alcohol use.[65] Also, one recent large experimental trial that focused on Native Americans showed a 20% relative reduction in recent alcohol use over a 3 1/2 follow-up period (see ref. 27), using a bi-culturally enhanced life skills training approach. Overall, little rigorously designed research on alcohol prevention has been completed with Native Americans.

Regarding rural region, seven studies were delivered in multiple regions that included rural regions (Projects CPRP, LST, MPP, ALERT, AMPS and MMCSHE in Table 1, and STARS for Families, in the text). Six studies were delivered only in rural regions [Northland, BLSP (for Native Americans), and PDFY in Table 1, and HLY2000 (see ref. 71), SFP+LST, and Families in Action, in the text]. In the rural regions-focused programming, however, rural-tailored materials were not developed. Among these 13 studies, seven programs showed effects on drinking at a 1-year follow-up (Projects BCSP, CPRP, LST, LST+SFP, MPP, Northland, and PDFY). Five studies failed to find lasting effects (Projects ALERT, HLY2000, MMCSHE, STARS for Families, ref. 71). One pilot study did not report behavioral data (Families in Action). Alcohol prevention programming as currently developed appears applicable for rural populations, though no rural-specific program has been evaluated.

5.1. *Summary of the Summary*

These studies also can be examined using "study" as a single, exchangeable unit, to explore effects on alcohol use at a 1-year follow-up. For Hispanics, 12 of 14 programs reported behavioral data. Of the 12 programs, 58% found preventive effects. For African-Americans, 12 of 15 programs reported behavioral data. Of these 12 programs, 58% found preventive effects. For Asian Americans, all five programs reported behavioral data and 60% of the programs found preventive effects. For Native Americans, five of 7 programs reported behavioral effects. All five programs found preventive effects. Finally, 58% of the programs conducted at least in part in rural regions showed preventive effects (12 of 13 programs reported behavioral data). The pattern of these findings suggests that approximately 60% of currently developed alcohol prevention programming show effects on the alcohol use behaviors of different special populations. Programs that include provision of bicultural education along with life skill material appear to be particularly promising.

Most of these 34 studies were school-based, though 15 involved family involvement or took a family-focus (MPP, Northland, BLSP, La Familia, Sembrando Salud, Soulbeat, NTU, Safe Haven, Project SAFE, Family Circle Prevention Program, HLY2000, LST+SFP, STARS for Families, T:S, and PDFY). In addition, five studies actively involved visual, auditory, or print media (MPP, La Esperanza del Valle, Northland, PDYF, and T:S). Finally, four programs also emphasized environmental strategies (MPP, Northland, BLSP, and Stiver's program).[68]

6. Future Research Needs

The impetus for studying special populations stems from health disparities. Minority groups, females, those in rural regions, those who are relatively poor, are persons for whom relatively less is known (etiology), less has been developed (effective prevention programming), and less has been delivered (reduced access or reach). By definition, etiology, prevention development, and implementation-related research are needed on special populations.

6.1. *Etiology*

When studies have examined the predictors of problem drinking, generally the same protective and risk factors operate across gender, ethnicity, region, and socioeconomic status (e.g., ref. 77). Relatively low expectations for success, low self-esteem, hopelessness, peer use, family use or tolerance of use, low school achievement, stress, tolerance of deviance, perceived availability and safety of alcohol, and lack of involvement in adult-supervised, pro-social activities predict drinking across groups. However, as presented previously in this review, their relative impact may differ as a function of the subject population (e.g., males have relatively worse refusal assertion skills than females). Also, currently used variables explain a lower percentage of the variance in the behavior of special populations than mainstream populations[78]. Importantly, there are some unique variables that should be considered. For example, ethnic pride may be important as a predictor (protective variable) of drinking in disadvantaged ethnic groups. A recent study found that ethnic identity (e.g., having a lot of pride in one's ethnic group and its accomplishments) moderated the effects of social skills on alcohol use. Also, in another statistical model in that study containing perceived competence (e.g., self-management and persistence) and ethnic identity as predictors, ethnic identity directly and inversely predicted alcohol use among a sample of young minority adolescents. In this sample, 60% were African-American and 40% were Latino[79].

Another consideration is that delineation of special populations is certain to change over time, as recognition of lack of access on the basis of different population groupings, or as changes in the social-geographical climate, come to pass. For example, most drug abuse prevention work has been completed with general population, middle school youth. Only a few researchers have investigated older teens that may be potential dropouts among a regular high school population, attending alternative schools, or otherwise are at the peak age for drug experimentation. Certainly, issues pertaining to formal education and work aspirations, family creation, and increasing self-identification with an alcohol-centered lifestyle, are of relative importance for the study of older teens. They may become formally recognized as a special population in the near future.[80]

6.2. *Prevention*

Social influences programming or comprehensive life skills training is considered the most effective programming currently available, and may be relatively effective for minority youth compared to whites.[17] However, as previously mentioned, the effectiveness of this programming on alcohol use is relatively weak compared with other drugs[2]. Also, most drug abuse prevention research has been conducted with white majority populations. For example, in Tobler and colleagues'[17] review of 207 drug abuse prevention program studies, only 42 studies involved greater than a 50% non-white majority (20% of the studies). Much research is needed on the prevention of alcohol use among special populations.

Since alcohol use is relatively widely available to youth, among drugs of abuse, there is a great need to evaluate further the effects of supply reduction approaches in special populations. Both nondiscriminatory policies and empowerment motives may be important mediators of the effects of these types of programs. In addition, it is not clear why culturally focused components added to effective demand reduction programs increase their efficacy. Potential mediators (e.g., increased receptivity versus increased ethnic pride) should be examined. Clearly, much more research is needed among minority populations both in mixed-ethnic group settings, and in mono-ethnic settings.

At this point in time, it is not clear what would be the most effective composition of ethnic group-oriented programming. One possibility is that deep structure culturally appropriate programming,[53] which considers critical values and traditions of a culture in specific social sectors, might be most effective. However, almost none of this type of programming has provided an evaluation of behavioral effects. A second possibility is that surface structure culturally appropriate programming, which considers and adapts graphic material and names, as examples, is sufficient to make ethnic-oriented programming maximally effective.[53] Current evaluations of such programming are promising (e.g., see refs. 30,31). One caveat is that there may be a tendency for implementers to add ethnic-specific elements of programming, while reducing the dosage provided of the evidence-based program material. This change in the programmatic soup's ingredients could reduce the program's overall effectiveness.[53]

A third possibility is that generic programming is relatively effective in the prevention of alcohol use, that interactive contents permit incorporation of ethnic-specific features.[78] Indeed, in any given community, diversity exists among members of ethnic groups and between ethnic groups, and sensitivity to each other's differences may be imperative to mobilize unifying action that prevents alcohol use. If a program can't address all groups involved in the programming, then perhaps a more generic form is needed. It would appear that generic programming is effective across gender, ethnicity, socioeconomic status, and region. Regarding any special population, a direct test of these three program formulations (deep structure, surface structure, or generic) has not yet been completed.

Also, most programs described have been delivered to young teens. Considerably more work should be entertained with preteen youth that involves long enough follow-ups to detect alcohol behavioral effects, as well as with older teens, and young adults. Programming for older teens as a new special population category needs continued thought. They tend to reject some of the strategies employed with young teens (e.g., refusal assertion training), and are more self-motivated than is assumed within social influence-type programming.[80] A different model of programming is needed. One such model is illustrated in Project TND. It might be referred to as a motivation-skills-decision model. Youths' motivations are harnessed against alcohol abuse. They learn that (a) they don't have to yield to stereotypes of others and use alcohol, (b) they learn to place partly-formed specific self-attitude ratings within a more general self-rating as a moderate, and (c) they learn to value their health as a means to achieving life goals. Youths are provided with skills to change, including (a) effective listening, (b) effective communication skills, and (c) self-control skills. Finally, youth learn to make a decision about their behavior, based on motivation, skills and consequences information. Consequences information includes (a) myths people hold about drug use, (b) the insidious nature of life consequences of alcohol abuse, and (c) the effects of alcohol abuse on others. Motivation and skills material is integrated by use of a decision-making process. While effects of TND are promising (i.e., 9% relative reduction of alcohol use has been observed across three experimental trials), effects do dissipate by two-year follow-up. Possibly, a mix of both prevention and cessation material are needed to maintain program effects among older teens.[28] Consideration of other special population types adds complexity, as these special populations might cross in various ways (e.g., poor rural African American older teens), and a wide spectrum of continued work is demanded.

6.3. *Implementation and Diffusion*

Ethnic minorities have relatively less access to effective programs,[78] as do poor sectors of society and rural populations.[67] Certainly, even with good contents, without the ability to reach a special population, programming will not be of any practical assistance. Funds are needed to be able to offer the programming, and institutionalization of programming is needed to be able to keep programming going a long time. Also, without ethnic-minority representation in program development or delivery, the target group may not be receptive to the program, and implementation will fail as well.[78] Very little implementation and dissemination research has been conducted on any drug (with any population) including alcohol use.[81]

7. Conclusions

Special population research is in its infancy. Consideration of unique variables relevant to gender (e.g., sex roles, hormonal expression), ethnic group (e.g., skin color, acculturation, discrimination, active coping), region (e.g., low density of institutional units, transportation issues), and socioeconomic factors (e.g., poverty, survival, crime) are needed to provide a more thorough assessment of etiologic factors. Participatory research involving extensive involvement of members of the special population is needed to make programming palatable, if not more effective, for its members. Consideration of how to make programming fresh and "hard wired" to special population delivery systems is needed. Certainly, a reconsideration of appropriate and inappropriate patterns of drinking is needed across groups to delineate more safe patterns of intake, or promote temperance.

ACKNOWLEDGMENTS: This study was supported by the Research Center for Alcoholic Liver and Pancreatic Diseases (P50 AA11999) funded by the National Institute on Alcohol Abuse and Alcoholism, and by grants from the National Institute on Drug Abuse (DA01070, DA07601, DA13814, and DA16094.

References

1. NIAAA: Report of a subcommittee of the National Advisory Council on Alcohol Abuse and Alcoholism on the review of the extramural research portfolio for prevention. 1998, Washington, D.C.: U.S. DHHS.
2. Komro KA, Toomey TL: Strategies to prevent underage drinking. *Alcohol Research & Health,* 26:5–14, 2002.
3. Dufour MC: What is moderate drinking?: Defining "drinks" and drinking levels. *Alcohol Research & Health,* 23:5–14, 1999.
4. Williams CL, Perry CL: Lessons from Project Northland: Preventing alcohol problems during adolescence. *Alcohol Research & Health,* 22:107–116, 1998.
5. Hansen WB: Prevention of alcohol use and abuse. *Preventive Medicine,* 23:683–687, 1994.
6. Millstein SG, Marcell AV: Screening and counseling for adolescent alcohol use among primary care physicians in the United States. *Pediatrics,* 111:114–122, 2003.
7. Gordis E: Contributions of behavioral science to alcohol research: Understanding who is at risk and why. *Experimental and Clinical Psychopharmacology,* 8:264–270, 2000.
8. Sussman S, Ames SL: *The social psychology of drug abuse.* Buckingham, GB: Open University Press, 2001.
9. Martin CS, Winters KC: Diagnosis and assessment of alcohol use disorders among adolescents. *Alcohol Research & Health,* 22:95–105, 1998.
10. Sussman S, Dent CW, Stacy AW, Burton D, Flay BR: Psychosocial variables as prospective predictors of violent events among adolescents. *Health Values,* 18: 29–40, 1994.
11. Molina B, Donovan J. (in press). High risk adolescents and young adult populations-Consumption and consequences. In: Marc Galanter (Ed.), Recent developments in alcoholism. Volume 17. Research on alcohol problems in adolescents and young adults. An official publication of the ASAM and the RSA. New York: Kluwer.
12. Tapert S: Cognitive and neuroimaging studies of the effects of chronic heavy drinking in adolescents. In: Marc Galanter (Ed.), Recent developments in alcoholism. Volume 17. Research on alcohol problems in adolescents and young adults. An official publication of the ASAM and the RSA. New York: Kluwer, (in press).
13. Windle M: Alcohol consumption and its consequences among adolescents and young adults. In: Marc Galanter (Ed.), Recent developments in alcoholism. Volume 17. Research on alcohol problems in adolescents and young adults. An official publication of the ASAM and the RSA. New York: Kluwer, (in press).
14. Pentz MA, Bonnie RJ, Shopland DR: Integrating supply and demand reduction strategies for drug abuse prevention. *American Behavioral Scientist,* 39: 87–910, 1996.
15. Wagenaar A: Environmental change to reduce underage drinking. In: Marc Galanter (Ed.), Recent developments in alcoholism. Volume 17. Research on alcohol problems in adolescents and young adults. An official publication of the ASAM and the RSA. New York: Kluwer, (in press).
16. Perry CL, Komro K: Comprehensive approaches to prevent adolescent drinking and related problems. In: Marc Galanter (Ed.), Recent developments in alcoholism. Volume 17. Research on alcohol problems in adolescents and young adults. An official publication of the ASAM and the RSA. New York: Kluwer, (in press).

17. Tobler NS, Roona MR, Ochshorn P, Marshall DG, Streke AV, Stackpole KM: School-based adolescent drug prevention programs: 1998 Meta-analysis. The *Journal of Primary Prevention*, 20:275–336, 2000.
18. Foxcroft DR, Lister-Sharp D, Lowe G: Alcohol misuse prevention for young people: A systematic review reveals methodological concerns and lack of reliable evidence of effectiveness. *Addiction*, 92:531–537, 1997.
19. Foxcroft DR, Ireland D, Lister-Sharp D, Lowe G, Breen R: Longer-term primary prevention for alcohol misuse in young people: A systematic review. *Addiction*, 98:397–411, 2003.
20. Gorman DM: Do school-based social skills training programs prevent alcohol use among young people? *Addiction Research*, 4:191–210, 1996.
21. Gorman DM, Speer PW: Preventing alcohol abuse and alcohol-related problems through community interventions: A review of evaluation studies. *Psychology and Health*, 11:95–131, 1996.
22. Werch CE, Owen DM: Iatrogenic effects of alcohol and drug prevention programs. *Journal of Studies on Alcohol*, 63:581–590, 2002.
23. Skara SN, Sussman S: A review of 25 long-term adolescent tobacco and other drug use prevention program evaluations. *Preventive Medicine*, 37:415–474, 2003.
24. Loveland-Cherry CJ, Ross LT, Kaufman SR. Effects of a home-based family intervention on adolescent alcohol use and misuse. *Journal of Studies on Alcohol-Supplement*, 13:94–102, 1999.
25. Park J, Kosterman R, Hawkins JD, Haggerty KP, Duncan TE, Duncan SC, Spoth R: Effects of the "Preparing for the Drug Free Years" curriculum on growth in alcohol use and risk for alcohol use in early adolescence. *Prevention Science*, 1:125–138, 2000.
26. Perry CL, Williams CL, Komro KA, Veblen-Mortenson S, Stigler MH, Munson KA, Farbakhsh K, Jones RM, Forster JL: Project Northland: Long-term outcomes of community action to reduce adolescent alcohol use. *Health Education Research: Theory & Practice*, 17:117–132, 2002.
27. Schinke SP, Tepavac L, Cole KC: Preventing substance use among Native American youth. *Addictive Behaviors*, 25:387–397, 2000.
28. Sussman S, Sun P, McCuller WJ, Dent CW: Project Towards No Drug Abuse: Two year outcomes of a trial that compares health educator delivery to self-instruction. *Preventive Medicine* 37:155–162, 2003.
29. Botvin GJ, Schinke SP, Epstein JA, Diaz T, Botvin EM: Effectiveness of culturally focused and generic skills training approaches to alcohol and drug abuse prevention among minority adolescents: Two-year follow-up results. *Psychology of Addictive Behaviors*, 9:183–194, 1995.
30. Botvin GJ, Griffin KW, Diaz T, Ifill-Williams M: Drug abuse prevention among minority adolescents: Posttest and one-year follow-up of a school-based preventive intervention. *Prevention Science*, 2:1–14, 2001a.
31. Botvin GJ, Griffin KW, Diaz T, Ifill-Williams M: Preventing binge drinking during adolescence: One- and two-year follow-up of a school-based preventive intervention. *Psychology of Addictive Behaviors*, 15:360–365, 2001b.
32. Elder JP, Litrownik AJ, Slymen DJ, Campbell NR, Parra-Medina D, Choe S, Lee V, Ayala GZ: Tobacco and alcohol use-prevention program for Hispanic migrant adolescents. *American Journal of Preventive Medicine*, 23:269–275, 2002.
33. Wynn SR, Schulenberg J, Kloska DD, Laetz VB: The mediating influence of refusal skills in preventing adolescent alcohol misuse. *Journal of School Health*, 67:390–395, 1997.
34. Duryea EJ, Okwumabua JO: Effects of a preventive alcohol education program after three years. *Journal of Drug Education*, 18:23–31, 1988.
35. Dielman T: School-based research on prevention of adolescent alcohol use and misuse: Methodological issues and advances. *Journal of Research on Adolescence*, 4:271–293, 1994.
36. Scheier S, Botvin GJ, Diaz T, Griffin KW: Social skills, competence, and drug refusal efficacy as predictors of adolescent alcohol use. *Journal of Drug Education*, 29:251–278, 1999.
37. Bevitt-Mills J: Gender differences in prevention strategies targeted to female adolescents. Paper presentation at the 129th Annual Meeting of the APHA, Atlanta, Georgia, 2001.

38. Opland EA, Winters KC, Stinchfield RD: Examining gender differences in drug-abusing adolescents. *Psychology of Addictive Behaviors*, 9:167–175, 1995.
39. Graham JW, Johnson CA, Hansen WB, Flay BR, Gee M: Drug use prevention programs, gender, and ethnicity: Evaluation of three seventh-grade Project SMART cohorts. *Preventive Medicine*, 19:305–313, 1990.
40. Sussman S, Dent CW, StacyAW: Project Towards No Drug Abuse: A review of the findings and future directions. *American Journal of Health Behavior*, 26:354–365, 2002.
41. Weiss F, Nicholson H: Friendly PEERsuation against substance use: The Girls Incorporated model and evaluation. *Drugs and Society*, 12:7–22, 1998.
42. Johnston LD, O'Malley PM, Bachman JG: National survey results on drug use from the Monitoring the Future Study, 1975–2001. Volumes 1 and 2. Rockville, MD: U.S.DHHS (NIH Publication No. 02–5106 & 02–5107), 2002.
43. Beauvais F: American Indians and alcohol. *Alcohol Research & Health*, 22:253–259, 1998.
44. Schinke S: Behavioral approaches to illness prevention for Native Americans. In: PM. Kato, T. Mann (Eds.), Handbook of diversity issues in health psychology. New York: Plenum Press, 1996.
45. Caetano R., Clark CL, Tam T: Alcohol consumption among racial/ethnic minorities: Theory and research. *Alcohol Research & Health*, 22:233–241, 1998.
46. De Lucio-Brock A: Our culture is not for sale. *Prevention Tactics*, 7: www.emt.org/publications, 2003
47. Sussman S, Dent CW, Skara S, deCalide P, Tsukamoto H: Alcoholic Liver Disease (ALD): A new domain for prevention efforts. *Substance Use & Misuse*, 37:1887–1904, 2002.
48. Lovato CY, Litrownik AJ, Elder J, Nunez-Liriano A, Suarez D, Talavera GA: Cigarette and alcohol use among migrant Hispanic adolescents. *Family and Community Health*, 16:18–31, 1994.
49. Forgey MA, Schinke S, Cole K: School-based interventions to prevent substance abuse among inner-city minority adolescents. In: DK Wilson, JR Rodriguez, WC Taylor (Eds.), Health-promoting and health-compromising behaviors among minority adolescents. Washington, D.C.: APA., pps 251–267, 1997.
50. Eisen M, Zellman GL, Murray DM: Evaluating the Lions-Quest "Skills for Adolescence" drug education program: Second-year behavior outcomes. *Addictive Behaviors*, 28:883–897, 2003.
51. Valentine J, Gottlieb B, Keel S, Griffith J, Ruthazer R: *The Journal of Primary Prevention*, 18:363–387, 1998.
52. Hernandez LP, Lucero E: DAYS La Familia community drug and alcohol prevention program: Family-centered model for working with inner-city Hispanic families. *The Journal of Primary Prevention*, 16:255–272, 1996.
53. Kumpfer KL, Alvarado R, Smith P, Bellamy N: Cultural sensitivity and adaptation in family-based prevention interventions. *Prevention Science*, 3:241–246, 2002.
54. Lalonde B, Rabinowitz P, Shefsky ML, Washienko K: La Esperanza del Valle: Alcohol prevention novelas for hispanic youth and their families. *Health Education Research*, 24:587–602, 1997.
55. Litrownik AJ, Elder JP, Campbell NR, Ayala GX, Slymen DJ, Parra-Medina D, Zavala FB, Lovato CY: Evaluation of a tobacco and alcohol use prevention program for Hispanic migrant adolescents: Promoting the protective factor of parent-child communication. *Preventive Medicine*, 31:124–133, 2000.
56. Stephenson JF, McMillan B, Mitchell RE, Blanco M: Project HOPE: Altering risk and protective factors among high risk Hispanic youth and their families. The *Journal of Primary Prevention*, 18:287–317, 1998.
57. Henderson G, Ma GX, Shive SE: African American substance users and abusers. In: GX Ma, G Henderson (Eds.): Ethnicity and substance abuse: Prevention and intervention. Springfield, Illinois: Charles C. Thomas, 2002.
58. Aktan FB: A cultural consistency evaluation of a substance abuse prevention program with inner city African-American families. *The Journal of Primary Prevention*, 19:227–239, 1999.

59. Cherry VR, Belgrave FZ, Jones W, Kennon K, Gray FS, Phillips F: NTU: An Africentric approach to substance abuse prevention among African American youth. *The Journal of Primary Prevention,* 18:319–339, 1998.
60. Maypole DE, Anderson RB: Culture-specific substance abuse prevention for Blacks. *Community Mental Health Journal,* 23:135–139, 1987.
61. Van Hasselt VB, Hersen M, Null JA, Ammerman RT, Bukstein OG, McGillivray J, Hunter A: Drug abuse prevention for high-risk African American children and their families: a review and model program. *Addictive Behaviors,* 18:213–234, 1993.
62. Harachi TW, Catalano RF, Kim S, Choi Y: Etiology and prevention of substance use among Asian American youth. *Prevention Science,* 2:57–65, 2001.
63. Moran JR: Preventing alcohol use among urban American Indian youth: The seventh generation program. *Journal of Human Behavior in the Social Environment,* 2:51–67, 1999.
64. May P, Moran J: Prevention of alcohol misuse: A review of health promotion efforts among American Indians. *American Journal of Health Promotion,* 9:288–298, 1995.
65. Moran JR, Reaman JA: Critical issues for substance abuse prevention targeting American Indian youth. *The Journal of Primary Prevention,* 22:201–233, 2002.
66. Parker-Langley L: Alcohol prevention programs among American Indians: Research findings and issues. In: P.D. Mail, S. Heurtin-Roberts, S.E. Martin, J. Howard (Eds.), Alcohol use among American Indians and Alaska Natives. Bethesda, MD: U.S. DHHS. (NIAAA Research Monograph #37) 2002.
67. D'Onofrio CN: The prevention of alcohol use by rural youth. In: Rural substance abuse: State of knowledge and issues. Rockville, MD: NIDA Research Monograph, Number 168, 1997.
68. Stivers C: Drug prevention in Zuni, New Mexico: Creation of a teen center as an alternative to alcohol and drug use. *Journal of Community Health,* 19:343–359, 1994.
69. Schinke S, Orlandi M, Botvin G, Gilchrist L, Trimble JE, Locklear VS: Preventing substance abuse among American-Indian adolescents: A bicultural competence skills approach. *Journal of Counseling Psychology,* 35:87–90, 1988.
70. Van Stelle KR, Allen GA, Moberg DP: Alcohol and drug prevention among American Indian families: The Family Circles Program. *Drugs & Society,* 12:53–60, 1998.
71. Stevens MM, Mott LA, Youells F: Rural adolescent drinking behavior: Three year follow-up in the New Hampshire substance abuse prevention study. *Adolescence,* 31, 159–1661996.
72. Spoth RL, Redmond C, Trudeau L, Shin C: Longitudinal substance initiation outcomes for a universal preventive intervention combining family and school programs. *Psychology of Addictive Behaviors,* 16:129–134, 2002.
73. Pilgram C, Abbey A, Hendrickson P, Lorenz S: Implementation and impact of a family-based substance abuse prevention program in rural communities. *The Journal of Primary Prevention,* 18:341–361, 1998.
74. Werch CE, Pappas DM, Carlson JM, DiClemente CC: Short- and long-term effects of a pilot prevention program to reduce alcohol consumption. *Substance Use & Misuse,* 33:2303–2321, 1998.
75. Schinke SP, Schwin TM, Ozanian AJ: Alcohol abuse prevention among high-risk youth via computer-based intervention. *Journal of Prevention and Intervention in the Community.* (in press).
76. Carpenter RA, Lyons CA, Miller WR: Peer-managed self-control program for prevention of alcohol abuse in American Indian high school students: A pilot evaluation study. *International Journal of the Addictions,* 20:299–310, 1985.
77. Costa FM, Jessor R, Turbin MS: Transition into adolescent problem drinking: The role of psychosocial risk and protective factors. *Journal of Studies on Alcohol,* 60: 480–490, 1999.
78. Dent CW, Sussman S, Ellickson P, Brown P, Richardson J: Is current drug abuse prevention programming generalizable across ethnic groups? *American Behavioral Scientist,* 39:911–918, 1996.

79. Scheier S, Botvin GJ, Diaz T, Ifill-Williams M: Ethnic identity as a moderator of psychosocial risk and adolescent alcohol and marijuana use: Concurrent and longitudinal analyses. *Journal of Child & Adolescent Substance Abuse*, 6:21–47, 1997.
80. Sussman S, Earleywine M, Wills TA, Biglan A, Newcomb M, Dent CW What are the implications of a motivation-skills-decision making approach on drug abuse prevention? Is this a transdisciplinary fusion approach? *Substance Use & Misuse*, (in press).
81. Rohrbach LA, D'Onofrio CN, Backer TE, Montgomery SB: Diffusion of school-based substance abuse programs. *American Behavioral Scientist*, 39:919–934, 1996.

12

Prevention of College Student Drinking Problems

A Brief Summary of Strategies and Degree of Empirical Support for Them

Robert F. Saltz

1. Introduction

The public's, or at least the mass media's attention to the problem of college student drinking have seemed to come and go over the past decades. This may be due to the periodic appearance of a cluster of student deaths related to drinking, perhaps due to some element of randomness in what captures the media's attention as a trend or newsworthy topic, or some of both, but it is unlikely to derive from sudden changes in student drinking itself. Wechsler and his colleagues have shown that student alcohol consumption (and the prevalence of heavy consumption) has held very steady over the decade or more that they have been conducting national surveys of student alcohol use (Wechsler & Isaac, 1992; Wechsler, et.al., 2000) and the Monitoring the Future followup of high school seniors into college has shown similar stability (with a slight downward trend) over a 20-year span that likely witnessed changes in the demographic composition of those attending college (O'Malley and Johnston, 2002). Indeed, the prevalence and stability of student drinking over the years gave Wechsler and his colleagues occasion to pessimistically conclude some time ago that "the scope of the problem makes immediate results of any interventions highly unlikely" (Wechsler, et. al., 1994: 1677).

In an effort to turn the latest peak of media attention into something positive, the National Institute on Alcohol Abuse and Alcoholism (NIAAA) formed

Robert F. Saltz • Pacific Institute for Research and Evaluation Prevention Research Center, Berkeley, California 94704.

a Task Force on College Drinking that reviewed the relevant epidemiological and prevention research, commissioned 18 review papers on specific areas of research and issued a report and recommendations for research and prevention strategies based on those reviews and the task force's deliberations (NIAAA, 2002). In this chapter, we will summarize and update the research that formed the basis of the task force report and that focused specifically on the prevention of college student drinking problems. We also provide some updated information on research that has been published since the task force report.

2. Why Focus on College Student Drinking?

News accounts of student tragedies and coverage of epidemiological research such as that cited above may make the question seem unnecessary, but in the service of basic research and for developing effective prevention interventions, one might wonder whether college students are at greater risk for alcohol-related harm than the general public or are subject to greater risk than other young adults who do not attend college. The question is complicated, of course, by the fact that college attendance is not a random event, so selection bias makes it difficult to determine what the risk of college students might be were they not to attend (and likewise non-students' risk were they to go to college).

O'Malley and Johnston (2002) report data from the Monitoring the Future study that compares college-bound students to their non-college bound peers during their senior year and after. Whereas the college-bound students rate of heavy drinking was below that of their peers during high school, the order was reversed when the one group entered college, with college students drinking more than their non-college peers. While the mechanism behind this reversal remains a question (e.g., whether delayed onset of heavy drinking among college students or an effect of the college environment or both), there is good reason to believe that entering college is associated with elevated risk for those students.

Apart from considerations of comparative risk, however, Hingson and his colleagues (2002) developed estimates of a variety of serious alcohol-related outcomes among college students based on data from the National Highway Traffic Safety Administration, national coroner studies, Department of Education college enrollment data, the National Household Survey on Drug Abuse (NHSDA), the CDC National College Health Risk Behavior Survey and the Harvard School of Public Health College Alcohol Survey (CAS). Using data from 1998 and 1999 that focused on 18–24 year olds and tying them with college enrollment data, the authors conservatively estimated an annual fatality rate of over 1,400 college students who died in alcohol-related events (primarily traffic crashes). The authors went on to estimate that over 2 million college students (of a total of 8 million) drove under the influence of alcohol, and over 3 million rode with a drinking driver. Furthermore, in addition to over 500,000 students who suffered unintentional injury with under the influence of alcohol, over 600,000 were hit or assaulted by another student who had been drinking. These estimates are alarming in themselves and even so are likely underestimates. The authors conclude by recommending improvements in epidemiological surveillance systems that can better track changes in college student injuries and deaths as well as urging many of the prevention strategies described below.

As we shall see, the empirical research on colleges interventions on which the NIAAA task force was able to base its recommendations was somewhat limited, with greater development for those interventions aimed at individual college students and fewer or no studies or evaluations of campus or community-level interventions. In the sections that follow, we will briefly summarize the evidence that the task force was able to consolidate, organized by the level of intervention (individual to campus and community) and the degree to which the task force felt there was empirical support for specific prevention strategies. Those recommended strategies will then also be described.

3. Interventions Aimed Directly at Individuals

Interventions that enhance individual cognitive and behavioral skills. Apart from minimum age laws, the prevention strategy with the longest history has likely been using some form of educational approach in an effort to either delay onset of alcohol consumption or moderate how much a person might drink. Coupled with the fact that prevention has long been seen as a province of particular interest to psychologists, and it is no surprise that this area is one of the best-developed among those reviewed by the NIAAA Task Force. While many school-based programs over the years have had limited or no effect on drinking or drinking problems, newer, multi-component approaches are demonstrating efficacy, especially among college students.

In their review of this area conducted for the task force, Larimer and Cronce (2002) gathered published evaluations, other review papers, and even a sample of model programs directed to college students over a period of 15 years. After filtering those reports for adequacy of evaluation design, they then distinguished between 1) educational or awareness programs; 2) cognitive-behavioral; and 3) motivational enhancement techniques.

Awareness programs, in turn, can be classified as focusing either on information per se, values clarification, or providing normative information on peer prevalence and levels of drinking. Larimer and Cronce found that of seven information interventions, most of which could show changes in knowledge or attitudes, only one (Kivlahan et. al., 1990)was associated with reductions in either consumption or problems. The impact of this 8-week curriculum (from 19.4 to 12.7 drinks per week) was greater than the control condition (which showed a slight increase in consumption 12 months later), but smaller than a decrease from 14.8 to 6.6 drinks per week in a skills training condition.

Larimer and Cronce then found that only two of five reports on programs based on values clarification (or a combination of values clarification with information) demonstrated a reduction in drinking, but all five studies were plagued by methodological, recruitment, or design problems that made it difficult to come to any conclusions regarding values clarification.

Finally (among the informational programs), only two studies were described that incorporated a normative re-education approach. In one (Barnett et. al., 1996), normative education was used alone or in combination with values clarification, with no significant effect of either condition on drinking. The students' perceptions of norms were indeed changed, however, and that change was greater than for conditions without the normative education. The other study (Schroeder and Prentice, 1998), ironically, found an effect of the re-education, but without seeing a change in perceived peer drinking. Larimer and Cronce speculate that the freshmen in this second study might have been more receptive to the intervention than the mixed-age students in the other normative study, but that still leaves the question of why no change in perception was observed.

In sum, then, Larimer and Cronce's summary of information-only programs is consistent with other reviews (e.g., Moskowitz, 1989) that have found such programs to be generally ineffective. We hasten to add that information-giving may well be a necessary component in other types of programs and interventions, and it may well be that future evaluations may identify informational programs that are efficacious, but the NIAAA Task Force would discourage colleges from adopting information-only campaigns based on current state-of-the-art.

Other approaches have fared better, however. Cognitive-behavioral skills training programs represent an enhancement of more traditional educational approaches in that they try to teach skills relevant to changing alcohol consumption in addition to other components that may include values clarification, information, and/or normative re-education. Those skills may be quite specific to drinking (e.g., monitoring one's consumption or gauging one's blood alcohol levels) to more general life skills such as stress management.

A particularly intriguing "skill" that can be conveyed to drinkers is to recognize that subjective effects of alcoholic beverages are largely determined by one's expectancies about those effects and not predominately (if at all) by the alcohol itself. Getting students to believe this is achieved by conducting what is called an "expectancy challenge." Here, as reported by Darkes and Goldman (1993; 1998), heavy-drinking male students were brought into a social environment and (by random assignment) given beverages that contained either alcohol or a placebo and given the task of guessing who had which beverage. These sessions (3 at 45 minutes each) were supplemented with information about placebo effects and expectancies, and students were to monitor their expectancies over the course of a 4-week period. There were other variations (e.g., whether the session included activities with a social vs. sexual component, or including problem-solving tasks), but at least in the short-term (2 to 6-

week follow ups), alcohol consumption had decreased significantly for those exposed to the expectancy challenge compared to control groups.

Larimer and Cronce (2002) also described a study by Jones et al (1995), in which students were randomly assigned to a condition in which they were given a beverage (either alcohol or placebo) without other students included in a social setting. The students were given information on expectancies and asked to monitor their own expectancies, but in the end, against a backdrop of reduced drinking overall, there was no effect by condition (the self-challenge). Further analysis suggested that only those involved in the self-challenge had significantly reduced their consumption. Larimer and Cronce conclude from these studies that the expectancy challenge procedure is quite promising for male drinkers at least, and more work should be done to better understand how the social and experiential aspects of the challenge may be key determinants of effectiveness. Further work would also be needed to explore this strategy's effectiveness for women, how long such preventive effects might last, and how such a strategy might be best adapted for whole college campuses.

An alternative strategy is to have students pay specific attention to their alcohol consumption and problems that it might lead to. This might be done in the form of a daily diary or via interactive prompting through a computer program. Larimer and Cronce found three studies evaluating such interventions (that met their inclusion criteria). In one, students who recorded how much alcohol they anticipated drinking over their spring break in fact reported fewer problems after that break than did a control group (Cronin, 1996). In another, fraternity pledges who were asked to record their daily alcohol consumption over a period of 7 weeks reported lower alcohol consumption 5 months later than students who received alcohol education or no intervention (Garvin, 1990). Miller (1999) employed a schedule of three computerized assessments and compared its effect to a two-session peer-led skills program and a two-session computerized peer-facilitated interactive program. All three interventions resulted in lower consumption and problems when compared to the control group, although the three assessments were all that one group had been exposed to.

There is no reason, of course, that these various skill-building techniques couldn't be combined into a comprehensive curriculum, and indeed, Larimer and Cronce (2002) found multi-component interventions to be the most common, accounting for seven studies comprising 10 treatment conditions. Of these, seven were found to be effective in reducing consumption or problems (Ametrano, 1992; Baer et al., 1992; Garvin et al., 1990; Jack, 1989; Kivlahan et al., 1990; Marcello et al., 1989; Miller, 1999) while the other three failed to show an impact on drinking or problems (Ametrano, 1992; Jack, 1989; Marcello et al., 1989).

School-based prevention curricula often focus on more general life skills, too, although Larimer and Cronce only found two studies that met methodological adequacy and were specific to college students (Murphy et al., 1986; Rohsenow et. al., 1985). The first study assigned students to either an exercise, meditation, or control condition, with reduction in alcohol use among the exercise group despite no direct linking of the intervention to alcohol use. Those in the meditation condition were less compliant, but showed similar reductions for those who did meditate. The second study focused on stress reduction, and reduced consumption after 2 months but not later at 5 months.

Brief motivational enhancement. Evolving out of treatment settings, researchers have developed techniques that help drinkers, especially those that may have already suffered negative consequences, bring their drinking into better alignment with professed desire to change that behavior. Although the number and length of sessions vary, a typical intervention might comprise a session of 45 minutes (in either an individual or group format) and include alcohol information, skills training, and personalized feedback to enhance motivation to change. The feedback stems from a formal assessment of the student's drinking and its consequences. A key aspect of the feedback is that it is presented to the student in a non-judgmental manner. Larimer and Cronce identified eight studies using this general strategy and involving college or college-age students (Aubrey, 1998; Baer et al., 1992; Borsari and Carey, 2000; D'Amico and Fromme, 2000; Dimeff, 1997; Larimer et al., 2001; Marlatt et al., 1998; Monti et al., 1999). All eight demonstrated efficacy in reducing alcohol consumption, problems, or both, and given that these reports were generally among the most controlled in the entire review of individual-level interventions, this strategy would appear to be strongly backed by empirical support for use with college students.

The kinds of subjects involved in these interventions included high-risk freshmen (Marlatt et. al., 1998), heavy drinkers (Baer et. al., 1992; Borsari & Carey, 2000, Dimeff, 1997); fraternity and sorority members (Anderson et. al., 1998; Larimer, et. al., 2001), outpatients in substance abuse treatment (Aubrey, 1998), and young adults appearing in emergency room for an alcohol-related event (Monti et. al., 1999). It also appears that the motivational enhancement and feedback may be effectively communicated via an interactive computer program (Dimeff, 1997) and even graphic personalized feedback delivered through the mail (Agostinelli et al., 1995; Walters et al., 1999, 2000), although Larimer and Conce regard the mail feedback studies as weaker methodologically due to small and ill-described samples and relatively short-term followup.

Forming recommendations for prevention of college student drinking problems. The studies summarized above generally comprise all the research the Task Force was able to identify that was specifically relevant to college student populations. In translating research into recommendations for prevention, the task force had the option of limiting its attention to just this body of research. To do so, however, was seen as negligent for a number of reasons. First, these studies focus primarily (but not exclusively) on students whose drinking puts them at risk of harm or has already created problems for them. Abstainers, for instance, would presumably not be an appropriate target for motivational enhancement (in its current format). Also, most of these studies were small in scale. Many research, cost, recruitment, and logistical questions remain unanswered were these strategies to be adopted for a campus-wide effort.

Secondly, limiting recommendations to those based on college student-specific interventions alone would ignore progress that has been made over the past decades in research on universal prevention efforts targeting general populations that could reasonably be expected to be relevant to college campus and community settings.

Third, a limited focus would tend to reinforce the attention now paid to individual-level interventions and perhaps postpone the development of complementary strategies for many years to come.

Finally, the task force was well aware that whatever recommendations it developed, new and untested prevention efforts are continually implemented throughout the country. Many of these strategies are well-reasoned and/or have had the benefit of limited evaluations. The task force wanted to acknowledge some of these approaches as well.

As a result of these considerations, the task force adopted a "tiered" set of recommendations to help college professionals, students, and other members of the campus community to make informed choices in adopting prevention interventions, and furthermore, to encourage colleges to contribute to its efforts by evaluating whatever strategies they did adopt. The recommendations were organized into four tiers based on the degree of evidence to support a given strategy for use in a college setting.

4. Tier 1: Evidence of Effectiveness among College Students

Stemming from the research described above, the task force identified the following strategies as falling into the first tier (best evidence for college application), but also noted that these strategies targeted individual problem, at-risk, or alcohol-dependent students and had not been tested for campus-wide applications. As the stragegies have already been describe above, we merely list them here:

- Combining cognitive-behavioral skills with norms clarification and motivational enhancement interventions
- Offering brief motivational enhancement interventions
- Challenging alcohol-expectancies

5. Tier 2: Evidence of Success with General Populations That Could Be Applied to College Environments

There are a number of prevention strategies that complement the individual-level interventions by focusing on the social, economic, legal, and even physical environments that can shape alcohol consumption and the degree of harm resulting from it. Many of these strategies, such as setting a minimum drinking age, are not new, but research (in non college-specific settings) has shown that their effectiveness can be enhanced to reduce drinking and problems. These strategies can be broadly classified as 1) restricting the availability of alcohol, and 2) creating conditions that would support these restrictions.

6. Reducing Specific and General Alcohol Availability

For convenience, we distinguish between strategies that restrict the sale or service of alcohol to specific populations or individuals from those that reduce availability overall. The most familiar and perhaps best-evaluated restriction, of course, is that prohibiting alcohol to minors. Because states have historically set their minimum drinking age, and those states had set different ages with many changing those ages until 1988 (as a result of federal legislation), researchers have had an excellent opportunity to evaluate the effect that changes in the minimum age have on alcohol consumption and subsequent problems, usually with an emphasis on motor vehicle crashes.

The task force commissioned a review of published studies on the effects of the minimum legal drinking age (MLDA) law. Wagenaar and Toomey (2002) began with 241 articles published between 1960 and 2000, which naturally comprised a range of methodological rigor and sophistication. Of these, 132 were deemed of sufficient methodological quality to use in the review. Forty-eight of these studies included one or more measures of alcohol consumption, and included a total of 78 separate analyses, still with varying degrees of methodological strength. Of these 78, 27 found significant changes in consumption inversely related to changes in the drinking age (i.e., lowered consumption with a rise in the drinking age, or higher consumption when the age was lowered). An additional 8 analyses found the same effect but did not specify statistical significance. Importantly, only 5 of the 78 analyses found opposite effects (rise in drinking age associated with higher consumption or lower age with lower drinking). All other results found no significant change either way. Wagenaar and Toomey go on to say that the results are even more supportive of MLDA effects when one looks at the highest quality studies on their own.

Wagenaar and Toomey (2002) then looked at 57 studies that reported on one or more measures of drunk driving and traffic crashes. These included 102 separate analyses, of which 52 demonstrated significant inverse effects of the MLDA and an additional 12 that reported the same thing but without significance tests. Only 2 of the 102 analyses found a significant positive relationship between changes in the MLDA and crashes or drunk driving (i.e., where raising the age was associated with an increase in crashes or lower age with reduction in crashes).

While the preponderance of evidence thus supports the effectiveness of a minimum age law, what is notable in these results is the fact that enforcement of minimum drinking age laws is spotty at best. Thus, as cited by Wagenaar and Toomey (2002), somewhere between over half and three-quarters of teens in surveys they summarized describe alcohol as easy to obtain. Studies testing retailers compliance with the law have found the prevalence of sales to underage buyers ranging from 44% to 97% (ibid).

Seeing an opportunity to enhance the effectiveness of MLDA, researchers have been able to show that increasing the enforcement of laws prohibiting sales to minors can cut the prevalence of sales to minors by at least half (Preusser et al., 1994; Lewis et al., 1996; Grube, 1997).

In addition to minors, there is another group to which service of alcohol is prohibited. Though these laws are less familiar to those outside the business, there exist criminal, administrative, and liability laws that require servers of alcohol to refuse service to anyone who is obviously intoxicated. Further more, to different degrees, state liquor liability laws hold servers and licensees responsible if they serve someone who is intoxicated who then in turn causes damage or injury to another party. Working from this legal precedent (and presumed incentive for servers), researchers have demonstrated the efficacy of Responsible Beverage Service programs and other interventions targeting bars and restaurants (Saltz, 1997; McKnight 1993). These programs typically include consultation with bar managers about setting house policies on serving practices and when to refuse service combined with training of bar and restaurant staff that comprises information on alcohol serving laws and skills in checking age identification and dealing with customers who have approached or exceeded their limit. McKnight and Streff (1993) have shown, though, that enforcement of serving laws alone can have as great an effect or more than such training provides. As described in Saltz (1997), there is a variety of other changes owners and managers can take to reduce the likelihood of intoxication in the first place, including the use of standard serving sizes and promotion of food and non-alcoholic drinks.

Besides targeted restrictions of alcohol service, there are more general strategies available, too. Research has shown that the density of alcohol outlets is associated with greater consumption and such problems as crime, violence and health problems (Scribner et. al., 1995, Gruenewald et. al., 1993; Toomey and Wagenaar, 2002). Chaloupka and Wechsler (1996) combined survey data from Wechsler's national sample of colleges with data on alcohol licensees within a mile of each campus and found higher levels of drinking and heavy ("binge") drinking where alcohol outlets were more numerous. The density of outlets may be set by local ordinances or fees associated with obtaining a license. General alcohol availability can also be shaped by laws affecting closing hours and days of sale, though results of research here are mixed (De Moira and Duffy, 1995; Ligon and Thyer, 1993; Smith, 1988).

Alcohol consumption and associated problems are also affected by the price of alcoholic beverages (Godfrey 1997; Chaloupka and Weschsler, 1996; Sutton and Godfrey, 1995; Kenkel, 1993; Williams et. al., 2002). While all drinkers seem to be affected by price, the size of that effect can vary by such factors as drinking level, age group, and type of alcohol (Coate and Grossman, 1988; Cook and Tauchen, 1982) Manning et. al. (1995) found heavy drinkers to be less affected than other drinkers, but the other studies noted above have found that young heavy drinkers are an exception in that they do seem more sensitive to price. An inverse relationship between price and a variety of problems (e.g., motor vehicle deaths, robberies, rapes, and liver cirrhosis mortality) has also been described (Cook and Tauchen, 1982; Cook and Moore, 1993; Ruhm, 1996). A variety of specific strategies related to using price as an intervention might include raising excise taxes on alcohol, setting local minimum pricing levels (either voluntarily or via ordinance), prohibiting certain drink promotions (e.g., two-for-one promotions or certain types of happy hour price reductions).

7. Community Interventions

Implementing any of these environmental strategies presents a challenge, of course. Unlike individual-level interventions, the unit for these is an entire campus, or more likely, the campus as well as the surrounding community. For this reason, the task force also reviewed research on community-level prevention trials. Such interventions have typically mobilized community attention and support on behalf of specific targets as adolescent drinking (e.g., Perry et al, 1996; Pentz et al, 1989), alcohol availability to minors (Wagenaar et al, 1999; 2000), traffic safety (including alcohol-related crashes) (Hingson et al, 1996), and alcohol-related injuries and death (Holder et al, 2000).

These community efforts can be quite comprehensive. As an example, the Massachusetts Saving Lives program targeted drunk driving and speeding through activities that included drunk driving checkpoints, establishing speed watch telephone hotlines, police training, alcohol-free prom nights, beer keg registration, business information campaigns, media campaigns, and increased surveillance of attempts of minors to buy alcohol. A great deal of attention was given to media advocacy to create and shape news stories in ways to support the prevention efforts (Hingson et al, 1996). The project reported that self-reported driving after drinking among those under 20 dropped from 19% to 9%, the prevalence of speeding was cut by half, and alcohol-related traffic deaths were reduced 45% more in the treatment cities by comparison to the rest of the state over the project's 5-year period.

Communities Mobilizing for Change on Alcohol (CMCA) focused on alcohol availability to youth in seven small to midsized communities in Minnesota and Wisconsin (with another 8 communities as comparison). A coordinator working with each community mobilized support for a variety of activities, including increased enforcement of laws prohibiting alcohol sales to minors and awareness of the problem and importance of enforcement to the community at large. As a result, alcohol sales to minors was reduced in the target communities, and surveys of youth showed a decline in attempts to purchase alcohol or provide alcohol to peers and to consume alcohol (Wagenaar et al, 1999; 2000). Drunk driving violations were also reduced in those communities. Interestingly, the program seemed to have the greatest affect on the oldest minors, i.e., those who were of traditional college age (though this study was not targeted to college students per se).

The Community Trials Project targeted alcohol-related injury and deaths in three communities (each with a matched community for comparison). Specific components included responsible beverage service training and enforcement; increased enforcement of drunk driving laws (and public perception of that increase); enforcement of underage sales laws; reduced alcohol availability via curtailing outlet density; and mobilizing the community and its leaders in support of these interventions. The intervention reduced alcohol-involved crashes by more than 10% over the comparison communities, and alcohol-related assaults appearing in emergency rooms declined by 43% (Holder, et. al., 2000).

Together, these studies demonstrate the efficacy of whole-community efforts. Much remains to be studied about what elements of community mobilization are necessary or sufficient, or indeed, to what extent such mobilizing efforts are required at all. In the meantime, these studies provide guidance and support for campus community coalitions that might be formed in support of environmental prevention strategies.

As a result of reviewing these and other findings, as well as through discussion and debate, the task force made the following Tier 2 recommendations:

- Increasing enforcement of minimum drinking age laws
- Implementation, increased publicity, and enforcement of laws to prevent alcohol-impaired driving
- Restrictions on alcohol retail outlet density
- Increased price and excise taxes on alcoholic beverages
- Responsible beverage service policies in social and commercial settings
- The formation of a campus and community coalition involving all major stakeholders may be critical to implement these strategies effectively

8. Tier 3: Evidence of Logical and Theoretical Promise, but Require More Comprehensive Evaluation

There are any number of creative ideas for college student drinking prevention, many with strong conceptual appeal and some that have been widely adopted by colleges based on that appeal or from reports of positive effects that have yet to be replicated using rigorous evaluation designs. The task force felt a need to recognize these alternative strategies while at the same time noting that strong empirical support is not currently available. Ideally, campuses that choose to implement these strategies would mount an adequate evaluation of them at the same time. These need not be "gold standard" evaluations, and most are unlikely to have the resources to meet that standard. Nevertheless, college programmers could do more in the way of evaluation than we see in current practice. To encourage these efforts, the task force commissioned a guide to college drinking prevention evaluation arguing the benefits of closely dovetailing program planning and evaluation for the mutual advantage of both (Saltz and DeJong; 2002).

As these (provisionally) recommended strategies do not have the same level of empirical research behind them as Tier 1 and 2 recommendations, they will be listed here with only brief description or commentary for the most part. Similarly, most of the references given for each are linked to descriptive pieces or reasoned arguments on their behalf rather than empirical results.

Conducting marketing campaigns to correct student misperceptions about alcohol use. This approach, sometimes called "social norms marketing" or normative education, has become especially popular among many campus prevention specialists. The approach stems from the universal finding that college students consistently over-estimate the frequency and amount of alcohol consumed by their peers (Baer and Carney, 1993; Baer et al., 1991; Perkins and Berkowitz, 1986, 1991; Perkins et al., 1999). As peer influence is especially salient among college students, it would be expected that this overestimate would encourage heavier alcohol use by students, and there is some evidence to support this connection (Lo, 1995; Perkins, 1986; Robinson et al., 1993). It is logical to believe, therefore, that correcting student misperceptions can lead to generally lower alcohol consumption, especially among those whose drinking is greater than the (corrected) perceived level of other students.

The strategy is especially appealing because it employs media campaign elements and techniques that many prevention programmers are familiar with from traditional awareness campaigns. Here, student survey data would be used to identify the correct level of student consumption (e.g., showing that a majority of students drink fewer than 5 drinks when they attend a party) and then publicizing that simple and direct message to the students themselves. In noted contrast to campaigns that might emphasize the danger of alcohol consumption or raise alarms about the widespread use alcohol, this approach leads to a more positive message about the relatively healthier practices that students engage in, in contrast to what they may have believed to be the case (see Berkowitz, 1997; Haines and Spear, 1996; Johannessen et al., 1999; Perkins, 1997, 2002).

As we have seen, correcting perceived peer use is often used in individual-level strategies and has been used for quite some time in k-12 school-based education programs. Supporters also note a good number of pre-post evaluation designs that have reported reductions in high-risk drinking of up to 20% (Berkowitz, 1997; DeJong and Linkenbach, 1999; Haines, 1996, 1998; Haines and Spear, 1996; Johannessen et al., 1999). While the task force decided that more rigorous evaluations would be required for stronger recommendation, many argue that the number of less-rigorous studies showing an impact should carry weight in itself. There are several federally-funded studies now in the field that may provide further insight into the merits of the normative education approach. In the meantime, Wechsler and colleagues (2003) used data from their national survey of colleges to compare those who reported the use of a social norms campaign with those that did not and found no difference in alcohol consumption or heavy consumption among the students. While thus issuing a cautionary message, this is not a direct test of the approach, of course, in that it was not possible to verify the administrators' reports of what they did, or of the intensity of the efforts. In addition, a study by Clapp and colleagues (2003) was the only one to date that found a negative impact of an intensive normative education campaign focused on one residential hall using another as a comparison. Clearly, there is much to learn about the effectiveness of this strategy and how best to implement it.

Increasing enforcement at campus-based events that promote excessive drinking. A logical extension of the responsible beverage service approach, campuses might turn their attention to raising the level of supervision and management of drinking events so as to reduce the availability of alcohol to minors and the likelihood of intoxication and other forms of disruptive behavior (DeJong and Langenbahn, 1996; Gulland, 1994). The task force noted that enforcement of policies at such events may require non-students to avoid placing students or even resident assistants in an awkward position.

Increasing publicity about and enforcement of underage drinking laws on campus and eliminating "mixed messages." While, as we have seen, increased enforcement of minimum drinking laws can be effective, this effectiveness might be further enhanced by creating a campus climate that reinforces the law (DeJong and Langford, 2002). Front-line prevention personnel often complain that their efforts are compromised by messages to the effect that underage drinking is condoned and sometimes encouraged.

Consistently enforcing disciplinary actions associated with policy violations. Again, inconsistent enforcement gives the implicit message that such policies are not important and may only be invoked for reasons other than a simple violation itself (DeJong and Langford, 2002).

Provision of "safe rides" programs. Another strategy that has been widely adopted to varying degrees is aimed at preventing alcohol-impaired driving by giving students access to alternative transportation via free or low-cost taxi or van services. Many campuses have found innovative ways to fund such programs and have refined logistical issues such as who can be given a ride and where and when such rides will be provided (DeJong, 1995). Though such programs have been criticized as "enabling" heavy drinking, such criticism (as well as claims of effectiveness) await empirical evidence.

Regulation of happy hours and sales and responsible social host policies. As noted above, higher prices can reduce alcohol consumption and subsequent problems, but more research could address the question of whether specific restrictions on price promotions at bars and restaurants can have significant effects (Chaloupka and Wechsler, 1996; Toomey and Wagenaar, 2002). Given how common such promotions are in areas proximate to college campuses, it behooves us all to know if consumption can be moderated by putting limits on them. Those non-commercial hosts for events that include alcoholic beverages (parties, events, celebrations) also need guidance on how best to plan such events so as to limit heavy alcohol consumption (e.g., by using servers instead of self-service, limiting the amount of free alcohol or promoting non-alcoholic beverages alongside them).

Informing new students and their parents about alcohol policies and penalties before arrival and during orientation periods. There is evidence that freshmen consume alcohol at higher peak levels than other students and are generally at higher risk (e.g., Pope et al., 1990). Anecdotal reports suggest that this risk is even higher at the beginning weeks after arriving on campus (e.g., during orientation and several weeks afterward). It seem reasonable, then, to initiate some form of intervention prior to the arrival of those new students, and perhaps including parents whose influence on their children's drinking, while diminishing, can still be significant.

Adopting the following campus-based policies and practices that appear to be capable of reducing high-risk alcohol use. This last recommendation is something of a residual category comprising a variety of ideas that might be amenable to experimentation on campuses with relatively lower cost for evaluation. They include:

- Reinforcing Friday classes and exams to reduce Thursday night partying; possibly scheduling Saturday morning classes.
- Implementing alcohol-free, expanded late-night student activities.
- Eliminating keg parties on campus where underage drinking is prevalent.
- Establishing alcohol-free dormitories.
- Employing older, salaried resident assistants or hiring adults to fulfill that role.
- Further controlling or eliminating alcohol at sports events and prohibiting tailgating parties that model heavy alcohol use.
- Refusing sponsorship gifts from the alcohol industry to avoid any perception that underage drinking is acceptable.
- Banning alcohol on campus, including at faculty and alumni events.

9. Tier 4: Evidence of Ineffectiveness

The task force took note that it is considered impossible to "prove a negative," in that there is always some possibility that a strategy that have failed to reduce alcohol consumption or problems may one day "work." Practically speaking, however, some strategies continue to be adopted when there has yet to be evidence for their effectiveness and the task force wanted to caution college administrators so as to draw attention to more proven strategies, or at least something from Tier 3, where one can remain more neutral with respect to likelihood of success.

As we described in the overview of individual-level approaches, there is little to recommend informational or values clarification interventions when used in isolation of any complementary components or strategies. Changes in knowledge and attitudes can often be accomplished, but there is little chance that they can change drinking behavior. Nevertheless, these kinds of campaigns remain the most widely-used prevention interventions on campuses today (DeJong and Langford, 2002; Larimer and Cronce, 2002; Ziemelis, 1998).

Another approach sometimes found on college campuses is to give students the opportunity to take a reading on their blood alcohol concentration (BAC) using a breathalyzer. The idea here is that students would gain information about their level of impairment and use this to moderate excessive consumption. The task force notes, however, that researchers who have made extensive use of breathalyzers in their prevention work have found that instead of moderating alcohol consumption, students will use the instrument to see who can reach the highest BAC (based on personal communication with those researchers). While this does not mean that breathalyzers could not be used in any format, the risks of providing instantaneous feedback to drinking students were judged great enough to urge caution.

The two Tier 4 recommendations, then, are to avoid these strategies until and unless new evidence of their value becomes available:

- Informational, knowledge-based, or values clarification interventions about alcohol and the problems related to its excessive use, when used alone; and
- Providing blood alcohol content feedback to students.

10. Putting It All Together

The NIAAA Task Force report on college drinking and its supporting documents and papers form an invaluable resource for those who want to learn what we know about student drinking problems and how to prevent them. There are other recommendations beyond the scope of this paper that are of specific interest to college administrators, researchers, parents, students and the general public and that should give hope to those who wonder whether anything substantial can be done at all.

References

Agostinelli G, Brown JM, Miller WR. Effects of normative feedback on consumption among heavy-drinking college students. Journal of Drug Education 25(1):31–40, 1995.

Ametrano, IM An evaluation of the effectiveness of a substance-abuse prevention program. Journal of College Student Development 33:507–515, 1992.

Anderson BK, Larimer ME, Lydum AR, Turner AP. Prevention of alcohol problems in college Greek systems. Poster presented at the conference for the American Psychological Association, January 1998.

Aubrey LL. Motivational interviewing with adolescents presenting for outpatient substance abuse treatment. Unpublished doctoral dissertation, University of New Mexico, Albuquerque, 1998.

Baer JS, Carney MM. Biases in the perceptions of the consequences of alcohol use among college students. Journal of Studies on Alcohol 54:54–60, 1993.

Baer JS, Marlatt GA., Kivlahan DR, Fromme K, Larimer ME ,Williams E An experimental test of three methods of alcohol risk reduction with young adults. Journal of Consulting and Clinical Psychology. 60:974–979, 1992.

Baer JS, Stacy A, Larimer M. Biases in the perception of drinking norms among college students. Journal of Studies on Alcohol 52:580–586, 1991.

Barnett LA, Far JM, Mauss AL, Miller JA. Changing perceptions of peer norms as a drinking reduction program for college students. Journal of Alcohol and Drug Education 41(2):39–62, 1996.

Berkowitz AD. From reactive to proactive prevention: promoting an ecology of health on campus. In: Rivers PC, Shore ER (eds), *Substance Abuse on Campus: A Handbook for* College and University Personnel. Westport, CT: Greenwood Press, 1997.

Borsari B, Carey KB. Effects of a brief motivational intervention with college student drinkers. Journal of Consulting and Clinical Psychology 68:728–733, 2000.

Chaloupka FJ, Wechsler H. Binge drinking in college: the impact of price, availability, and alcohol control policies. Contemporary Economic Policy 14:112–124, 1996.

Clapp JD, Lange JE, Russell C, Shillington A, Voas RB. Failed norms social marketing campaign. Journal of Studies on Alcohol 64(3):409–414, 2003.

Coate D, Grossman M. Effects of alcoholic beverage prices and legal drinking ages on youth alcohol use. Journal of Law and Economics 31(1):145–171, 1988.

Cook PJ, Moore MJ. Violence reduction through restrictions on alcohol availability. Alcohol Health & Research World 17:151–156, 1993.

Cook PJ, Tauchen G. The effect of liquor taxes on heavy drinking. Bell Journal of Economics 13:379–390, 1982.

Cronin C. Harm reduction of alcohol-use related problems among college students. Substance Use and Misuse 31:2029–2037, 1996.

D'Amico EJ, Fromme K. Implementation of the risk skills training program: A brief intervention targeting adolescent participation in risk behaviors. Cognitive and Behavioral Practice, 7(1):101–117, 2000.

Darkes J, Goldman MS. Expectancy challenge and drinking reduction: experimental evidence for a meditational process. Journal of Consulting and Clinical Psychology 61:344–353, 1993.

Darkes J, Goldman MS. Expectancy challenge and drinking reduction: Process and structure in the alcohol expectancy network. Experimental and Clinical Psychopharmacology 6(1):64–76, 1998.

DeJong W. Preventing Alcohol-Related Problems on Campus: Impaired Driving: A Guide for Program Coordinators. Newton, MA: Higher Education Center for Alcohol and Other Drug Prevention, 1995.

DeJong W, Langenbahn S. Setting and Improving Policies for Reducing Alcohol and Other Drug Problems on Campus: A Guide for Administrators. Newton, MA: The Higher Education Center for Alcohol and Other Drug Prevention, 1996.

DeJong W, Langford LA. Typology for campus-based alcohol prevention: Moving toward environmental management strategies. Journal of Studies on Alcohol Supplement 14:140–147, 2002.

DeJong W, Linkenbach J. Telling it like it is: Using social norms marketing campaigns to reduce student drinking. American Association for Higher Education Bulletin 32(4):11–16, 1999.

De Moira ACP, Duffy JC. Changes in licensing law in England and Wales and alcohol-related mortality. Addiction Research, 3(2):151–164, 1995.

Dimeff LA. Brief Intervention for Heavy and Hazardous College Drinkers in a Student Primary Health Care Setting, Ph.D. Dissertation, University of Washington, Seattle, 1997.

Dimeff LA, Baer JS, Kivlahan DR, Marlatt GA. Brief alcohol screening and intervention for college students (BASICS). Substance Abuse 21(4):283–285, 2000.

Garvin RB, Alcorn JD, Faulkner KK. Behavioral strategies for alcohol abuse prevention with high risk college males. Journal of Alcohol and Drug Education 36(1):23–34, 1990.

Godfrey C. Can tax be used to minimise harm? A health economist's perspective. In: Plant M, Single E, Stockwell T (eds), Alcohol: Minimising the Harm. London: Free Association Books, 1997.

Grube J. Preventing sales of alcohol to minors: Results from a community trial. Addiction 92(Suppl 2):S251–S260, 1997.

Gruenewald PJ, Ponicki WR, Holder HD. The relationship of outlet densities to alcohol consumption: A time series cross-sectional analysis. Alcoholism, Clinical and Experimental Research 17:38–47, 1993.

Gulland E. Developing Effective and Legally Sound Alcohol Policies. Washington, DC: National Association of College and University Business Officers, 1994.

Haines MP. A Social Norms Approach to Preventing Binge Drinking at Colleges and Universities. Newton, MA: The Higher Education Center for Alcohol and Other Drug Prevention, 1996.

Haines MP. Social norms in a wellness model for health promotion in higher education. Wellness Management 14(4):1–10, 1998.

Haines MP, Spear SF. Changing the perception of the norm: A strategy to decrease binge drinking among college students. Journal of American College Health 24(3):134–140, 1996.

Hingson R, Heeren T, Zakocs R, Kopstein A, Wechsler H. Magnitude of alcohol-related morbidity, mortality, and alcohol dependence among U.S. college students age 18–24. Journal of Studies on Alcohol 63(2):136–144, 2002.

Hingson R, McGovern T, Howland J, Hereen T, Winter M, Zakocs R. Reducing alcohol-impaired driving in Massachusetts: The Saving Lives Program. American Journal of Public Health 86:791–797, 1996.

Holder HD, Gruenewald PJ, Ponicki WR, Treno AJ, Grube JW, Saltz RF, Voas RB, Reynolds R, Davis J, Sanchez L, Gaumont G, Roeper P. Effect of community-based interventions on high-risk drinking and alcohol-related injuries. Journal of the American Medical Association 284(18):2341–2347, 2000.

Jack LW. The educational impact of a course about addiction. Journal of Nursing Education 28:22–28, 1989.

Johannessen K, Collins C, Mills-Novoa B, Glider P. A Practical Guide to Alcohol Abuse Prevention: A Campus Case Study in Implementing Social Norms and Environmental Management Approaches. Tucson, AZ: Campus Health Service, University of Arizona, 1999.

Jones LM, Silvia LY, Richman CL. Increased awareness and self-challenge of alcohol expectancies. Substance Abuse 16(2):77–85, 1995.

Kenkel DS. Prohibition versus taxation: Reconsidering the legal drinking age. Contemporary Policy Issues July:48–57, 1993.

Kivlahan D., Marlatt GA., Fromme K, Coppel DB, Williams E. Secondary prevention with college drinkers: Evaluation of an alcohol skills training program. Journal of Consulting and Clinical Psychology 58:805–810, 1990.

Larimer M, Cronce J. Identification, prevention and treatment: A review of individual-focused strategies to reduce problematic alcohol consumption by college students. Journal of Studies on Alcohol Supplement 14: 148–163, 2002.

Larimer ME, Turner A.P, Anderson BK, Fader JS, Kilmer JR, Palmer RS, Cronce J.M. Evaluating a brief alcohol intervention with fraternities. Journal of Studies on Alcohol 62:70–380, 2001.

Lewis RK, Paine-Andrews A, Fawcett SB, Francisco VT, Richter KP, Copple B, Copple JE. Evaluating the effects of a community coalition's efforts to reduce illegal sales of alcohol and tobacco products to minors. Journal of Community Health 21:429–436, 1996.

Ligon J, Thyer BA. The effects of a Sunday liquor sales ban on DUI arrests. Journal of Alcohol and Drug Education 38:33–40, 1993.

Lo CC. Gender differences in collegiate alcohol abuse. Journal of Drug Issues 25(4):817–836, 1995.

Manning WG, Blumberg L, Moulton LH. The demand for alcohol: The differential response to price. Journal of Health Education 14:123–148, 1995.

Marcello RJ, Danish SJ, Stolberg AL. An evaluation of strategies developed to prevent substance abuse among student-athletes. Sport Psychologist 3:196–211, 1989.

Marlatt GA, Baer JS, Kivlahan DR, Dimeff LA, Larimer ME, Quigley LA, Somers JM, Williams E. Screening and brief intervention for high-risk college student drinkers: Results from a two-year follow-up assessment. Journal of Consulting and Clinical Psychology 66:604–615, 1998.

McKnight AJ. Server Intervention: Accomplishments and Needs. Alcohol Health & Research World 17(1):76–83, 1993

McKnight A.J, Streff FM. The Effect of Enforcement upon Service of Alcohol to Intoxicated Patrons of Bars and Restaurants. In: Alcohol, Drugs and Traffic Safety—T92. Proceedings of the 12th International Conference on Alcohol, Drugs, and Traffic Safety. Cologne, Germany: Verlag TÜV Rheinland, pp. 1296–1302, 1993

Miller ET. Preventing alcohol abuse and alcohol-related negative consequences among freshman college students: using emerging computer technology to deliver and evaluate the effectiveness of brief intervention efforts. Unpublished doctoral dissertation, University of Washington, Seattle, 1999.

Monti PM, Colby SM, Barnett NP, Spirito A, Rohsenow DJ, Myers M, Wollard R, Lewander W. Brief intervention for harm reduction with alcohol-positive older adolescents in a hospital emergency department. Journal of Consulting and Clinical Psychology 67:989–994, 1999.

Moskowitz JM. The primary prevention of alcohol problems: A critical review of the research literature. Journal of Studies on Alcohol 50:54–88, 1989.

Murphy TJ, Pagano RR, Marlatt GA. Lifestyle modification with heavy alcohol drinkers: Effects of aerobic exercise and meditation. Addictive Behavior 11:175–186, 1986.

NIAAA. A Call to Action: Changing the Culture of Drinking at U.S. Colleges Final Report of the Task Force on College Drinking. NIH Publication No: 02–5010 Printed Date: April 2002

O'Malley PM, Johnston LD. Epidemiology of alcohol and other drug use among American college students. Journal of Studies on Alcohol (Suppl 14):S23–S39, 2002.

Pentz M, Dwyer J, MacKinnon D, Flay B, Hansen W, Wang E, Johnson A. A multi community trial for primary prevention of adolescent drug abuse. Journal of the American Medical Association 261(22):3259–3265, 1989.

Perkins HW. College student misperceptions of alcohol and other drug norms among peers: Exploring causes, consequences, and implications for prevention programs. In: Designing Alcohol and Other Drug Prevention Programs in Higher Education. Newton, MA: The Higher Education Center for Alcohol and Other Drug Prevention, 1997.

Perkins HW. Social norms and the prevention of alcohol misuse in collegiate contexts. Journal of Studies on Alcohol Supplement 14:164–172, 2002.

Perkins HW, Berkowitz AD. Perceiving the community norms of alcohol use among students: Some research implications for campus alcohol education programming. International Journal of the Addictions 21(9/10):961–976, 1986.

Perkins HW, Berkowitz AD. Collegiate COAs and alcohol abuse: Problem drinking in relation to assessments of parent and grandparent alcoholism. Journal of Counseling and Development 69(3):237–240, 1991.

Perkins HW, Meilman PW, Leichliter JS, Cashin JS, Presley CA. Misperceptions of the norms for the frequency of alcohol and other drug use on college campuses. Journal of American College Health 47:253–258, 1999.

Perry CL, Williams CL, Veblen-Mortenson S, Toomey TL, Komro KA, Anstine PS, McGovern P, Finnegan JR, Forster JL, Wagenaar AC, Wolfson M. Project Northland: Outcomes of a community-wide alcohol use prevention program during early adolescence. American Journal of Public Health 86:956–965, 1996.

Pope HG, Ionescu-Pioggia M, Aizley HG, Varma DK. Drug use and life style among college undergraduates in 1989: A comparison with 1969 and 1978. American Journal of Psychiatry 147:998–1001, 1990.

Preusser DF, Williams AF, Weinstein HB. Policing underage alcohol sales. Journal on Safety Research 25:127–133, 1994.

Robinson SE, Roth SL, Gloria AM, Keim J. Influence of substance abuse education on undergraduates' knowledge, attitudes and behaviors. Journal of Alcohol and Drug Education 39:123–130, 1993.

Rohsenow DJ, Smith RE, Johnson S. Stress management training as a prevention program for heavy social drinkers: cognitions, affect, drinking, and individual differences. Addictive Behaviors 10:45–54, 1985.

Ruhm CJ. Alcohol policies and highway vehicle fatalities. Journal of Health Economics 15:435–454, 1996.

Saltz RF. Prevention where alcohol is sold and consumed: Server intervention and responsible beverage service. In: M. Plant, E. Singer, and T. Stockwell (eds.) Alcohol: Minimising the Harm. London: Free Association Books, Ltd., 1997.

Saltz R, DeJong W. Reducing Alcohol Problems on Campus: A Planning and Evaluation Guide. Paper prepared for the Panel on Prevention and Treatment, National Advisory Council on Alcohol Abuse and Alcoholism, National Institute on Alcohol Abuse and Alcoholism, Bethesda, MD, 2002.

Schroeder CM, Prentice DA. Exposing pluralistic ignorance to reduce alcohol use among college students. Journal of Applied Social Psychology 28:2150–2180, 1998.

Scribner RA, MacKinnon DP, Dwyer JH. Risk of assaultive violence and alcohol availability in Los Angeles County. American Journal of Public Health 85:335–340, 1995.

Smith DI. Effect on traffic accidents of introducing Sunday alcohol sales in Brisbane, Australia. International Journal of the Addictions 23:1091–1099, 1988.

Sutton M, Godfrey CA. Grouped data regression approach to estimating economic and social influences on individual drinking behavior. Health Economics 4:237–247, 1995.

Toomey TL, Wagenaar AC. Environmental policies to reduce college drinking: Options and research findings. Journal of Studies on Alcohol Supplement 14:193–205, 2002.

Wagenaar A, Gehan J, Jones-Webb R, Toomey T, Forster J. Communities mobilizing for change lessons and results from a 15 community randomized trial. Journal of Community Psychology 27(3):315–326, 1999.

Wagenaar AC, Murray DM, Gehan JP, Wolfson M, Forster JL, Toomey TL, Perry CL, Jones-Webb R. Communities mobilizing for change on alcohol: outcomes from a randomized community trial. Journal of Studies on Alcohol 61(1):85–94, 2000a.

Wagenaar AC, Murray DM, Toomey TL. Communities mobilizing for change on alcohol (CMCA): Effects of a randomized trial on arrests and traffic crashes. Addiction 95(2):209–217, 2000b.

Wagenaar A, Toomey T. Effects of minimum drinking age laws: Review and analyses of the literature from 1960 to 2000. Journal of Studies on Alcohol Supplement 14:206–225, 2002.

Walters ST. In praise of feedback: Notes on an effective intervention for heavy drinking college students. Journal of American College Health 48(5):235–238, 2000.

Walters ST, Martin JE, Norto J. A controlled trial of two feedback-based interventions for heavy drinking college students. Poster session at annual meeting of Research Society on Alcoholism, Santa Barbara, CA, June 1999.

Wechsler H, Davenport A, Dowdall G, Moeykens B, Castillo S. Health and behavioral consequences of binge drinking at colleges: A national survey of students at 140 campuses. Journal of the American Medical *Association* 272(21):1672–1677, 1994.

Wechsler H, Dowdall G, Maenner G, Gledhill-Hoyt J, Lee H. Changes in binge drinking and related problems among American college students between 1993 and 1997: Results of the Harvard School of Public Health College Alcohol Study. Journal of American College Health 47:57–68, 1998.

Wechsler H, Lee JE, Kuo M, Lee H. College binge drinking in the 1990s: A continuing problem. Results of the Harvard School of Public Health 1999 College Alcohol Study. Journal of American College Health 48:199–210, 2000.

Wechsler H, Lee JE, Kuo M, Seibring M, Nelson TF, Lee H. Trends in college binge drinking during a period of increased prevention efforts: Findings from 4 Harvard School of Public Health College Alcohol Study Surveys: 1993–2001. Journal of American College Health 50(5):203–217, 2002.

Wechsler H, Isaac N. 'Binge'drinkers at Massachusetts colleges: Prevalence, drinking style, time trends, and associated problems. JAMA: Journal of the American Medical Association, 267(21):2929- 2931, 1992.

Wechsler H, Nelson, TF, Lee JE, Seibring M, Lewis C, Keeling RP. Perception and reality: A national evaluation of social norms marketing interventions to reduce college students' heavy alcohol use. Journal of Studies on Alcohol, 64(4):484–494, 2003.

Williams J, Chaloupka FJ, Wechsler H. Are there differential effects of price and policy on college students' drinking intensity? Cambridge, MA: National Bureau of Economic Research, 2002.

Ziemelis A. Drug prevention in higher education: Efforts, evidence, and promising directions. Paper presented at The Higher Education Center for Alcohol and Other Drug Prevention Center Associates Annual Meeting, January 1998.

13

Policies to Reduce Underage Drinking
A Review of the Recent Literature

Alexander C. Wagenaar, Kathleen M. Lenk, and Traci L. Toomey

1. Introduction

Drinking behavior is influenced by many factors in the social and policy environment, such as messages in media programming, advertising, community norms, public laws, policies and practices of public and private institutions, and economic factors (Wagenaar & Perry, 1994). Even the best-designed and most effective programs to change knowledge, attitudes, perceptions, expectancies, intentions to drink, and to teach refusal skills typically have modest or temporary effects because people continue to be exposed to a multidimensional environment that encourages risky alcohol use (Holder & Edwards, 1995). Changing the environment through public and institutional policies is an important approach to achieving permanent reductions in underage drinking. Our working definition of 'policy' is: standards for behavior or practices that are formalized to some degree (i.e., written), and embodied in rules, regulations, or operating procedures.

In this paper, we review the scientific literature on numerous alcohol control policies that may affect underage drinking and related problems. For each policy, we first summarize all published studies on the effectiveness of that particular policy in reducing drinking and drinking-related problems among the general population. We then provide a more detailed review of published studies that specifically address the effectiveness of the policy on reducing underage drinking and drinking-related problems (Table 1). We group policies

Alexander C. Wagenaar • Department of Epidemiology and Health Policy Research, University of Florida School of Medicine, Gainesville, Florida 32608.
Kathleen M. Lenk and Traci L. Toomey • Alcohol Epidemiology Program, University of Minnesota, School of Public Health, Minneapolis, Minnesota 55454-1015.

into four categories based on the number of published studies available: extensive research (more than 100 studies); moderate research (10 to 30 studies); minimal research (fewer than 10 studies); or no research (no studies to date). We do not cover here all alcohol control measures, but rather limit this review to policies that are most likely to directly affect youth drinking and drinking-related outcomes.

2. Policies with Extensive Research

Minimum Legal Drinking Age. The most well-studied policy aimed at reducing underage drinking is the minimum legal drinking age (MLDA). Since 1988, all 50 U.S. states legally prohibit individuals under the age of 21 from consuming, purchasing, or possessing alcohol, and prohibit adults from selling or giving alcohol to those under age 21 (exact legal language varies from state to state). During the 1970s, many states lowered the MLDA from 21 to either 18 or 19, and then increased the MLDA back to 21 in the late 1970s and early 1980s. These shifts in the MLDA led many researchers to study the effects of the changes. We previously conducted a comprehensive review of research on the MLDA, where we identified and examined 132 published studies from 1965 through 2000 (Wagenaar & Toomey, 2002). We also evaluated the methods used in each study, and identified studies with higher-quality designs and statistical methods. The review showed strong evidence that the age-21 MLDA is associated with reductions in drinking and traffic crashes among 18- to 20-year-olds. We also found some evidence that the age-21 MLDA reduces other alcohol-related problems, such as suicide and vandalism, among young people.

For this paper, we identified ten studies, with twelve separate analyses, evaluating the MLDA that were published since our comprehensive review (Table 1). Six studies examined effects of changes in the MLDA on alcohol consumption, and five of these were high-quality, using multivariate analyses of census or nationally representative samples across several years. All but one of the high-quality studies showed a statistically significant inverse relationship between the MLDA and alcohol consumption. Recent analyses of data from Monitoring the Future, a national annual survey of high school seniors in the U.S., showed increases in the MLDA from 1980 to 1989 were associated with slight reductions in the prevalence of alcohol consumption (DiNardo & Lemieux, 2001), and from 1977 to 1992, increases in the MLDA were associated with lower probabilities of both moderate (10 or more drinks in past month) and heavy (five or more drinks in a row in past two weeks) drinking (Dee & Evans, 2003). Two studies used overall sales figures as measures of alcohol consumption, so outcomes reflect consumption across the general population, rather than among youth specifically. Among 45 states from 1982 to 1997, a higher MLDA was associated with lower beverage-specific and total alcohol

Table 1. Research Articles on Alcohol Policies Aimed at Reducing Youth Drinking and Drinking-Related Problems

Authors	Year	Jurisdiction/Sample	Data Source	Probability Sample	Design	Comparison Group	Analysis Method	Outcome Measure
Minimum Legal Drinking Age (MLDA)								
Dee	1999b	High school seniors in 44 states	Survey 1977–92	Yes	Longitudinal	Yes	Regression	Smoking rates
Mast et al.	1999	48 states	Traffic records 1984–92	Census	Longitudinal	Yes	Regression	Traffic fatalities
Kaestner	2000	Youth ages 17–21 in US	Surveys 1982 & 1985	Yes	Repeated cross-sectional	Yes	Regression	Consumption
Xie et al.	2000	All Canadian provinces	Sales figures 1968–86	Census	Longitudinal	Yes	Regression	• Consumption • Cirrhosis mortality
Dee	2001	50 states & DC	Vital statistics 1977–92	Census	Longitudinal	Yes	Regression	Teen child-bearing rates
DiNardo & Lemieux	2001	High school seniors in 43 states	Survey 1980–89	Yes	Longitudinal	Yes	Regression	Consumption
Everitt & Jones	2002	1 emergency dept. in New Zealand	ER records 1998–2000	Census	Pre-post	Yes	Chi-square	Intoxicated persons
Kuo et al.	2002	US & Canadian college students	Surveys 1998 & 1999	Yes	Cross-sectional	Yes	Bivariate	Consumption
Dee & Evans	2003	• High school seniors in 44 states • Adults (1960–69 birth cohorts)	• Survey 1977–92 • 1990 Census	Yes	Longitudinal	Yes	Regression	• Consumption • Educational attainment
Nelson	2003	45 states	Sales figures 1982–97	Census	Longitudinal	Yes	Regression	Consumption

(continued)

Table 1. Research Articles on Alcohol Policies Aimed at Reducing Youth Drinking and Drinking-Related Problems *(continued)*

Authors	Year	Jurisdiction/Sample	Data Source	Probability Sample	Design	Comparison Group	Analysis Method	Outcome Measure
Taxes/Price								
Saffer & Grossman	1987a	48 states	Traffic records 1975–81	Census	Longitudinal	Yes	Regression	Traffic fatalities
Saffer & Grossman	1987b	48 states	Traffic records 1975–81	Census	Longitudinal	Yes	Regression	Traffic fatalities
Coate & Grossman	1988	1,761 youth age 16–21 in US	Survey 1976–80	Yes	Longitudinal	Yes	Regression	Consumption
Chaloupka et al.	1993	48 states	Traffic records 1982–88	Census	Longitudinal	Yes	Regression	Traffic fatalities
Cook & Moore	1993	Cohort of 753 youth in US	Survey 1979–88	Yes	Longitudinal	Yes	Regression	• Consumption • College graduation rates
Kenkel	1993	Youth ages 18–21 in US	Survey 1985	Yes	Cross-sectional	Yes	Regression	• Consumption • Drunk-driving
Laixuthai & Chaloupka	1993	>10,000 high school seniors in US	Survey 1982 & 1989	Yes	Repeated cross-sectional	Yes	Regression	Consumption
Lockhart et al.	1993	1,360 students at 1 MD high school	Survey 1991	Census (83%)	Cross-sectional	Yes	Descriptive	Consumption
Chaloupka & Wechsler	1996	Students at 140 US colleges	Survey 1993	Yes	Cross-sectional	Yes	Regression	Consumption
Ruhm	1996	48 states	Traffic records 1982–88	Census	Longitudinal	Yes	Regression	Traffic fatalities
Yamada et al.	1996	672 high school seniors in US	Survey 1982	Yes	Cross-sectional	Yes	Regression	• Consumption • High school graduation rates
Grossman et al.	1998	7,140 high school seniors in US	Survey 1976–85	Yes	Longitudinal	Yes	Regression	Consumption

Dee	1999a	High school seniors in 44 states	Survey 1977–92	Yes	Longitudinal	Yes	Regression	• Consumption • Traffic fatalities
Wechsler et al.	2000	Students at 116 US colleges	Survey 1997	Yes	Cross-sectional	Yes	Regression	Consumption
Whetten-Goldstein et al.	2000	50 states	Traffic records 1984–95	Yes	Longitudinal	Yes	Regression	Traffic fatalities
Young & Likens	2000	48 states	Traffic records 1982–90	Census	Longitudinal	Yes	Regression	Traffic fatalities
DiNardo & Lemieux	2001	High school seniors in 43 states	Survey 1980–89	Yes	Longitudinal	Yes	Regression	Consumption
Dee & Evans	2003	High school seniors in 44 states	Survey 1977–92	Yes	Longitudinal	Yes	Regression	Consumption
Weitzman et al.	2003	Students at 119 US colleges	Survey 1999	Yes	Cross-sectional	Yes	Regression	Consumption
Server/Management Training								
Gliksman et al.	1993	Thunder Bay, Ontario—On-sale outlets	Survey Observation	No	Pre-post	Yes	T-tests ANOVA	Knowledge Behaviors
Lang et al.	1996	Perth, Australia—On-sale outlets	Purchase attempts	No	Pre-post	Yes	Not reported	ID checks
Grube	1997	1 SC & 2 CA cities—Off-sale outlets	Purchase attempts	No	Pre-post	Yes	Regression	Sales rates
Toomey et al.	2001	One metro area—On-sale outlets	Purchase attempts	No	Pre-post	Yes	ANCOVA	Sales rate
Compliance Checks								
Preusser et al.	1994	Denver, CO—Off-sale outlets	Purchase attempts	Yes	Longitudinal	No	Descriptive	Sales rates
Grube	1997	1 SC & 2 CA cities—Off-sale outlets	Purchase attempts	Yes	Pre-post	Yes	Regression	Sales rates

(continued)

Table 1. Research Articles on Alcohol Policies Aimed at Reducing Youth Drinking and Drinking-Related Problems *(continued)*

Authors	Year	Jurisdiction/Sample	Data Source	Probability Sample	Design	Comparison Group	Analysis Method	Outcome Measure
Willner et al.	2000	2 cities in UK— On- & off-sale outlets	Purchase attempts	No	Pre-post	Yes	Chi-square	Sales rates
Cohen et al.	2001	107 cities in 38 states	Traffic records 1995–97	Census	Longitudinal	Yes	Regression	Traffic fatalities
Scribner & Cohen	2001	New Orleans, LA— Off-sale outlets	Purchase attempts	Yes	Longitudinal	No	Not reported	Compliance rates
Seller/Server Liability								
Chaloupka et al.	1993	48 states	Traffic records 1982–88	Census	Longitudinal	Yes	Regression	Traffic fatalities
Ruhm	1996	48 states	Traffic records 1982–88	Census	Longitudinal	Yes	Regression	Traffic fatalities
Whetten-Goldstein et al.	2000	50 states	Traffic records 1984–95	Census	Longitudinal	Yes	Regression	Traffic fatalities
Young & Likens	2000	48 states	Traffic records 1982–90	Census	Longitudinal	Yes	Regression	Traffic fatalities
Community/Public Event Restrictions								
Spaite et al.	1990	U of AZ football games	Medical records 1983–86	Census	Longitudinal	No	Chi-square	Illnesses/injuries
Gliksman et al.	1995	Ontario, Canada— 107 municipal facilities	Administrator survey 1995	Census (88%)	Cross-sectional	No	Descriptive	• Underage drinking • Fights • Vandalism
Bormann & Stone	2001	U of CO football games	Police records 1995–99	Census	Longitudinal	No	Chi-square	Crime incidents
Johannessen et al.	2001	U of AZ homecoming events	Police records 1992–98	Census	Longitudinal	No	Descriptive	Police calls

Happy Hour Restrictions								
Christie et al.	2001	1 US university—189 undergraduate students	Survey (simulation)	No	Cross-sectional	Yes	MANOVA	Consumption
Social Host Liability								
Whetten-Goldstein et al.	2000	50 states	Traffic records 1984–95	Census	Longitudinal	Yes	Regression	Traffic fatalities
Keg Registration								
Cohen et al.	2001	107 cities in 38 states	Traffic records 1995–97	Census	Longitudinal	Yes	Regression	Traffic fatalities

consumption (Nelson, 2003). Similarly, Xie and associates (2000), using alcohol sales data from all Canadian provinces over a 19-year period (1968 to 1986), found that a lower MLDA was associated with increased consumption. Using several different types of analyses of U.S. national survey data from 1982 and 1985, Kaestner (2000) found that a higher MLDA was not consistently associated with reduced consumption among male or female 17- to 21-year olds.

Using a weaker study design (i.e., cross-sectional; descriptive statistics only), Kuo and colleagues (2002) compared drinking rates among college students in Canada in 1998, where the MLDA was either 18 or 19, to the U.S. in 1999 where the MLDA was 21. Underage Canadian students (under age 18 or 19) were significantly more likely than underage U.S. students (under age 21; 43% vs. 35% respectively) to report heavy episodic drinking (defined as five or more drinks in one sitting for men; four or more for women) in the past month.

Six of the recent MLDA studies examined the effects of changes in the MLDA on various other outcomes. Results are mixed among the five high-quality studies. In analyses of several alcohol control policies, Mast and colleagues (1999) found that from 1984 to 1992 in the U.S., a higher MLDA was associated with reduced traffic fatalities among persons 16 and older. Dee (2001), analyzing U.S. Vital Statistics from 1977 to 1992, found the MLDA was inversely associated with childbearing among black teens but not necessarily among white teens. Analyses of Monitoring the Future data for the same time period showed that a higher MLDA was associated with a 3% to 5% decrease in teen smoking (Dee, 1999). Xie and associates (2000) found lowering the MLDA did not affect liver cirrhosis mortality in Canada from 1968 to 1986. Also, Dee and Evans (2003) found, through analyses of MTF data combined with data on adult birth cohorts (1960–69) from the 1990 U.S. Census, that changes in the MLDA were not associated with educational attainment.

Using a weaker pre-post design, a smaller study of a hospital emergency department (ED) in New Zealand one year after the MLDA was lowered from 21 to 18 found that among all 18- and 19-year-old patients who presented to the ED, the proportion who were found to be intoxicated increased 50% (2.9% to 4.4%), while the proportion of patients over age 19 who were intoxicated did not change significantly (Everitt and Jones, 2002).

Evidence from recent studies, along with cumulated evidence from the 132 studies we previously reviewed (Wagenaar & Toomey, 2002), clearly shows that increases in the legal age for drinking from 18 to 21 were effective in reducing teen drinking and rates of alcohol-related traffic crashes in the U.S among 18- to 20-year-olds. The National Highway Traffic Safety Administration (NHTSA) estimates that age-21 policies have reduced traffic fatalities and saved over 21,000 lives since 1975 (NHTSA, 2003). The substantial effects of the MLDA were achieved with only modest efforts to enforce the policy (Wagenaar & Wolfson, 1994). States and communities that more actively enforce the age-21 policy may be even more likely to achieve significant reductions in youth access to alcohol, drinking and alcohol-related problems (Holder et al., 2000; Wagenaar et al., 2000a; b).

Alcohol Taxes/Prices. The next most-studied policies are those that affect alcohol consumption and related problems by changing the price of alcohol (Wagenaar & Toomey, 2000). We reviewed over 100 studies on the effects of alcohol prices on alcohol consumption and related problems among the general population. Although we did not assess the quality of each study, we found that 85% (75 of 85) of the studies examining price effects on alcohol consumption showed that as the price of alcohol increased, consumption decreased. Several studies also showed that as the price of alcohol increased, numerous types of alcohol-related problems, including motor vehicle fatalities, robberies, rapes, and liver cirrhosis mortality, among the general population decreased. See literature reviews by Cook and Moore (2002) and the National Institute on Alcohol Abuse and Alcoholism (2000) for further discussion of the effects of changes in alcohol prices on the general drinking population.

Nineteen studies, including 21 separate analyses, examined price effects on alcohol consumption and alcohol-related problems among youth, specifically (Table 1). Most studies (10 of 13) examining effects of alcohol prices/taxes on youth alcohol consumption concluded that increases in price were associated with decreases in consumption. Four of seven of the high-quality studies (i.e., multivariate analyses of probability samples across two or more years) found this inverse relationship between price/tax and consumption. Monitoring the Future data on high school seniors were analyzed in five of the high-quality studies. Laixuthai and Chaloupka (1993), using data from 1982 and 1989, found increased beer taxes were associated with reduction in the frequency of beer consumption in the past month and past year, and in the probability of heavy episodic drinking in past two weeks. Similarly, Grossman and colleagues (1998) analyzed data from 1976 to 1985 and found that increased beer prices were associated with a decrease in reported number of drinks consumed per year. In contrast, analyses of data from 1980 to 1989 (DiNardo & Lemieux, 2001) and 1977 to 1992 (Dee, 1999a; Dee & Evans, 2003) showed that variation in alcohol taxes did not correlate with teen drinking rates.

The two other high-quality studies to find that increases in price were associated with decreases in consumption also used national youth survey data. Based on a cohort of 753 youth from 1979 to 1988, Cook and Moore (1993) found that those who went to high school in states with higher beer taxes tended to drink fewer drinks per week, and were less likely to be frequent drinkers (two or more occasions in last week) or frequently drunk (six or more drinks on four or more occasions in last month), compared to youth in other states. Coate and Grossman (1988) determined that among 16- to 21-year olds from 1976 to 1980, an increase in beer prices significantly lowered the probability of frequent (4–7 times/week) and fairly frequent (1–3 times/week) drinking.

Six studies also used probability or census samples, but used cross-sectional, rather than longitudinal, designs. Three of these studies analyzed data from the Harvard School of Public Health College Alcohol Study, an annual nationally representative survey of college students. Analyses of data from 1993 showed that equating the federal tax on beer to that of spirits in 1951, and then indexing the tax to the rate of inflation, would have led to a 15% reduction in the number of underage female drinkers, and a 21% reduction in heavy episodic drinking among underage females (Chaloupka & Wechsler, 1996). Alcohol consumption among male students was not affected by changes in the beer tax in these data. Analyses of 1997 data showed that the ability to obtain drinks at low prices (drinks < $1.00 each or a set fee for unlimited drinks) was associated with increased heavy episodic drinking in past two weeks among underage students (Wechsler et al., 2000). Weitzman and colleagues (2003), analyzing data from students age 19 or younger in 1999, also found that ability to obtain drinks at low prices increased heavy episodic drinking in past two weeks. A 1982 survey showed that a 10% increase in beer taxes reduced the probability of being a frequent drinker (drinking on two or more days in past week) by 2.8% among high school seniors (Yamada et al., 1996). Similarly, a study of 1985 data showed higher alcohol prices were associated with reductions in the number of days in past year that 18- to 21-year olds reported consuming five or more drinks (Kenkel, 1993). A smaller study of 1,360 students at one high school in Maryland found that 24% of drinkers reported drinking less (quantity) and 35% reported drinking less frequently following a federal excise tax increase in 1991 (Lockhart et al., 1993).

Ten studies examined how changes in alcohol prices and/or taxes affected other outcomes among youth, all including multivariate analyses of probability or census samples. Researchers examined effects of alcohol prices on traffic crash mortality or drunk driving rates in eight of the ten studies. Using data from 48 states from 1975 to 1981, simulation models showed that increases in beer tax rates would result in significant declines in motor vehicle fatalities among youth ages 15 to 20 (Saffer & Grossman, 1987a; b), and analyses of a cross-sectional sample of youth ages 18 to 21 in 1985 showed higher alcohol prices were associated with reductions in drunk driving (Kenkel, 1993). Similarly, two studies that analyzed data from 1982 to 1988 across 48 states found increased beer taxes were associated with significant reductions in total, nighttime and alcohol-related traffic fatalities among 18- to 20-year olds (Chaloupka et al., 1993; Ruhm, 1996). In contrast, other analyses of traffic data from the 1970s through the early 1990s revealed that alcohol prices did not affect total, alcohol-related or single-vehicle nighttime traffic fatalities among underage youth (Dee, 1999b; Whetten-Goldstein et al., 2000; Young & Likens, 2000).

Two studies examined alcohol tax effects on school graduation rates. Cook and Moore (1993) found that students who went to high school in states with higher beer taxes were more likely to graduate from college compared to students in lower tax states. Yamada and colleagues (1996) found that among a national cross-sectional sample of high school seniors in 1982, a 10% increase in beer taxes would raise the probability of high school graduation by about 3%.

The preponderance of research evidence suggests that drinking behavior is responsive to price, and that youth are particularly sensitive to price changes. Increased alcohol taxes and prices reduce rates of drinking and a range of alcohol-related problems among youth, as well as among adults.

Despite the extensive evidence of the beneficial effects of increased alcohol prices, federal excise taxes have not been not adjusted for inflation over time and the "real" (inflation-adjusted) price of alcohol continues to decrease. State alcohol taxes also have rarely increased significantly in the past few decades (AEP, 2000).

In summary, large bodies of scientific evidence clearly indicate that a minimum drinking age of 21 and increased taxes on alcoholic beverages are effective policy options to significantly reduce youth drinking and associated morbidity, mortality and social disruption.

3. Policies with Moderate Research

Server/Manager Training. To reduce the likelihood that underage youth can buy alcohol at commercial establishments such as bars, restaurants or liquor stores, servers, managers and owners of alcohol establishments can be trained on ways to reduce illegal underage sales. Training programs include topics such as checking age identification, detecting and handling false age identification documents, offering food and non-alcoholic beverage options and refusing alcohol service. Participation in sever/manager training programs can be either voluntary or required by local or state laws.

We identified 15 studies, including 16 separate analyses, on the effectiveness of server/management training programs and policies. Ten of these studies focused on how participation in a server training program affected servers' knowledge and attitudes, patrons' drunkenness or blood-alcohol content (BAC) levels, or traffic crashes among the general population (Buka & Birdthistle, 1999; Coutts et al., 2000; Hennessy & Saltz, 1989; Howard-Pitney et al., 1991; Lang et al., 1998; McKnight, 1991; Riccelli, 1986; Russ & Geller, 1987; Saltz, 1987; Simons-Morton & Cummings, 1997). While results across the studies were mixed, some showed that participation in server training programs was associated with improving servers' attitudes, knowledge and behaviors in handling intoxicated customers. Only one of the 15 studies analyzed the effectiveness of a state-level policy mandating server training. Holder and Wagenaar (1994), using interrupted time-series analyses, found that a mandated 1987 server training law in Oregon was associated with a 11% decrease in single-vehicle nighttime crashes by the end of the first year of implementation.

Four studies examined how server/management training affects outcomes related to youth drinking, specifically (Table 1). All of the studies used pre-post study designs and comparison or control groups, although none used probability samples. Among servers at four on-sale alcohol establishments in Ontario, Canada, trained servers demonstrated increased knowledge and improved serving behaviors, such as checking age identification of pseudo-underage patrons (i.e., individuals at or above the legal drinking age but who appear to be younger), compared to servers at comparison establishments (Gliksman et al., 1993). In contrast, three studies concluded that server/management training was not effective in reducing underage alcohol sales. Lang and colleagues (1996), for example, found that among seven on-sale alcohol establishments in Perth, Australia, staff who received training did not check age identification of pseudo-underage buyers significantly more often than staff at comparison establishments. In South Carolina and California, training programs for servers, managers, and owners were conducted in 59 outlets in three cities (Grube, 1997), and in a small demonstration project in Minnesota, managers from five bars in one metropolitan area received one-on-one consultation on the implementation of policies to promote responsible beverage service (Toomey et al., 2001). In both studies, sales rates to underage or pseudo-underage buyers were not significantly different in establishments that received training compared to those that had not.

An obvious possible explanation for mixed results across studies on the effectiveness of server/management training on reducing youth access to alcohol is the small sample sizes in these studies. Another possible explanation is the inconsistent quality of server training programs and recommended alcohol policies. Toomey and colleagues (1998) analyzed the quality of existing server training programs and found high variability across programs, with few programs adequately covering underage sales issues and even fewer using science-based behavior-change techniques to improve server skills and confidence to refuse alcohol sales. Similarly, detailed analyses of 23 state server training laws across the U.S. found the quality of laws highly variable, with few meeting minimum standards (Mosher et al., 2002).

Advertising Restrictions. Federal, state and community regulations can be used to control the types, placement or amount of alcohol advertisements in a given area. Regulations might also address advertising that specifically appeals to youth, as well as alcohol industry sponsorship of events that focus on youth. We found 13 studies that examined effects of bans or restrictions on alcohol advertising; however, none specifically pertained to advertising aimed at youth nor included youth drinking-related outcomes. Ten studies evaluated how advertising restrictions affect alcohol consumption among the general population. While four of the ten studies found that restrictions on advertising did not affect consumption (Nelson, 2003; Ogborne & Smart, 1980; Smart & Cutler, 1976; Stout et al., 2000), the remaining six studies found that restrictions were associated with reductions in consumption of alcohol (Ornstein, 1984; Ornstein & Hannsens, 1985; Makowsky & Whitehead, 1991; Saffer, 1991; Saffer & Dave, 2002; Tremblay & Okuyama, 2001). In addition, Saffer (1991; 1997) found that alcohol advertising bans were associated with lower rates of motor vehicle fatalities, and Stout and colleagues (2000) found that restrictions on liquor store advertising significantly reduced probability of drunk driving. Finally, Markowitz and Grossman (1998; 2000) found no effects of advertising restrictions on rates of domestic violence toward children.

In summary, several scientific studies have examined server training policies and policies that restrict or regulate alcohol advertising, but most of these studies did not focus on youth. To learn whether these types of policies are effective in reducing underage drinking and related problems, additional research studies are needed.

4. Policies with Minimal Research

Compliance Checks. Enforcement of minimum legal drinking age laws is an important strategy in preventing alcohol sales to young people. Using data from 1988 to 1990, Wagenaar and Wolfson (1994) estimated that only two out of every 1,000 instances of underage drinking resulted in an arrest or citation of a teen drinker, and only five out of every 100,000 instances of underage drinking resulted in any action against an establishment that provided the alcohol. A compliance check is an enforcement technique in which an underage person attempts to purchase alcohol under the supervision of police. If an alcohol sale is made, police apply warnings or penalties to the server and/or the license holder of the establishment. Compliance checks can be voluntarily conducted by local or state law enforcement agencies, or mandated by either local- or state-level laws.

Four studies evaluated the effectiveness of compliance checks in reducing youth access to alcohol via alcohol purchase attempts by underage or pseudo-underage buyers (Table 1). Three of these studies used probability samples and provided evidence that compliance checks were effective in reducing alcohol sales to minors. Among over 400 off-sale outlets in California and South Carolina, multivariate analyses showed that sales rates to pseudo-underage patrons decreased in cities where police compliance checks and a corresponding media campaign were conducted, compared to matched comparison cities that did not receive interventions (Grube, 1997). In two studies, several waves of compliance checks were conducted among probability samples of outlets, but comparison groups were not used. Results of four waves of compliance checks at approximately six-month intervals at 88 off-sale establishments in Denver, Colorado, showed sales to underage buyers reduced from 59% at baseline to 32% at wave two, and to 26% at waves three and four (Preusser et al., 1994). At 143 off-sale outlets in New Orleans, Louisiana, three waves of compliance checks with 17- to 22-year-olds (judged to look 18 or under) were conducted in conjunction with the State Alcoholic Beverage Control agency, along with a corresponding media event between the first and second waves. Sales rates to buyers reduced from 89% at baseline to 60% five months later; however, one year after the initial compliance checks, sales rates returned to 80% (Scribner & Cohen, 2001).

One study in the United Kingdom found that compliance checks were not effective in reducing underage alcohol sales, although researchers did not use a probability sample or multivariate analyses. Willner and colleagues (2000) found, during initial purchase attempts, 83% of on- and off-sale alcohol outlets in two cities in the U. K., where the legal drinking age is 18, sold alcohol to 16-year-olds. The sales rate did not change significantly following police compliance checks and a corresponding media campaign, compared to cities that did not receive the intervention.

Cohen and colleagues (2002) analyzed the effectiveness of state- and city-level compliance check policies, along with numerous other alcohol policies, across 97 U.S. cities in 38 states from 1995–1997. They found that cities that rated higher on an index of several enforcement policies, including compliance checks, had lower rates of total traffic fatalities (youth and adults).

Seller/Server Liability. Practices associated with selling and serving alcohol may also be altered by legal liability emerging from laws passed by state legislatures or from court cases. Such statutory or case law enables individuals to sue alcohol establishments for injuries or fatalities that occur due to illegal or negligent alcohol sales. We identified nine studies evaluating the effectiveness of such "dram shop" liability. Based on analyses of a national U.S. survey of persons 18 or older, dram shop liability was associated with decreased probability of drinking and driving, but had no effect on heavy episodic drinking in the last month or driving after heavy episodic drinking (Sloan et al., 1995; Stout et al., 2000). Seven studies analyzed national statistics to examine effects of dram shop liability on alcohol-related incidents and fatalities in the U.S. Dram shop laws were shown to reduce alcohol-related, overall traffic and single-vehicle nighttime fatalities, and mortality from homicides, falls, fires, and alcohol-related diseases (Chaloupka et al., 1993; Mast et al., 1999; Ruhm, 1996; Sloan et al., 1994; Wagenaar & Holder, 1991; Whetten-Goldstein et al., 2000; Young & Likens, 2000). In contrast, dram shop liability had no effect on total fatalities per mile driven or mortality from suicides (Ruhm, 1996; Sloan et al., 1994).

Four studies examined effects of dram shop liability on alcohol-related traffic fatalities among underage youth, specifically, and all were of high quality (i.e., longitudinal designs using multivariate analyses, comparison groups and data across several years; Table 1). Analyses of traffic data from 48 states in the 1980s showed that dram shop laws were associated with reductions in alcohol-related, total and nighttime traffic fatalities—but not traffic fatalities per capita—among 18- to 20-year olds (Chaloupka et al., 1993; Ruhm, 1996; Young & Likens, 2000). Analyses of traffic data from across all 50 states from 1984 to 1995 revealed that dram shop laws reduced total and alcohol-related fatalities, but not single-vehicle nighttime fatalities among underage youth (Whetten-Goldstein et al., 2000).

Community/Public Event Restrictions. Alcoholic beverages are often available to underage youth at community festivals or public events. Limits on drinks per person per order, restrictions on where alcohol can be consumed, and use of wristbands to identify customers over age 21 are examples of policies that can be used to reduce youth access to alcohol at community events. We identified six studies examining alcohol policies at public and community events. Two of the six studies examined effects of alcohol policies at sports stadiums on traffic crashes among the general population. Following introduction of beer sales at a Toronto stadium, no significant changes occurred in the number of alcohol-related motor vehicle crashes recorded in the area (Vingilis et al.,

1992). In a much larger study examining stadium policies in 97 U.S. cities in 38 states from 1995–1997, 36% of cities had restrictions on alcohol consumption at sporting events, and cities with more regulations controlling access to alcohol, including alcohol restrictions at sporting events, had significantly lower rates of traffic fatalities than cities with fewer regulations on alcohol access (Cohen et al., 2002).

Four of the six studies examined effects of restrictions on alcohol at community/public events on alcohol-related problems among youth. Three of the four studies were conducted in college settings using longitudinal designs and census samples, but none used comparison groups or multivariate analyses (Table 1). After a ban on beer sales at University of Colorado football games in 1996, arrests, assaults, ejections from the stadium and student referrals to the judicial affairs office decreased (Bormann & Stone, 2001). A study of an alcohol ban in the football stadium at the University of Arizona found no changes in injury or illness rates following the ban, although baseline rates of injuries and illness were very low (Spaite et al., 1990). Another study at the University of Arizona found that after new alcohol control policies were put into effect for 1995 homecoming events (e.g., alcohol restricted to certain areas; ban on beer kegs; liability insurance required), neighborhood complaint calls were reduced but no consistent change was found in arrests or other law enforcement actions (Johannessen et al., 2001).

Finally, one study assessed the perceived effects of alcohol policies on youth-related outcomes across 107 municipally owned facilities in Ontario. Forty-four (24%) of facility administrators perceived a reduction in alcohol-related problems, including underage drinking, fights and vandalism, following adoption of new alcohol policies (Gliksman et al., 1995).

Happy Hour Restrictions. In addition to taxes, other policies can affect the retail price of alcohol, including restrictions on "happy hours" or other special price promotions. Three studies examined effects of happy hours or discount pricing on alcohol consumption in the general population and one study examined effects of the price discounts on consumption among college students (Table 1)—three were conducted in experimental versus actual settings, and all used small samples. Babor and associates (1978; 1980) found that among 34 male drinkers, subjects in experimental happy hour conditions drank twice as much and at a faster rate than those in non-happy hour conditions. In Ontario, Canada, a ban on happy hours did not affect alcohol consumption among 49 patrons across five establishments, and did not affect overall sales figures; however, the ban was associated with a decrease in drinking-driving charges (Smart & Adlaf, 1986). Another study, with a sample of 189 undergraduate college students in an experimental lab setting, found that students exposed to advertised price discounts on alcohol and a longer duration of the discounts were more likely than comparison students to estimate higher rates of personal alcohol consumption (Christie et al., 2001).

Social Host Liability. Social host liability laws stipulate that if a person illegally gives alcohol to an underage person, and the underage person injures him/herself or another person, a third party can sue the provider of alcohol for damages. In a study of survey data across all 50 states, social host liability laws were associated with reduced probability of drinking and driving and reduced heavy episodic drinking among the general population (Stout et al., 2000). Whetten-Goldstein and associates (2000) examined laws across all 50 states from 1984 to 1995 and found that social host liability laws were associated with lower total traffic fatalities among youth and alcohol-related traffic fatalities among adults; however, social host laws were not associated with single-vehicle nighttime fatalities among youth or adults, or with alcohol-related fatalities among youth (Table 1).

Keg Registration. Youth often have access to large quantities of alcohol at drinking parties where beer is served in kegs at no charge or at very low cost (Wagenaar et al., 1993). One strategy to reduce this type of youth access to alcohol is through keg registration laws· Keg registration laws require alcohol retailers to affix a unique identification number to each beer keg and/or tap that is sold, then record the number, as well as the name and address of the keg purchaser. Keg registration policies enable law enforcement officers to identify and cite adults who purchase kegs and allow underage individuals to consume alcohol from the kegs. Keg registration policies are implemented at the local or state level, although implementing a keg law in only one area will likely be ineffective because buyers can go to adjacent communities to purchase kegs. A detailed analysis of keg laws in 20 states and the District of Columbia revealed that many of the laws were poorly written and implementation of the laws was limited in many states (Wagenaar et al., under review). Poorly written and implemented policies are less likely to be effective—an important issue for many alcohol control policies.

Cohen and colleagues (2002) analyzed effects of keg registration laws, along with numerous other alcohol policies, across 97 U.S. cities in 38 states from 1995–1997. They found that 31% of the cities had a keg registration law, and cities with more regulations on alcohol accessibility, including keg registration laws, had lower rates of total traffic fatalities (for both youth and adults) compared to cities with fewer regulations.

Warning Signs. State or local policies can require alcohol establishments to post warnings signs to inform customers of the minimum legal drinking age, identification checking policies, or penalties for selling or providing alcohol to underage youth. No studies of effects of warning signs pertaining to underage drinking have been published; however, studies of the effects of laws mandating warning signs to inform customers about risks of fetal injury from alcohol consumption during pregnancy show that warning signs increased awareness of risks, but did not change beliefs (Fenaughty & MacKinnon, 1993; Prugh, 1986).

Public Drinking Restrictions. Youth drinking and drinking-related problems often occur in public places, such as beaches, parking lots and parks. Two studies examined public drinking restrictions, although neither specifically addressed youth drinking. Cohen and colleagues (2002) found that 85% of 97 cities in 38 states prohibited public drinking, and cities with more regulations on alcohol accessibility, including public drinking restrictions, had lower rates of total traffic fatalities (for youth and adults) compared to cities with fewer alcohol accessibility regulations. Following a ban on alcohol at beaches in a New Zealand community, the number of crime incidents in the community decreased from 46 in the year prior to the ban to 20 after the ban, and police calls also declined (Conway, 2002).

In summary, while some policies—such as those affecting compliance checks and seller/server liability—show promise in reducing alcohol-related problems among youth, further research is needed to ascertain the effects of such policies on youth drinking and alcohol-related problems.

5. Policies with No Research

Home Delivery Restrictions. Youth may choose to have alcohol delivered to their homes to avoid attempting illegal purchases in public. To prevent such deliveries to underage people, communities or states can prohibit or restrict home deliveries of alcohol. One study found that over half the states in the U.S. allow home delivery of alcohol, and 7% of 18- to 20-year-olds and 10% of 12th graders in 15 mid-sized, Midwestern communities indicated drinking alcohol that had been delivered to their homes from retail establishments (Fletcher et al., 2000). In addition to home deliveries from local retail outlets, concern has also recently increased over delivery of alcoholic beverages that are ordered via the Internet.

Restricting Specific Products. Federal, state and local regulations can be used to restrict sales of products that particularly appeal to youth, such as sweet-flavored drinks or drinks packaged as single servings. Studies show that sweet-flavored alcoholic drinks appeal to teens (Hughes et al., 1997), and introduction of sales of these beverages in Sweden was associated with increased consumption among underage youth (Romanus, 2000).

Server Minimum Age. Laws can specify a minimum age for alcohol servers and store clerks to prevent individuals who are under the legal drinking age from selling or serving alcohol. Forster and colleagues (1994; 1995) found that younger servers are more likely to sell alcohol to underage youth.

Shoulder-Tap Enforcement. Some youth obtain alcohol by loitering outside alcohol establishments and asking adults to buy alcohol for them. To deter such sales, "shoulder tap" enforcement campaigns, in which underage individuals under the supervision of law enforcement approach adults outside alcohol establishments and ask adults to purchase alcohol for them, are implemented in some communities. In such a campaign, if an adult purchases alcohol for an underage youth, the adult is warned, cited, or arrested.

False Age-Identification Regulations. One difficulty in preventing youth purchases of alcohol may be the use of false age identification. To reduce use of false age identification, states and provinces may enhance the design of drivers' licenses (e.g., use holographic images, different colors, picture placement/profile for underage drivers) so that alterations or unofficial replications are difficult to achieve and easier to detect. States and communities may also increase penalties for producing, selling, or using false age identification cards.

In summary, many policies that have not yet been scientifically studied may be important for future efforts to reduce youth drinking and related problems.

6. Discussion

Understanding of the effects of alcohol control policies has been greatly advanced in the past two decades. Significant resources have been invested to gain understanding of two alcohol control policies—the MLDA and increased in excise taxes on alcohol. Many methodologically robust studies have evaluated effects of these policies on alcohol use and problems, such as traffic crashes, among underage youth. The preponderance of evidence from higher-quality studies indicates that the age-21 MLDA and higher prices of alcohol are associated with lower rates of alcohol consumption and related health and social problems among individuals under age 21.

Although less developed, we have also gained considerable knowledge in the past decade about several other alcohol control policies, including server/manager training, compliance checks, server/seller and social host liability, and advertising and happy hour restrictions. While sufficient research evidence is not yet available to reliably estimate the magnitude of the effects of each individual alcohol control policy, enough evidence has accumulated to suggest that taking action to decrease the availability of alcohol can prevent alcohol-related problems among the adult population, as well as reduce drinking and related problems among youth. As always, however, further research will be beneficial. While in the first few studies to assess promise of a specific policy we may be more accepting of weaker study designs (Holder et al., 1999), rigorous evaluations of alcohol control policies require studies with comparison groups, baseline data, representative samples, sufficient statistical power, and strong internal validity (e.g., randomized trials, time-series designs). Absence of observed policy effects in many studies may be the result of poorly developed or implemented policies, and particularly weak study designs. We must not prematurely reject prevention policies before policy implementations are evaluated using quality study designs; on the other hand, however, there comes a point when additional studies add little to our knowledge (e.g., MLDA) and research resources should be directed to other policies.

While effective policies, such as the MLDA and excise taxes, create large enough changes when implemented by themselves to affect alcohol-related problems, some alcohol control policies may only be effective when implemented in combination with other policies. Further research is needed to determine the optimal combination of alcohol control policies necessary to achieve sustained reductions in alcohol-related problems among youth.

As evaluation of alcohol control policies continues to evolve, we also need examinations of the multidimensionality of policies, specification of key policy components, and means for measuring the quality of policies and their implementation. In many policy evaluations, policies are treated dichotomously (present vs. absent), when in reality almost all are continua. Moreover, each policy includes many components or dimensions, and the importance or weight of each dimension for achieving the policy's aims varies. For example, a recent analysis of server training laws across 23 U.S. states determined 23 specific components logically grouped into five broader dimensions (Mosher et al., 2002). A similar analysis of keg registration laws across 20 U.S. states identified 91 specific components logically grouped into seven dimensions (Wagenaar et al., under review). Future policy evaluations will benefit from taking such complexity into account. In addition, even before rigorous evaluations are available, specification of "best practices" based on theory and that which has been found in analogous domains will advance the quality of policy design and implementation.

References

Alcohol Epidemiology Program (AEP). Alcohol Policies in the United States: Highlights from the 50 states. University of Minnesota: Minneapolis, MN, 2000.

Babor TF, Mendelson JH, Greenberg I, Kuehnle J. Experimental analysis of the "happy hour:" effects of purchase price on alcohol consumption. Psychopharmacology 1978;58:35–41.

Babor TF, Mendelson JH, Uhly B, Souza E. Drinking patterns in experimental and barroom settings. Journal of Studies on Alcohol 1980;41(7):635–51.

Bormann CA, Stone MH. The effects of eliminating alcohol in a college stadium: The Folsom Field beer ban. Journal of American College Health 2001 Sep;50(2):81–8.

Buka SL, Birdthistle I. Long-term effects of a community-wide alcohol server training intervention. Journal of Studies on Alcohol 1999;60:27–36.

Chaloupka FJ, Saffer H, Grossman M. Alcohol-control policies and motor-vehicle fatalities. Journal of Legal Studies 1993;22:161–86.

Chaloupka FJ, Wechsler H. Binge drinking in college: The impact of price, availability, and alcohol control policies. Contemporary Economic Policy 1996;14:112–24.

Christie J, Fisher D, Kozup JC, Smith S, Burton S, Creyer EH. The effects of bar-sponsored alcohol beverage promotions across binge and nonbinge drinkers. Journal of Public Policy & Marketing 2001 Fall;20(2):240–53.

Coate D, Grossman M. Effects of alcoholic beverage prices and legal drinking ages on youth alcohol use. Journal of Law & Economics 1988 Apr;31(1):145–71.

Cohen DA, Mason K, Scribner R. The population consumption model, alcohol control practices, and alcohol-related traffic fatalities. Preventive Medicine 2002 Feb;34(2):187–97.

Conway K. Booze and beach bans: turning the tide through community action in New Zealand. Health Promotion International 2002 Jun;17(2):171–7.

Cook PJ, Moore MJ. Drinking and schooling. Journal of Health Economics 1993;12:411–29.

Cook PJ, Moore MJ. The economics of alcohol abuse and alcohol-control policies. Health Affairs 2002;21(2):120–33.

Coutts MC, Graham K, Braun K, Wells S. Results of a pilot program for training bar staff in preventing aggression. Journal of Drug Education 2000;30(2):171–91.

Dee TS, Evans WN. Teen drinking and educational attainment: Evidence from two-sample instrumental variables estimates. Journal of Labor Economics 2003 Jan;21(1):178–209.

Dee TS. State alcohol policies, teen drinking and traffic fatalities. Journal of Public Economics 1999a May;72(2):289–315.
Dee TS. The complementarity of teen smoking and drinking. Journal of Health Economics 1999b Dec;18(6):769–93.
Dee TS. The effects of minimum legal drinking ages on teen childbearing. Journal of Human Resources 2001 Fall;36(4):823–38.
DiNardo J, Lemieux T. Alcohol, marijuana, and American youth: the unintended consequences of government regulation. Journal of Health Economics 2001 Nov;20(6):991–1010.
Everitt R, Jones P. Changing the minimum legal drinking age - its effect on a central city Emergency Department. New Zealand Medical Journal 2002 Jan;115(1146):9–11.
Fenaughty AM, MacKinnon DP. Immediate effects of the Arizona alcohol warning poster. Journal of Public Policy & Marketing 1993;12(1):69–77.
Fletcher LA, Toomey TL, Wagenaar AC, Short B, Willenbring ML. Alcohol home delivery services: A source of alcohol for underage drinkers. Journal of Studies on Alcohol 2000 Jan;61(1):81–4.
Forster JL, McGovern PG, Wagenaar AC, Wolfson M, Perry CL, Anstine PS. The ability of young people to purchase alcohol without age identification in northeastern Minnesota, USA. Addiction 1994;89:699–705.
Forster JL, Murray DM, Wolfson M, Wagenaar AC. Commercial availability of alcohol to young people: Results of alcohol purchase attempts. Preventive Medicine 1995;24(4):342–7.
Gliksman L, Douglas RR, Rylett M, Narbonne-Fortin C. Reducing problems through municipal alcohol policies: The Canadian experiment in Ontario. Drugs: Education, Prevention and Policy 1995;2(2):105–18.
Gliksman L, McKenzie D, Single E, Douglas R, Brunet S, Moffatt K. The role of alcohol providers in prevention: An evaluation of a server intervention programme. Addiction 1993;88(9):1195–203.
Grossman M, Chaloupka FJ, Sirtalan I. An empirical analysis of alcohol addiction: Results from the monitoring the future panels. Economic Inquiry 1998;36(January):39–48.
Grube JW. Preventing sales of alcohol to minors: Results from a community trial. Addiction 1997;92(Supplement 2):S251-S260.
Hennessy M, Saltz RF. Adjusting for multimethod bias through selection modeling. Evaluation Review 1989;13(4):380–99.
Holder HD, Edwards G. Alcohol and public policy: Evidence and issues. New York: Oxford University Press, 1995.
Holder H, Flay B, Howard J, Boyd G, Voas R, Grossman M. Phases of alcohol problem prevention research. Alcoholism: Clinical and Experimental Research 1999;23(1):183–94.
Holder HD, Gruenewald PJ, Ponicki WR, Treno AJ, Grube JW, Saltz RF, Voas RB, Reynolds R, Davis J, Sanchez L, Gaumont G, Roeper P. Effect of community-based interventions on high-risk drinking and alcohol-related injuries. Journal of the American Medical Association 2000 Nov; 284(18):2341–7.
Holder HD, Wagenaar AC. Mandated server training and reduced alcohol-involved traffic crashes: A time series analysis of the Oregon experience. Accident Analysis and Prevention 1994;26(1):89–97.
Howard-Pitney B, Johnson MD, Altman DG, Hopkins R, Hammond N. Responsible alcohol service: A study of server, manager, and environmental impact. American Journal of Public Health 1991 Feb;81(2):197–9.
Hughes K, Mackintosh AM, Hastings G, Wheeler C, Watson J, Inglis J. Young people, alcohol, and designer drinks - quantitative and qualitative study. British Medical Journal 1997 Feb;(7078):414–8.
Johannessen K, Glider P, Collins C, Hueston H, DeJong W. Preventing alcohol-related problems at the University of Arizona's homecoming: An environmental management case study. American Journal of Drug & Alcohol Abuse 2001;27(3):587–97.
Kaestner R. A note on the effect of minimum drinking age laws on youth alcohol consumption. Contemporary Economic Policy 2000 Jul;18(3):315–25.

Kenkel DS. Drinking, driving, and deterrence: The effectiveness and social costs of alternative policies. Journal of Law and Economics 1993;36(October):877–913.

Kuo M, Adlaf EM, Lee H, Gliksman L, Demers A, Wechsler H. More Canadian students drink but American students drink more: Comparing college alcohol use in two countries. Addiction 2002 Dec;97(12):1583–92.

Laixuthai A, Chaloupka FJ. Youth alcohol use and public policy. Contemporary Policy Issues 1993 Oct;11:70–81.

Lang E, Stockwell T, Rydon P, Beel A. Use of pseudo-patrons to assess compliance with laws regarding under-age drinking. Australian and New Zealand Journal of Public Health 1996;20(3):296–300.

Lang E, Stockwell T, Rydon P, Beel A. Can training bar staff in responsible serving practices reduce alcohol-related harm? Drug and Alcohol Review 1998;1:39–50.

Lockhart SJ, Beck KH, Summons TG. Impact of higher alcohol prices on alcohol-related attitudes and perceptions of suburban, middle-class youth. Journal of Youth and Adolescence 1993;22(4):441–53.

Makowsky CR, Whitehead PC. Advertising and alcohol sales: A legal impact study. Journal of Studies on Alcohol 1991;52:555–67.

Markowitz S, Grossman M. Alcohol regulation and domestic violence towards children. Contemporary Economic Policy 1998 Jul;(3):309–20.

Markowitz S, Grossman M. The effects of beer taxes on physical child abuse. Journal of Health Economics 2000 Mar;19(2):271–82.

Mast BD, Benson BL, Rasmussen DW. Beer taxation and alcohol-related traffic fatalities. Southern Economic Journal 1999 Oct;66(2):214–49.

McKnight J. Factors influencing the effectiveness of server-intervention education. Journal of Studies on Alcohol 1991;52(5):389–97.

Mosher JF, Toomey TL, Good C, Harwood E, Wagenaar AC. State laws mandating or promoting training programs for alcohol servers and establishment managers: An assessment of statutory and administrative procedures. Journal of Public Health Policy 2002;23(1):90–113.

National Institute on Alcohol Abuse and Alcoholism. Tenth Special Report to the U.S. Congress on Alcohol and Health. Rockville, MD: U.S. Department of Health and Human Services, National Institutes of Health, 2000. Report No.: NIH Publication No. 00–1583.

National Highway Traffic Safety Administration. Traffic Safety Facts 2002. Alcohol. Washington, DC: U.S. Department of Transportation, 2003 Aug. Report No.: DOT HS 809 606.

Nelson JP. Advertising bans, monopoly, and alcohol demand: Testing for substitution effects using state panel data. Review of Industrial Organization 2003 Feb;22(1):1–25.

Ogborne AC, Smart RG. Will restrictions on alcohol advertising reduce alcohol consumption? British Journal of Addiction 1980;75:293–6.

Ornstein SI. A survey of findings on the economic and regulatory determinants of the demand for alcoholic beverages. Substance Abuse and Alcohol Actions/Misuse 1984;5:39–44.

Ornstein SI, Hannsens DM. Alcohol control laws and the consumption of distilled spirits and beer. Journal of Consumer Research 1985;12(2):200–13.

Preusser DF, Williams AF, Weinstein HB. Policing underage alcohol sales. Journal of Safety Research 1994;25(3):127–33.

Prugh T. Point of purchase health warning notices. Alcohol Health and Research World 1986;10(4):36.

Riccelli C. Alcohol dispenser training in Amherst Massachusetts. Journal of Alcohol and Drug Education 1986;31(3):1–5.

Romanus G. Alcopops in Sweden - a supply side initiative. Addiction 2000 Dec;95(12 Suppl 4):S609-S619.

Ruhm CJ. Alcohol policies and highway vehicle fatalities. Journal of Health Economics 1996;15:435–54.

Russ NW, Geller ES. Training bar personnel to prevent drunken driving: A field evaluation. American Journal of Public Health 1987 Aug;77(8):952–4.

Saffer H, Dave D. Alcohol consumption and alcohol advertising bans. Applied Economics 2002 Jul;34(11):1325–34.

Saffer H, Grossman M. Beer taxes, the legal drinking age, and youth motor vehicle fatalities. Journal of Legal Studies 1987a;16(2):351–74.

Saffer H, Grossman M. Drinking age laws and highway mortality rates: Cause and effect. Economic Inquiry 1987b;25(3):403–17.

Saffer H. Alcohol advertising bans and alcohol abuse: An international perspective. Journal of Health Economics 1991;65–79.

Saffer H. Alcohol advertising and motor vehicle fatalities. Review of Economics and Statistics 1997;79(3):431–42.

Saltz RF. The roles of bars and restaurants in preventing alcohol-impaired driving: An evaluation of server intervention. Evaluation and Health Professions 1987;10(1):5–27.

Scribner R, Cohen D. The effect of enforcement on merchant compliance with the minimum legal drinking age law. Journal of Drug Issues 2001 Fall;31(4):857–66.

Simons-Morton BG, Cummings SS. Evaluation of a local designated driver and responsible server program to prevent drinking and driving. Journal of Drug Education 1997;27(4):321–33.

Sloan FA, Reilly BA, Schenzler C. Effects of prices, civil and criminal sanctions, and law enforcement on alcohol-related mortality. Journal of Studies on Alcohol 1994;55(4):454–65.

Sloan FA, Reilly BA, Schenzler C. Effects of tort liability and insurance on heavy drinking and drinking and driving. Journal of Law and Economics 1995;38(April):49–77.

Smart RG, Adlaf EM. Banning happy hours: the impact on drinking and impaired-driving charges in Ontario, Canada. Journal of Studies on Alcohol 1986;47(3):256–8.

Smart RG, Cutler RE. The alcohol advertising ban in British Columbia: Problems and effects on beverage consumption. British Journal of Addiction to Alcohol and other Drugs 1976;71:13–21.

Spaite DW, Meislin HW, Valenzuela T, Criss EA, Smith R, Nelson A. Banning alcohol in a major college stadium: Impact on the incidence and patterns of injury and illness. Journal of American College Health 1990;39:125–8.

Stout EM, Sloan FA, Liang L, Davies HH. Reducing harmful alcohol-related behaviors: Effective regulatory methods. Journal of Studies on Alcohol 2000 May;61(3):402–12.

Toomey TL, Kilian GR, Gehan JP, Perry CL, Jones-Webb R, Wagenaar AC. Qualitative assessment of training programs for alcohol servers and establishment managers. Public Health Reports 1998;113(2):162–9.

Toomey TL, Wagenaar AC, Gehan JP, Kilian G, Murray DM, Perry CL. Project ARM: Alcohol risk management to prevent sales to underage and intoxicated patrons. Health Education & Behavior 2001 Apr;28(2):186–99.

Tremblay VJ, Okuyama K. Advertising restrictions, competition, and alcohol consumption. Contemporary Economic Policy 2001 Jul;19(3):313–21.

Vingilis E, Liban CB, Blefgen H, Colbourne D, Reynolds D. Introducing beer sales at a Canadian ball park: The effect on motor vehicle accidents. Accident Analysis & Prevention 1992;24(5):521–6.

Wagenaar AC, Finnegan JR, Wolfson M, Anstine PS, Williams CL, Perry CL. Where and how adolescents obtain alcoholic beverages. Public Health Reports 1993;108(4):459–64.

Wagenaar AC, Harwood EM, Silianoff C, Toomey TL. Beer keg registration laws in the U.S.: Statutory, regulatory, and implementation issue. Under review.

Wagenaar AC, Holder HD. Effects of alcoholic beverage server liability on traffic crash injuries. Alcoholism: Clinical and Experimental Research 1991; 15(6):942–7.

Wagenaar AC, Murray DM, Gehan JP, Wolfson M, Forster JL, Toomey TL, Perry CL, Jones-Webb R. Communities Mobilizing for Change on Alcohol: Outcomes from a randomized community trial. Journal of Studies on Alcohol 2000a;61(1):85–94.

Wagenaar AC, Murray DM, Toomey TL. Communities Mobilizing for Change on Alcohol (CMCA): Effects of a randomized trial on arrests and traffic crashes. Addiction 2000b;95(2):209–17.

Wagenaar AC, Perry CL. Community strategies for the reduction of youth drinking: Theory and application. Journal of Research on Adolescence 1994;4(2):319–45.

Wagenaar AC, Toomey TL. Alcohol policy: Gaps between legislative actions and current research. Contemporary Drug Problems 2000;27:681–733.

Wagenaar AC, Toomey TL. Effects of minimum drinking age laws: Review and analyses of the literature from 1960 to 2000. Journal of Studies on Alcohol 2002 Mar;(Suppl 14):206–25.

Wagenaar AC, Wolfson M. Enforcement of the legal minimum drinking age in the United States. Journal of Public Health Policy 1994;15(1):37–53.

Wechsler H, Kuo MC, Lee H, Dowdall GM. Environmental correlates of underage alcohol use and related problems of college students. American Journal of Preventive Medicine 2000 Jul;19(1):24–9.

Weitzman ER, Nelson TF, Wechsler H. Taking up binge drinking in college: The influences of person, social group, and environment. Journal of Adolescent Health 2003 Jan;32(1):26–35.

Whetten-Goldstein K, Sloan FA, Stout E, Liang L. Civil liability, criminal law, and other policies and alcohol-related motor vehicle fatalities in the United States: 1984–1995. Accident Analysis & Prevention 2000 Nov;32(6):723–33.

Willner P, Hart K, Binmore J, Cavendish M, Dunphy E. Alcohol sales to underage adolescents: An unobtrusive observational field study and evaluation of a police intervention. Addiction 2000 Sep;95(9):1373–88.

Xie X, Mann RE, Smart RG. The direct and indirect relationships between alcohol prevention measures and alcoholic liver cirrhosis mortality. Journal of Studies on Alcohol 2000 Jul;61(4):499–506.

Yamada T, Kendix M, Yamada T. The impact of alcohol consumption and marijuana use on high school graduation. Health Economics 1996;5:77–92.

Young DJ, Likens TW. Alcohol regulation and auto fatalities. International Review of Law & Economics 2000 Mar;20(1):107–26.

14

Prevention for Children of Alcoholics and Other High Risk Groups

Robert A. Zucker and Maria M. Wong

1. Introduction

Median age of onset of alcohol use nationally is age 14 and median age of first drunkenness is 17 (Johnston et al., 2003). Thus, it is not surprising that the greatest public concern about drinking among young people begins with a focus on adolescence. It does not necessarily follow that the problems of risk for children of alcoholics[1] (COAs) and other children at high risk for the eventual development of alcohol use disorder (AUD) are the problems of adolescence. In fact, a now substantial body of evidence indicates that the drinking problems and other difficulties of adolescent and young adult COAs are predicted by much earlier markers. Thus the prevention question for this population becomes one of dealing with when the most appropriate time is to begin the intervention (i.e., what age to target) as well as how best to dampen or eliminate risk. Similarly, what is known about the adult disorder can also be informative about what to prevent, and what some of the prevention issues may be, given that this is the parenting generation. This chapter applies a developmental lens to the problem of prevention of risk among these very high risk populations.

1. We use the generic term "alcoholism" as well as the term "alcohol use disorder" interchangeably in this chapter to refer to what is more precisely designated in DSM-IV (American Psychiatric Association, 1994) as alcohol abuse and alcohol dependence. The more differential terminology is used when a more fine grained distinction is called for.

Robert A. Zucker and Maria Wong • Addiction Research Center, Department of Psychiatry, University of Michigan, Ann Arbor, Michigan 48105-2194.

2. Scope of the Problem

According to National Longitudinal Alcohol Epidemiologic Survey (NLAES) data (Grant, 2000), approximately 9.7 million children age 17 or younger, or 15 percent of the child population in that age range, were living in households with one or more adults classified with an alcohol abuse or dependence diagnosis during the past year (Table 1). Approximately 70 percent of these children were biological, foster, adopted, or step-children. That is, 6.8 million children meet the formal definition of COA, although, as noted below, not all are exposed to the same level of risk. In addition, 12 percent of the 66 million children in this age range were younger siblings of the alcoholic adult, 9 percent were other biological relatives (e.g., cousins, grandchildren) and approximately 6 percent were nonrelatives with or without their own relatives in the household, or were in an unspecified relationship. All of these other children and youth likewise fall under the umbrella of elevated socialization risk, although degree of biologic risk is probably lower.

Table 1. Number and Percentage of Children Living in Households with One or More Adults Who Abused or Were Dependent on Alcohol

	Parent AUD	
	During Past Year No.[a] (%)	During Child's Lifetime No.[a] (%)
Sex		
Male	4.7 (48.4)	14.3 (51.1)
Female	4.9 (50.5)	13.7 (48.9)
Race/ethnicity		
Black	1.1 (11.3)	2.4 (8.6)
Non-Black	8.5 (87.6)	25.7 (91.8)
Age (Years)		
0-2	1.8 (18.6)	5.3 (18.9)
3-5	1.7 (17.5)	5.1 (18.2)
6-8	1.7 (17.5)	5.0 (17.9)
9-11	1.5 (15.5)	4.6 (16.4)
12-14	1.4 (14.4)	4.3 (15.4)
15-17	1.5 (15.5)	4.0 (14.3)
Total Exposed	9.7 (100)	28.0 (100)
Total US Child Population	66 (15)	66 (43)

[a] In millions

Note: Adapted from Grant, B.F. (1997). Estimates of U.S. Children Exposed to Alcohol Abuse and Dependence in the Family. Am. J. Pub. Health, 90: 112-115.

Given that these figures concern *past year* exposure to at least one alcoholic adult, from the perspective of socialization risk they only reflect acute exposure. Other data from the NLAES provide estimates of magnitude of overall child risk pertaining to exposure to an either currently or previously alcoholic adult; the figure is 43 percent of the under-18 population, or slightly less than half of all children (also Table 1). The figure for COAs is only 30 percent, but this is still a literally enormous population of risk. Taken together, these figures speak to the social complexity, and likely risk variability among the families and households in which risk has the potential to unfold. At the same time, they also speak to the enormity of the social problem.

A second point needs to be underscored. COA status is heavily used as a proxy for "alcoholism risk" on the one hand, and socialization risk on the other, but the COA designation more precisely is a proxy for multiple causal inputs, not all of which may be present in the individual case. Thus, being a COA implies elevated genetic risk, on the average, although the alcoholic genetic diatheses may not have been passed on to a particular child. One may be a COA without being undercontrolled, having an attention deficit hyperactivity disorder (ADHD) diagnosis, etc. Moreover, the genetic risk is polygenic, and the alleles conveying risk are not always the dominant ones so that additivity of risk to produce problem outcomes is the rule rather than the exception (Rutter, 1982; Stoltenberg and Burmeister, 2000). Socialization risk involves exposure, but given the heavy divorce rates found in this population, evaluating level of socialization risk is complex, involving quantification not only of how long the exposure has been, but also the developmental period during which the socialization took place. Some developmental periods have the potential to be more vulnerability-producing than others (Fuller *et al.*, 2003). In addition, a substantial amount of marital assortment occurs in alcoholic families (Hall *et al.*, 1983). When assortment is present, risk exposure is multiplied, and COA effects become a function of genetic risk(s), individual parent risk, and the synergistic risk created by marital interaction (Fuller *et al.*, 2003).

Third, COA risk is not simply risk for the development of AUD. Given what is known about the elevated comorbidities found among offspring of alcoholics, this designator is also a marker of elevated risk for behavioral and cognitive deficits. These include attention deficit disorder, behavioral undercontrol/conduct disorder, delinquency, lower IQ, poor school performance, low self esteem, etc. (Noll *et al.*, 1992; Nigg *et al.*, 1998; Poon *et al*, 2000; Sher, 1991; West and Prinz, 1987). Furthermore, the evidence strongly implicates some of these nonalcohol specific characteristics as causal to both problem alcohol use and elevated risk for AUD (Caspi *et al*, 1996; Donovan and Jessor, 1985, Nigg *et al.*, 1998). The converse is also true; the nonalcohol specific characteristics among nonCOA children are markers of elevated risk for alcohol problems, alcoholism, and other drug involvement, hence the title of this chapter and the necessary focus on "other high risk groups" (Biglan *et al.*, 2004; Zucker and Gomberg, 1986).

3. Early Development Origins of Risk among COAS

One of the historically most important findings of the past generation has been the documentation of a link between delinquent and aggressive activity in adolescence and earlier onset of alcohol use, as well as more problematic use (Jessor and Jessor, 1977; Kandel, 1978; Donovan and Jessor, 1985; Ellickson et al., 2003). An extensive body of work has documented how these behaviors emerge from a matrix of personality and temperament influences, attitudes, and parental socialization practices and modeling, that encourage the development of independent and rebellious behavior. (Colder & Chassin, 1999; Tarter et al, 1985; Tarter & Vanukov, 1994;) This in turn produces more exposure to a deviant peer network, which then drives the emergence of earlier and more problem alcohol use (Blackson & Tarter, 1994; Blackson et al, 1994; Blackson, 1997; Zucker et al., 1995a).

Until recently, only the adolescent version of these linkages had been established. However, within the past decade three prospective studies beginning in early childhood have shown a direct link between the early child manifestations of these attributes, specifically behavioral undercontrol and aggressiveness, and AUD and other alcohol problem outcomes in adolescence and early adulthood (Caspi et al., 1996; Masse and Tremblay, 1997; Zucker et al., 2000; Mayzer et al., 2001, 2002, 2003). These studies join with two earlier reports of projects beginning in middle childhood (Cloninger et al, 1988; Eron et al, 1987) with similar childhood markers at baseline, and with alcoholism and drunk driving outcomes in adulthood. Three of the studies, the Dunedin Health and Development Study (Caspi et al, 1996), the Columbia County Study (Eron et al, 1987), and the Montreal Longitudinal Study (Masse and Tremblay, 1997) involve general population samples, and two involve COA samples (Cloninger et al., 1988; Zucker et al., 2000; Mayzer et al, 2001, 2002). Table 2 describes the ages at baseline and follow-up, and the baseline behaviors and adolescent/adult outcomes of the study. The level of replication shown across these studies must be taken as definitive evidence that an early childhood behavior-adulthood AUD relationship exists. Combined with the adolescent studies noted above, findings indicate that a continuity pathway exists from very early childhood to an alcoholism outcome in adulthood.

Equally importantly, both the COA studies (Cloninger et al, 1988; Mayzer et al, 2002) and the Dunedin study (Caspi et al., 1996) find a behavioral inhibition/shyness/social fearfulness cluster predicted alcoholism and alcohol problem outcomes in adolescence and early adulthood. These latter characteristics have only sporadically been reported in the adolescent literature (Kaplan, 1975) but they are consistent with the known adult relationship between social phobia and AUD (Kushner et al., 1990), and they also have been reported in some historically earlier prospective studies begun in early childhood. Thus Werner (1986), observed a relationship between a low sociability temperament in infancy and early childhood with the greater likelihood of an alcoholic outcome in early adulthood, and Kellam et al, (1980; 1983) observed a relationship

Table 2. Longitudinal Studies Connecting Early Child Behavior to AUD and Alcohol Problem Outcomes in Adolescence and Adulthood

Study	Early Child Behavior	Baseline Age (Yrs)	Follow-Up Age (Yrs)	Outcome Behavior
General Population Studies				
Dunedin Health & Development Study	Behavioral Undercontrol	3	21	Alcohol Dependence
Dunedin Health & Development Study	Behavioral Inhibition	3	21	More Alcohol Problems
Montreal Longitudinal Study	Low Fearfulness; Hyperactivity	6 and 10	11 to 15	Earlier Drunkenness Onset
Columbia County Study	Aggression	8	30	Driving While Intoxicated
COA Studies				
Michigan Longitudinal Study	Externalizing Behavior	3 to 5	12–14	Early drinking Onset
Michigan Longitudinal Study	Internalizing Behavior	3 to 5	12–14	Early drinking Onset
Swedish Adoption Study-2	High Novelty Seeking; Low Harm Avoid	11	27	Alcoholism
Swedish Adoption Study	High Harm Avoid; Low Novelty Seek	11	27	Alcoholism

Note: See text for study citations.

between shyness/social inhibition in 1st grade and greater alcohol and drug use in adolescence.

It is noteworthy that in all of this work, parallel findings are reported out of both the COA and the general population studies, suggesting that it is the risk factor(s) rather than COA status in particular, that is driving these relationships. At the same time, the socialization environment is virtually uncharacterized in most of the studies. Thus it is not possible to determine the degree to which contextual factors may be moderating or mediating the relationship. Moreover, even in the nonCOA samples, one cannot automatically assume a more benign environment. In fact, in two of the general population studies reviewed above, the Montreal Longitudinal Study (Masse and Tremblay, 1997) and the Woodlawn Study (Kellam et al, 1980), the population sampling was deliberately set to provide a group of families of low socioeconomic status and high social adversity. Thus even in the nonCOA studies, the level of environmental adversity may be sufficiently damaging and sufficiently similar to what exists in alcoholic homes to produce the parallel effects.

In terms of relevance of these findings to prevention activity, one final observation is called for: these studies in toto, are potentially a call to arms for preventionists because they provide easily identifiable targets for preventive programming at an early age. The etiologic data pertaining to behavioral undercontrol clearly indicate continuity of risk over the course of development, and therefore strongly suggest that change in the risk factor should lead to change in the outcome. Interestingly however, although these findings are dramatic and have now been in the literature for between 8 and 17 years, they remain almost totally neglected in the prevention literature. To my knowledge, only one just published policy book (Biglan et al, 2004), a recent report following families from birth to age 18 (Garnier and Stein, 2002), and a very brief summary in the most recent NIAAA Report to Congress (NIAAA, 2000) begin to address the prevention implications they raise. I will return to this issue at the end of the chapter.

4. Heterogeneity of Risk Pathways

In the previous section, I noted that characterization of environmental adversity has been relatively ignored in most of the long term, early-starting high risk studies. This is a significant omission because of the need to understand the potential for environmental adversity to exacerbate individual risk on the one hand, and for its absence to alleviate individual risk on the other. For the same reason, within the nonCOA population it is important to understand the degree to which environmental adversity, or its absence, makes a difference in producing an adverse outcome. Our group has examined this issue using data from an ongoing longitudinal family study of alcoholic men, their spouses, their initially 3 to 5 year old sons, other siblings, and a suitably matched set of contrast families drawn from the same high risk neighborhoods where the alcoholic families lived, but where neither parent had a lifetime diagnosis for any substance use disorder (Zucker et al, 1996; 2000). Families were followed at 3-year intervals beginning when the target boy was 3 to 5 years of age.

We used a person-centered approach in examining the interactive nature of family adversity and child risk vulnerability over the interval between 3 and 14 years of age.[2] The adversity index used was one that assessed level of exposure to a highly pathological family environment. A summative family psychopathology measure was created that scaled both currency and severity of AUD as well as the presence/absence of antisocial behavior in each of the parents, then added them together (cf. Wong et al, 1999; Zucker et al, 2003). High family adversity involved having two parents with currently active alcoholism, or one parent with an antisocial alcoholism diagnosis, or both. This index, although established by way of parental psychopathology, is an effective proxy for a number of other pertinent indicators of family adversity, including conflict, violence, economic difficulty, family crises, other psychiatric comorbidity,

2. Findings described in this section are based on data originally reported in Zucker et al, 2003, and the reader is referred to that source for more precise details of measures and analyses.

and trouble with the law (Zucker et al., 1996). In addition, on the basis of national Epidemiologic Catchment Area Study alcoholism comorbidity rates (Helzer et al, 1991) and national familial alcoholism figures (Grant, 2000; Huang et al, 1998), these cutoff criteria would yield a population encompassing slightly less than 1 percent of U.S. households, but approximately 20 percent of alcoholic families (the severest subset).

The child's initial risk status at age 3 to 5 was described by a global socio-behavioral psychopathology measure that was nationally normed. Low risk was defined as being within normal limits on this global index, high risk was defined as being at the 80th percentile or higher on the measure (0.84 SDs above the norm). A two by two grid was created by cross cutting these dimensions. Initially *Resilient children* were defined by having normal to high adaptation (i.e., low "risk" scores) even though they were living in the high family adversity environment. The normal risk under conditions of low family adversity group was labeled *Non-challenged* to emphasize that their behavior was unremarkable, within a family context involving low parent psychopathology that exerted no pressure for deviance, and that was more likely to be nurturant and encouraging. The high risk (high psychopathology) under conditions of high family adversity group was labeled *Vulnerable,* in order to emphasize the continuing exposure to family trouble that took place here. Other evidence from the study shows that these children had been negatively impacted by this exposure (Wong, et al. 1999). Finally, those children with high risk (high psychopathology) under conditions of low family adversity were characterized as *Troubled* in order to emphasize that, even without the familial adversity, they still showed a poor behavioral adaptation. In other words, they showed up as already symptomatic, even with a lack of environmental press.

Figure 1a shows the trajectory of externalizing problems for each of the groups and Figure 1b shows the trajectory of internalizing problems. Overall across-age group differences were significant for both externalizing and internalizing problem trajectories. The non-challenged group sustained the lowest level of externalizing problems over the course of childhood and early adolescence, followed by the resilient group, the troubled group, and the vulnerable group. At all ages, the vulnerable group sustained the highest level of externalizing problems. The figure also shows a consistent pattern of decline in externalizing behavior over childhood, a pattern that is normative for this age range. In addition, there is increasing convergence in level of externalizing difficulties through middle childhood. At the transition to adolescence we again see the normative pattern of a developmental shift, involving increasing externalizing (aggressive/delinquent/impulsive) behavior (cf. Jessor and Jessor, 1977). The individual difference data indicate that whereas the resilient children were not distinguishable from their non-challenged peers as pre-schoolers, they showed a small but reliably higher level of externalizing problems as they grew older. At the same time, they still occupied an intermediate place, having a lower level of these behaviors than did their vulnerable peers. In addition, the divergence of slopes between ages 9 to 11 and 12 to 14 depicts a significant interaction between child individual differences in initial risk and level of experienced environmental adversity during a period of life when the overall norm is for increasing deviant and impulsive activity. This interactional

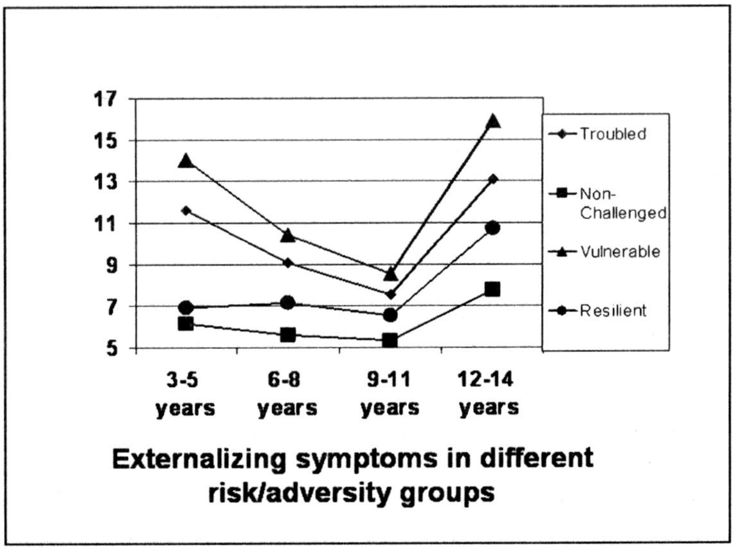

Figure 1a. Externalizing symptoms over time in groups differing on risk and adversity. (*Source:* p. 88 in Zucker, R.A., Wong, M.M., Puttler, L. I. and Fitzgerald, H.E. (2003). Resilience and vulnerability among sons of alcoholics: Relationship to developmental outcomes between early childhood and adolescence. In S. Luthar (Ed.), *Resilience and Vulnerability: Adaptation in the Context of Childhood Adversities.* Cambridge University Press, New York. Reprinted with permission.)

relationship had previously been observed cross-sectionally among these children when they were 3 to 5 years of age (Wong et al., 1999). The trajectory data indicate the pattern is sustained developmentally; they depict continuity over time in group positioning vis a vis level of undercontrolled behavior, and the positioning is sustained across the risk-adversity groups even though level of group differentiation varies, as does absolute level of undercontrolled activity.

Figure 1b shows the trajectories for internalizing problems; here also the non-challenged group shows the lowest level of problems, followed by the resilient group. The troubled group was similar to the vulnerable group. The figure also shows important pattern variations. During preschool and up through the early school years, an identical individual difference pattern exists. Non-challenged and resilient children are significantly lower in internalizing symptoms than both the vulnerable and troubled groups, and there are no differences between the resilient and the non-challenged children. The pattern begins to diverge following 2nd-3rd grade, and by early adolescence the non-challenged group is significantly lower than all others, and no differences exist between any of the other three groups. In other words, at this juncture the resilient children have developed a level of internalizing symptoms that is similar to both the vulnerable and the troubled children. Here also we tested this group by time interaction with a repeated measures analysis of variance. A significant interaction effect of time and adaptation group indicates that the developmental trajectories of internalizing problems varied differently among

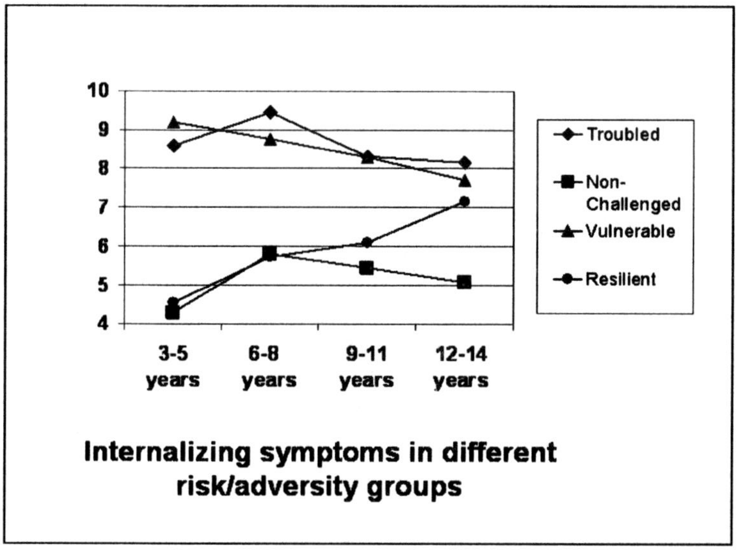

Figure 1b. Internalizing symptoms over time in groups differing on risk and adversity. (*Source:* p. 88 in Zucker, R.A., Wong, M.M., Puttler, L. I. and Fitzgerald, H.E. (2003). Resilience and vulnerability among sons of alcoholics: Relationship to developmental outcomes between early childhood and adolescence. In S. Luthar (Ed.), *Resilience and Vulnerability: Adaptation in the Context of Childhood Adversities.* Cambridge University Press, New York. Reprinted with permission.)

the adaptation groups, with three of the four showing a continuity pattern, and one a discontinuity pattern.

These patterns of trajectory variation in both externalizing and internalizing problems are more than simply patterns of risk variation over time. As already noted in Table 2, they also are proxies for differences in probability of problem drinking, other problem behavior, and also alcohol dependence (Ellickson et al, 2003; Grant and Dawson, 1997; Pederson and Skrondal, 1998). In the Michigan study, Mayzer and colleagues (2000, 2002, 2003) have already confirmed the first step in this chain of effect, by showing that higher levels of early externalizing and internalizing behavior are predictive of both early onset of drinking, as well as higher levels of externalizing and internalizing behavior and delinquent activity in adolescence. On both these grounds, the results indicate that the children identified as vulnerable are at highest risk, the non-challenged group is of lowest risk, and the resilient group is of intermediary risk, in particular because of the increasing experience of internalizing problems as they move into adolescence.

Finally, it is instructive to remind ourselves who the COAs are in this matrix of individual and contextual risk. They are the youth labeled as Vulnerable and Resilient, the children who were born into, and reared in families with high alcoholism density and high parental antisocial comorbidity. Conversely, the nonCOAs are comprised of the Non-Challenged and the Troubled groups yet they have strikingly different pathways of risk. Given what has already been established about the utility of the externalizing and internalizing behavior measures as proxy indicators of alcohol problems and elevated risk for later AUD, these findings make clear that an understanding of both familial risk and individual risk is essential to an understanding of pathways into problem alcohol use (also see Garnier and Stein, 2002). When individual vulnerability is present early, even a nonchallenging family environment is insufficient to moderate the child's vulnerability. Conversely, from the perspective of risk for externalizing problems, a subset of COAs moves through childhood relatively trouble free, while another subset, showing early risk, is the highest risk subgroup.

This pattern is tempered to a considerable degree for internalizing risk. For one subgroup of young COAs, their early behavior indicates they are relatively free of sadness, anxiety, depression and worry. Exposure to the adversity of an actively alcoholic home, with its attendant strain and conflict (Loukas et al, 2003) leads to a gradual degradation of their affective status, such that by the time adolescence is reached, their level of internal trouble is equivalent to that of their more obviously less fortunate peers.

5. The Timing and Dosing of Prevention Programming: Toward a Hypothetic-Deduction Science of Prevention

A science of timing and dosing for prevention activity does not yet exist. Earlier is perhaps better, but earlier is more expensive, and effects delivered early, if not sustained by boosters, have the potential to decay over time. The variations in externalizing and internalizing trajectories documented above suggest some interesting, and to our knowledge previously undescribed preventive intervention strategies. They also suggest some interesting hypotheses. The trajectory data indicate that the critical timing points for intervention for externalizing and internalizing behaviors may be different. For externalizing problems, despite the variation in level over time, grouping based on early risk and early family adversity holds its order. At the same time, the later elementary school years appear to be the point of greatest subsidence of these risky characteristics. If the hypothesis is that the best way-point to intervene is when the problem behavior is most quiescent, then late elementary school would be the timing point of choice. If the hypothesis is that the point of greatest impact will be when the problem behavior is most active, because there is more to engage with and potentially change, then an early childhood start would appear to be the timing point of choice. These two alternative strategies need to be pitted against each other and evaluated.

For internalizing problems, for three of the four risk/adversity groups a pattern of continuity exists from early childhood onward, with an essentially flat trajectory over that interval. For the resilient group however, the point of greatest quiescence is either preschool or the earlier elementary school years. "Quiescence" theory does not provide a clear choice about whether it would be more efficacious to begin early, or to begin around the time when higher levels of internalizing problems begin to manifest themselves. One might speculate that an intervention in this content arena that is done too early might have little effect. Conversely, if one's choice is driven by "Activation" theory, then an intervention at the latter part of elementary school, or even at the transition to middle school or junior high might be the most appropriate intervention point. Again, these alternatives should be evaluated.

What about dosing? For vulnerable and troubled children, the long term presence of both sets of risk factors, at the highest levels vis a vis the other groups, points to the need for a multilevel intervention regimen that is based upon a chronic disease model (McLellan et al, 2000). Such programming would involve initial evaluation and dosing, addressed both to the child's difficulties as well as the difficulties of the family in which he/she is grouping up. Periodic check-ups, that provide an opportunity for renewed intervention when called for, would be a part of such a regimen. It would also be expected that such programming be available over a substantial portion of the childhood life course, although not necessarily required at all times. For resilient children, it is not at all clear how long such a developmentally timed intervention would be required. The presence of other coping skills in this group has already been documented (Zucker et al, 2003). These skills (e.g. reading) are suggestive that the intervention would be facilitated by the child's own orthogenic competence, and that the dosing would not need to be as prolonged.

One last point: With the exception of the change in internalizing symptoms among the low child risk/high family adversity resilient children, the mean trajectory patterns are stable, and remain in the same risk rank ordering over time. This is the case as much for the "off-diagonal" groups—where one might anticipate that individual risk-variability and social environmental stress would work at cross purposes, as it is for the "on-diagonal" groups. Although the study design was never set up to evaluate the relative role of environmental and genetic influences, we have elsewhere suggested that the strong auto-stability of risk is consistent with the hypothesis of a substantial genetic contribution to risk (Fuller et al., 2003). Should this ultimately prove to be the case, then it would open the door to considering more physiological and pharmacologic methods for risk reduction.

6. Current Prevention Strategies

In 1994 the Institute of Medicine proposed a revised set of definitions of prevention programming. Refining the earlier distinction between Primary, Secondary, and Tertiary Prevention, new categories of activity were again proposed at three levels. *Universal prevention activity* targets entire populations, and involves working with a group that has not been identified on the basis of individual risk. *Selective intervention* targets individuals or subgroups whose risk is known to be higher than the population at large, but where the disorder or problem has not yet manifested itself. *Indicated preventive intervention* targets individuals who have already shown prodromal signs or symptoms, but who do not yet meet diagnostic criteria (Institute of Medicine, 1994).

Given the evidence just reviewed that indicates risky behaviors prodromal to AUD can be identified in COA and other high risk populations at a very early age, one might conclude that the data are sufficient to require a level of programming that is at the least at the Selective level, and perhaps even the Indicated level for most COA and other designated high risk populations. Moreover, the sheer magnitude of the at risk population, involve 15 percent of children under 17, suggests that preventive programming targeted at COAs should be regarded as a major public health effort. Interestingly, it is not.

In the literature review conducted for this report, I was able to identify only two selective programs focusing on COAs, that have been (or are in the process of being) subjected to the rigorous evaluation of the randomized clinical trial. The first, carried out by the author and colleagues in the late '80s and early '90s (Maguin et al, 1994; Nye et al., 1999; Zucker and Noll, 1987) used a population based recruitment protocol to recruit families with active alcoholism in the father at the time of first contact. The project used a manualized 10 month parent training and marital problem solving protocol modeled after Patterson et al.'s (1975) social learning therapy. The child focus was reduction in conduct problems and development of prosocial behaviors, a focus that was theoretically selected as a precursive pathway to later alcoholism risk. At end of treatment and 6 month follow-up, as predicted, positive changes in child behavior and parenting style occurred. Unfortunately, later evaluation of potential drinking offsets were not conducted. The second program, a joint U.S./Canadian program still in progress, is being conducted by Nochajski, DeWit, and colleagues at the Research Institute on Addictions in Buffalo and the Centre for Addiction and Mental Health in London, Ontario. The intervention makes use of Kumpfer's (1998) Strengthening Families Program (SFP) and enrolls families with an alcohol abusing parent and their school aged children. The intervention involves a 14 session group therapy program that combines parent training with family communication skills training and child social skills training. Results to date show that as compared to a minimal attention control group, SFP produced significant improvements in child externalizing behavior problems (Maguin, et al., 2003) and family functioning (Safyer, et al., 2003). A longer term delay of onset of alcohol use, as well as reduction in alcohol problems among the children is eventually anticipated, but the study has not been running long enough to determine whether this effect occurs. Nonetheless, the robustness of externalizing problems as an early proxy for alcohol problem outcomes is such that the anticipated outcome is a highly plausible one.

One other selective early intervention program, while not specifically alcohol focused, also has shown long term alcohol prevention effects; it is David Olds' Nurse Visitation Program. The program initially involved home visits with high risk, high poverty, primarily teen mothers during pregnancy; reassessments were at 2 years, and again at a 15 year follow-up. At the 15 year follow-up, the visited group of mothers reported fewer days drinking, and fewer cigarettes smoked per day in the prior six months than did their no treatment control group (Olds et al., 1998).

The programs just described involve families whose parents are from clinical or quasi-clinical populations, where level of risk for problem alcohol outcomes among offspring is substantially elevated. However, several hundred universal programs focusing on delay of substance use, or alternatively, delay or reductions in delinquent behavior, have been carried out, and a number of those have demonstrated specific alcohol related prevention effects (Biglan et al, 2004). Programs have rarely been simply child focused, but rather have chosen interventions to address *systems interacting with the child* (parent behavior, family interactions and relationships*), systems interacting around the child* (teacher training and curriculum development, parent training, working with the courts and legal system), *systems acting at the community level* (community action programs, changes in the rigorousness of enforcement of alcohol and cigarette access, and *systems addressing policy* (establishment of drug courts, zero tolerance drivers' license programs, changes in pricing, etc.). Although there is a plethora of such programming, relatively few protocols have been subjected to rigorous process and outcome evaluation. The reader is referred to a recent comprehensive review of this spectrum of offerings by Biglan and colleagues (2004) for detailed descriptions and evaluations of the most rigorous of these programs. Following, we briefly describe four of the most comprehensive, that have been rigorously developed and carefully evaluated:

(1) A truncated (7 session) version of the Strengthening Families Program has been used as a universal prevention program involving initially 6th grade (ca. age 12) children from rural elementary schools in Iowa. The program is of special interest because of its promise to ultimately impact new cases of AUD as program participants grow into adulthood. (The study also evaluated another program, Preparing for the Drug Free Years (PDFY), a 5 session family competency program based on the Social Development Model (Hawkins et al, 1999), but since PDFY effects were always weaker than the SFP arm of the study, only findings from the SFP protocol are discussed here.) Remarkably strong improvements both in parenting skills and in family relations (Kumpfer, Alvarado, Tait, Turner and Alder, 2002) were demonstrated both 4 years out and 6 years out from the intervention (Spoth, Redmond and

Chin, 2001; Spoth, 2003). More importantly from the standpoint of this chapter, the program successfully delayed onset of alcohol use as well as dampened increases in level of consumption over time (Guyll et al, in press; Spoth, 2003), and also slowed the rate of initiation into tobacco, marijuana, and other illicit drug use. Benefit-cost calculations relating to projected rates of AUD prevented indicated a return of $9.60 per dollar invested, and net benefits per family of $5,923 (Spoth et al, 2002).

Other preventive intervention programs, all universal in focus, have been able to demonstrate impact upon early drinking behavior during adolescence, although none have evaluated their ultimate impact on a later AUD outcome. Several are noteworthy for their comprehensive focus on individual, school and community, their relatively early initial contact with the child, and/ or their impressive impact on alcohol related behaviors.

(2) Project Northland (Perry et al, 1996) is currently the only specifically alcohol focused program addressing the distal domains as well as the child's micro-social environmental domains, as part of a unified effort to delay onset of use as well as reduce problems once drinking has begun. Results have included significantly lower prevalence of alcohol use after three years of intervention, with strongest effects among those who were nonusers at baseline. The magnitude of effects in this program was small, but because of the low initial base rates of drinking at younger ages, the comparative effects were substantial. Looking only at students who were nondrinkers at the 6th grade baseline, 15.3 % in the treatment sites at 8th grade follow-up had past month alcohol use, while 21.2 percent had use in the control sites. The protocol also showed effects in reducing marijuana use (3.1 vs. 6.2 percent) and cigarette use (15.5 vs. 24.6 percent). All of these effects were confined to the baseline nondrinker group. No significant changes were found among those who had already begun drinking. This work was not able to parse out the reasons for these differential effects on initial nonusers vs. users, but youth who are already using at 6th grade are very much an early onset group, given that median age of onset of first use is 14. Given also what is known about the impulsivity, heavier drinking of parents, and conflicted family backgrounds of early onset users (Ellickson et al, 2003; Mayzer et al, 2001, 2002, 2003) it is likely that the social micronetworks within which the early onset drinkers moved would have insulated them to a greater degree from program effects. Effects decayed after the intervention was no longer active (Perry et al, 1998, reported in Wagenaar, 2000).

(3) In another long term and very comprehensive universal prevention program, the Seattle Social Development Project (Hawkins et al, 1992) targeted a high risk community sample in a program that involved individual, school/teacher, and family interventions. The program emphasized the creation and maintenance of strong family and school bonds, and also had a component focused on cognitive and social skills training in the early school years and refusal and life skills training in late elementary school. One subset of youngsters received all levels of the program (the Full Intervention Group), a second Late Intervention Group received only the later programming, and a

third subset was a No Intervention Control. Long term follow up at age 18 showed a number of differences for the full intervention group on school attachment and achievement, no differences on lifetime prevalence of alcohol use, cigarettes or other drug use, but reduced past year heavy alcohol use at this point. In other words, the problem level of alcohol use was impacted downstream but overall use was not (Hawkins et al, 1999). The late-dosing-only group did not show this effect.

(4) Another universal program, with its point of entree and raison d'etre being the reduction of bullying and related problems was implemented by Olweus (1989) in a national program conducted in Norway in the mid'80s. The evaluation for this work utilized a quasi-experimental design, and a subset of students initially in grades 4 to 7 in a large number of elementary and middle schools in Bergen, Norway in 1984–1985 to conduct the evaluation. This extraordinarily comprehensive program incorporated a number of levels: first a questionnaire to increase awareness as well as gauge severity, then feedback to the schools and discussion, then setting up structures to monitor level of the problem and effectiveness of solutions at the school and classroom levels, conduct of classroom discussions, as well as individual discussion with perpetrators victims, and their parents, etc. The program produced significant reductions in antisocial/delinquent activity, as well as drunkenness as far out as two years from baseline. This is but one of a host of examples in the universal focus literature where a focus on the undercontrolled aspects of behavior also has an effect on drinking.

The Olweus program involved a large number of individuals and groups in a multi-tiered framework of interventions involving interwoven, "across level" relationships. Moreover, the rule structure legislating this prevention activity was at the political, community leader, as well as the educational policy levels, given that the program was community wide (in actuality, the entire project, not all of which was subject to formal evaluation, was the country of Norway), and the educational system had agreed to modify itself, by conducting all day conferences, changing monitoring practices for the bullying behavior in and outside of class, setting up coordinating committees, etc.

One final note: Population generalizability for those treated (i.e., those participating in a program) against those eligible is not well documented in existing studies. However, the available data across studies indicates that the selectivity of who is being treated vis a vis who is high risk is a potentially significant problem given that programs routinely have very high initial nonparticipation rates. Thus, the Iowa program reported a 51% completion rate of the baseline assessment among all 6th graders in the schools they recruited from (Spoth et al, 2001), the New York/ Ontario program reports a 70% treatment entry rate for those who completed the baseline assessment (rate of involvement in the baseline assessment vis a vis the population of those eligible was not available) , and participation rates more generally in indicated as well as universal programs have hovered around the 60 to 70 % range (Tremblay et al, 1995; Dishion et al, 2002) . Much like the Project Northland program issue of only having impact on initial nondrinkers, this is a critical policy concern if one's interest is in addressing risk among the most disadvantaged. It is such families, with high rates of family disorganization and lack of child involvement that are the ones most likely to not initially engage (Ary et al, 1999; Chilcoat et al, 1996). Some researchers have attempted to demonstrate that the problem is a minor one (e.g., Spoth, 2003) because the limited contrast data comparing participants to nonparticipators suggests minimal differences. However, the problem is a difficult one to address because nonparticipators do not provide the same level of descriptive data as do the enrollees. The jury must still remain out on this issue.

7. Unresolved Issues and Next Steps

Two questions persist as meta-issues in this review. We address each in turn, with some observations about how the issues might be resolved.

(1) Why are so few selective programs focused on the COA population, given what is known about short and long term risk?

There are two issues here: The problem of preventing AUD in a nation where 32 percent of its men and 15 percent of its women will at some point in their lives make the diagnosis (Kessler et al, 1997) is a problem that initially requires placing a diagnostic label on the activity. In so doing, the potential to produce shame and stigmatization is a much larger one than would be the case if prevalence were confined to only 5 percent of the population. Grouping the problem with the abuse of other drugs, behavior that is more clearly regarded as negative, and including it as part of a larger category rather than giving it its own name effectively diffuses the issue of what is actively being prevented. This is at least part of the difficulty.

The second issue is that from a public health standpoint, the prevention of instances of abuse, single events, rather than the prevention of diagnoses (changing the behavior of individuals) , is a more effective strategy because the total of problem events created by persons without AUD is greater than the total of those with it. Thus, in terms of solving health problem issues at the community level, it is more cost effective to work at preventing the single events, which moves the discourse away from AUD.

(2) Why have not the clearly replicated findings of the predictability of AUD risk entered the mainstream of early identification and prevention programming? The findings remain largely unknown to alcohol researchers, they have not been disseminated to health educators, and family practice and pediatric physicians are also largely unacquainted with them.

Undoubtedly part of the explanation of why it has been difficult to make this work visible is the same as what has just been described; it is the problem that labeling creates shame and stigma. There is also another, more practical reason. It is extraordinarily difficult to face a painful experience and not be able to remediate it. Knowing that a youngster is at high risk for later AUD without having any way to address the problem is to create a considerable amount of pain and despair in the observer. This is a part of the dilemma that any health professional or educator must grapple with in attempting to assimilate this new knowledge. If programming can be created that provides some effective plan of action, it is reasonable to expect that this resistance to understanding will dissipate.

What are some of the barriers, and how might they be resolved? In an era of managed care, escalating health costs, and carve out medical plans that provide little reimbursement for behavioral health, it is utopian to believe that any new long term identification and treatment program would be embraced by the health care system. This is especially so for a condition such as alcoholism, which is realistically regarded as a chronic and recurring disorder (McLellan et al., 2000). In contrast, identification (and treatment) have more likelihood of being sustained if they are piggybacked onto an already existing and compensated program. There are currently a number of venues where such a plan would be feasible: regular check up time in a managed care pediatric or family medicine program would be one readily accessible access point for screening, and possibly also for brief intervention programming if it were not too costly. Another point of access would be screening at pediatric emergency medicine facilities. Impulsive sensation seeking and aggressiveness are both markers of high AUD risk. They also are more likely to get the youngster into the Emergency Department. A third would involve family contact and brief family screening for all adults who come in for outpatient alcoholism or other drug treatment. A child and family focused brief intervention package would be simple to implement once agency staff were accepting of such a new, extended family model of treatment. Furthermore, the health care context is one that routinely expects repeat checkups and follow through. This would permit a program of booster sessions, on an as needed bases. There are undoubtedly other natural settings where such a spin off assessment and brief treatment could be carried out.

8. Epilogue

In a 1997 review and critique of prevention efforts for substance abuse programs, the eminent developmental psychologist and initiator of Head Start, Edward Zigler, and his colleague Nancy Hall observed the following:

> "Thirty years of research findings indicate that the most promising intervention/prevention efforts are likely to be those that are truly ecological in nature—programs that target children within the context of families (e.g., two generation programs such as Head Start. . . . and that address children and families within the context of their communities. . . .
>
> Myriad attempts to inoculate children against later substance abuse. . . . have sprung up in direct response to current policy mandates. If these ini-

tiatives are to make inroads in the nation's battle against drug abuse, however, the next wave of such programs must reflect greater understanding of the knowledge base with respect to the development and socialization of young children, the onset of delinquent behavior, and the importance of implementing and applying both process and outcome evaluations" (Hall & Zigler, 1997, p. 141).

These observations seem are as true today as they were in 1997. Contextually based interventions still show the greatest promise, and a number of them have been evaluated and shown to be efficacious. But the field is still in its infancy in conceptually and practically addressing the problems of COAs and other high risk populations before they become manifest. Alcohol is the nation's most common drug of abuse, but those children who have the greatest potential to abuse it still remain a hidden and untended population. The technology and the knowledge base now exists to remedy that situation.

ACKNOWLEDGMENTS: Preparation of this chapter was supported in part by National Institute on Alcohol Abuse and Alcoholism grants R37 AA07065 and R01 AA12214, and National Institute on Drug Abuse grant U10 DA13710. Correspondence may be addressed to zuckerra@umich.edu.

References

American Psychiatric Association (1994). *Diagnostic and statistical manual of mental disorders,* 4th ed. Author, Washington, D. C.

Ary, D.V., Duncan, T.E., Duncan, S. C. and Hops, H. (1999). Adolescent problem behavior: The influence of parents and peers. *Behav Res Ther,* 37: 217–230.

Biglan, A., Brennan, P.A., Foster, S.L., Holder, H.D., Miller, T.L., Cunningham, P.B., Derzon, J.H., Flay, B.R., Goeders, N.E., Kelder, S.H., Kenkel, D., and Zucker, R.A. (2004). *Multi-problem youth: Prevention, intervention, and treatment.* Guilford, New York.

Blackson, T.C., & Tarter, R.E. (1994). Individual, family, and peer affiliation factors predisposing to early-age onset of alcohol and drug use. *Alcohol Clin Exp Res,* 18: 813–821.

Blackson, T.C., Tarter, R.E., Martin, R.E., & Moss, H.B. (1994). Temperament-induced father-son family dysfunction: Etiologic implications for child behavior problems and substance abuse. *Am J Orthopsychiat,* 64: 280–292.

Blackson, T.C. (1997). Temperament: A salient correlate of risk factors for alcohol and drug abuse. *Drug and Alcohol Depend,* 36: 205–214.

Bronfenbrenner, U. (1977). Toward an experimental ecology of human development. *Am Psychol.* 32: 513–531.

Caspi, A., Moffitt, T.E., Newman, D.L., and Silva, E.A. (1996). Behavioral observations at age 3 years predict adult psychiatric disorders: Longitudinal evidence from a birth cohort. *Arch Gen Psychiat,* 53:1033–1039.

Chassin, L., Rogosch, F., and Barrera, M. (1991). Substance use and symptomatology among adolescent children of alcoholics. *J Abnorm Psychol.* 100:449–463.

Chilcoat, H.D., Breslau, N. & Anthony, J.C. (1996). Potential barriers to parent monitoring: Social disadvantage, marital status and maternal psychiatric disorder. *J Am Acad Child Adolescent Psychiat,* 35:1673–1682.

Cloninger,C.R., Sigvardsson, S. & Bohman, M. (1988). Childhood personality predicts alcohol abuse in young adults. *Alcohol Clin Exp Res,* 12:494–505.

Colder, C.R. and Chassin, L. (1999). The psychosocial characteristics of alcohol users versus problem users: Data from a study of adolescents at risk. *Dev Psychopathol*, 11:321–348.

Dishion, T. J., Kavanaugh, K. Schneiger, A. Nelson, S. and Kaufman, N. (2002). Preventing early adolescent substance abuse: A family centered strategy for the public, middle-school ecology. *Prevention Science*, 3: 191–201.

Donovan, J.E. & Jessor, R. (1985) Structure of problem behavior in adolescence and young adulthood. *J Consult Clin Psychol*, 53:890–904.

Ellickson, P. L., Tucker, J. S., and Klein, D. J. (2003). Ten-year prospective study of public health problems associated with early drinking. *Pediatrics*. 111:949–955.

Eron, L. D., Huesmann, L. R., Dubow, E., Romanoff, R. & Yarmel, P.W. (1987). Aggression and its correlates over 22 years. In Crowell, D. H., Evans, I. M. & O'Donnell, C.R. (eds.) *Childhood aggression and violence*. Plenum, New York, pp. 249–262.

Fitzgerald, H. E., Sullivan, L. A., Ham, H. P., Zucker, R. A., Bruckel, S., and Schneider, A. M. (1993). Predictors of behavioral problems in three-year-old sons of alcoholics: Early evidence for onset of risk. *Child Dev*, 64:110–123.

Fuller, B.E., Chermack, S.T., Cruise, K.A., Kirsch, E., Fitzgerald, H.E., and Zucker, R.A., (2003). Predictors of aggression across three generations among sons of alcoholics: Relationships involving grandparental and parental alcoholism, child aggression, marital aggression and parenting practices. *J Stud Alcohol*, 64:472–483.

Garnier, H. E., and Stein, J.A. (2002). An 18-year model of family and peer effects on adolescent drug use and delinquency. *J Youth Adolesc*, 31:45–56.

Grant, B.F. (2000) Estimates of US children exposed to alcohol abuse and dependence in the family. *Am J Public Health*, 90:112–115.

Grant, B. F., and Dawson, D.A. (1997). Age at onset of alcohol use and its association with DSM-IV alcohol abuse and dependence:Results from the National Longitudinal Alcohol Epidemiologic Survey. *J Substance Abuse*, 9: 103–110.

Hall, R.L., Hesselbrock, V.M., and Stabenau, J.R. (1983). Familial distribution of alcohol use: II. Assortative mating of alcoholic probands. *Behav Genet*, 13:361–372.

Hall, N.S., and Zigler, E. (1997). Drug-abuse prevention efforts for young children: A review and critique of existing programs. *Am J Orthopsychiatry*, 67:134–143.

Hawkins, J. D. and Catalano, R. F. (1992). *Communities that care: Action for drug abuse prevention*. Jossey-Bass, San Francisco.

Hawkins, J.D., Catalano, R.F., Kosterman, R., Abbott, R., and Hill, K.G. (1999). Preventing adolescent health-risk behaviors by strengthening protection during childhood. *Arch Pediatr Adolesc Med*, 153:226–234.

Helzer, J.E., Burnam, A., and McEvoy, L.T. (1991). Alcohol abuse and dependence. In Robins, L. (ed.) *Psychiatric disorders in America: The epidemiologic area catchment studies*. Free Press, New York, pp. 81–115.

Hogue, A., and Liddle, ,H. A. (1999). Family-based preventive intervention: An approach to preventing substance use and antisocial behavior. *Am J Orthopsychiatry*, 69:278–293.

Hussong, A. M., and Chassin, L. (1994). The stress-negative affect model of adolescent alcohol use: Disaggregating negative affect. *J Stud Alcohol*, 55:707–718.

Huang, L. X., Cerbone, F. G., and Gfroerer, J. C. (1998). Children at risk because of substance abuse. In: Office of Applied Studies, Substance Abuse and Mental Health Services Administration (eds.) *Analyses of substance abuse and treatment need issues*, DHHS Publication Document No. (SMA) 98–3227, Rockville, pp. 5–18.

Institute of Medicine (1994). *Reducing risks for mental disorders: Frontiers for preventive intervention research*. National Academy Press, Washington, D.C.

Jessor, R. and Jessor, S. L. (1977). *Problem behavior and psychosocial development: A longitudinal study of youth*. Academic Press, New York.

Johnston, L.D., O'Malley, P.M., & Bachman, J.G.(2003). *Monitoring the Future national results on adolescent drug use: Overview of key findings, 2002*. NIDA, Bethesda, MD.

Kandel, D. (1978). Convergences in prospective longitudinal surveys of drug use in normal populations. In D. B. Kandel (ed). *Longitudinal research on drug abuse.* Hemisphere, Washington, D.C., pp. 3–38.

Kaplan, H.B. (1975). Increase in self-rejection as an antecedent of deviant responses. *J Youth Adolescence,* 4:281–292.

Kellam, S.,G., Ensminger, M.E., and Simon, M.B. (1980). Mental health in first grade and teenage drug, alcohol, and cigarette use. *Drug Alcohol Dep,* 5:273–304.

Kellam, S.G., Brown, C.H., Rubin, B.R., and Ensminger, M.E. (1983). Paths leading to teenage psychiatric symptoms and substance use: Developmental epidemiological studies in Woodlawn. In S.B. Guze, F.J. Earls, and J.E. Barrett, eds., *Childhood psychopathology and development.* Plenum, New York, pp. 17–47.

Kumpfer, K. (1998). Selective preventive interventions: The Strengthening Families program. In: Asher, R.S., Robertson, E.B., and Kumpfer, K.L. (eds.) *Drug abuse prevention through family interventions. National Institute on Drug Abuse: Research Monograph No. 177.* National Institute on Drug Abuse, Rockville, MD, pp. 160–207.

Kushner, M. , Sher, K. J., and Beitman, B. (1990). The relation between alcohol problems and the anxiety disorders. *Am J Psychiat,* 147: 685–695.

Lerner, J. V. and Vicary., J. R. (1984). Difficult temperament and drug use: Analyses from the New York Longitudinal Study. *J Drug Educ,* 14:1–8.

Maguin, E., Safyer, A., Nochajski, T., DeWit, D. and Macdonald, S. (2003). The impact of a family-based alcohol prevention program on children's externalizing behavior problems (Abstract). *Alcohol:Clin Exp Research, 27,* 72A (No. 401).

Maguin, E., Zucker, R.A. and Fitzgerald, H.E. (1994). The path to alcohol problems through conduct problems: A family based approach to very early intervention with risk. *J Research Adolesc, 4,* 249–269.

Masse, L. C. and Tremblay R. E. (1997). Behavior of boys in kindergarten and the onset of substance use during adolescence. *Arch Gen Psychiatry,* 54:62–68.

Mayzer, R., Wong, M.M., Puttler, L.I., Fitzgerald, H.E., and Zucker, R.A. (2001, November). Onset of alcohol use: Profiling adolescents characterized as "Early Drinkers" (Abstract). Annual meeting of the American Society of Criminology, Atlanta.

Mayzer, R., Puttler, L.I.,Wong, M.M., Fitzgerald, H.E., and Zucker, R.A. (2002). Predicting early onset of first alcohol use from behavior problem indicators in early childhood. *Alcohol Clin Exp Res Suppl,* 26:124A.

Mayzer, R., Puttler, L.I., Wong, M.M., Fitzgerald, H.E., and Zucker, R.A. (2003). Development constancy of social misbehavior from early childhood to adolescence as a predictor of early onset of alcohol use. (Abstract). *Alcohol Clin Exp Res Suppl.* 27:65A.

McLellan, A.T., Lewis, D.C., O'Brien, C.P. and Kleber, H.D. (2000). Drug dependence, a chronic medical illness: implications for treatment, insurance, and outcomes evaluation. *JAMA.* 284: 1689–1695.

Merriam-Webster, Inc. (1994) *Merriam-Webster's Collegiate Dictionary; 10th edition.* Author, Springfield, MA.

National Institute on Alcohol Abuse and Alcoholism (2000). Alcohol involvement over the life course. In Author, *Tenth special report to the U.S. Congress on alcohol and health: Highlights from current research.* Bethesda: Dept Health and Human Services, pp.28–53.

Nigg, J.T., Hinshaw, S.P., Carte, E., and Treuting, J. (1998). Neuropsychological correlates of antisocial behavior and comorbid disruptive behavior disorders in children with ADHD. *J Abnorm Psychol,* 107:468–480.

Noll, R.B., Zucker, R.A., Fitzgerald, H.E., & Curtis, W.J. (1992). Cognitive and motoric function of sons of alcoholic fathers: The early childhood years. *Dev Psychol,* 28:665–675.

Nye, C.L., Zucker, R.A., and Fitzgerald, H.E. (1999). Early family-based intervention in the path to alcohol problems: Rationale and relationship between treatment process characteristics and child and parenting outcomes. *J Stud Alcohol Suppl,* 13:10–21.

Olweus, D. (1989) Bully/victim problems among school children: Basic facts and the effects of a school based intervention program. In Rubin, K., and Heppler, D. (eds.) *The development and treatment of childhood aggression.* Erlbaum, Hillsdale, NJ, pp. 411–448.

Pandina, R. J., and Johnson, V. (1989). Familial drinking history and a predictor of alcohol and drug consumption among adolescent children. *J Stud Alcohol*, 50:245–254.

Patterson, G. R., Forgatch, M. S., Yoerger, K. L., and Stoolmiller, M. (1998) Variables that initiate and maintain an early-onset trajectory for juvenile offending. *Dev Psychopathol*, 10:531–547.

Patterson, G. R., Reid, J.D., Jones, R. R., and Conger, R.R. (1975). *A social learning approach to family intervention, Vol. 1.* Castalia Publishing Co., Eugene, OR

Pederson, W. and Skrondal, A. (1998). Alcohol consumption debut: Predictors and consequences. *J Stud Alcohol*, 59: 32–42.

Perry, C.L., Williams, C.L., Veblen-Mortenson, S., Toomey, T.L., Komro, K.A., Anstine, P.S., McGovern, P.G., Finnegan, J.F., Forster, J.L., Wagenaar, A.C., and Wolfson, M. (1996). Project Northland: Outcomes of a community-wide alcohol use prevention program during early adolescence. *Am J Public Health*, 86:956–965.

Perry, C.L., Williams, C.L., Kumro, K. A., Veblen-MOrtenson, S., Forster, J. L, Bernstein-Lachter, R., Pratt, L. K., Munson, K. A., and Farbakhsh, K. (1998). Project Northland-Phase II: Community action to reduce adolescent alcohol use. Presented at the Kettil Bruun Society Fourth Symposium on Community Action Research and the Prevention of Alcohol and Other Drug Problems, Russell, Bay of Islands, New Zealand, February 8–13.

Poon, E., Ellis, D.A., Fitzgerald, H.E., and Zucker, R.A. (2000). Intellectual, cognitive and academic performance among sons of alcoholics during the early elementary school years: differences related to subtypes of familial alcoholism. *Alcohol Clin Exp Res*, 24:1020–1027.

Russell, M. (1990). Prevalence of alcoholism among children of alcoholics. In: Windle, M. (ed.), *Children of alcoholics: Critical perspectives.* Guilford, New York, pp. 9–38.

Rutter, M. (1982). Prevention of children's psychosocial disorders: Myth and substance. *Pediatrics*, 70:883–894.

Safyer, A., Maguin, E., Nochajski, Dewit, D. & Macdonald, S. (2003). The impact of a family based alcohol prevention program on family functioning. *Alcohol Clin Exp Res, 27*, 72A (No. 400).

Sher, K. J. (1991). *Children of alcoholics: A critical appraisal of theory and research.* University of Chicago Press, Chicago.

Smith, S.(1991). Two-generation program models: A new intervention strategy. *Soc Policy, Rep 5*

Spoth, R., Redmond, C., & Shin, C, (2001). Randomized trial of brief family interventions for general populations: Adolescent substance use outcomes 4 years following baseline. *J Consult Clin Psychol*, 69: 627–642.

Spoth, R., Guyll, M. and Day, S.X. (2002). Universal family-focused interventions in alcohol-use disorder prevention: Cost effectiveness and cost-benefit analyses of two interventions. *J. Stud. Alcohol*, 63: 219–228.

Spoth, R. (2003). Final Progress Report for 5R01MH49217 (Rural Youth at Risk: Extension-based Prevention Efficacy). Author: Institute for Social and Behavioral Research, Ames, IA.

Stoltenberg. S.F. and Burmeister, M. (2000) Recent progress in psychiatric genetics—some hope but no hype. *Hum Mol Genet*, 9:927–935.

Tarter, R.E., Alterman, A.L. and Edwards, K.L. (1985). Vulnerability to alcoholism in men: A behavior-genetic perspective. *J Stud Alcohol*, 46:329–356.

Tarter, R.E. and Vanyukov, M.M. (1994). Stepwise developmental model of alcoholism etiology. In Zucker, R.A., Howard, J., and Boyd, G.M. (eds.), *The development of alcohol problems: Exploring the biopsychosocial matrix of risk* (NIAAA Research Monograph No. 26). U.S. Department of Health and Human Services, Rockville, MD, pp. 303–330.

Tremblay, R. E., Pagani-Kurtz, L, Masse, L. C., Vitaro, F. and Pihl, R. O. (1995). A bi-modal preventive intervention for disruptive kindergarten boys: Its impact through mid-adolescence. *J Consult Clin Psychol,* 63: 560–568.

Wagenaar, A.C., Murray, D.M., Gehan, J.P., Wolfson, M., Forster, J.L., Toomey, T.L., Perry, C.L., and Jones-Webb, R. (2000). Communities Mobilizing for Change on Alcohol: Outcomes from a randomized community. *J Stud Alcohol,* 61(1):85–94.

Werner, E. E. (1986). Resilient offspring of alcoholics: A longitudinal study from birth to age 18. *J Stud Alcohol,* 47:34–40.

West, M. O. and Prinz, R. J. (1987). Parental alcoholism and childhood psychopathology. *Psychol Bull,* 102:201–218.

Wong, M. M., Zucker, R. A., Puttler, L. I., and Fitzgerald, H. E. (1999). Heterogeneity of risk aggregation for alcohol problems between early and middle childhood: Nesting structure variations. *Dev Psychopathol,* 11:727–744.

Zucker, R. A., Ellis, D. A., Fitzgerald, H. E., Bingham, C. R., and Sanford, K. (1996). Other evidence for at least two alcoholisms II: Life course variation in antisociality and heterogeneity of alcoholic outcome. *Dev Psychopathol,* 8:831–848.

Zucker, Fitzgerald, H. E. & Moses, H. M. (1995). Emergence of alcohol problems and the several alcoholisms: A developmental perspective on etiologic theory and life course trajectory. In: D. Cicchetti & D.J. Cohen (eds.). *Developmental Psychopathology, Volume 2: Risk, disorder and adaptation.* Wiley. , New York, pp. 677–711.

Zucker, R. A., Fitzgerald, H. E., Refior, S. K., Puttler, L. I., Pallas, D. M., and Ellis, D. A. (2000). The clinical and social ecology of childhood for children of alcoholics: Description of a study and implications for a differentiated social policy. In: Fitzgerald, H.E., Lester, B.M., and Zuckerman, B.S. (eds.), *Children of addiction: Research, health, and policy issues.* Garland Press, New York, pp. 1–30.

Zucker, R.A., & Gomberg, E.S.L. (1986). Etiology of alcoholism reconsidered: The case for a biopsychosocial process. *Am Psychol,* 41:783–793.

Zucker, R. A. and Noll, R. B.(1987)The interaction of child and environment in the early development of drug involvement: A planned very early intervention. *Drugs Soc,* 2: 57–97.

Zucker, R.A., Wong, M.M., Puttler, L.I., & Fitzgerald, H.E. (2003). Resilience and vulnerability among sons of alcoholics: Relationship to developmental outcomes between early childhood and adolescence. In Luthar, S. (ed.), *Resilience and vulnerability: Adaptation in the context of childhood adversities.* Cambridge University Press, New York, pp. 76–103.

IV

Treatment

Cherry Lowman, *Section Editor*

The purpose of the treatment section is to highlight several emerging trends in treatment research on adolescent alcohol use disorders. In 1997, the NIAAA initiated a program of adolescent treatment research. Since then, 20 clinical projects have been funded, the majority of which are clinical trials. Fifteen of these are behavioral projects and three are pharmacotherapy projects. These are the first controlled, manualized, and randomized studies to specifically assess the efficacy of interventions for the treatment of alcohol use disorders in adolescents. The objective of this initial wave of studies is to design and test innovative developmentally tailored interventions that provide evidence-based knowledge to improve treatment outcomes in adolescents.

Results for most of these projects will be forthcoming over the next few years, and will yield a broad perspective on the potential efficacy of family-based, cognitive behavioral, brief motivational, and guided self-change interventions in a range of settings and subgroups of adolescents, including homeless and runaway youth, high school students, juvenile justice-involved youth, and minority youth. In the meantime, new emphases are beginning to emerge in adolescent treatment research related to what research questions are important to pursue next. A research approach is emerging which unifies developmental and transdisciplinary perspectives on the etiology, development, and course of substance abuse disorders in order to better understand alcohol effects in youth, and ultimately to use this knowledge to design more effective interventions for youth.[1,2,3]

In most adolescent alcohol research treatment studies, developmental criteria have been limited to age and grade as indicators of position along the developmental continuum. There is now a nascent trend to adopt more devel-

Cherry Lowman • National Institute on Alcohol Abuse and Alcoholism, Division of Treatment and Recovery Research, Bethesda, Maryland 20892-9034. This introduction was written in a personal capacity amd does not represent the opinions of the NIH, DHHS, or the Federal Government.

opmentally specific models and methods from developmental psychology, developmental psychopathology, and developmental neuropsychology as a means to improve design and outcomes of adolescent treatment interventions. The translational approach to research in the health sciences represents a major paradigm shift in the way research is conducted, one supported by the U.S. National Institutes of Health. The aim of this approach is to solve major public health problems by bringing together scientists from relevant disciplines in the basic, clinical, and social sciences to develop transdisciplinary, integrated theoretical models and interventions based upon them that can resolve the target problem.[4,5,6,7] The authors who have contributed chapters to the treatment section provide both direct and indirect empirical evidence of this emerging research approach.[8,9,10,11,12]

Brown and colleagues[8] examine the complex interactions across and changes over time in four major domains of functioning during adolescent development. These include biological (puberty, neurological development), socioemotional (family influence, emotionality, intimate relations), cognitive (executive functioning, spatial operations, and attention), and behavioral (self-regulation and risk management) domains. Adolescent long-term risk pathways (i.e., trajectories) for alcohol use appear to be influenced by these factors, particularly developmental dysregulation and family- and experience-based psychopathologies. The authors distinguish three pathways of risk for underage alcohol use and disorders—normative risk, personality/temperament risk, and psychopathological risk—and illustrate each of these with empirical data. They also discuss the long-term as well as acute health consequences of adolescent alcohol use and how these along with developmental stage need to be taken into consideration in the design of treatment outcome studies. Guidelines to development of substance abuse interventions for adolescents are provided, and a number of evidence-based adolescent treatments are reviewed. In addition, the authors recommend that developmental and environmental specificity be assessed by including variables which represent environmental constraints on alcohol consumption, developmental milestones and transitions (and delays in these), age-normed neurocognitive functioning, family functioning, and job performance.

The authors conclude with a summary of alcohol treatment outcome evaluations from the perspective of the four domains of development considered in this chapter. They note, for example, that different domains of functioning post treatment have been observed to improve at different rates and therefore, to adequately assess treatment effectiveness, evaluation needs to be timed such that all salient improvements are assessed. Evaluation also needs to take into account the reciprocal influences between positive change in one domain and positive changes in other interdependent domains. This discussion of outcome evaluation from a longitudinal, developmental perspective should be invaluable not only to those planning future research in this area but also to inform clinicians, educators, and parents about the nature, interdependence, and sources of change in long-term adolescent developmental pathways related to alcohol and drug disorder treatment outcomes.

Winters and Kahnhorst provide an overview of assessment issues in adolescent substance abuse research from a developmental perspective.[9] They discuss the importance of early assessment of alcohol and other drug (AOD) use in order to distinguish normative from problematic use. They also discuss barriers to early assessment, indicators of progression in use (e.g., age of onset, regular use, polydrug use), and issues related to valid diagnosis of alcohol abuse and dependence in adolescents whose use patterns and consequences of use often vary from those of adults. Also emphasized is the importance of identifying comorbid psychiatric disorders, which may contribute to AOD relapse as may emotional dysregulation which can occur during this developmental stage.

The emerging human developmental and translational research trends are augmented by increasing emphasis on the importance of evaluating and treating psychiatric comorbidity and polydrug use associated with alcohol and drug use disorders. Longitudinal developmental research has shown that severe adolescent alcohol disorders have been, in the majority of cases, chronologically preceded by psychiatric and other disorders or symptomology and are often associated with multiple concurrent substance use disorders.[2,3,13,14] It has become increasingly clear that effective treatment for adolescents with advanced alcohol use disorders will require a multifaceted and possibly transdisciplinary treatment approach.

The chapter contributed by Cornelius[10] and colleagues reviews state-of-the-art approaches to treating comorbid adolescents with an emphasis on medications, knowledge gaps, and future research needs. Prescription of medications for substance use comorbidities has been increasing over the past ten years despite an absence of evidence-based knowledge on their safety, side effects, and efficacy in this population. To address this important medical issue, the authors provide a useful review (see also Dawes and Johnson)[15] of potential pharmacological approaches to treating concurrent alcohol use and other psychiatric disorders including major depression, bipolar disorder, anxiety disorders, conduct disorder, and attention deficit hyperactivity disorder. The authors stress that this area of research is in its infancy and needs to begin with the basics, including conduct of safety and sequencing studies followed by double-blind, placebo-controlled pharmacotherapy trials to establish long term efficacy and optimal combinations of pharmacotherapies and behavioral therapies in comorbid youth.

Another emerging emphasis involves efforts to deconstruct complex treatment processes in order to better understand and evaluate the mechanisms of positive change associated with particular components. Even brief interventions are sufficiently complex that their mechanisms of action are not yet fully understood.[16] Once achieved, this knowledge can be utilized to customize, combine, and sequence treatment components such that they meet the specific needs of youth as identified through both developmental and environmental assessments.

Kaminer and Slesnick[11] discuss the varied and complex nature of cognitive behavioral therapies, interventions based on classical and operant conditioning models, and social learning models. This has resulted in the creation of distinctive cognitive behavioral treatments (CBT)—integrated multicomponent strategies which focus on unique aspects of substance abuse. Among the active ingredients of CBT identified to date in adolescent studies are training in coping skills, problem solving skills, identification of high-risk situations, and role playing. The authors acknowledge that establishing the effectiveness of cognitive behavioral therapies is challenged by lack of comparability across clinical trials. Despite the analytic challenge, they note significantly more rapid overall response of subjects to CBT as a whole in early weeks of a clinical trial as compared with other credible psychotherapies.

The different types of family therapy discussed by Kaminer and Slesnick reveal similar issues in comparing treatment results across family intervention clinical trials. CBT and family therapies not only lack a standard battery of outcome assessment instruments, they both comprise complexes of interventions, particularly the ecologically focused multisystemic and multidimensional family therapies, which include community components in the treatment as well. Clearly needed is treatment process research that has as its aims (1) the parsing of specific treatment components and evaluation of the processes that underly their independent effects on treatment outcomes and (2) discrimination of unspecified treatment effects (e.g., assessment effects in the placebo group) and evaluation of their overall contributions to treatment outcome.

Godley and White[12] provide in their chapter a comprehensive overview of youth substance abuse treatment service systems and report current data on the number and distribution of adolescents receiving treatment for alcohol and drug use in both public and private programs. Included in their discussion is a summary of the current status of existing adolescent evidence-based substance abuse treatments. The authors also discuss the need for aftercare services to maintain treatment gains during recovery.

The need for post-treatment continuing care introduces the final emerging research trend to be discussed in this introduction to the treatment section—the extension of the chronic model of alcohol use disorders to a subset of adolescent substance abusers. For most adolescent drinkers, alcohol-related problems are likely to be transient and to resolve with maturation. But for those adolescents most likely to be seen in substance abuse treatment settings, alcohol-related problems can be chronic in nature. The chronic model is based on the recognition that recovery from addiction to substance use may be a long and complex biopsychosocial process during which some adolescents in recovery may need further intervention to achieve long-term sobriety.[17,18] The authors report that nearly 75% of adolescents treated for marijuana abuse/dependence in clinical trials conducted in five outpatient settings reported having experienced multiple treatment episodes, either before or after the current treatment episode.

Godley and White discuss the need for post-treatment interventions to address the longer-term recovery process in which recovery and relapse to alcohol use and related problems are "precariously balanced." Among the stabilizing post-treatment interventions which the authors recommend are formalized programs of continuing care such as those that include proactive linkages to youth-specific recovery groups. The authors also provide evidence for the effectiveness of assertive continuing care services that give responsibility for maintaining contact with aftercare services (e.g., monitoring, support, recovery education, re-intervention) to the treatment professional (for example, by telephone or home visits) rather than to the client.[19] In addition, Godley and White point to the importance of developing environmental interventions to reduce adolescents' risks of relapse, often attributable to peer or familial influences.

In sum, a number of new emphases and trends characterize emerging research related to improving the effectiveness of treatments for youth with alcohol use disorders. This emerging research includes the adoption and integration of human developmental and transdisciplinary research perspectives and methodologies.[8] Adoption of a transdisciplinary human developmental framework in epidemiologic and natural history studies can be expected to yield salient and specific knowledge on the origins and causes of alcohol abuse and dependence in youth, and on variations in the nature of associated biopsychosocial problems in this subgroup. To achieve these results, it will be critical to develop core batteries of instruments tailored to a developmental perspective.[8,9] Adoption of this approach in research to develop more effective prevention and treatment interventions should improve ability to match treatments to developmental subtypes of adolescents. Another emerging research area focuses on testing the effectiveness of pharmacotherapies in subtypes of youth characterized by comorbid alcohol use and psychiatric disorders.[10] Yet another emerging research target is to identify mechanisms of positive change in complex interventions in order to better guide improvement in treatment effects through customization, combination, and sequencing of treatment components.[11] The final emerging area discussed here is development of post-treatment interventions designed to maintain treatment gains during the recovery phase by providing continuing care monitoring and services.[12] Overall, research findings arising from these new directions in youth treatment research could provide even more developmentally sensitive and specific interventions with associated gains in both short- and long-term treatment outcomes.

References

1. Chung, T, Martin, CS, Grella, CE, Winters, KC, Abrantes, AM, Brown, SA: Course of alcohol problems in treated adolescents. *Alcoholism: Clinical and Experimental Research* 27:253–261, 2003.

2. Tarter, RE, Vanyukov, MM, Giancola, P, Dawes, M, Blackson, T, Mezzich, A, Clark, DB: Etiology of early onset substance use disorder. A maturational perspective. *Development and Psychopathology* 11: 657–683, 1999.
3. Zucker, RA, Wong, MM, Puttler, LI, Fitzgerald, HE: Resilience and vulnerability in sons of alcoholics. Relationship to development and outcomes between early childhood and adolescence, in Luthar, SS (ed): *Resilience and Vulnerability.* New York: Cambridge University Press, 2003, pp. 77–103.
4. Curtis, JW, Cicchetti, D: Moving research on resilience into the 21st century. Theoretical and methodological considerations in examining biological contributors to resilience. *Development and Psychopathology* 15: 773–810, 2003.
5. Cicchetti, D, Cannon, TD: Neurodevelopmental processes in the ontogenesis and epigenesis of psychopathology. *Development and Psychopathology* 11:375–393, 1999.
6. Rutter, Michael: Psychosocial influence. Critiques, findings, and research needs. *Development and Psychopathology* 12: 375–405, 2000.
7. Steinberg, L, Dahl, R, Keating, D, Kupfer, DJ, Masten, AS, Pine, D: The study of developmental psychopathology in adolescence: Integrating affective neuroscience with the study of context, in Cicchetti, D (ed): *Handbook of Developmental Psychopathology.* New York: John Wiley & Sons, in press.
8. Brown, SA, Anderson, KG, Ramo, DE, Tomlinson, KL: Treatment of adolescent alcohol related problems, in Galanter, M (ed): *Recent Developments in Alcoholism,* New York: Klumer Academic/Plenum, 2005, pp. 325–346.
9. Winters, K, Fahnhorst, T: Assessment issues in adolescent alcohol and drug abuse treatment research, in Galanter, M (ed): *Recent Developments in Alcoholism Research,* New York: Klumer Academic/Plenum, 2005, pp. 405–423.
10. Cornelius, JR, Clark, DB, Bukstein, OG, Salloum, IM: Treatment of co-occurring alcohol, drug, and psychiatric disorders, in Galanter, M: *Recent Developments in Alcoholism,* New York: Klumer Academic/Penum, 2005, pp. 347–363.
11. Kaminer, Y, Slesnick, N: Evidence-based cognitive-behavioral and family therapies for adolescent alcohol and other substance use disorder, in Galanter, M (ed): *Recent Developments in Alcoholism,* New York: Klumer Academic/Plenum, 20005, pp. 381–403.
12. Godley, MD, White, WL: A brief history and some current dimensions of adolescent treatment in the United States, in Galanter, M (ed) *Recent Developments in Alcoholism,* New York: Klumer Academic/Plenum, pp. 365–380.
13. Abrantes, AM, Brown, SA,Tomlinson, B.S.: Psychiatric comorbidity among inpatient substance abusing adolescents. *Journal of Child and Adolescent Substance Abuse,* in press.
14. Wong, MM, Brower, KJ, Fitzgerald, HE, Zucker, RA: Sleep problems in early childhood and early onset of alcohol and other drug use in adolescence. *Alcoholism: Clinical and Experimental Research,* in press.
15. Dawes, MA & Johnson, BA: Pharmacotherapeutic trials in adolescent alcohol use disorders. Opportunties and challenges. *Alcohol and Alcoholism* 39, in press.
16. Drummond, DC: Alcohol interventions: do the best things come in small packages? Addiction 92: 375–379, 1997.
17. McLellan, AT: Have we evaluated addiction treatment correctly? Implications from a chronic care perspective.
18. Kaminer, Y, Napolitano, C: Dial for therapy. Aftercare for adolescent substance use disorders. *Journal of the American Academy of Adolescent Psychiatry,* in press.
19. Godley, M, Godley, S, Dennis, M et al.: Preliminary outcomes from the assertive continuing care experiment for adolescents discharged from residential treatment. *Journal of Substance Abuse Treatment* 23: 21–32, 2002.

15

Treatment of Adolescent Alcohol-Related Problems

A Translational Perspective

Sandra A. Brown, Kristen G. Anderson, Danielle E. Ramo, and Kristin L.Tomlinson

Adolescence is a period of remarkable change and challenge. Development during this period can be characterized by growth within four major domains of functioning: biological, socioemotional, cognitive and behavioral. Changes within and across these domains provide a framework from which the complex interactions of adolescent alcohol problems and normal development can be understood. Variations in functioning in these domains can lead to increased risk for drinking and alcohol problems, just as alcohol can modify the developmental trajectories of youth. Thus, multidimensional developmental adolescent alcohol use disorders are a consequence of an interactive system of pre-existing characteristics, maturational changes and the environment. In this chapter we seek to exemplify how a developmental perspective translates to adolescent alcohol treatment and outcome evaluation.

Although developmental domains of functioning are related, each can produce unique as well as synergistic alcohol effects. Regarding biological changes of adolescence, research demonstrates that transitions in sexual development (puberty), neuroendocrine systems and neuroanatomical development are impacted by and can influence alcohol use. For example, the timing of

Sandra A. Brown • University of California San Diego, Department of Psychology, Veterans Affairs San Diego Healthcare System, La Jolla, California 92093-0109.
Kristen G. Anderson • University of California San Diego, La Jolla, California 92093-0109.
Danielle E. Ramo • San Diego State University/University of California, San Diego, Joint Program in Clinical Psychology, La Jolla, California 92093-0109.
Kristin L. Tomlinson • University of California, San Diego, La Jolla, California 92093-0109.

pubertal development has been shown to influence adolescent drinking with early maturing girls more likely to associate with older males, leading to earlier onset of alcohol involvement (Caspi, Lynam, Moffitt, & Silva, 1993). Throughout adolescence, neuroendocrine changes and neuroanatomical development move at a rapid pace producing shifts in stress reactivity, and increased regional specialization and myelenation of brain structures. Consequently, youth during this period may experience stage specific problems and potentially be at greater risk for long-term detrimental effects of heavy drinking (Brown & Tapert, in press).

Changes in family influence, emotionality and intimate relations are common socioemotional transitions for youth. As adolescence progresses, there is a move away from a dominance of familial influences on behavior towards greater impact from peers. Thus, peer characteristics and use are better predictors of adolescent alcohol use than parental or family influences (Newcomb & Bentler, 1986). Emotionality also undergoes maturation during adolescence. In addition to the elevated rates of stage specific and environmentally contingent life stress, trait negative affectivity is substantially higher than at other points in the life span (Jorm, 1987). The increased negative affect and emotional lability of adolescence serve as risks for teens to drink in response to interpersonal stress (Colder & Chassin, 1993). Risk taking also increases across species during adolescence (Spear, 2002). Youth experiment with new behaviors in more diversified situations. For example, adolescents are more likely to engage in risky sexual behavior (e.g., unprotected sex) particularly during drinking episodes resulting in unwanted pregnancies and sexually transmitted diseases (Fergusson & Lynskey, 1996). Additionally, alcohol use is involved in two-thirds of sexual assault and date rape cases among teens (Office of Inspector General, 1992).

The cumulative impact of early life experiences and aberrations in functioning can most easily be seen in the cognitive domain of functioning of youth. Cognitive development in adolescence is characterized by improved executive functioning including planning, abstract reasoning, behavioral inhibition and problem solving. These developmental changes coincide with more diversified expectations and greater academic demands at school. However, young heavy drinkers perform more poorly on tests of planning and executive functioning (Giancola & Mezzich, 2000), memory (Brown, Tapert, Granholm, & Delis, 2000), spatial operations, and attention (Tapert & Brown, 1999) compared to matched controls. These problems have a cumulative effect, producing poorer academic performance and reduced involvement at school, which can lead to limitations on future achievement in occupational domains.

Behaviorally, adolescence is a time when teens are exposed to increasing diversity in the environment and social experiences and experiment with various adult roles. Drinking and engagement in high risk behaviors often characterizes this role experimentation. However, as teens move further from the influence of their parents, there is an increasing need for them to manage and monitor their own behavior in changing contexts. Drinking alcohol can diminish their ability to manage fluid social situations and assess risk in the environment (Myers & Brown, 1990).

These transitions in function occur within the context of pre-existing characteristics, personal experiences and the environment of youth. Individual differences in temperament, cognitive abilities and exposure to alcohol dependence in the family interact with developmental demands to alter the trajectories of adolescent alcohol use. These pre-existing characteristics of the individual and environment influence the progression of use, as well as the ability and opportunities to change behavior and maintain these changes. Unfortunately, risk factors "cluster" together or are "nested" within one another, building a trajectory of psychopathology in the form of alcohol use disorders (Zucker, Chermack & Curran, 2000). This cumulative disadvantage (Elder, 1998) can limit the developing adolescent's ability to initiate and maintain change behaviors, and benefit from intervention efforts.

Because multidimensional developmental models consider transitions in the context of individual and environment influences, they support equifinality. Equifinality is the notion that one developmental outcome can be attained through a variety of divergent paths (Cummings, Davies & Campbell, 2000). The expanding social and behavioral repertoire of the adolescent is the growth medium for multiple pathways into and out of alcohol use disorders (AUDs). Thus, adolescent AUDs are not simply the cumulative result of independent or even correlated risks (e.g., genetic, environmental), but rather reflect the emergence and persistence of problematic behaviors related to networks of risks producing different trajectories into and out of AUDs. While the concept of multiple risk patterns for the development of substance use disorders (SUDs) is not new, it may be equally relevant to the resolution of alcohol problems. This chapter highlights the importance of several developmental influences on alcohol involvement and problems, treatment, and youth efforts at behavior change.

1. Lessons from Basic and Applied Alcohol Research

Adolescent risk for AUDs progresses through a network of multiply determined pathways. At least three pathways can be identified within the network (developmentally normative risk; temperament/personality risk; psychopathology risk) that have implications for treatment planning, implementation and outcome assessment of youth with AUDs. The first pathway begins as developmentally normative risk taking and experimentation, leading to maladaptive and pathological use. Autonomy can be seen as an adolescent's search for separation from parents, self-governance or agency (Beyers, Goossens, Vansant, & Moors, 2003). Increased autonomy facilitates experimentation with social roles in the search for a unique identity. This common cross-species adolescent stage increase in risk-taking behaviors for humans includes experimentation with alcohol and other drugs (Baumrind, 1987). Clearly, not all alcohol use by youth is pathological since the vast majority of high school students have alcohol experience by graduation (Johnston, O'Malley, & Bachman, 2004). However, a subset of youth engage in developmentally limited alcohol abuse and dependence where pathological alcohol use is embedded within stage-limited adolescent problem behavior (Zucker et al., 2000). Fortunately, many youths who exhibit these and other problems during adolescence will mature out of the disorders in young adulthood (e.g., Moffitt, 1993). For this group, the progression into and out of AUDs may be driven by normal adolescent development in high risk environments. Consequently, treatment planning and implementation needs to be informed by the need for autonomy and role experimentation in youth within the context of obtaining and maintaining sobriety.

Independence, the ability to take responsibility for one's actions and fulfill role expectations without direct parental monitoring, is a major developmental goal of adolescence. Two hallmarks of the move toward independence are obtaining a drivers license and moving out of the home of origin. Many adolescents obtain drivers licenses in middle adolescence, modifying the personal and social contexts associated with alcohol use. For example, driving an automobile can provide opportunities for exposure to new environments with fewer drinking constraints, decreased parental monitoring and unsupervised activities, potentially leading to increased risks for alcohol consumption (McCarthy & Brown, 2003). Considering teen and peer driving status may provide opportunities to gather useful information about exposure specific situations, strategies to circumvent parental monitoring, as well as the dynamics of these relationships, and potential areas for intervention regarding drunk driving.

In late adolescence, moving away from home is a tangible step toward independence for youth from their families. The move away from home exposes the adolescent to new environments requiring new behavioral management skills. Difficulties in the transition from home to independent living have been shown to predict adjustment problems in young adulthood (O'Connor, Allen, Bell, & Hauser, 1996). Drinking alcohol can contribute to the difficulties associated with this developmental transition as well as be a consequence of poor adjustment. Kypri, McCarthy, Coe and Brown (2004) found that transition into independent living was associated with an increase of 35% in monthly drinking episodes and a 46% increase in drinks per week for both community adolescents with no history of alcohol abuse and those with a history of alcohol treatment. Lower levels of autonomy might be a consequence of increased drinking; one study saw teens who drank heavily as less autonomous in young adulthood (Chassin, Pitts, & DeLucia, 1999). Post-treatment environment has implications for the success of abstinence-maintenance. For youth returning to independent living after substance use treatment, the behavioral management requirements for sobriety should be made explicit. Aftercare planning, involving frank discussions of the importance of sober living environments, might be necessary for this age group.

Longitudinal developmental studies consistently find certain temperamental and personality characteristics to be associated with AUDs which emerge during adolescence. Personality pathways to adolescent AUDs begin well before exposure to alcohol and can be considered more generalized risk factors for various forms of psychopathology. One such pathway is characterized by sensation-seeking/behavioral disinhibition. High sensation seeking and low harm avoidance in childhood has been shown to be predictive of early-onset alcoholism (Cloninger, Sigvardsson & Bohman, 1988). Disinhibition, low impulse control, and hyperactivity are also traits consistent with this pathway (e.g., Goodwin, Knop, Jensen, Gabrielli, & Pennick, 1994). Youth characterized as being defiant towards authority figures, exhibiting disruptive behavior, and being aggressive are also more likely to develop an alcohol problem during adolescence than youth without these personality characteristics (e.g., Loeber & Dishion, 1983). As disinhibited youth navigate the developmental transitions of adolescence, particularly those requiring behavioral management (e.g., sexual activity, driving, substance involvement), impulsive decision-making and preference for heightened sensation puts them at greater risk for negative outcomes (e.g., unwanted pregnancy, drunk driving, addiction). This disinhibition pathway has different implications for treatment and outcome assessment. The realistic goal of treatment is not to eradicate these traits, but rather to assist the teen in navigating the developmental transitions of adolescence. Thus, measurement regarding these transitions should be incorporated in this research.

A second potential personality pathway to adolescent AUDs is through anxiety sensitivity or behavioral inhibition. For example, behaviorally inhibited 12 to 14 year olds, more often girls, were found to have higher levels of anxiety, worry and depression than their non-inhibited peers (Muris, Merckle-bach, Wessel, & van de Ven, 1999). Some studies show elevated risk for alcohol involvement in anxiety-disordered youth (e.g., Neighbors, Kempton, & Forehand, 1992), while others suggest that anxiety may protect against initial adolescent alcohol use (e.g., Stice, Myers, and Brown, 1998). An important contextual precipitant to the emergence of psychiatric disorders and AUDs in adolescence is childhood victimization, including physical and sexual abuse (e.g., Edwall, Hoffman, & Harrison, 1989). These traumatic experiences might serve as a stress to the diathesis of anxiety sensitivity in some cases. Treating youth with difficulties managing negative affect might benefit from the diathesis-stress perspective (Monroe & Simons, 1991). The developmental challenges of adolescence are stressful and require substantial coping resources. Interventions targeting stress management and coping might have greater success with this type of individual.

Childhood and adolescent onset psychiatric disorders can modify trajectories into and out of AUDs. Youth with certain childhood-onset psychiatric disorders accelerate their alcohol use more rapidly than youth without concomitant psychopathology (White, Xie, Thompson, Loeber, & Stouthamer-Loeber, 2001). For example, adolescents with ADHD evidence higher rates and earlier onset of AUDs than youth without ADHD (Milberger, Biederman, Faraone, Wilens, & Chu, 1997). In a recent review of the literature, Abrantes and Brown (2003) report high rates of conduct and/or oppositional defiant disorder, mood disorders, and anxiety disorders among adolescents in treatment for AUDs. This co-occurrence of Axis I psychopathology and AUDs reflects a nesting or clustering of risks; effective treatment of one type of disorder may not be possible without treating the other.

While certain risk pathways can be seen as influencing the movement into AUDs, the use of alcohol has reciprocal effects on the developing adolescent. Although the chronic health problems commonly observed in adults (e.g., liver problems, hypertension) are less often seen in AUD adolescents, youth with AUDs suffer a number of serious health consequences due to their drinking-related behavior. The leading cause of death for teenagers is unintentional injury, primarily due to motor vehicle accidents, and 20% of all traffic crashes involving teenage drivers are alcohol-related (Yi, Williams, & Dufour, 2001). Animal studies have revealed that adolescents experience less of the sedating effects (Silveri & Spear, 2002), and more memory impairment (White, Ghia, Levin, & Swartzwelder, 2000) during alcohol intoxication compared to adults. These developmental differences in alcohol-induced cognitive impairment may account for the findings that youth are more likely to continue risky behaviors during a drinking episode that leads to physical injury (Bonomo et al., 2001).

Above and beyond acute health consequences for teens, chronic alcohol use for adolescents may add complexity to the assessment of AUDs, time to remission and maintenance of treatment gains. Recent findings from animal research indicate that alcohol exposure during adolescence produces greater memory impairments and alcohol-induced motor coordination impairments compared to results from initial exposure during adulthood (White et al., 2000). Frontal brain regions in particular are more damaged when exposed to alcohol during adolescence than when exposed in adulthood (Crews, Braun, Hoplight, Switzer, & Knapp, 2000). Several recent studies with humans support these neuroanatomical and neuroadaptive findings. An MRI study found that youth with AUDs had significantly smaller hippocampi, a region of the brain critical for the formation of new memories, compared to non-abusing youth (De Bellis et al., 2000). Brown, Tapert, Granholm and Delis (2000) found 10% poorer retention of verbal and nonverbal information among heavy alcohol using teens compared to their nonusing counterparts. These cognitive effects secondary to heavy alcohol use may influence youth perception of problems as well as their ability to attend and retain information presented in treatment.

Finally, youth who develop AUDs in adolescence may become impaired in their ability to successfully transition into adult roles, which alters the trajectory of development and reduces potential adult functioning. For example, adolescent alcohol abuse compromises school performance, which can impair youths' ability to get into college or obtain the career of their choice (O'Malley, Johnston, & Bachman, 1998). AUDs are also associated with socialization into deviant peer groups, who are less likely to participate in school, family, or community activities. These individuals are disadvantaged in adult social skills, and may fail to complete goals regarding marriage, education, employment, and financial independence (Schulenberg, O'Malley, Bachman, Wadsworth, & Johnston, 1996). Early transition into adult family roles also carries risks for poorer long-term outcomes (Newcomb & Bentler, 1986).

Clinical and basic research on the negative consequences of AUDs on adolescent health and continuing development clearly indicate that the presence of AUDs in this population severely impacts all domains of functioning, and can disadvantage youth when facing challenges which emerge as they move into young adulthood. Furthermore, there are unique risks in this population for both the development and consequences of AUDs that emerge during adolescence. For these reasons it is critical that the unique risks and problems of adolescents with AUDs are considered and incorporated into the measurement of AUDs and related problems for at-risk youth, so that crucial domains of functioning in this age group are assessed in order to be accurately attended to during treatment. Additionally, clinicians and researchers involved in the design, implementation and evaluation of interventions for adolescents with AUDs need to be aware of the differences and special needs of this population in order to optimally treat these individuals.

2. Role of Developmental Stage in Design and Implementation of Alcohol Treatment for Youth

As basic and applied research continue to identify salient predictors of youth treatment outcome, the role of developmental stage becomes increasingly important in design and implementation of effective alcohol treatment for youth. Interventions should consider family factors associated with use (e.g., family history of alcohol abuse, youth exposure to family use, family relations and communication pathways), peer substance involvement, and patterns associated specifically with adolescent drinking behavior. For example, the majority of adolescents who enter treatment programs rarely use only alcohol (Brown, Tapert, Tate & Abrantes, 2000). The rule rather than the exception among adolescents with alcohol and drug use disorders is multiple substance involvement that generally starts with alcohol and nicotine and progresses to marijuana. The "gateway" theory of substance involvement suggests that this progression to marijuana use may be a key factor in the progression to other illicit drug use (Kandel, Yamaguchi, & Chen, 1992). This pattern seems to hold after treatment at least for some youth, in that alcohol is the substance most likely to be involved in relapse after treatment, even among youth who do not report alcohol as their substance of choice (Brown, Tapert, Tate et al., 2000), and relapse to alcohol use was found to predict gradual progression to other substance use whereas relapse to "drug of choice" resulted in a more rapid return to polysubstance involvement. Other use patterns that seem to be specific to adolescents are that, while adults drink more often, adolescents drink about as much in terms of sheer quantity per occasion, show high levels of mood and conduct disorder comorbidity, and show an early onset of drinking that leads to rapid symptom acquisition and early identification as alcohol dependent (Deas, Riggs, Langenbucher, Goldman, & Brown, 2000).

Brown (in press), Wagner and Kassel (1995) and others have suggested several guidelines to follow when developing an alcohol and drug abuse intervention for adolescents. First, interventions should focus on salient concerns of and for youth to facilitate and maintain their motivation for a nonabusing lifestyle. Failure to consider these developmentally related problems and the therapeutic alliance related issues diminish youth engagement and retention in treatment (Brown, in press; Liddle, Dakof, Diamond, Barrett, & Tejeda, 2001). Second, interventions must consider the unique developmental issues and problems characteristic of adolescents (e.g., ascendancy of the peer group, identity formation issues, propensity toward limit-setting), rather than applying unmodified versions of interventions designed for adults (e.g., Wagner, Dinklage, Cudworth, & Vyse, 1999). Third, active efforts should be made to identify the mechanisms of change that underlie positive behavioral change (e.g., motivation, self-efficacy; see for example Kelly, Myers, & Brown, 2000) to improve adolescent alcohol and drug abuse interventions and sustain improvements in functioning. Fourth, consideration must be given to the fact that the modal adolescent patient in alcohol and drug treatment has multiple problems (Brown & Ramo, in press; Hoffmann, Sonis, & Halikas, 1987). Thus, multiple functional domains (e.g., family functioning, peer network, stress coping) should be assessed, and when necessary, treated. Finally, treatment plans should emphasize the individual needs and preferences of teens (Metrik, Frissell, McCarthy, D'Amico, & Brown, 2003). For example, family-based interventions are likely to be more effective for younger adolescents whose alcohol and other drug abuse appears to be related to family problems (Brown, 1993). In contrast, treatment based on cognitive-behavioral coping skills development is likely to be more effective for abusing youth who have poor interaction and drug refusal skills.

Diverse forms of psychosocial treatments have already shown success in reducing alcohol and drug use among adolescents. These include, but are not limited to: family therapies such as multisystemic therapy (MST; Henggeler, Clingempeel, Brondino, & Pickrel, 2002), functional family therapy (FFT; Waldron, Slesnick, Brody, Turner, & Peterson, 2001), brief strategic family therapy (BSFT; Santisteban et al., 1997), and multidimentional family therapy (Liddle, Roll, Ledgerwood, and Schuster, 2001) as well as behavioral therapy (Azrin et al., 2001), cognitive behavioral therapy (CBT; Kaminer, Burleson, & Goldberger, 2002), motivational interviewing (Monti, 1999), Minnesota 12-step model (Winters, Stinchfield, Opland, Weller, & Latimer, 2000), contingency management reinforcement (Corby et al., 2000), and integrative models of treatment (Kaminer, 2001). Kaminer and Slesnick, and Cornelius review these treatment modalities in detail in chapters in this text.

Recent work in our laboratory has focused specifically on the dominant model of addiction relapse for the last two decades, the cognitive-behavioral model (Witkiewitz & Marlatt, 2004). Although modifications have been suggested (e.g., incorporating craving, cue reactivity), the basic premise is that when individuals are in situations with elevated risk for relapse, those who adequately cope with these situations without using addictive substances experience more confidence in their ability to abstain (increased self-efficacy) and are more likely to abstain in the future. By contrast, if abusers do not attempt to cope or do not cope successfully, and expect more positive outcomes with use, the likelihood of substance use in these situations is high. Once drinking or drug use is initiated, negative cognitive states (e.g., guilt, self-blame) ensue, thereby reducing self-efficacy and likelihood of future abstinence. As highlighted in Figure 1, this developmental specificity enhances the model's applicability for youth (Brown, in press; Brown, & Ramo, in press). One of the most important modifications of this model for youth is the key role of motivation. Motivation will dictate the extent to which youth make effortful coping responses in risk situations and is critical to sustained success following treatment (Kelly et al., 2000). Among youth, motivation for abstinence varies across types of substances (Brown, Tapert, Tate et al., 2000), and while teens are typically motivated to resolve use-related problems, they are seldom motivated to abstain from all addictive substances (Brown, 1999).

The dominant contextual features of high-risk situations are substantially different for AUD teens than for adults. For example, the majority of episodes of adult alcoholic relapse are precipitated by situations of anger or frustration, social pressure to drink, or interpersonal conflict (Marlatt & Gordon, 1985). In contrast, youth relapse most often in unsupervised social settings in which there is direct social pressure to drink, while negative affect or interpersonal conflict is seldom reported (Brown, Vik & Creamer, 1989). Exposure to substances in the environment, particularly through peer networks, is associated with reduced length of initial abstinence and measures of severity of post treatment use (Vik, Grissel, & Brown, 1992). As noted in Figure 1, these differences may in part reflect reduced vigilance for relapse risks, greater cue reactivity, lower anticipation of consequences associated with neuroanatomical development or other temperamental or genetic risks. They may also be consequences of concomitant psychopathology (e.g., Tomlinson, Brown, & Abrantes, 2004) or reflect reduced mobility and control over risks in their environment (Brown, 1993). Finally, developmental differences in social information processing may result in perceptions of greater use than is the norm and less differentiation of options to manage the emotional consequences of initial use (Brown, Stetson, & Beatty, 1989).

A number of youth oriented interventions have considered these cognitive behavioral model adjustments in efforts to engage youth in treatment, sustain behavioral change, and reduce relapse risk. These approaches focus less on issues of alcohol or other drug dependence, and more on the immediate positive and negative (perceived and actual) consequences of use and abstinence. For example, Monti and colleagues (Monti et al., 1999) used a brief youth specific motivational intervention of those entering a hospital emergencey department.

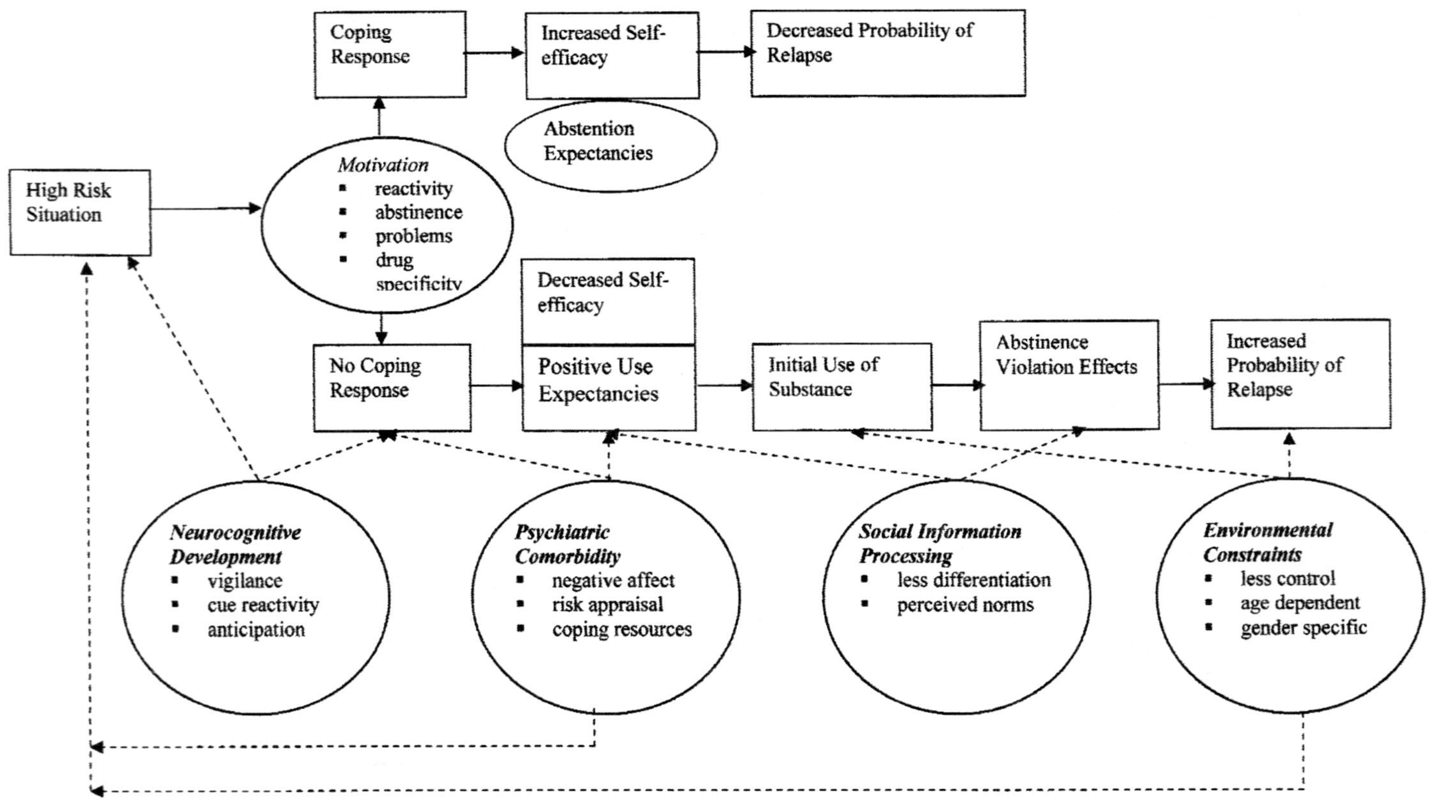

Figure 1. Modified cognitive behavioral model of adolescent addiction relapse. (From "Measuring youth outcomes from alcohol and drug treatment," by S.A. Brown, in press, *Addictions*. Cognitive behavioral model of relapse from "Relapse Prevention: Maintenance Strategies in the Treatment of Addictive Behaviors," by G.A. Marlatt & J.A. Gordon, 1985. Copyright 1985 by Guilford Press. Reprinted with permission.)

Results of their work suggest that targeting teens at a youth specific "teachable moment" can reduce alcohol intake and problems (especially for older teens). Since a low proportion of teens with alcohol problems seek treatment, identifying contexts and strategies most conducive to motivational enhancement are critical to enhancing treatment engagement and optimal treatments for youth. Motivationally focused interventions for other youth addictive disorders demonstrate the importance of factors such as timing and therapeutic style in determining the effectiveness of adolescent interventions (Brown, in press). In another series of studies, Waldron (e.g., Waldron et al., 2001) has provided evidence for the efficacy of an intervention that combines family therapy and cognitive-behavioral therapy for reducing the frequency of alcohol and drug use among adolescent substance abusers. Integrative Behavioral Family Therapy (IBFT) incorporates key facets of the cognitive-behavioral model (e.g., cognitive problem-solving and substance refusal skills) with family-based motivation enhancement and skill building that recognizes the importance of the family environment in helping teens to reduce alcohol and drug use. This treatment makes a particular effort to account for the competing sources of influence that adolescents struggle with in the teen years, such as parents' external limit setting and demands for conformity from both traditional and more deviant peer groups.

Based on perceived barriers and facilitators to treatment for youth (Metrik et al., 2003) and salient concerns of youth, we have developed interventions in the high school setting (e.g., Brown, 2001). This line of research suggests that optimal strategies to reduce/stop alcohol involvement and maintain behavior change for adolescents should consist of low-threshold, multiple-option packages ("toolbox for potential remitters"), which offer diverse forms of engagement, confidentiality, self-selected preferences, broad availability and strategies perceived by youth as socially acceptable and helpful for change. Our "Project Options" intervention allows youth with limited motivation for alcohol reduction to engage in self-selected group discussions, individual sessions or an interactive website which focuses on diverse but salient alcohol related problems (Brown, 2001). Motivational interviewing-based techniques are used to highlight common problems and positive solutions reached by peers as well as accurate normative alcohol use data, thereby incorporating the social aspects found to be most influential for youth in the early intervention process. Wagner and colleagues (e.g., Wagner et al., 1999) have used a Student Assistance Program approach to identify students that are at risk for developing a substance abuse problem. The approach uses a manualized group treatment to educate teens about their use and helps to motivate changes in use and maintenance of those changes. Each of the interventions described above has incorporated lessons learned from both adult literature and developmental literature to create programs that are particularly effective for youth. Future studies about the adolescent relapse process and the changes that occur in the adolescent brain will continue to contribute to the design and development of effective treatment programs.

3. Mapping Measurement onto Critical Domains of Adolescent Functioning

As seen above, adolescence is a stage of development where alcohol has specific and, in some cases, unique biological, cognitive and psychosocial effects on youth functioning compared to adults. In this section we attempt to exemplify ways in which measurement of adolescents in treatment and following treatment may be advantaged by increasing developmental specificity. Prior to designing, implementing and evaluating youth treatment programs, it is important to consider the domains and developmental expectations most negatively affected by alcohol abuse in youth. While certain developmental tasks are specific to adolescents (i.e., getting a drivers license, leaving home for the first time, initiation of dating or sexual relationships), many arenas are not unique but rather new to adolescents (i.e., alcohol specific) and may require alternative assessment techniques to address the specific social, environmental and developmental considerations of this time period.

A variety of environmental constraints (e.g., parental monitoring, inability to legally purchase alcohol) influence the topography of youth drinking patterns. Table 1 presents examples of measurement domains used in the adult research and suggests specific or additional measures for adolescents. For example, when assessing the quantity and frequency of adult drinking, mean drinks per drinking day is often used to measure consumption. However, for adolescents, consumption is often constrained by environmental factors ranging from parental monitoring to school constraints to supervised residential placement or incarceration. When measuring consumption in youth, quantitative measures need to be placed within the context of these environmental constraints. There are a number alcohol use measures available for adolescents (Brown, 1999; Deas et al., 2000). The Customary Drinking and Drug Use Questionnaire (CDDR; Brown et al., 1998) and Adolescent Diagnostic Interview (ADI; Winters & Henly, 1993) are two examples of available alcohol use measures that assist with this developmental specificity.

Axis I psychopathology is a fundamental clinical change in assessment of alcohol abusing youth (Tomlinson et al., in press). A number of clinical assessment tools are available to assess Axis I psychopathology in adolescents such as the Diagnostic Interview Schedule for Children (DISC; Shaffer, Fisher, Lucas, Dulcan, & Schwab-Stone, 2000), however few consider the sequence of symptom onset or exacerbation in relation to alcohol and drug use (Tomlinson et al., 2004). Given the high rates of concomitant psychopathology among youth presenting for treatment, the ability to assess adolescent psychopathology which is secondary to alcohol and drug use is central to adequate treatment planning and to understanding differing outcome trajectories for youth.

The attainment of developmental milestones can be indicators of decreasing or increasing risk for alcohol involvement or can be hallmarks of delayed development as a function of alcohol use. Thus, measurement of the timing and success of these transitions are useful adjuncts to assessment of youth. For

Table 1. Examples of Alternative Measures for Outcome Domains in Adolescent Alcohol and Drug Treatment

Standard Adult Domains	Proposed Domain Modifications to Match Topography of Youth
Alcohol-Specific Treatment Outcome Measures	
Percent Days Using	—Percent days use with and without environmental constraints*
Mean Drinks Per Drinking Day	—Mean drinks per unconstrained drinking day
Maximum Drinks Per Occasion	—Number of heavy drinking episodes (5+ Drinks)
	—Percent of heavy drinking episodes for drinking days
Drug Use Frequency	—Number of types of drugs used
	—Multiple substance use episodes
Withdrawal	—Types of withdrawal symptoms
	—Number of distinct withdrawal episodes
Episodic Drinking	—Longitudinal Trajectories
Developmental Stage-Specific Treatment Outcome Measures/Life Events	
Physical Health	
Injuries/Accidents	—Injuries/Accidents
Chronic Ailments	
High risk sexual behavior	—Early initiation of sexual activity
Unwanted sexual activity/date rape	—Unwanted sexual activity/date rape
Contraction of STDs/Pregnancy	—Contraction of STDs/Pregnancy
Cognitive Processes	
Neuropsychological functioning	—Developmental delays in functioning
Alcohol-related biological/physiological brain injuries	—Maturational growth deficits in the brain
Alcohol Expectancies	—Alcohol use expectancies
	—Alcohol cessation expectancies
Emotional Functioning	
Depression/Anxiety	—Emotional liability
	—Intensity of affect
Employment	
Job Functioning	—School Functioning:
—Absenteeism	—Attendance
	—Class Participation
—Job Loss	—Academic performance
	—Preparedness (Homework, Tests)

(continued)

Table 1. Examples of Alternative Measures for Outcome Domains in Adolescent Alcohol and Drug Treatment *(continued)*

Standard Adult Domains	Proposed Domain Modifications to Match Topography of Youth
Developmental Stage-Specific Treatment Outcome Measures/Life Events *(continued)*	
Interpersonal Relations	
Quality of relationships with children	—Quality of relationships with family of origin
—Parent/child relations	—Parental monitoring
—Parenting style	—Sibling relationships
	—Parental conflict
Quality of intimate relationships	—New primary relationships
—Level of Intimacy	—Peer conflict and changes
	—Initiation of sexual activity
	—Acquisition of romantic partner
—Abuse/discord in partner relationship	—Abuse/discord in partner relationship
—Separation/Divorce	—Breakup of relationship with boy/girlfriend
—Death of spouse	—Death of friend
Other Life Events	
Legal Problems	—Warnings and arrest
	—Police contact without arrests
	—Curfew violations
Children moving out of the home	—Transition to independent living
Job/Career change	—Graduating high school/going to college
	—Obtaining driver's license

Note: Constraint refers to Inpatient/Residential Treatment, Incarceration, etc. Reprinted from Brown (2003).

example, the success of transitions to independent living may reflect: 1) timing or age of leaving home, 2) reasons reported by youth for leaving, 3) the extent to which consultation occurred with parents and 4) affective reactions to leaving home (Hussong & Chassin, 2002). With the increasing rates of alcohol use after leaving home (Kypri et al., 2004), the impact of this transition on alcohol use and alcohol use's impact on this developmental transition is an important area to measure. Similarly, autonomy and social role transitions are related aspects of an individual's movement from adolescence into young adulthood. The measurement of autonomy in adolescence varies (Beyers et al., 2003) but appears to reflect the shared influence of connectedness (close parent-adolescent relationships), separation (interpersonal distance between parent and adolescent), detachment (mistrust and alienation from parents) and agency (possibility of self-directed behavior). This framework may show promise in examining the influence of autonomy on progressions in drinking behavior in youth.

Another area in which assessment might benefit from developmental specificity is in the area of process measures. For example, measurement of relapse to alcohol use should consider how negative affect can influence situation selection and subsequent alcohol risk. This idea comes from research demonstrating that for teens with concurrent AUDs and Axis I psychopathology, drinking in contexts involving temptation and stress (e.g., life and social) is commonly endorsed (Anderson, Frissell, & Brown, 2004). While many relapse-related measures have been developed for use with adults, there are instruments available to measure responses in adolescent relapse situations (ARCQ; Myers & Brown, 1990) and negative affectivity (e.g., PANAS-C; Laurent et al., 1999) in children and adolescents.

Another process area is assessment of cognitive abilities as they are influenced by and affect alcohol use. As discussed in the previous section, neurocognitive differences (e.g., social information processing, memory, problem solving) emerge during adolescence as function of development and as a consequence of alcohol use. Measures such as California Verbal Learning Test for Children (Delis, Kramer, Kaplan, & Ober, 1994), Wechsler Memory Scale (Wechsler, 1991) and Rey-Osterrieth Complex Figure Copy (Osterrieth, 1944) are age-normed instruments developed to assess dimensions of neurocognitive functioning associated with alcohol involvement. Many other instruments are available to assess specific aspects of neuropsychological functioning, many with age-norms for adolescents (e.g., Lezak, 1995).

Measuring treatment outcomes for adolescent AUDs often requires the creation of new measures to capture aspects unique to adolescent functioning. For example, family functioning and job performance are domains often assessed in treatment outcome research. The Family Environment Scale (FES; Moos & Moos, 1986) is often used as an index of family functioning in adulthood. For adolescents, parental monitoring is an aspect of family functioning related to alcohol and other drug use not often assessed by instruments developed for adults. In the area of work, employment status is often an indicator treatment success. For youth, school is the closest equivalent. Measuring proxies for school functioning (e.g., GPA) may provide useful information regarding treatment outcome. When designing treatment outcome assessments, adolescent development must inform the selection of constructs and instruments used to monitor the progression of AUDs.

4. Alcohol Treatment Outcome Evaluations with Youth

Evaluating treatment outcomes for youth requires attention to the impact of treatment on a variety of aspects of adolescent functioning (Brown & D'Amico, 2001). The majority of treatment outcome studies have focused on relapse rates as a measure of treatment success (for review of adolescent treatment outcomes, please see Brown & Ramo, in press; Brown, 1999). While the primary goal of alcohol treatment is total cessation of drinking, measures of quantity, frequency and problems are also considered core. A broader view of treatment outcome incorporates improvements across many domains of functioning often associated with alcohol use, particularly those implicated in the successful attainment of developmental goals. As discussed above, social, emotional, cognitive and behavioral functioning are aspects of adolescent development that should be taken into consideration when assessing teens entering treatment and when evaluating their outcomes. Particularly important are those areas where use seems to have reciprocal effects on development (e.g., independence, autonomy, social role transitions). In addition, motivations to change and contextual features differ between adults and teens, which have implications for engagement in treatment and relapse prevention.

For adults, aside from abstinence, treatment gains are often related to domains pertinent to adult functioning such as employment and relationship status (e.g., Tate, Brown, Unrod, & Ramo, in press). Specific to adolescent treatment outcome evaluation, the domains of school functioning (attendance, academic performance and behavioral problems), family relations (e.g., cohesion, conflict), social functioning (interpersonal conflict, peer group changes), activities (work, illegal behavior) and health (physical/emotional) are areas that are affected by alcohol abuse. Examining treatment effects on these domains are additional venues for evaluating success (Brown, 1993).

For adolescents, improved functioning in several psychosocial domains has been associated with decreased alcohol involvement following treatment. Better school functioning (increased attendance, fewer academic problems) and fewer interpersonal problems are evident among abstinent youth and those with low levels of use immediately following treatment. Teens who abstained from alcohol use also demonstrated gradual improvements in family relations (e.g., cohesion and expressiveness) over time (Brown, Myers, Mott & Vik, 1994). In the interpersonal arena, long term abstainers demonstrated the highest level of social functioning during young adulthood, whereas youth with trajectories of more frequent use of alcohol in the 8 years following adolescent treatment evidenced the poorest interpersonal outcomes (Abrantes, McCarthy, Aarons, & Brown, 2002). Adolescents who predominantly maintained abstinence over a four-year period after treatment showed greater educational attainment and higher occupational status than their using peers (Brown, D'Amico, McCarthy, & Tapert, 2001). Longer term (4 year) outcome evaluation of the MST program indicated that decreases in aggressive criminal behavior were a positive outcome from their intervention, despite mixed findings for substance use (Henggeler et al., 2002). Youth with heavy intermittent or chronic drinking evidence poorer outcomes across a variety of emotional and physical health domains (Brown & Tapert, in press).

These findings emerging from longitudinal trajectory analyses not only highlight that different domains of functioning improve at different rates, but demonstrate that to measure improvement in youth functioning following treatment the timing and sequencing of the assessments needs to be appropriate for the rates of change feasible for these improvements (Brown, in press). Thus, if school attendance must improve prior to academic performance improvement, the outcome assessment time points should match this pattern. Similarly, if decreases in family conflict necessarily precede improvements in cohesion, then the measurement of these aspects of functioning should parallel the pattern of improvement and should temporally coincide with time needed for these slower interpersonal changes.

From the brief summary above, it is clear that treatment impacts adolescent functioning on a variety of levels. Treatment gains with adolescents need to be viewed from a perspective of sequential change—one area of improvement can affect other aspects of the teen's system, fostering more positive subsequent outcomes. Thus, outcome assessments of youth should consider potential reciprocal developmental influences on outcomes (e.g., autonomy, independence) as well as psychosocial outcomes for the developing adolescent (e.g., onset of sexual behavior, family cohesion). For example, a teen has maintained sobriety for one month post-treatment. As a consequence of sobriety, the teen is more alert during school hours and more engaged in the learning environment. With the improvement in her attendance, her parents begin to praise her accomplishments, rather than focus on past failures. This reinforcement fosters youth perception of parental acceptance which facilitates family cohesion. Conversely, the improved family relations and the reinforcement derived from academic gains may diminish affiliation with substance abusing peers and relapse risk situations. An understanding of the multiple dimensions in which problematic youth drinking is embedded, allows for greater awareness of how modifications in one aspect of a system can have cumulative consequences for teens.

One means to examine models of these diverse sequential and reciprocal relations is through post-treatment trajectory patterns. Specifically, the utilization of mixed modeling procedures with longitudinal data is consistent with the presumption that divergent pathways and mechanisms can result in success following treatment (Brown, 1993) Articulating these naturally occurring alcohol and drug use patterns over time and evaluations of fluctuations in the trajectories of use can clarify: 1) the sequencing of use and abuse of multiple substances (trajectories can define progressions into and out of use of individual substances), and 2) use patterns in relation to developmentally important changes such as obtaining a driver's license, marital engagement, or coming of legal age to purchase alcohol (Abrantes et al., 2002). Just as the conceptual model of equifinality lends understanding to ways in which developmentally influenced risk pathways may intersect and interact in the emergence of AUDs, a similar statistical approach may help articulate the divergent pathways to success (or failure) following treatment for distinct subgroups of youth. Approaching outcome evaluation from this longitudinal modeling perspective will be useful in bringing uniformity to the developmental alcohol treatment outcome literature as well as help clinicians in treatment planning for youth during developmental risk periods.

5. Summary

In the present chapter we have sought to articulate a translational perspective linking development during adolescence to alcohol treatment and its evaluation. Clearly adolescents with alcohol use disorders cannot be treated as younger versions of adults. The unique demands of their developmental stage permeate all aspects of their behavior, including alcohol use and abuse. Multidimensional developmental models help inform the design, implementation, and evaluation of alcohol and drug treatment programs. While an understanding of individual risk factors is informative, only through models integrating multiple risk pathways embedded in the context of adolescent development can we hope to build more efficacious and effective systems of intervention for youth with AUDs. Effective treatment of adolescent AUDs not only urges translation of the developmental perspective into pre-existing treatment approaches but argues for a paradigm shift towards alternative intervention designs and evaluation procedures and foci.

References

Abrantes, A.M. & Brown, S.A. (2003). *Psychiatric comorbidity among substance abusing adolescents: Assessment issues in clinical research.* Manuscript submitted for publication.

Abrantes, A., McCarthy, D.M., Aarons, G., & Brown, S.A. (2002, June). *Long-term trajectories of alcohol involvement following addictions treatment in adolescence.* Symposium presented at the Research Society on Alcoholism, San Francisco, California.

Anderson, K.G., Frissell, K.C., & Brown, S.A. (2004). *Contexts of first post-treatment use for substance abusing adolescents with comorbid psychopathology.* Manuscript submitted for publication.

Azrin, N.H., Donohoe, B., Teicher, G.A., Crum, T., Howell, J., & DeCato, L.A. (2001). A controlled evaluation and description of individual-cognitive problem solving and family-behavior therapies in dually-diagnosed conduct-disordered and substance-dependent youth. *Journal of Child and Adolescent Substance Abuse, 11*, 1–43.

Baumrind, D. (1987). A developmental perspective on adolescent risk taking in contemporary America. *New Directions in Child Development, 37*, 93–125.

Beyers, W., Goossens, L., Vansant, I., & Moors, E. (2003). A structural model of autonomy in middle and late adolescence: Connectedness, separation, detachment, and agency. *Journal of Youth and Adolescence, 32*(5), 351–365.

Bonomo, Y., Coffey, C., Wolfe, R., Lynskey, M., Bowes, G., & Patton, G. (2001). Adverse outcomes of alcohol use in adolescents. *Addiction, 96*, 1485–1496.

Brown, S.A. (1993). Recovery patterns in adolescent substance abuse. In J.S. Baer & G.A. Marlatt (Eds.), *Addictive Behaviors Across the Life Span: Prevention, Treatment, and Policy Issues* (pp. 161–183). CA: Sage Publications.

Brown, S.A. (1999). Treatment of adolescent alcohol problems: Research review and appraisal. In National Institute on Alcohol Abuse and Alcoholism extramural scientific advisory board (Ed.), *Treatment* (pp. 1–26). Bethesda, MD.

Brown, S.A. (2001). Facilitating change for adolescent alcohol problems: A multiple options approach. In E.F. Wagner & H.B. Waldron (Eds.), *Innovations in Adolescent Substance Abuse Interventions* (pp. 169–187). Oxford: Elsevier Science Ltd.

Brown, S.A. (in press). Measuring youth outcomes from alcohol and drug treatment. *Addictions.*

Brown, S.A. & D'Amico, E.J. (2001). Outcomes for alcohol treatment for adolescents. In Galanter, M. (Ed.), *Recent Developments in Alcoholism Vol. 17: Selected Treatment Topics.* New York: Plenum.

Brown, S.A., D'Amico, E.J., McCarthy, D.M., & Tapert, S.F. (2001). Four-year outcomes from adolescent alcohol and drug treatment. *Journal of Studies on Alcohol, 63*(3), 381–388.

Brown, S.A., Myers, M.G., Lippke, L.F., Stewart, D.G., Tapert, S.F., & Vik, P.W. (1998). Psychometric evaluation of the Customary Drinking and Drug Use Record (CDDR): A measure of adolescent alcohol and drug involvement. *Journal of Studies on Alcohol, 59*, 427–439.

Brown, S.A., Myers, M.G., Mott, M.A., & Vik, P.W. (1994). Correlates of success following treatment for adolescent substance abuse. *Applied and Preventive Psychology, 3*(2), 61–73.

Brown, S.A. & Ramo, D.E. (in press) Clinical course of youth following treatment for alcohol and drug problems. In H. Liddle & C. Rowe (Eds.), *Treating Adolescent Substance Abuse: State of the Science.* Cambridge: Cambridge University Press.

Brown, S.A., Stetson, B.A., & Beatty, P. (1989). Cognitive and behavioral features of adolescent coping in high risk drinking situations. *Addictive Behaviors, 14*, 43–52.

Brown, S.A. & Tapert, S.F. (in press). Health consequences of adolescent alcohol involvement. In *Health Consequences and Costs of Adolescent Alcohol Use.* Washington, D.C.: National Academy Press.

Brown, S. A., Tapert, S. F., Granholm, E., & Delis, D. C. (2000). Neurocognitive functioning of adolescents: effects of protracted alcohol use. *Alcoholism: Clinical and Experimental Research, 24*, 164–171.

Brown, S.A., Tapert, S.F., Tate, S.R., & Abrantes, A.M. (2000). The role of alcohol in adolescent relapse and outcome. *Journal of Psychoactive Drugs, 32*, 107–115.

Brown, S.A., Vik, P.W., & Creamer, V.A. (1989). Characteristics of relapse following adolescent substance abuse treatment. *Addictive Behaviors, 14*(3), 291–300.

Brownell, K. D., Marlatt, G.A., Lictenstein, E., Wilson, G.T. (1986). Understanding and preventing relapse. *American Psychologist, 41*, 765–782.

Caspi, A., Lynam, D., Moffitt, T.E., Silva, P.A. (1993). *Unraveling girls' delinquency: Biological, dispositional, and contextual contributions to adolescent misbehavior.* Developmental Psychology, 29*(1), 19–30.*

Chassin, L., Pitts, S.C., & DeLucia, C. (1999). The relation of adolescent substance use to young adult autonomy, positive activity involvement, and perceived competence. *Development and Psychopathology, 11*, 915–932.

Cloninger, C. R., Sigvardsson, S., & Bohman, M. (1988). Childhood personality predicts alcohol abuse in young adults. *Alcoholism: Clinical and Experimental Research, 12*, 494–505.

Colder, C.R. & Chassin, L. (1993). The stress and negative affect model of adolescent alcohol use and the moderating effects of behavioral undercontrol. *Journal of Studies on Alcohol, 54*(3), 326–333.

Corby, E.A., Roll, J.M., Ledgerwood, D.M., Schuster, C.R. (2000). Contingency management interventions for treating the substance abuse of adolescents: A feasibility study. *Experimental and Clinical Psychopharmacology, 8*, 371–376.

Crews, F. T., Braun, C. J., Hoplight, B., Switzer, R. C., 3rd, & Knapp, D. J. (2000). Binge ethanol consumption causes differential brain damage in young adolescent rats compared with adult rats. *Alcoholism: Clinical and Experimental Research, 24*, 1712–1723.

Cummings, E.M., Davies, P.T., & Campbell, S.B. (2000). *Developmental psychopathology and family process: Theory, research and clinical implications.* New York: Guilford Press.

Deas, D., Riggs, P., Langenbucher, J., Goldman, M., & Brown, S. (2000). Adolescents are not adults: Developmental considerations in alcohol users. *Alcoholism: Clinical and Experimental Research, 24*, 232–237.

De Bellis, M. D., Clark, D. B., Beers, S. R., Soloff, P. H., Boring, A. M., Hall, J., Kersh, A., & Keshavan, M. S. (2000). Hippocampal volume in adolescent-onset alcohol use disorders. *American Journal of Psychiatry, 157*, 737–744.

Delis, D.C., Kramer, J., Kaplan, E., & Ober, B.A. (1994). *California Verbal learning Test for Children.* New York: The Psychological Corporation.

Edwall, G.E., Hoffmann, N.G., & Harrison, P.A. (1989). Psychological correlates of sexual abuse in adolescent girls in chemical dependency treatment. *Adolescence, 24*, 279–288.

Elder, G. H. (1998). The life course and human development. In W.Damon (Series ed.) & R.M. Lerner (Vol. ed.), *Handbook of Child Psychology: Volume 1. Theoretical Models of Human Development* (5th ed., pp. 939–992). New York: Wiley.

Fergusson, D. M., & Lynskey, M. T. (1996). Alcohol misuse and adolescent sexual behaviors and risk taking. *Pediatrics, 98,* 91–96.

Giancola, P. R., & Mezzich, A. C. (2000). Neuropsychological deficits in female adolescents with a substance use disorder: better accounted for by conduct disorder? *Journal of Studies on Alcohol, 61,* 809–817.

Goodwin, D.W., Knop, J., Jensen, P., Gabrielli, Jr., W.F., & Pennick, E.C. (1994). Thirty-year follow-up of men at high risk for alcoholism. *Annals of the New York Academy of Science, 708,* 97–101.

Henggeler, S.W., Clingempeel, W.G., Brondino, M.J., & Pickrel, S.G. (2002). Four-year follow-up of multisystemic therapy with substance-abusing and substance-dependent juvenile offenders. *Journal of the American Academy of Child and Adolescent Psychiatry, 41,* 868–874.

Hoffmann, N.G., Sonis, W.A., & Halikas, J.A. (1987). Issues in the evaluation of chemical dependency treatment programs for adolescents. *The Pediatric clinics of North America, 34,* 449–459.

Hussong, A.M. & Chassin, L. (2002). Parent alcoholism and the leaving home transition. *Development & Psychopathology, 14,* 139–157.

Johnston, L.D., O'Malley, P.M., Bachman, J.G., & Schulenberg (2004). *Monitoring the future national results on adolescent drug use: Overview of key findings, 2003* (NIH Publication No. 04–5506). Bethesda, MD: National Institute on Drug Abuse.

Jorm, A.F. (1987). Sex and age differences in depression: A quantitative synthesis of published research. *Australian & New Zealand Journal of Psychiatry, 21,* 46–53.

Kaminer, Y. (2001). Adolescent substance abuse treatment: Where do we go from here? *Psychiatry Service, 52,* 147–149.

Kaminer, Y., Burleson, J., & Goldberger, R. (2002). Cognitive-behavioral coping skills and psychoeducation therapies for adolescent substance abuse. *Journal of Nervous and Mental Disease, 190,* 737–745.

Kandel, D., Yamaguchi, K., & Chen, K. (1992). Stages of progression in drug involvement from adolescence to adulthood: Further evidence for the gateway theory. *Journal of Studies on Alcohol, 53,* 447–457.

Kelly, J.F., Myers, M.G., & Brown, S.A. (2000). A multivariate process model of adolescent 12-step attendance and substance use outcome following inpatient treatment. *Psychology of Addictive Behaviors, 14,* 376–389.

Kypri, K., McCarthy, D.M., Coe, M.T., & Brown, S.A. (in press). Transition to independent living and substance involvement of treated and high risk youth. *Journal of Child and Adolescent Substance Abuse.*

Laurent, J., Catanzaro, S. J., Joiner, T. E., Jr., Rudolph, K. D., Potter, K. I., Lambert, S. et al., (1999). A measure of positive and negative affect for children: Scale development and initial validation. *Psychological Assessment, 11,* 326–338.

Lezak (1995). *Neuropsychological Assessment (3rd Edition).* New York: Oxford University Press.

Liddle, H.A., Dakof, G.A., Diamond, G.S., Barrett, K., Tejeda, M. (2001). Multidimentional family therapy for adolescent substance abuse: Results of a randomized clinical trial. *American Journal of Drug and Alcohol Abuse, 27,* 651–687.

Loeber, R., & Dishion, T. (1983). Early predictors of male delinquency: a review. *Psychological Bulletin, 94,* 68–99.

Marlatt, G.A., & Gordon, J.R. (1980). Determinants of relapse: Implications for the maintenance of behavior change. In P. Davidson & S.M. Davidson (Eds.), *Behavioral medicine: Changing health lifestyles* (pp. 410–452). Elmsford, NY: Pergamon.

Marlatt, G.A., & Gordon, J.A. (1985). *Relapse prevention: Maintenance strategies in the treatment of addictive behaviors.* New York: Guilford Press.

McCarthy, D.M. & Brown, S.A. (2003). *The influence of obtaining a drivers license on alcohol and drug involvement, alcohol-related cognitions and drinking and driving behavior.* Manuscript submitted for publication.

Metrik, J., Frissell, K.C., McCarthy, D.M., DAmico, E.J., & Brown, S.A. (2003). Strategies for reduction and cessation of alcohol use: Adolescent preferences. *Alcoholism: Clinical & Experimental Research, 27*, 74–80.

Milberger, S., Biederman, J., Faraone, S. V., Wilens, T., & Chu, M. P. (1997). Associations between ADHD and psychoactive substance use disorders: Findings from a longitudinal study of high-risk siblings of ADHD children. *American Journal on Addictions, 6*, 318–329.

Moffitt, T. E. (1993). Adolescence-limited and life-course-persistent antisocial behavior: a developmental taxonomy. *Psychological Review, 100*, 674–701.

Monroe, S.M. & Simons, A.D. (1991). Diathesis stress theories in the context of life stress research: Implications for the depressive disorders. *Psychological Bulletin, 110*, 406–425.

Monti, P.M. (1999). Innovations in adolescent substance abuse intervention. *Alcoholism: Clinical and Experimental Research, 23*, 236–249.

Monti, P.M., Colby, S.M., Barnett, N.P., Spirito, A., Rohsenow, D.J., Myers, M., et al. (1999). Brief intervention for harm reduction with alcohol-positive older adolescents in a hospital emergency department. *Journal of Consulting & Clinical Psychology, 67*, 989–994.

Moos, B.R. & Moos, B.S. (1986). *The Family Environment Scale manual* (Rev. ed.). Palo Alto, CA: Consulting Psychologists Press.

Muris, P., Mercklebach, H., Wessel, I., & van de Ven, M. (1999). Pathological correlates of self-reported behavioral inhibition in normal children. *Behavioral Research and Therapy, 37*, 575–584.

Myers, M.G., & Brown, S.A. (1990). Coping and appraisal in relapse risk situations among adolescent substance abusers following treatment. *Journal of Adolescent Chemical Dependency, 1*, 95–115.

Neighbors, B. Kempton, T., & Forehand, R. (1992). Co-occurrence of substance abuse with conduct, anxiety, and depression disorders in juvenile delinquents. *Addictive Behaviors, 17*, 379–386.

Newcomb, M. D., & Bentler, P. M. (1986). Frequency and sequence of drug use: a longitudinal study from early adolescence to young adulthood. *Journal of Drug Education, 16*, 101–120.

O'Connor, T.G., Allen, J.P., Bell, K.L., & Hauser, S.T. (1996). Adolescent-parent relationships and leaving home in young adulthood. In J.A. Graber & J.S. Dubas (Eds.), *New directions for child development: Vol. 71. Leaving home: Understanding the transition to adulthood* (pp. 39–52). San Francisco: Jossey-Bass.

Office of Inspector General. (1992). *Youth and Alcohol: Dangerous and Deadly Consequences*. Washington D.C.: U.S. Department of Health and Human Services.

O'Malley, P.M., Johnston, L.D., & Bachman, J.G. (1998). Alcohol use among adolescents. *Alcohol Health and Research World, 22*, 85–93.

Osterrieth, P.A. (1944). Le test de copie d'une figure complexe. *Archive de Psychologie, 30*, 206–356; translated by J. Corwin and F.W. Blysma (1993), *The Clinical Neuropsychologist, 7*, 9–15.

Santisteban, D. A., Coatsworth, D., Perez-Vidal, A., Mitrani, V., Jean-Gilles, M., & Szapocznik, J. (1997). Brief structural/strategic family therapy with African American and Hispanic youth. *Journal of Community Psychology, 25*, 453–471.

Schulenberg, J., O'Malley, P. M., Bachman, J. G., Wadsworth, K. N., & Johnston, L. D. (1996). Getting drunk and growing up: trajectories of frequent binge drinking during the transition to young adulthood. *Journal of Studies on Alcohol, 57*, 289–304.

Shaffer, D., Fisher, P., Lucas, C.P., Dulcan, M. K. & Schwab-Stone, M.E. (2000). NIMH Diagnostic Interview Schedule for Children Version IV (NIMH DISC-IV): Description, differences from previous versions, and reliability of some common diagnoses. *Journal of the American Academy of Child & Adolescent Psychiatry, 39*, 28–38.

Silveri, M. M., & Spear, L. P. (2002). The effects of NMDA and GABA(A) pharmacological manipulations on ethanol sensitivity in immature and mature animals. *Alcoholism: Clinical and Experimental Research, 26*, 449–456.

Spear, L. (2002). The adolescent brain and the college drinker: Biological basis of propensity to use and misuse alcohol. *Journal of Studies on Alcohol. Special Issue: College drinking, what it is, and what do to about it: Review of the state of the science*, Suppl 14, 71–81.

Stice, E., Myers, M.G., & Brown, S.A. (1998). A longitudinal grouping analysis of adolescent substance use escalation and de-escalation. *Psychology of Addictive Behaviors* 12, 14–27.

Tapert, S. F., & Brown, S. A. (1999). Neuropsychological correlates of adolescent substance abuse: four-year outcomes. Journal of the International Neuropsychological Society, 5, 481–493.

Tate, S., Brown, S.A., Unrod, M. & Ramo, D. (in press). *Context of relapse for substance abusers with and without comorbid psychiatric disorders. Addictive Behavior.*

Tomlinson, K.L., Brown, S.A., & Abrantes, A. (2004). Psychiatric Comorbidity and Substance Use Treatment Outcomes of Adolescents. *Psychology of Addictive Behaviors, 18,* 160–169.

Vik, P.W., Grissel, K., & Brown, S.A. (1992). Social resource characteristics and adolescent substance abuser relapse. *Journal of Adolescent Chemical Dependency, 2,* 59–74.

Wagner, E.F., Dinklage, S., Cudworth, C., & Vyse, J. (1999). A preliminary evaluation of the effectiveness of a standardized Student Assistance Program. *Substance Use & Misuse, 34,* 1571–1584

Wagner, E.F. & Kassel, J.D. (1995). Substance use and abuse. In RT Ammerman and M. Hersen (Eds.): Handbook of Child Behavior Therapy in the Psychiatric Setting. New York: John Wiley & Sons, pp. 367–388.

Waldron, H.B., Slesnick, N., Brody, J.L., Turner, C.W., & Peterson, T.R. (2001). Treatment outcomes for adolescent substance abuse at 4- and 7-month assessments. *Journal of Consulting and Clinical Psychology, 69,* 802–813.

Wechsler, D. (1991). *Wechsler Memory Scale Revised Manual.* San Antonio, TX: The Psychological Corporation.

White, A. M., Ghia, A. J., Levin, E. D., & Swartzwelder, H. S. (2000). Binge pattern ethanol exposure in adolescent and adult rats: differential impact on subsequent responsiveness to ethanol. *Alcoholism: Clinical and Experimental Research, 24,* 1251–1256.

White, H. R., Xie, M., Thompson, W., Loeber, R., & Stouthamer-Loeber, M. (2001). Psychopathology as a predictor of adolescent drug use trajectories. *Psychology of Addictive Behaviors, 15,* 210–218.

Winters, K. & Henly, G. (1993). *The Adolescent Diagnostic Interview Schedule and User's Manual.* Los Angeles: Western Psychological Services.

Winters, K.C., Stinchfield, R.D., Opland, E., Weller, C., Latimer, W. W. (2000). The effectiveness of the Minnesota Model approach in the treatment of adolescent drug abusers. *Addiction, 95,* 601–6.

Witkiewitz, k, & Marlatt, G.A. (2004). Relapse prevention for alcohol and drug problems: That was Zen, this is Tao. *American Psychologist, 59,* 224–235.

Yi, H.-y., Williams, G.D., & Dufour, M.C. (2001). *Surveillance report # 56: Trends in alcohol-related fatal traffic crashes, United States, 1977–99.* Bethesda, MD: National Institute on Alcohol Abuse and Alcoholism.

Zucker, R.A., Chermack, S.T., & Curran, G.M. (2000). Alcoholism: A life span perspective on etiology and course. In A.J. Sameroff, M. Lewis, and S.M. Miller (Eds.), *Handbook of Developmental Psychopathology* (2nd ed., pp. 569–587). New York: Kluwer Academic/Plenum Publishers.

16

Treatment of Co-occurring Alcohol, Drug, and Psychiatric Disorders

Jack R. Cornelius, Duncan B. Clark, Oscar G. Bukstein, and Ihsan M. Salloum

Abstract. Comorbid psychiatric disorders and drug use disorders (DUDs) are common among adolescents with alcohol use disorders (AUDs). These comorbid disorders have a large potential significance on the clinical course of the AUDs among adolescents, and can predict a shorter time to relapse of alcohol use. The use of medication for treatment of the various comorbid adolescent populations has increased dramatically in recent years, despite the lack of double-blind, placebo-controlled studies that demonstrate their safety and efficacy. Consequently, to date, no empirically proven treatment exists for most of these comorbid disorders. This chapter reviews the state of the art regarding the treatment of comorbid adolescents. This chapter also identifies gaps in knowledge regarding the treatment of comorbid adolescents, and outlines directions for future research in this field.

1. Introduction

The comorbidity of alcohol use disorders (AUDs) with psychiatric disorders and with other substance use disorders (SUDs) is now recognized as a common problem among both adolescents and adults. AUDs (alcohol abuse and alcohol dependence) typically begin in late adolescence or young adulthood, with a median age of onset of 21 years, as shown by data from the Epidemiologic Catchment Area (ECA) study (Christie et al., 1988). Data from that same large epidemiologic study also demonstrated that 45% of all persons with an AUD also had some other drug or mental disorder (Regier et al., 1990), including 37% of those AUD individuals who demonstrated a comorbid mental disorder and 22% who demonstrated another SUD in their lifetime. Of those

Jack R. Cornelius, Duncan B. Clark, Oscar G. Bukstein, and Ihsan M. Salloum • School of Medicine, University of Pittsburgh, Pittsburgh, Pennsylvania 15213-2593.

with comorbid disorders, 80% reported an onset before the age of 20 (Christie et al., 1988), suggesting that comorbidity typically begins during adolescence. Data from the National Comorbidity Survey (NCS), demonstrate that that the vast majority of lifetime disorders in their sample (79%) were comorbid disorders (Kessler et al., 1994), and also show that comorbidity is the rule rather than the exception among young people (Kessler & Walters, 1998). A number of studies have demonstrated an even stronger association between AUDs and comorbid psychiatric disorders in clinical samples of adolescents (Bukstein et al., 1989; Clark, Pollock, et al., 1997; Rohde et al., 1991). Data from the NCS also demonstrated that the presence of co-occurring disorders is significantly associated with persistence of alcohol abuse (Kessler et al., 1997). This comorbidity has a large influence on the clinical course of the AUDs among adolescents, as was recently shown by a study which demonstrated that comorbid major depression predicts earlier alcohol relapse among teenagers with an AUD (Cornelius, Maisto, et al., 2004).

Adolescents with comorbid disorders have unique treatment needs both because of their stage of development and because of their comorbid disorders (Deas et al., 2000; Hird et al., 1997). The use of psychotropic medications among adolescents has increased dramatically in the last ten years, and is now widespread (Zito et al., 2003; Clark et al., 2003). However, few studies have been conducted that involve alcoholics with comorbid disorders, and even fewer involve adolescents with comorbid disorders (Clark, Bukstein, et al., 2002), despite the prevalence of these comorbid disorders among adolescents. Double-blind, placebo-controlled studies are particularly scarce involving comorbid adolescent populations, though open label studies have been conducted on most of these populations. Consequently, no empirically proven treatment exists for most of these comorbid disorders among adolescents.

This chapter will review the state of the art regarding the treatment of adolescents with an AUD in combination with a comorbid drug or psychiatric disorder. Because research in this area is in its relative infancy, we will also review relevant lessons from the adult literature. Because of space limitations, this chapter will focus on the most common and clinically relevant comorbid conditions among adolescents. This chapter will identify gaps in knowledge regarding the treatment of comorbid adolescents, and will outline issues for future research in this field.

2. Comorbidity with Non-Alcohol Drug Use Disorders

Data from the NCS (Kessler et al., 1997) demonstrated that DUDs are the group of disorders that is most likely to co-occur with AUD, as they are present in 30% of these individuals. The Methods for the Epidemiology of Child and Adolescent Mental Disorders (MECA) study provides population estimates concerning patterns of SUDs among children and adolescents (Kandel et al., 1997). That study demonstrated that the prevalence of DUDs increases with age, from 1.5% at age 14 to 8.7% at age 17. The most common DUD in that study was alcohol abuse or dependence, while the most common illicit SUD was marijuana abuse or dependence. Other SUDs were substantially less prevalent. In that study, only three groups of psychiatric disorders were more prevalent than DUDs: anxiety disorders (13%), mood disorders (7%), and disruptive behavior disorders (10%).

More data are available regarding levels of drug use among adolescents than are available regarding levels of DUDs among this age group. This data concerning adolescent drug use is available from sources such as the National Household Survey on Drug Abuse (Summary, 2002). According to that survey, current (in the last 30 days) illicit drug use among youth 12 to 17 years of age was prevalent, being present in 11% of persons in that age group. In contrast, 29% of youth age 12 to 20 drank alcohol in the last month (10.1 million adolescents). Of that total, 6.8 million were binge drinkers, and 2.1 million were heavy drinkers (Summary, 2002). Thus, according to the National Household Survey, alcohol is the most common substance used by adolescents. In 2001, almost two of every three teenagers, ages 12 to 17, who demonstrated frequent drinking binges also abused drugs. In contrast, only about one in 20 teenagers who did not drink at all used drugs. These findings demonstrate that drug addiction and alcohol addiction are strongly linked in adolescents.

Despite the prevalence of DUDs and AUDs among adolescents, relatively little research has been conducted to assess the effectiveness of treatment for these disorders in that age group, and most literature on treatment outcome has been based on adult patients (Bukstein & Cornelius, in press; Hser et al., 2001). Two of the early major studies of drug treatment outcomes included NIDA's National Follow-Up Study of Drug Abuse Treatment in Drug Abuse Reporting Program (the DARP Study) (Sells & Simpson, 1979), and NIDA's Treatment Outcome Prospective Study (the TOPS study) (Hubbard et al., 1985). These early large-scale studies focused primarily on adults treated with a variety of psychotherapy modalities, and included only small samples of adolescents. These early studies generally reported less favorable outcomes among adolescents than adult patients, with substantial residual levels of drug and alcohol use, despite some reductions in level of drug use (Hubbard et al., 1985; Sells & Simpson, 1979). Subsequently, a SAMHSA study was conducted entitled the Services Research Outcomes Study, which showed less positive outcomes (National Opinion Research Center, 1997). That study found an increase of 13% in alcohol use and a doubling of crack cocaine use in the five years following treatment of their patients.

Recently, the first large scale study was completed which had been designed to evaluate drug abuse treatment outcomes among adolescents. That study was called the Drug Abuse Treatment Outcome Studies for Adolescents (DATOS) (Hser et al., 2001), and studied 1167 adolescents in 4 American cities, using a naturalistic, non-experimental study design. The results of that study suggested that drug treatment programs can effectively decrease drug and alcohol use, and can decrease criminal activity as well, in addition to improving school performance and psychological adjustment. However, a substantial prevalence of alcohol and drug use persisted at the end of the one-year follow-up period. Also, because of a lack of a control group, it was unclear to what extent the decreases in drug and alcohol use were the result of treatment versus being the result of other factors.

Some very recent studies have suggested promise for several forms of psychotherapy in treating adolescent AUDs and DUDs. These forms of psychotherapy include several forms of family therapy, such as functional family therapy (Waldron et al., 2001), multildimensional family therapy (Liddle et al., 2001) multisystemic therapy (MST) (Henggeler et al., 2002), and community reinforcement (Cannabis Youth Treatment Group, 2000). Other promising forms of treatment in this population include motivational interviewing (MI) (Wagner et al., 1999), cognitive-behavioral therapy (CBT) (Kaminer et al., 1998), the 12-step approach (Winters et al., 2000), contingency management reinforcement (CM) (Corby et al., 2000), and integrative treatment models employing CBT combined with MI or with a family intervention (Cannabis Youth Treatment Group, 2000; Waldron et al., 2001).

A recent review of adolescent substance abuse treatment studies evaluated the effectiveness of five main treatment modalities: family-based and multi-systemic intervention, behavioral therapy, cognitive behavioral therapy, pharmacotherapy, and twelve step approaches (Deas & Thomas, 2001). The authors of that review concluded that the results of those studies looked promising for cognitive behavioral therapy and family-based multi-systemic therapies for adolescents with SUDs, but said that various methodological limitations made it difficult to evaluate whether one treatment approach is clearly more effective than another. Similarly, Kaminer (1994) concluded that virtually no studies have yet documented the differential efficacy of various therapies for treating adolescent DUDs, and also concluded that no clear optimal dosage or length of treatment has been identified (Kaminer, 2002). Kaminer (1995) also concluded that the literature on treatment of adolescents diagnosed with SUDs is replete with descriptions of treatment philosophies, modalities, and programs, but said that little empirical research on treatment outcome has been reported. In addition, the study samples in most of the treatment samples tend to be heterogeneous, and the treatments have generally not been evaluated in specific comorbid populations, so their effectiveness in comorbid populations is unclear. Another review (Hird et al., 1997) concluded that it is difficult to draw conclusions about the effectiveness of various treatments based on the literature, because of variations between studies in operational definitions, terminology, and measures of outcome effectiveness. Pharmacotherapy studies have been particularly scarce among adolescents with DUDs or with DUDs in combination with AUDs or other disorders (Kaminer, 1994).

Perhaps because of this lack of data regarding effectiveness of treatment for DUDs, and for those with comorbid disorders, varying degrees of skepticism still exist regarding the effectiveness of drug treatment among the general public, policymakers, third-party payers, researchers, and journalists (Apsler, 1994;

Pendergast et al., 2002). However, as noted above, the literature in the last five years is somewhat more positive regarding the effectiveness of treatment of adolescent DUDs, and the methodology of these more recent studies is more rigorous that that of previous studies. The results of the recent DATOS study are particularly convincing regarding the effectiveness of treatment of this population. Therefore, it can be concluded that several psychotherapy treatment approaches suggest promise for treating adolescent DUD, including DUDs associated with AUDs and other comorbid disorders, but none has been proven to be more effective than other treatment modalities.

3. Comorbidity with Major Depression

Depression and other psychiatric disorders are common among adolescents with alcohol and drug disorders, as has been shown by data from national surveys (Fleming & Offord, 1990; Kandel et al., 1997) and from a variety of clinical populations (Bukstein et al., 1989; Clark, Pollock, et al., 1997; Fleming & Offord, 1990). Adolescent-onset depression has been shown to be associated with a higher level of comorbidity than adult-onset depression (Rohde et al., 1991). Major depression has also been shown to be a predictor of earlier alcohol relapse in adolescents (Cornelius, Maisto, et al., 2004) and among adults (Greenfield et al., 1998).

To date, few studies have been conducted involving adolescents with comorbid AUDs and major depression. Indeed, only recently have double-blind, placebo-controlled studies been completed involving any SSRI antidepressant in an adolescent population with major depression alone (Emslie et al., 1997). That study, involving 96 child and adolescent outpatients, demonstrated efficacy for fluoxetine for decreasing the depressive symptoms of child and adolescent outpatients with major depression. That study was the first double-blind, placebo-controlled trial of any antidepressant medication, whether SSRI or tricyclic antidepressant, to demonstrate efficacy for treating major depression among children and adolescents. Subsequently, that same research group conducted a first long-term (one-year) naturalistic follow-up study of a SSRI medication (fluoxetine), involving the patients who had participated in their acute phase trial (Emslie et al., 1998). The results of that study demonstrated long-term efficacy for fluoxetine for decreasing the depressive symptoms of adolescents with major depression who do not display comorbid alcohol or substance abuse. The results of that study also demonstrated a high rate of recurrence of major depression (40%) among their participants in the year following their treatment trial. The authors of that study also concluded that this high rate of recurrence of major depression among adolescents was even higher than that which is typically reported for adults. The results of that study were replicated in a recent double-blind, placebo-controlled multi-site study involving fluoxetine in 122 children and 97 adolescents with major depression (Emslie, 2002). On the basis of those two double-blind, placebo-controlled studies, the Food and Drug Administration (FDA) approved fluoxetine for treatment of major depression in children and adolescents on January 3, 2003. Fluoxetine thus became the first SSRI medication (and the first antidepressant medication of any kind, including tricyclic antidepressants, SSRI antidepressants, etc.) to receive approval from the FDA for treating major depression in adolescents and children (FDA, 2003).

Recent double-blind placebo-controlled studies have also suggested efficacy for the SSRI medications sertraline (Wagner et al., 2003) and paroxetine (Keller et al., 2001) for treating major depression among children and adolescents, though these results have not been replicated. In contrast, tricyclic medications have not demonstrated efficacy for treating major depression among children and adolescents with major depression (Hazell et al., 1995), and tricyclic antidepressants have been shown to be associated with sudden death when taking therapeutic dosages (Varley, 2001).

To date, only two open label studies and one very small double-blind study have assessed the efficacy of any SSRI medication among adolescents with a comorbid AUD and major depression (Riggs et al., 1997; Cornelius, Bukstein, et al., 2001; Deas-Nesmith et al., 1998). The first of these two studies involved the open-label use of fluoxetine in eight adolescent subjects with major depression, conduct disorder, and an AUD, generally in combination with other DUDs (Riggs et al., 1997). This study demonstrated within-group efficacy of fluoxetine in decreasing depression. Potential effects on drug or alcohol use could not be assessed in this study because it was conducted in a controlled environment.

The second of these two open label studies was a 12-week trial that involved the SSRI medication fluoxetine in a sample of 13 adolescents with comorbid major depression and an AUD, most (10) of whom also demonstrated cannabis abuse. All participants also received motivation enhancement therapy (MET) (Miller et al., 1992) for their AUD and cognitive behavioral therapy CBT) (Birmaher et al., 2000) for their depressive disorder. A significant decrease was noted during the course of the study in both depressive symptoms and level of drinking. A significant decrease was also noted in suicidal ideations over the course of the study. A significant association was noted between alcohol use and cannabis use during the course of the study. No subjects made a suicide attempt during the course of the study. The medication was well tolerated during the study. Those findings suggest promise for fluoxetine, in combination with CBT and MET, for decreasing both the depressive symptoms and the drinking of adolescents with comorbid major depression and an AUD.

The investigators of that study then conducted the first naturalistic one-year follow-up evaluation of adolescent comorbid participants. That study involved 10 of the 13 subjects who had participated in the 12-week acute phase trial (Cornelius, Bukstein, et al., 2004). All 10 subjects who had signed informed consent for the follow-up study participated in the one-year assessment. At the one-year follow-up evaluation, the group continued to demonstrate significantly less depressive symptoms and less frequency of drinking than they had demonstrated at the baseline of the acute phase study. Surprisingly, all of the subjects had chosen to discontinue their antidepressant medication by the second month of their naturalistic follow-up period, saying that they felt that they no longer needed treatment with an antidepressant medication because their symptoms had decreased. Three of the subjects had experienced a recurrence of their major depression during the follow-up period, and three others demonstrated a persistence of their original depressive episode throughout the follow-up period. Also, the number of drinks per drinking day continued to be high (about five per day), which was not significantly different from their level at baseline. Thus, the long-term therapeutic effects of an acute phase trial of fluoxetine plus psychotherapy were limited, when fluoxetine was discontinued shortly after the acute phase trial. The high rate of recurrence or persistence of major depression in that comorbid sample was consistent with the rate that had been reported by Emslie et al. (1998) in a non-comorbid sample of adolescents with major depression.

The investigators of that study then conducted a three-year naturalistic follow-up assessment involving those same 10 individuals who had participated in the one-year naturalistic follow-up evaluation (Cornelius et al., 2003). At the three-year follow-up evaluation, the group continued to demonstrate fewer DSM alcohol dependence criteria and fewer depressive symptoms than at the baseline of the acute phase study, and also consumed fewer standard drinks. However, they no longer demonstrated significantly fewer diagnostic criteria for major depression or for cannabis dependence than they had demonstrated at the baseline of the acute phase study. In the three years since the completion of the 12-week acute phase study, 7 subjects had utilized psychiatric outpatient treatment, 2 had utilized outpatient alcohol or drug treatment, and 4 had restarted fluoxetine. The presence of an AUD at the three-year follow-up assessment was significantly associated with the presence of major depression, as had also been true at the one-year follow-up evaluation, suggesting a continued link between the AUD and the major depression following acute phase treatment.

One pilot study has evaluated the efficacy of the SSRI antidepressant sertraline for treating adolescents with concurrent major depression and alcohol dependence (Deas-Nesmith et al., 1998). That double-blind, placebo-controlled study, which involved only 10 subjects, demonstrated a significant reduction in both drinking and depressive symptoms in both treatment groups, though no significant difference between groups was noted in this very small study.

It should be noted that all SSRI antidepressants are not necessarily the same in their effectiveness and their side effect profile among comorbid or non-comorbid adolescents with major depression, despite the fact that the various SSRI antidepressants have been shown to be similar in their effectiveness in adults treated in primary care settings (Kroenke et al., 2001). For example, the Food and Drug Administration recently warned of an increased suicide risk when using the SSRI antidepressant paroxetine in children and adolescents with major depression (Rosack, 2003). Specifically, on June 19, 2003, the

FDA warned that the antidepressant paroxetine may be linked to "a possible increased rate" of self-harming behaviors, including suicidal behavior in children and adolescents. The FDA concluded that there is currently no evidence that paroxetine is effective in children or adolescents with major depression, and that paroxetine is not currently approved for use in children and adolescents. The FDA also noted that other approved treatment options are available for treating major depression in children and adolescents. As a result, the FDA stated that the medication paroxetine should not be prescribed to that population for the treatment of major depression. Also, on March 22, 2004, the FDA issued a Public Health Advisory that asked the manufacturers of ten antidepressant medications to include in their labeling a warning statement that recommends close observation of adult and pediatric patients treated with those agents (Food and Drug Administration, 2004). To date, the results of no other studies have been published involving adolescents with comorbid AUDs and depressive disorders. No studies have been conducted involving tricyclic antidepressants in adolescent populations with comorbid major depression and an AUD, possibly because of concerns about sudden death and overdose risk among adolescents receiving tricyclic antidepressants (Varley, 2001).

In both the ECA study and the NCS study, it has been shown that bipolar disorder has a particularly high rate of co-occurrence with AUD. In the ECA study, the odds of having a bipolar disorder were five times greater if one had an AUD than if one did not have an AUD (Regier et al., 1990). In the NCS study, the odds of having a diagnosis of alcohol dependence were 12 times greater among those with a bipolar disorder than among those without a bipolar disorder, which was the highest odds ratio noted for any Axis I disorder (Kessler et al., 1997). However, despite increased awareness in recent years of the common co-occurrence of bipolar disorder and AUDs, no epidemiological studies have addressed this comorbid population among adolescents, and only one double-blind study has addressed the efficacy of lithium or any other mood stabilizer medication in this adolescent dual diagnosis population (Geller et al., 1999). That double-blind, placebo-controlled study involved 25 adolescents with bipolar disorder and alcohol or cannabis dependence who were treated with lithium for 6 weeks. The results of the study demonstrated a significant difference between the medication group and the placebo group for both psychopathology measures and weekly random urine drug assays.

4. Comorbidity with Anxiety Disorders

Anxiety disorders are the most common psychiatric disorders among children and adolescents, being present in 13% of that age group, according to the Methods for the Epidemiology of Child and Adolescent Mental Disorders (MECA) study (Kandel et al., 1997). Similarly, according to the National Comorbidity survey (Kessler et al., 1994), one in every four Americans reports a history of at least one anxiety disorder, making anxiety disorders roughly equivalent in prevalence to DUDs. That study also reported that anxiety disorders, as a group, are considerably more likely to occur in the 12 months before the interview (17%) than either DUDs (11%) or affective disorders (11%). In that study, 61% of women and 36% of men with any lifetime anxiety disorder reported a lifetime diagnosis of alcohol dependence, and these disorders were significantly correlated with each other.

Anxiety disorders are also commonly present in clinical populations of adolescents, including adolescents being treated for AUDs (Clark et al., 1995). Social phobia and posttraumatic stress disorder (PTSD) are the most common anxiety disorders among adolescents treated for AUDs (Clark et al., 1995). PTSD is present in higher rates in adolescents with alcohol dependence than among community controls (Clark, Pollock, et al., 1997). AUDs are strongly associated with physical and sexual abuse history among adolescents (Clark, Lesnick & Hegedus, 1997).

Despite the prevalence of anxiety disorders among children and adolescents, few treatment trials have been conducted in this population. Recently, the SSRI medication fluoxetine has been demonstrated to be effective for the treatment of childhood anxiety disorders in a double-blind, placebo-controlled study (Birmaher et al., 2003). No medications studies involving any anxiolytic medication have been conducted to date among adolescents with comorbid anxiety disorders and an AUD.

Other classes of pharmacotherapeutic agents, such as tricyclic antidepressants, SSRI antidepressants, monoamine oxidase inhibitors, and benzodiazepines have been studied for treating anxiety disorders in patients without comorbid alcoholism. However, to date, none of these classes of medications has been studied in adolescent or adult alcoholics with anxiety disorders (Litten & Allen, 1995). Consequently, the efficacy of these medications, in adolescent or adult alcoholics with comorbid anxiety disorders remains unclear. Also, to date no studies have been conducted involving manualized psychotherapy for adolescents with comorbid AUDs and an anxiety disorder.

5. Comorbidity with Conduct Disorder

According to the Methods for the Epidemiology of Child and Adolescent Mental Disorders (MECA) Study (Kandel et al., 1997), the disruptive behavior disorders, including conduct disorder and antisocial personality disorder, are the second most prevalent category of psychiatric disorder in children and adolescents, being present in 10% of that population. The disruptive behavior disorders are the most common comorbid conditions in adolescents afflicted with an AUD (Bukstein et al., 1989; Clark, Pollock, et al., 1997). Conduct disorder is significantly more common among adolescents with alcohol dependence than in a community control group (Clark, Pollock, et al., 1997). Indeed, a recent study found that nearly three-quarters of alcohol-dependent adolescents had at least one disruptive behavior disorder diagnosis (Kuperman et al., 2001).

The presence of antisocial personality disorder appears to modify the course of alcoholism (Bukstein et al., 1989). For example, alcoholic individuals with antisocial personality disorder have an earlier onset of alcohol use and a more rapid course to alcohol-related problems than alcoholic individuals without antisocial personality disorder (Hesselbrock et al., 1985). Antisocial behaviors during childhood have been shown to predict AUDs during adolescence (Clark et al., 2002).

Despite the prevalence of conduct disorder among adolescents, little is known about the treatment of this condition. Lewis (1996) concluded that no single treatment modality for conduct disorder has proven itself to be especially effective. Armentano & Solhkhah (2003) concluded that adolescents with conduct disorders and antisocial personality disorder need a strong behavioral program with clear limits, but did not cite empirical data to support that assertion. That same author also stated that no treatment programs have yet evolved to address this set of behaviors. Also, it has been reported that grouping high-risk youths for preventative group psychotherapy of adolescents may harm more than help those individuals, with increased cigarette smoking and increased delinquency (Dishion et al., 1999; Poulin et al., 2001). However, more recently, prevention programs targeting childhood antisocial behaviors have reportedly met with some success (Clark, Vanyukov, et al., 2002). Also, Henggeler et al., (2002) reported that multisystemic therapy (MST), a family-based treatment, was associated with significant long-term treatment effects for aggressive criminal activity, but showed only mixed effects for illicit drug use, and no clear effects on psychiatric symptoms. No controlled empirical studies to date have assessed the treatment of individuals with comorbid conduct disorder and an AUD. Thus, despite the widespread co-occurrence of conduct disorder and AUD, the field of treatment of this comorbid condition is in its infancy.

6. Comorbidity with Attention Deficit Hyperactivity Disorder

Attention Deficit Hyperactivity Disorder (ADHD) is common among children and adolescents, though the prevalence figures given for ADHD vary greatly (Weiss, 1996). A review of several studies found that 3% to 9% of children have ADHD (Szatmari, 1992). Szatmari, Offord, and coworkers determined the prevalence of ADHD from data from the Ontario Child Health Study (Szatmari et al., 1989). They found a peak prevalence of 8% between the ages of 6 and 9 years in a representative community sample, with lower rates for preschoolers and adolescents. The condition was more prevalent among boys (9%) than among girls (3%). At least half of children and adolescents with ADHD demonstrate a variety of comorbid disorders, such as AUDs, DUDs, conduct disorder, mood and anxiety disorders, and learning disabilities (Weiss, 1996). Most children "grow out" of the diagnosis of ADHD, in that they do not meet full criteria in adulthood (Mannuzza & Klein, 2000). Klein and Mannuzza

(1991) concluded that about 30% of children diagnosed with ADHD will still demonstrate ADHD at age 18, and about 8% will continue to demonstrate ADHD at 26 years of age. However, clinical experience suggests that most persons with this diagnosis in childhood continue to demonstrate significant impairment as a result of persistent ADHD symptoms (Levin et al., 2003). Unfortunately, prevalence rates of adult ADHD have not been obtained in large community surveys such as the National Comorbidity Study (NCS) (Kessler et al., 1994) or the Epidemiologic Catchment Area (ECA) Study (Regier et al., 1990).

A variety of studies have demonstrated an association between ADHD and alcohol dependence and other SUDs. For example, elevated rates of childhood ADHD have been found among various groups of person with DUDs (Eyre et al., 1982). Furthermore, Wood and colleagues (1983) found that 33% of persons with alcohol dependence seeking treatment had residual attention deficit disorder.

The most common pharmacotherapies for ADHD are stimulant medications, particularly methylphenidate, dextroamphetamine, and pemoline. Several studies have shown that these medications are highly effective in increasing attentiveness, reducing hyperactivity and destructive behavior, and improving classroom behavior and academic performance (King & Ellinwood, 1997). However, methylphenidate and dextroamphetamine are classified as schedule II medications by the Drug Enforcement Administration (DEA), thus indicating a high potential for abuse of these medications. Because of the abuse potential of the stimulant medication, some authors have concluded that their risks may outweigh potential benefits in some persons, such as some persons with DUDs (Brady et al., 1999). Other medication side effects may also limit the use of stimulant medications. For example, stimulants cannot be easily used late in the day or in the evening because of their activating effects, and they may have adverse effects on mood (King & Ellinwood, 1997). Also, some researchers believe that it is common clinical practice to discontinue the use of stimulants during the adolescent growth spurt to avoid growth retardation (Weiss, 1996).

Few studies have been conducted involving persons with comorbid ADHD and an AUD or DUD, and studies involving adolescent dual diagnosis populations are particularly scarce. Riggs et al. (2001) conducted a randomized double-blind placebo-controlled trial of the schedule IV stimulant medication pemoline in adolescents with a DUD and ADHD. They found that subjects in the pemoline group (n=35) had significantly lower hyperactivity scores, but no differences in substance use from those in the placebo group (n=34). Some case reports suggest that treatment of ADHD with stimulants or with the dopamine agonist bromocriptine can lessen substance use (Khantzian, 1983). Consequently, controversy remains regarding the use of stimulant medications among adolescents or adults with AUDs or DUDs.

A variety of non-stimulant medications have been used to treat ADHD with some success, such as tricyclic antidepressants, the antidepressant medications bupropion and venlafaxine, the antihypertensive medications clonidine and propranolol, and the noradrenergic medication atomoxitine (Weiss, 1996; King & Ellinwood, 1997; Brady et al., 1999; Michelson et al., 2001). However, to date, no controlled studies have been conducted involving ADHD in adults or adolescents with AUDs or DUDs (Levin et al., 2003).

Compared to the pharmacologic treatment literature for ADHD, there are fewer clinical studies that have assessed psychotherapeutic approaches for persons with ADHD and an AUD or DUD (Levin et al., 2003). It has been suggested that psychotherapy for ADHD should address psychoeducation surrounding ADHD, SUDs, interpersonal difficulties, low self-esteem, impulsivity, and time management (Brady et al., 1999). However, it has been noted that compared with other patients with DUDs, individuals with ADHD may have greater difficulties in processing information and may have greater problems in sitting through group meetings, which is a common format for addiction treatment (Levin et al., 2003). Medication and psychotherapy are often used concurrently in the treatment of persons with ADHD and an AUD or DUD (Levin et al., 2003).

7. Conclusions

Co-occurring disorders are the norm rather than the exception among adolescents with AUDs. The use of medications for the treatment of this population has increased dramatically in the last ten years, despite the relative paucity of empirical evidence to support or refute the safety and effectiveness of these treatments. Inadequate data are available in the adult literature to fully assess the safety and efficacy of the various treatments of AUDs in combination with various comorbid disorders, and the data available are particularly scarce in the literature concerning adolescents with these dual diagnoses. This lack of data is particularly problematic because treatments that are effective for comorbid adults are not necessarily safe and effective for comorbid adolescents. Studies are clearly warranted to clarify the safety and efficacy of various treatments for comorbid adolescents, in the areas listed below:

1. Studies are warranted to clarify the safety, optimal dose, duration, and sequence of treatment of various treatments involving comorbid populations of adolescents.
2. To date, few if any double-blind, placebo-controlled pharmacotherapy studies have been conducted for many large populations that are comorbid with AUD in adolescents. Controlled studies with these populations that are comorbid with alcoholism are clearly warranted.
3. Longer term treatment studies are warranted to assess the longer-term efficacy of various treatments.
4. Combination medication studies are warranted, such as studies involving the use of a psychotropic medication in combination with naltrexone or acamprosate.

5. Studies assessing the optimal combination of pharmacotherapy in combination with psychotherapy are warranted among the populations of alcoholics with various comorbid disorders.
6. Studies are warranted to determine the predictors and interactive effects of treatment response.

References

Apsler, R. (1994). Is drug abuse treatment effective? *American Enterprise* March/April, 46–53.

Armentano, M.E., & Solhkhah, R. (2003). Co-occurring disorders in adolescents, In Principles of Addiction Medicine, Third Ed, Section 13, Chapter 8, pp. 1573–1584, 2003.

Birmaher, B., Brent, D.A., Kolko, D., Baugher, M., Bridge, J., Holder, D., Iyengar, S., & Uloa, R.E. (2000). Clinical outcome after short-term psychotherapy for adolescents with major depressive disorder. *Archives of General Psychiatry 57*, 29–36.

Birmaher, B., Axelson, D.A., Monk, K., Kalas, C., Clark, D.B., Ehmann, M., Bridge, J., Heo, J., & Brent, D.A. (2003). Flouxetine for the treatment of childhood anxiety disorders. *Journal of the American Academy of Child and Adolescent Psychiatry 42*, 415–423.

Brady, K.T., Halligan, P., & Malcolm, R.J. (1999). Dual diagnosis. In M. Galanter & H.D. Kleber (Eds.), *Textbook of Substance Abuse Treatment*, 2nd ed., Washington, DC: The American Psychiatric Press, pp. 475–483.

Bukstein, O.G., & Cornelius, J. (in press). Psychopharmacology of adolescents with substance use disorders: using diagnostic specific treatments. In H. Liddle & C. Rowe (Eds.) *Treating Adolescent Substance Abuse: State of the Science.*

Bukstein, O.G., & Kaminer, Y. (1994). The nosology of adolescent substance abuse and dependence. *Alcohol Health and Research World 18*, 296–301.

Cannabis Youth Treatment (CYT) Group (2000). Cannabis youth treatment (CYT) experiment: preliminary findings. A report presented to the Center for Substance Abuse Treatment (CSAT). U.S. Department of Health and Human Services, Substance Abuse and Mental Health Services Administration, Rockville, MD.

Christie, K.A., Burke, J.D., Regier, D.A., Rae, D.S., Bod, J.H., & Locke, B.Z. (1988). Epidemiologic evidence for early onset of mental disorders and higher risk of drug abuse in young adults. *American Journal of Psychiatry 145*, 971–975.

Clark, D.B., Bukstein, O., & Cornelius, J. (2002). Alcohol use disorders in adolescents: epidemiology, diagnosis, psychosocial interventions, and pharmacological treatment. *Pediatric Drugs 4*, 493–502.

Clark, D.B., Bukstein, O.G., Smith, M.G., Kaczynski, N.A., Mezzich, A.C., & Donovan, J.E. (1995). Identifying anxiety disorders in adolescents hospitalized for alcohol abuse or dependence. *Psychiatric Services 46*, 618–620.

Clark, D.B., Lesnick, L., & Hegedus, A.M. (1997). Traumas and other adverse events in adolescents with alcohol abuse or dependence. *Journal of the American Academy of Child and Adolescent Psychiatry 36*, 1744–1751.

Clark, D.B., Pollock, N.K., Bukstein, O.G., Mezzich, A.C., Bromberger, J.T., & Donovan, J.E. (1997). Gender and comorbid psychopathology in adolescents with alcohol dependence. *Journal of the American Academy of Child and Adolescent Psychiatry 36*, 1195–1203.

Clark, D.B, Vanyukov, M., & Cornelius, J. (2002). Childhood antisocial behavior and adolescent alcohol use disorders. *Alcohol Research and Health 26*, 109–115.

Clark, D.B., Wood, D.S., Cornelius, J.R., Bukstein, O.G., & Martin, C.S. (2003). Clinical practices in the pharmacological treatment of comorbid psychopathology in adolescents with alcohol use disorders. *Journal of Substance Abuse Treatment*. 25:293–295.

Corby, E.A., Roll, J.M., Ledgerwood, D.M., & Schuster, C.R. (2000). Contingency management interventions for treating the substance abuse of adolescents: a feasibility study. *Experimental Clinical Psychopharmacology 8*, 371–376.

Cornelius, J.R., Bukstein, O.G., Birmaher, I.M., Salloum, I.M., Kelly, T.M., Walters, M.C., Wood, S.D., & Clark, D.B. (2003). Fluoxetine in depressed AUD adolescents: a three-year follow-up evaluation. *Alcoholism: Clinical and Experimental Research* 27(5) Suppl. 145A.

Cornelius, J.R., Bukstein, O.G., Birmaher, B., Salloum, I.M., Lynch, K., Pollock, N.K., Gershon, S., & Clark, D.B. (2001). Fluoxetine in adolescents with major depression and an alcohol use disorder: An open label trial. *Addictive Behaviors 26*, 735–739.

Cornelius, J.R., Bukstein, O.G., Salloum, I.M., Kelly, T.M, Wood, D.S., & Clark, D.B. (2004). Fluoxetine in depressed AUD adolescents: a one-year follow-up evaluation. *Journal of Child and Adolescent Psychopharmacology*. 14:35–40.

Cornelius, J.R., Maisto, S.A., Martin, C.S., Bukstein, O.G., Salloum, I.M., Daley, D.C., Wood, D.S., & Clark, D.B. (2004). Major depression associated with earlier alcohol relapse in treated teens with AUD. *Addictive Behaviors*. 29:1035–1038.

Deas, D., Riggs, P., Langenbucher, J., Goldman, M., & Brown, S. (2000). Adolescents are not adults: developmental considerations in alcohol users. *Alcoholism: Clinical and Experimental Research 24*, 232–237.

Deas, D., & Thomas, S.E. (2001). An overview of controlled studies of adolescent substance abuse treatment. *The American Journal on Addictions 10*, 178–189.

Deas-Nesmith, D., Randall, C., Roberts, J., & Anton, R. (1998). Sertraline treatment of depressed adolescent alcoholics: a pilot study. *Alcoholism: Clinical and Experimental Research 22*, 74A.

Dishion, T.J., McCord, J., & Poulin, F. (1999). When interventions harm: Peer groups and problem behavior. *American Psychologist 54*(4), 755–764.

Emslie, G.J. (2002). Second controlled study finds efficacy of fluoxetine in pediatric depression. *Brown University Child and Adolescent Psychopharmacology Update* 4(12) 1–3.

Emslie, G.J., Rush, A.J., Weinberg, W.A., Kowatch, R.A., Hughes, C.W., Carmody, T., & Rintelmann, J. (1997). A double-blind, randomized, placebo-controlled trial of fluoxetine in children and adolescents with depression. *Archives of General Psychiatry 54*, 1031–1037.

Emslie, G.J., Rush, A.J., Weinberg, W.A., Kowatch, R.A., Carmody, T., & Mayes, T.L. (1998). Fluoxetine in child and adolescent depression: acute and maintenance treatment. *Depression and Anxiety 7*, 32–39.

Eyre, S.L., Rounsaville, B.J., & Kleber, H.D. (1982). History of childhood hyperactivity in a clinic population of opiate addicts. *Journal of Nervous and Mental Disorders 170*, 522–529.

Fleming, J.E., & Offord, D.R. (1990). Epidemiology of childhood depressive disorders: a critical review. *Journal of the American Academy of Child and Adolescent Psychiatry 29*, 571–580.

Food and Drug Administration (FDA) Approvals (2003). Fluoxetine Supplemental NDA. *Medscape Pharmacists* 4(1), 2.

Food and Drug Administration (2004). Worsening depression and suicidality in patients being treated with antidepressant medications.
http://www.fda.gov/cder/drug/antidepressants/default.htm

Geller, B., Cooper, T.B., Sun, K., Zimerman, B., Frazier, J., Williams, M., & Heath, J. (1999). Double-blind and placebo-controlled study of lithium for adolescent bipolar disorders with secondary substance dependency. *Journal of the American Academy of Child and Adolescent Psychiatry 37*, 171–178.

Greenfield, S.F., Weiss, R.D., Muenz, L.R., Vagge, L.M., Kelly, J.F., Bello, L.R., & Michael, J. (1998). The effect of depression on return to drinking. *Archives of General Psychiatry 55*, 259–265.

Hazell, P., O'Connell, D., Heathcote, D., Robertson, J., & Henry, D. (1995). Efficacy of tricyclic drugs in treating child and adolescent depression: a meta-analysis. *British Medical Journal 310*, 897–901.

Henggeler, S.W., Clingempeel, W.G., Brondino, M.J., & Pickrel, S.G. (2002). Four-year follow-up of multisystemic therapy with substance-abusing and substance-dependent juvenile offenders. *Journal of the American Academy of Child and Adolescent Psychiatry 41*, 868–874.

Hesselbrock, M.N., Meyer, R.E., & Keener, J.J. (1985). Psychopathology in hospitalized alcoholics. *Archives of General Psychiatry 42*, 1050–1055.

Hird, S., Khuri, E.T., Dusenbury, L., & Millman, R.B. (1997). Adolescents. In J.H. Lowinson, P. Ruiz, R.B. Milman, & J.G. Langrod (Eds.) *Substance Abuse: A Comprehensive Textbook 3rd ed.*, Williams & Wilkins, Baltimore, pp. 683–692.

Hser, Y.I., Grella, C.E., Hubbard, R.L., Hsieh, S.C., Fletcher, B.W., Brown, B.S., & Anglin, D. (2001). An evaluation of drug treatments for adolescents in 4 US cities. *Archives of General Psychiatry 58*, 689–695.

Hubbard, R.L., Cavanaugh, E.R., Craddock, S.G., & Rachal, J.V. (1985). Characteristics, behaviors, and outcomes for youth in the TOPS. In A.S. Friedman & G. Beschner (Eds.), *Treatment Services for Adolescent Substance Abusers*, Rockville, MD: U.S. Department of Health and Human Services, pp. 49–65.

Kaminer, Y. (1994). *Understanding and Treating Adolescent Substance Abuse.* New York: Plenum Press.

Kaminer, Y. (1995). Pharmacotherapy for adolescents with psychoactive substance use disorders. In E. Rahdert & D. Czechowicz (Eds.), *National Institute of Drug Abuse Research Monograph 156, Adolescent Drug Abuse: Clinical Assessment and Therapeutic Interventions*, U.S. Department of Health and Human Services, Public Health Service, National Institutes of Health, Rockville, MD, pp. 291–324.

Kaminer, Y. (2002). Adolescent substance abuse treatment: evidence-based practice in outpatient services. *Current Psychiatry Reports 4*, 397–401.

Kaminer, Y., Burleson, J.A., Blitz, C., Sussman, J., & Rounsaville, B.J. (1998). Psychotherapies for adolescent substance abusers: a pilot study. *Journal of Nervous and Mental Disorders 186*, 684–690.

Kandel, D.B., Johnson, J.G., Bird, H.R, Canino G., Goodman, S.H., Lahey, B.B., Regier, D.A., & Schwab-Stone, M. (1997). Psychiatric disorders associated with substance use among children and adolescents: findings from the methods for the epidemiology of child and adolescent mental disorders (MECA) study. *Journal of Abnormal Child Psychology 25*,121–132.

Keller, M.B., Ryan, N.D., Strober, M., Klein, R.G., Stan, K., Birmaher, B., Hagino, O., Koplewicz, H., Carlson, G., Clarke, G., Emslie, G., Feinberg, D., Geller, B., Kusumakar, V., Papatheodoro, G., Wagner, K.D., Weller, E.B., Winters, N.C., Oakes, R., & McCafferty, J.P. (2001). Efficacy of paroxetine in the treatment of adolescent major depression: a randomized, controlled trial. *Journal of the American Academy of Child and Adolescent Psychiatry 40*, 762–772.

Kessler, R.C., Crum, R.M., Warner, L.A., Nelson, C.B., Schulenberg, J., & Anthony, J.C. (1997). Lifetime co-occurrence of DSM-III-R alcohol abuse and dependence with other psychiatric disorders in the National Comorbidity Survey. *Archives of General Psychiatry 54*, 313–321.

Kessler, R.C., McGonagle, K.A., Zhao, S., Nelson, C.B., Hughes, M., Eshleman, S., Wittchen, H.U., & Kendler, K.S. (1994). Lifetime and 12-month prevalence of DSM-III-R psychiatric disorders in the United States. Results from the National Comorbidity Survey. *Archives of General Psychiatry 51*, 8–19.

Kessler, R.C., & Walters, E.E. (1998). Epidemiology of DSM-III-R major depression and minor depression among adolescents and young adults in the national comorbidity survey. *Depression and Anxiety 7*, 3–14.

Khantzian, E.J. (1983). An extreme case of cocaine dependence and marked improvement with methylphenidate treatment. *American Journal of Psychiatry 140*, 784–785.

King, G.R., & Ellinwood, E.H. (1997). Amphetamines and other stimulants. In J.H. Lowinson, P. Ruiz, R.B. Milman, & J.G. Langrod (Eds.) *Substance Abuse: A Comprehensive Textbook 3rd ed.* Baltimore: Williams & Wilkins, pp. 207–223.

Klein, R.G., & Mannuzza, S. (1991). Long-term outcome of hyperactive children: a review. *Journal of the American Academy of Child and Adolescent Psychiatry 30*, 383–387.

Kroenke, K, West, S.L., Swindle, R., Gilsenan, A., Eckert, G.J., Dolor, R., Stang, P., Zhou, X., Hays, R., & Weinberger, M. (2001). Similar effectiveness of paroxetine, fluoxetine, and sertraline in primary care: a randomized trial. *Journal of the American Medical Association 286*, 2947–2955.

Kuperman, S., Schlosser, S.S., Kramer, J.R., Bucholz, K., Hesselbrock, V., Reich, T., & Reich, W. (2001). Developmental sequence from disruptive behavior diagnosis to adolescent alcohol dependence. *American Journal of Psychiatry 158,* 2022–2026.

Levin, F.R., Sullivan, M.A., Donovan, S.J. (2003). Co-occurring addictive and attention deficit/hyperactivity disorder and eating disorder. In A.W. Graham, T.K. Schultz, M.F. Mayo-Smith, R.K. Ries, & B.B. Wilford (Eds.), *Principles of Addiction Medicine, Third Edition,* American Society of Addiction Medicine, Inc., Chevy Chase, MD, pp. 1321–1346.

Lewis, D.O (1996). Conduct disorder. In M. Lewis (Ed.), *Child and Adolescent Psychiatry: A Comprehensive Textbook, Second Edition,* Williams & Wilkins, Baltimore, MD, pp. 564–574.

Litten, R.Z., & Allen, J.P. (1995). Pharmacotherapy for alcoholics with collateral depression or anxiety: An update of research findings. *Experimental and Clinical Psychopharmacology 3,* 87–93.

Liddle, H.A., Dakof, G.A., Parker, K., Diamond, G.S., Barrett, K., & Jejeda, M. (2001). Multidimensional family therapy for adolescent drug abuse: results of a randomized clinical trial. *American Journal of Drug and Alcohol Abuse 27,* 651–687.

Mannuzza, S., & Klein, R.G. (2000). Long-term prognosis in attention-deficit/hyperactivity disorder. *Child and Adolescent Psychiatric Clinics of North America 9*(3), 711–726.

Michelson, D., Faries, D., Wernicke, J., Kelsey, D., Kendrick, K., Sallee, F.R., Spencer, T., & The Atomoxetine ADHD Study Group (2001). Atomoxetine in the treatment of children and adolescents with ADHD: a randomized, placebo-controlled, dose-response study. *Pediatrics 108,* e83.

Miller, W.R., Zweben, A., DiClemente, C.C., & Rychtarik, R.G. (1992). *Motivational Enhancement Therapy Manual: A Clinical Research Guide for Therapists Treating Individuals with Alcohol Abuse and Dependence.* NIAAA Project MATCH Monograph Series, Volume 2, Editor: Margaret E. Mattson, Ph.D., U.S. Department of Health and Human Services, Public Health Service, NIH.

National Opinion Research Center (1997). *National Treatment Improvement Evaluation Study, Final Report.* Rockville, MD: Center for Substance Abuse and Treatment, US Department of Health and Human Services.

Pendergast, M. ., Podus, D., Chang, E., & Urada, D. (2002). The effectiveness of drug abuse treatment: A meta-analysis of comparison group studies. *Drug and Alcohol Dependence 67,* 53–72.

Poulin, F., Dishion, T.J, & Burraston, B. (2001). 3-year iatrogenic effects associated with aggregating high-risk adolescents in cognitive-behavioral preventive interventions. *Applied Development Science 5*(4), 214–224.

Regier, D.A., Farmer, M.E., Rae, D.E., Locke, B.Z., Keith, E.J., Judd, L.L., & Goodwin, F.K. (1990). Comorbidity of mental disorders with alcohol and other drug abuse: Results from the Epidemiologic Catchment Area (ECA) study. *Journal of the American Medical Association 264,* 2511–2518.

Riggs, P.D., Mikulich, S.K., Coffman, L.M., & Crowley, T.J. (1997). Fluoxetine in drug-dependent delinquents with major depression: An open trial. *Journal of Child and Adolescent Psychopharmacology 7,* 87–95.

Riggs, P.D., Mikulich, S.K., & Hall, S.K. (2001). Effects of pemoline on ADHD, antisocial behaviors, and substance use in adolescents with conduct disorder and substance use disorder. *Drug and Alcohol Dependence 63,* S131.

Rohde, P., Lewinsohn, P.M., & Seeley, J.R. (1991). Comorbidity of unipolar depression: II. Comorbidity with other mental disorders in adolescents and adults. *Journal of Abnormal Psychology 100,* 214–221.

Rosack, J. (2003). FDA warns of suicide risk with paroxetine. *Psychiatric News 38,* 1,37.

Sells, S.B., & Simpson, D.D. (1979). Evaluation of treatment outcome for youths in the Drug-Abuse Reporting Program (DARP): a follow-up study. In G.M. Beschner & A.S. Friedman (eds.) *Youth Drug Abuse: Problems, Issues, and Treatment.* Lexington Books, Lexington, MA, pp. 571–628.

Szatmari, P. (1992). The epidemiology of attention deficit hyperactivity disorder. In G. Weiss (ed.) *Child and Adolescent Psychiatric Clinics of North America.* Philadelphia, PA: W.B. Saunders, pp. 361–384.

Szatmari, P., Offord, D.R., & Boyle, M.N. (1989). Ontario child health study: Prevalence of attention deficit disorder with hyperactivity. *Journal of Child Psychology and Psychiatry 30*, 205–218.

Varley, C.K., (2001). Sudden death related to selected tricyclic antidepressants in children: epidemiology, mechanisms, and clinical implications. *Paediatric Drugs 3*, 613–627.

Wagner, E.F., Brown, S.A., Monti, P.M., Myers, M.G., & Waldron, H.B. (1999). Innovations in adolescent substance abuse intervention. *Alcoholism: Clinical and Experimental Research 23*, 236–249.

Wagner, K.D., Ambrosini, P., Rynn, M., Wohlberg, C., Yang, R., Greenbaum, M.S., Childress, A., Donnelly, C., & Deas, D. (2003). Efficacy of sertraline in the treatment of children and adolescents with major depressive disorder. *Journal of the American Medical Association 290*, 1033–1041.

Waldron, H.B., Slesnick, N., Turner, C.W., Brody, J.L., & Peterson, T.R. (2001). Treatment outcomes for adolescent substance abuse at 4- and 7-month assessments. *Journal of Consulting and Clinical Psychology 69*, 802–813.

Weiss, G. (1996). Attention deficit hyperactivity disorder. In M. Lewis (ed.) *Child and Adolescent Psychiatry: A Comprehensive Textbook, 2nd Ed.* Baltimore: Williams & Wilkins, pp. 544–563.

Winters, K.C., Stinchfield, R.D., & Opland, E. (2000). The effectiveness of the Minnesota Model approach in the treatment of adolescent drug abusers. *Addiction 95*, 601–612.

Wood, D., Wender, P.H., & Reimherr, F.W. (1983). The prevalence of attention deficit disorder, residual type, or minimal drain dysfunction, in a population of male alcoholic patients. *American Journal of Psychiatry140*, 95–98.

Zito, J.M., Safer, D.J., DosReis, S., Gardner, J.F., Soeken, K., Boles, M., & Lynch, F. (2002). Rising prevalence of antidepressants among US youth. *Pediatrics 109*, 721–727.

Zito, J.M., Safer, D.J., DosReis, S., Gardner, J.F., Magder, L., Soeken, K., Boles, M., Lynch, F., & Little, M.A. (2003). Psychotropic practice patterns for youth: a 10-year perspective. *Archives of Pediatric and Adolescent Medicine 157*, 17–25.

17

A Brief History and Some Current Dimensions of Adolescent Treatment in the United States

Mark D. Godley and William L. White

1. Introduction

The development of a national system for treating adolescent substance use disorders actually began more than a century ago. In this chapter, we will provide a brief history of adolescent substance use and its clinical management, an overview of the state of adolescent treatment system development in the United States, describe the characteristics of substance-involved adolescents entering specialty treatment and the levels of care within which they are treated, and discuss how recent research findings are beginning to influence clinical responses to alcohol and other drug problems among adolescents.

A Brief History of Adolescent Treatment. Growing concerns about "drunkard children" in the late eighteenth and early nineteenth centuries fueled minimum drinking age and temperance education laws, the inclusion of young people in cadet branches of recovery-oriented societies such as the Washingtonians and the Ribbon Reform Clubs, and the admission of adolescents into the nation's first inebriate homes and asylums (Mosher, 1980; White, 1998). Opiate addiction among disaffiliated urban youth garnered early twentieth century attention via reports of rising juvenile arrests and the rejection in thousands of World War I draftees due to heroin addiction (Musto, 1973; Terry & Pellens, 1921). Efforts to treat juvenile addiction included hospital detoxification and enrolling addicted adolescents in the morphine maintenance clinics that operated across the nation between 1919–1924 . During this time approximately

Mark D. Godley and William L. White • Director, Research and Development, Chestnut Health Systems, Bloomington, Illinois 61701.

7,500 narcotic addicts were registered at the Worth Street Clinic in New York City and 743 of these were under the age of 19 (Hubbard, 1920).

Juvenile narcotic addiction declined in the 1930s and 1940s but rose again in the early 1950s. Admissions of persons under age 21 at the two U.S. Public Health Hospitals (narcotics farms) in Lexington, Kentucky and Forth Worth, Texas increased from 22 in 1947 to 440 in 1950. In the 1950s, alarm over juvenile narcotic use triggered the opening of addiction wards in some urban community hospitals (e.g., Chicago's Bridewell Hospital, Detroit Receiving Hospital, and New York City's Manhattan General) and sparked faith-based addiction counseling ministries (e.g., St. Mark's Clinic in Chicago, the Addicts Rehabilitation Center and Exodus House in New York City, and Teen Challenge (Conferences, 1953; White, 1998). Adolescents and adults were treated in these programs together as only one specialized adolescent treatment facility existed in the 1950s.

The opening of Riverside Hospital in New York City in 1952 marked the birth of specialized treatment for adolescent substance use disorders. Riverside's 140-bed facility offered a multidisciplinary staff to provide detoxification; psychiatric and medical evaluation; psychological testing; and an inpatient program of therapeutic, educational, vocational and recreational activities followed by outpatient visits at community clinics. In spite of its "state-of-the-art" status, Riverside was closed in 1961 after a follow-up study of former patients documented a 97 percent relapse rate (Gamso & Mason, 1958). Other mid-century events that influenced the future evolution of adolescent treatment included the development of "young peoples' meetings" within Alcoholics Anonymous and Narcotics Anonymous, the development of modified therapeutic communities for adolescents (Jainchill, 1997), and the appearance of adolescent chemical dependency programs based on the "Minnesota Model" (Winters et al., 2000).

Alarm about polydrug experimentation by adolescents in the 1960s undergirded federal and state support for the expansion of treatment services in the 1970s, but support for specialized adolescent treatment services waned as youthful drug experimentation declined in the 1980s (National Institute of Drug Addiction [NIDA], 1999). Between the 1960s and mid-80s, the treatment of adolescent substance use disorders continued to be provided primarily in adult substance use units using adult models of treatment. A 1985 federal report on adolescent treatment services lamented the lack of treatment programs in the U.S. designed specifically for adolescents (Friedman & Beschner, 1985).

This situation changed as adolescent experimentation with marijuana, LSD, methamphetamine, "club drugs" (MDMA/"ecstasy," GHB, rohypnol), and dissociative anesthetics (PCP, ketamine) rose in the 1990s. Between 1991 and 1999, past year illicit drug use rose from 29% to 42% among high school seniors and from 11% to 21% among eighth grade students. National high school survey data also revealed high rates of binge drinking (consuming five or more drinks in one drinking episode): 15% of 8th graders, 26 percent of 10th graders, and 31% of 12th graders (NIDA, 1999). At the height of this surge in drug use (1992–1998), the number of youth admitted to substance treatment in the U.S. increased 53% (from 96,787 to 147,899), fueled by marijuana-related juvenile arrests and treatment referrals from the criminal justice system (Office of Applied Studies [OAS], 2003).

The resurgence in youthful polydrug experimentation led to a greater emphasis on systems of prevention (Drug Free Schools and Community Act-1986), early intervention (the proliferation of student assistance programs via the National Association of Student Assistance Professionals-1994), an expansion of public and private programs that specialized in the treatment of adolescent substance use disorders, and an increase in the number of controlled studies evaluating the efficacy and effectiveness of adolescent treatment. This surge in treatment and research activity was guided by the collective efforts of the National Institute on Alcohol Abuse and Alcoholism, the National Institute on Drug Abuse, and the Center for Substance Abuse Treatment. In the opening decade of the twenty-first century, the treatment of adolescent substance use disorders is transitioning from folk art status to a subspecialty of the larger addiction treatment effort. Increasingly it is noted that adolescent treatment is becoming a professionalized, and science-guided endeavor (White, Dennis & Tims, 2002).

2. The Adolescent Treatment System

Adolescents experiencing substance-related problems in the United State can be found in multiple health and social service systems. They are served by a host of child welfare and juvenile justice youth service agencies, publicly funded addiction treatment agencies, private addiction treatment agencies that cater to insured and private pay insured families, and by more than one third of the juvenile correctional facilities (37%) that provide on-site substance abuse treatment (Office of Applied Studies [OAS], 2002).

More than 145,000 adolescents each year are treated in publicly funded addiction treatment programs in the United States (Office of Applied Studies [OAS], 2000). The number of adolescent specialty programs and overall adolescent admissions rose rapidly through the late 1980s and 1990s. A comparison of Substance Abuse and Mental Health Services Administration's (SAMHSA) national treatment center directories reveals that the number of self-identified adolescent specialty programs increased from 2,874 to 4,291 (a 49% increase) between 1987 and 2003. The growth of adolescent treatment was not the same across different regions of the country. While the number of adolescent specialty units actually decreased in seven states between 1987 and 2003, figure 1 shows that growth occurred across each region of the U.S., ranging from an 84% increase in the Pacific Region to only 2% in the New England.

The 2002 National Survey of Substance Abuse Treatment Services (N-SSATS; SAMHSA, 2003) provides a window into the current status of adolescent treatment in the United States. The survey identified 18,204 institutions

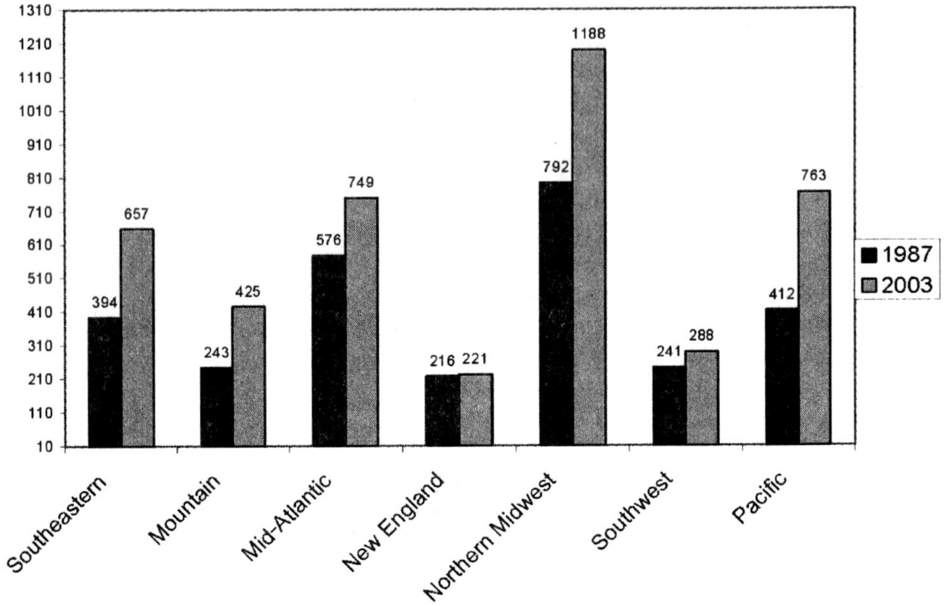

Southeastern Region; Alabama, Florida, Georgia, Kentucky, Mississippi, North Carolina, South Carolina, Tennessee, Virginia, West Virginia: **Mountain Region**; Arizona, Colorado, Idaho, New Mexico, Montana, Nevada, Utah, Wyoming: **Mid-Atlantic Region**; Delaware, District of Columbia, Maryland, New Jersey, New York, Pennsylvania: **New England Region**; Connecticut, Maine, Massachusetts, New Hampshire, Rhode Island, Vermont: **Northern Midwest**; Illinois, Indiana, Iowa, Kansas, Michigan, Minnesota, Nebraska, North Dakota, Ohio, South Dakota, Wisconsin: **Southwest Region**; Arkansas, Louisiana, Okalahoma, Texas: **Pacific Region**; Alaska, California, Hawaii, Oregon, Washington:

Figure 1. Increase in Adolescent Treatment Programs from 1987–2003.

that provide substance abuse treatment services and 13,720 participated in the survey. Services to adolescents were provided by 37 % of the surveyed facilities. Adolescent substance abuse treatment services were provided by private non-profit facilities (37% survey response rate), private for profit facilities (36% responded); local government facilities (42% responded), 167 of 441 state-operated facilities (38% responded), federal facilities (8% responded), and tribal owned facilities (64% responded). Substance abuse treatment services for adolescents were more likely to be provided in facilities that offered both substance abuse treatment and mental health services (50%) than in substance abuse treatment only (33%), mental health services only (34%), or general health care facilities (22%).

Most of what we know about adolescent treatment in the United States is based on surveys and studies of the publicly funded programs. Surveys of private sector treatment programs documented a dramatic growth in private for-profit addiction treatment during the 1980s but did not segregate data for adolescent specialty units (Yahr, 1988). While many private treatment programs closed in the early 1990s in the face of an aggressive system of managed behavioral health care, the private sector continues to provide a significant source of specialized adolescent treatment. The most recent data on private programs is contained in the National Treatment Center Study (NTCS) conducted by the University of Georgia and the Georgia Institute of Technology (Roman, Blum, Johnson, & Neal, 2002).

The NTCS surveyed 400-private programs specializing in addiction treatment during three waves of data collection between 1997–98 and 2000–01. The survey findings revealed considerable institutional turnover in the private sector with approximately one fourth of the 1996 programs surveyed closed by the 2001 survey. (Roman et al., 2002). The number of private programs providing adolescent treatment only remained at four programs between the 1996 and 2001 surveys; however 38% of the programs offered a separate treatment track for adolescents by the 2000–01 survey. For the preparation of this chapter Johnson (2003) has contributed several adolescent program findings from the NTCS survey results. While the small number of programs specializing in adolescent treatment should be interpreted with caution, the NTCS survey provides a better understanding of current private treatment and allows us to compare some dimensions of private programs to publicly funded programs.

Private Sector Adolescent Treatment. Adolescents constitute more than half of admissions in only four percent of the 450 private programs surveyed; only one percent of private addiction treatment facilities specialize exclusively in adolescent treatment. There has been considerable growth in the number of private programs treating adolescents (38% of total) but the number of designated adolescent beds to total facility beds is actually declining (Johnson, 2003). Similarly, 40% of publicly funded treatment programs admit adolescents, with two thirds of these offering a specialized treatment track for adolescents (OAS, 2003).

The number of beds devoted to adolescent treatment within private centers averages 17 and ranges from 2 to 88. Utilization rates (daily census divided by number of beds) for specialized adolescent units ranges between 33% and 36% within the surveys. The average length of stay within private inpatient adolescent specialty units increased from 17.6 days in 1995 to 21.1 days in 2000. Daily rates for inpatient treatment ranged from $357-$1045 per day (Roman and Blum, 1997; Roman et al., 2002). Payor sources in the specialty adolescent programs (when compared to private adult addiction treatment units) have a higher percentage of Medicaid reimbursement and charity write-offs and a lower percentage of self-pay (Medicaid 45%; Private Indemnity Insurance 2%; HMOs 10.2%; POSs-7.5%; Self-Pay 17.5%; and Charity 17.5%) (Johnson, 2003).

Referral Source. The primary referral sources of adolescents into private specialty treatment are the legal system (36%), schools (34%), and social service agencies (29%). In contrast, the primary referral sources for adolescents into publicly funded treatment are the: legal system (41%), school/community agencies (22%), and self/family (17%), other substance abuse providers (6%) (OAS, 2000).

Characteristics of Clients Entering Treatment. While national data is lacking on demographic characteristics of adolescents entering private treatment, those entering public treatment are primarily male (70%), racially diverse (63% Caucasian/non-Hispanic, 15% African American, 11% Hispanic, and 5% other races), and range in age from early to late adolescence (25% age 14 or younger; 75% ages 15–17) (Dennis, Dawud-Noursi, et al, 2002).

Presenting Problems. Adolescents are entering private addiction treatment due to dependence upon cannabis (66%), alcohol (34%), cocaine (15%) and opiates (6.5%) (exceeds 100% because of multiple drug choices). These findings compare to the following drug choices for adolescents entering publicly funded treatment: cannabis (54%), alcohol (24%), cocaine (2%), opiates (1%), and stimulants (3%) (Johnson, 2003; OAS, 2000). Dennis and his colleagues (2003) summarized changes in drug of choice characteristics between 1992 and 1998 adolescent treatment admissions. Especially noteworthy is the reversal between alcohol as the dominant drug in 1992 (56% of admissions) decreasing to 24% of admissions in 1998 while marijuana increased as the drug of choice for admissions during this period, from 23% to 54% . Just over half (54.5%) of adolescents admitted to private treatment programs have a co-occurring psychiatric disorder. Studies of youth admitted to public sector treatment programs (e.g, Dennis, Godley, & Titus, 1999) have found higher rates of co-morbid problems, e.g., other substance use disorders, internal emotional disorders (major depression, generalized anxiety, suicidal thoughts or actions, traumatic stress disorders), and external behavioral disorders (conduct disorder, attention deficit-hyperactivity disorder), and high rates of victimization. In terms of prior treatment for substance use disorders, 71% of adolescents admitted to private programs compared to 29% of adolescents admitted to public treatment have one or more prior episodes of treatment (Johnson, 2003; OAS, 2000).

Levels of Care. Addiction specialists recommend that placement in a level of care (e.g., outpatient, intensive outpatient, residential) should be based on a number of presenting characteristics including the adolescent's substance use diagnosis/severity, intoxication and withdrawal risk, biomedical issues, psychological problems, treatment acceptance and resistance, relapse potential, environmental risk, legal pressure, and school or vocational pressure (American Society of Addiction Medicine [ASAM], 1996). Adolescents presenting with complex problems across multiple ASAM dimensions are more likely to be placed in residential treatment while those with fewer/less severe problems are placed in a lower level of care such as outpatient treatment. Levels of care provided were not broken out for the adolescent programs within the NTCS surveys but public surveys reveal the following adolescent admission pattern to adolescent treatment: outpatient (69%), intensive outpatient (11%), long-term residential (9%), short-term residential (6%), and detoxification (6%), (Dennis, Dawud-Noursi, et al, 2003). Changing reimbursement policies that required greater justification for costlier treatment and the introduction of the ASAM Patient Placement Criteria (1996) encouraged adolescent treatment providers in both the private and public sector to move from providing a single level of care (e.g., residential only) to providing multiple levels of care.

ASAM placement recommendations support the practice of continuing or "step down" care in the treatment of substance use disorders (both adult and adolescent). Under this plan, a client successfully discharged from residential treatment would be referred to a "lower" level of care such as Intensive Outpatient or Outpatient treatment and so on.

Treatment Approach. Descriptions of private programs for adolescent treatment center around a 12-step foundation that involves confrontational group therapy, family and individual psychotherapy, and pharmacological adjuncts (Johnson, 2003). Funded by SAMHSA's Center for Substance Abuse Treatment, Stevens and Morral (2003) provide a description of current best practice approaches for ten outpatient, intensive outpatient, and residential treatment programs. Unlike private programs the Minnesota Model/12 step programs are likely to be viewed as one of several approaches used with adolescents in treatment rather than the foundation of the treatment experience. Social learning theory, self-efficacy, social skills training within group and individual treatment is evident. Cultural appropriateness is frequently mentioned in the training and therapeutic approaches in the publicly funded programs, however pharmacotherapy, while evident, appears to be used less than in the private programs. The lower use of pharmacotherapy in public programs may be due to less affiliation with medical resources than private programs. Whatever the reasons for this trend, it is disturbing given the higher rates of co-occurring disorders noted in the publicly funded programs. Continuing care services exist in public and private programs to the extent that they follow an ASAM placement model and make "step down" referrals to less intensive levels of care when clients are successfully discharged. The extent to which such transfers are successful is not fully known but one study indicates a need for greater attention to this (Godley et al., 2002). Except to the extent that clients participate in mutual aid support groups, long-term disease management strategies (e.g., recovery monitoring and support) do not appear to be available in either private or public treatment models.

Treatment Staff. Staff working in private specialty adolescent units (compared to staff working in private adult units) are less likely to be in recovery, less likely to be a certified counselor, but more likely to have a Master's degree and more likely to turnover (29% versus 19% annual turnover). There are no comparable national studies of publicly funded facilities regarding treatment staff. Although little national information is available on treatment staff qualifications and stability in publicly funded programs, McLellan (2003) recently reported annual counselor turnover in these programs as high as 50%. High rates of staff turnover in publicly funded programs due to low salaries and difficult working conditions have also been noted in state evaluation reports (Carlson, Deck, & Wadeson, 2001; Northrup & Heflinger, 2000).

Summary. Several conclusions can be drawn comparing public and private treatment using the N-SSSATS, TEDS and NTCS data. The overwhelming majority of adolescents treated for substance use disorders in the United States are treated within the network of publicly funded programs, but the differences between public and private treatment (e.g., characteristics of clients, staff qualifications and staffing patterns, treatment duration and outcomes) remain relatively unexplored. It does appear, from available data, that adolescents entering publicly funded treatment are less likely to have had prior treatment episodes, but are more likely to be referred from the criminal justice system or by self/family referral, and more likely to present with a co-occurring disorder.

3. From Science to Service

The past 30 years of adolescent treatment evaluation spans early studies that included adolescents (the Drug Abuse Reporting Program (DARP) in the early 1970s, the Treatment Outcome Perspective Study (TOPS) in the late 1970s and early 1980s, the Service Research Outcome Study (SROS) and National Treatment Improvement Evaluation Study (NTIES) that extended into the 1990s. All of these studies evaluated adolescents as a small subset of the larger treatment population. Over the past 15 years increased attention to adolescent treatment evaluation and research has resulted in a host of adolescent-specific, longitudinal outcome studies and randomized clinical trials (Hser, Grella, Hubbard et al., 2001; Brown et al., 2001; Williams & Chang, 2000; Deas & Thomas, 2001; Muck et al., 2001). While not perfect, the recent generation of studies are methodologically more rigorous than their predecessors. The cumulative effect of these studies has been a growing body of scientific knowledge that is slowly influencing funding policy and practice. Considerable efforts are underway by various federal agencies, scientific committees, and professional associations to forge an evidence-based system of adolescent treatment. Led by the National Institute on Alcoholism and Alcohol Abuse, the National Institute on Drug Abuse, the Robert Wood Johnson Foundation, and the Center for Substance Abuse Treatment each of these national organizations have funded major initiatives designed to improve clinical practice.

With increasing frequency treatment provider associations (e.g., The National Association of Addiction Treatment Providers), trade publications (e.g., *The Counselor*) and provider agencies across the country are exploring the practical implications of available scientific studies. Some of the most significant of these findings (for reviews, see Deas and Thomas, 2001; Muck, et al., 2001; Williams & Chang, 2000; Winters, 1999) and their implications for clinical practice include the following:

Early Age of Onset. A significant factor affecting adolescent substance use disorders and their treatment is the lowered age of onset of alcohol and other drug use (White, 1999). Several recent studies have documented progressive declines in the age of substance use initiation during the second half of the twentieth century (Presley, Meilman, & Lyerla, 1991; Dennis, Babor, Roebuck, & Donaldson, 2002; National Institute on Drug Abuse, 1999; Substance Abuse and Mental Health Services Administration, 1999). A tri-generational study of those born before 1930, between 1930 and 1949, and after 1949 found a progressive decline in the age of onset of regular alcohol consumption and a parallel increase in the probability of developing an alcohol-related problem before age 25 (Stoltenberg, Hill, Mudd, Blow, & Zucker, 1999). Lowered age of onset of drug use is particularly prominent among juveniles entering the criminal justice system and addiction treatment programs (U.S. Department of Justice, 1994). In a national study of the treatment of adolescent substance use disorders, 80% of the 600 youth admitted to the study began regular substance use between the ages of 12 and 14 (Dennis, Titus, et al., 2002).

Concern about lowered age of onset of substance use springs from studies suggesting that precocious drug experimentation is related to: juvenile offending and school failure (Fergusson, Lynskey and Horwood, 1996), risk of adult alcohol dependence (Chou and Pickering, 1992; Grant & Dawson, 1997; Dennis, et al., 2000), faster progression of substance-related problems (Kreichbaun & Zering, 2000), greater problem severity (Chen & Millar, 1998; National Institute on Alcohol Abuse and Alcoholism, 2003), increased health risk behaviors (DuRant, Smith, Kreiter, and Krowchuk, 1999), greater medical and psychiatric comorbidity (Fergusson, Lynskey and Horwood, 1996; Warren, et al, 1997; Sobell, Sobell, Cunningham, & Agrawal, 1998), and increased risk of future alcohol-related accidents and violence (Hingson, Heeren, Jananka, & Howland, 2000; Hingson, Heeren, & Zakocs, 2001). There is also evidence suggesting that early age of onset may be linked to poorer treatment outcomes (Keller, Lavori, Beardslee, Wunder, & Hasin, 1992; Kessler, et al., 2001; Chen & Millar, 1998).

In summary, the evidence suggests that decreased age of onset leads to increased risk of a subsequent substance use disorder, increases in the developmental speed and severity of substance-related problems and compromises treatment outcomes. The practical implications of this research auger for the need to intensify prevention programs as well as youth-oriented outreach and early intervention programs. Realization of the risks associated with precocious substance use has contributed to the development of a growing national network of school-based student assistance programs and the development of more effective youth screening instruments and brief interventions. In 2003 the Center for Substance Abuse Treatment (CSAT) funded 22 adolescent grants to implement standardized screening, assessment and brief treatment for low problem severity youth to test the effectiveness of an early intervention model.

Course and Outcome. There is growing evidence that adolescent substance use disorders can appear as transient or chronic problems. Where the former are amenable to resolution through maturation or relatively brief intervention (Temple and Fillmore, 1985–86), the latter constitute problems characterized by escalating severity and prolonged duration. In the recently completed Cannabis Youth Treatment (CYT) study of outpatient interventions, 41% of adolescent participants diagnosed with cannabis abuse or dependence reported they had failed prior attempts to stop drug use, 25% had prior episodes of formal treatment, and 33% were re-admitted to treatment during the year following their treatment in the CYT study (Dennis, et al, 2000). Those suffering more chronic substance use disorders can be distinguished by greater personal vulnerability (e.g., lower age of onset, family history of addiction), greater medical and psychiatric co-morbidity, and less personal, family and social assets to support recovery and resolve problems (Babor et al., 2002). This suggests the need to differentiate these two populations and to develop intervention modalities more appropriate for this high problem severity/duration group. Interventions for the latter will likely address a broad spectrum of problems and involve interventions of greater intensity and duration.

Other problems of youth and families interact (as causes and consequences) of adolescent substance use disorders to compromise clinical outcomes. Unfortunately, co-morbidity is the norm among adolescent admissions to treatment (Hoffmann, Mee-Lee, and Arrowood, 1993; Hser, et al., 2001). Of the 600 adolescents admitted to the CYT study, 95% reported one or more (83% had three or more) other problems, e.g., alcohol use disorders, other substance use disorders, internal emotional disorders (major depression, generalized anxiety, suicidal thoughts or actions, traumatic stress disorders), external behavioral disorders (conduct disorder, attention deficit-hyperactivity disorder), victimization, and violence (Dennis, et al, 2000). These findings reinforce the need for multidimensional screening and assessment procedures, and the need for multi-disciplinary, if not multi-agency intervention models that can provide an integrated response to adolescent clients who present with multiple, co-occurring problems.

Engagement. The earlier noted roles of courts, schools and parents in the referral of adolescents to treatment suggest that most adolescents enter treatment under coercive influences. Voluntarily engaging adolescents and eliciting positive involvement of those coerced to treatment is a considerable challenge. Findings from the DATOS-A studies suggest that such engagement and involvement is enhanced by building rapport between the adolescent and the service team, enhancing the adolescent's confidence in his or her ability to change and encouraging and strengthening the adolescent's commitment to change (http://www.datos.org). Outreach services (e.g., home visits) and case management services have also been found to exert a positive influence on treatment engagement and retention (Szapocznik et al., 1988; Henggeler, Borduin, Melton et al., 1991; Godley et al., 1994; Garner, Godley & Funk, 2002).

Variability of Treatment Effectiveness. All treatment programs are not the same. Friedman and Glickman (1986) conducted one of the first studies that attempted to link clinical outcomes to characteristics of particular treatment programs. They found that programs with the best clinical outcomes: a) treat a larger number of adolescents, b) have a larger budget, c) use evidence-based therapies, d) offer specialized educational, vocational, and psychiatric services, e) employ counselors with two or more years experience working with adolescents, f) offer a larger menu of youth-specific services (e.g., art therapy, recreational, and other prosocial activities and services), and g) are perceived by clients as empathic allies in the recovery process (Friedman and Glickman, 1986).

Lack of Theoretical Superiority. No theoretical model or clinical protocol of adolescent treatment has proven itself superior to others in the treatment of all adolescent substance use disorders. While some reviews attributed slight superiority to family therapies (Williams & Chang, 2001) more recent randomized trials have not shown a clearly superior treatment approach for substance-involved adolescents (Dennis, et al, in press). In the absence of superior outcomes for a particular model, communities may be encouraged to develop a menu of early intervention, treatment, and post-treatment recovery support services that meet other criteria, e.g., cultural viability, cost-effectiveness.

Post-treatment Functioning. Following treatment, most adolescents are precariously balanced between recovery and reactivation of substance use and related problems. The percentage of treated adolescents in stable recovery erodes in the years following treatment while others who relapsed and continued to use relatively early after treatment move into stable recovery in the years following treatment (Brown, A'Amico, McCarthy, and Tapert, 2001). Also noteworthy is the relatively low percentage of treated adolescents who participate in professionally directed aftercare groups or mutual aid groups such as Alcoholics Anonymous (AA) or Narcotics Anonymous (NA) relative to adults (Godley, Godley, & Dennis, 2001; Donovan, 1998). Recovery mutual aid groups can help support long-term recovery following primary treatment (Hoffman and Miller, 1992; Hoffman, et al, 1993), but they suffer from low post-treatment affiliation and high attrition rates. These findings suggest the need for more formalized programs of continuing care, the creation of more indigenous, youth-specific recovery support groups, and more active linkage to such resources during the treatment process.

Post-treatment Support. Post-treatment monitoring and recovery support services can enhance the stability and durability of recovery, however, there is little evidence from controlled studies to support this clinical and correlational observation (Donovan, 1998). In practice, step-down continuing care is recommended by ASAM and is considered to be standard practice. Retrospective studies of statewide datasets (Godley et al., 2003) as well as prospective follow-up studies of post residential functioning and services (Godley, Godley, & Dennis, 2001) suggests that the actual rate of linkage to a continuing care service within 90 days of discharge from residential treatment is less than 40 percent. These findings suggest the need for improved approaches to step-down care linkage. Assertive continuing care approaches that shift the responsibility for continued contact from the client to the treatment professional and involve extended telephone follow-up and/or home visits for monitoring, recovery education, support, and early re-intervention are currently being tested. In a randomized study of adolescent post-residential continuing care services, 94% of an assertive continuing care (ACC) group received monitoring and other continuing care services compared to 54% of the "usual continuing care"(UCC) group. During a 90 day continuing care test phase the median number of face-to-face contacts for the ACC group was 10 compared to 2 for the UCC group. At the end of the active continuing care phase, 52% of ACC group members were still abstinent from marijuana compared to 32% in the UCC group (Godley, Godley, Dennis, Funk & Passetti, 2002). Organizing post-treatment recovery support services within the adolescent's natural environment (e.g., recovery home rooms, in-school recovery meetings, recovery schools) also offers promise for preventing relapse and boosting post-treatment recovery. More research is needed to evaluate proactive continuing care and recovery management to strategies to determine if this approach results in long-term improved clinical outcomes and a better stewardship of community resources

Post-treatment Environment. Peer group, social networks, and family environment have high salience to most adolescents. It is, therefore, not surprising that treatment outcome is heavily influenced by the adolescent's post-treatment family and social environment. Adolescents who experience major relapse experience higher rates of parental substance use and family conflict and a higher density of drug users in their post-treatment social milieu (Hoffman, et al, 1993; Brown et al., 2001; Godley et al., in press). This suggests the need for models of intervention that can alter these family and peer environments. Few treated adolescents completely change their social networks. Future research is needed to find ways to lessen the risk in the adolescent's recovery environment. Additionally, creative methods of working with the adolescent's peer network are also needed. For example, is it possible to recruit close using peers into treatment as well as the primary client? Could one or more close peers be enlisted to attend recovery support meetings to assist the primary client? Finding new ways to work with the adolescent's social and peer networks is an outstanding need to further support and maintain treatment gains experienced during treatment.

4. Summary

Resources for the treatment of adolescent substance use disorders have increased over the past century in tandem with the increased visibility and cultural alarm regarding adolescent substance-related problems. The United States now has a multi-branched and growing system of adolescent treatment services that spans public and private sectors and offers services in both specialty and non-specialty service settings. Most adolescents are entering treatment due to alcohol and/or cannabis-related problems (and, to a lesser degree, other illicit drugs), but present with a wide array of co-occurring problems and obstacles to recovery. Multiple levels of specialized care are available but most adolescents being treated via outpatient counseling. The number and methodological rigor of adolescent treatment outcome studies have increased dramatically in recent years. The findings of these studies suggest the need for earlier systems of problem identification and intervention, a model of sustained recovery support for adolescents presenting with high problem severity and complexity, and sustained interventions with the adolescent's post-treatment family and social environment. In the opening decade of the twenty-first century, the treatment of adolescent substance use disorders is itself maturing into a professionalized and science-guided service arena.

References

American Society of Addiction Medicine (ASAM) (1996). *Patient placement criteria for the treatment of psychoactive substance disorders* (second Edition). Checy Chase, MD: Author.

Babor, T. R., Webb, C. P. M., Burleston, J. A., & Kaminer, Y. (2002). Subtypes for classifying adolescents with marijuana use disorders: Construct validity and clinical implications. *Addiction, 97*, 58–69.

Brown, S. A., D'Amico, E. J., McCarthy, D. M., & Taggart, S. F. (2001). Four year outcomes from adolescent alcohol and drug treatment. *Journal of Studies on Alcohol, 62*, 381–388.

Carlson, K., Deck, D. and Wadeson, K. (2001). *School-based Outpatient Treatment for Adolescent Substance Abuse*. Portland, Oregon: RMC Research Corporation.

Chen, J., & Millar, W. (1998). Age of smoking initiation: Implications for quitting. *Health Reports*, 9(4), 39–46.

Chou, S. P., & Pickering, R. P. (1992). Early onset of drinking as a risk factor for lifetime alcohol-related problems. *British Journal of Addiction, 87*, 1199–1204.

Conferences on Drug Addiction Among Adolescents. (The New York Academy of Medicine) (1953). New York: The Blakiston Company.

Deas, D. and Thomas, S.E. (2001). An overview of controlled studies of adolescent substance abuse treatment. *American Journal of Addictions*, 10, 178–189.

Dennis, M.L., Godley, S. & Titus, J. (1999). Co-occurring Psychiatric Problems Among Adolescents: Variations by Treatment, Level of Care and Gender. *TIE Communiqué* (pp.5–8 &16). Rockville, MD: Substance Abuse and Mental Health Services Administration, Center for Substance Abuse Treatment.

Dennis, M.L., Babor, T.F., Diamond, G., Donaldson, J, Godley, S.H., Tims, F., et al. (2000). *The Cannabis Youth Treatment (CYT) experiment: Preliminary findings*. Rockville, MD: Substance Abuse and Mental Health Services Administration, Center for Substance Abuse Treatment. [Available online at http://www.chestnut.org/li/cyt/findings].

Dennis, M. L., Babor, T., Roebuck, M. C., & Donaldson, J. (2002). Changing the focus: The case for recognizing and treating marijuana use disorders. *Addiction, 97* (Suppl. 1), S4-S15.

Dennis, M.L., Dawud-Noursi, S., Muck, R., and McDermeit, M. (2002). The need for developing and evaluating adolescent treatment models. In S.J. Stevens & A.R. Moral (Eds.) *Adolescent drug treatment in the United States: Exemplary models from a National Evaluation Study*, pp. 3–334. Binghamton, NY: Haworth Press.

Dennis, M. L., Godley, S. H., Babor, T., Diamond, G., Tims, F. M., Donaldson, J., Liddle, H., Titus, J. C., Kaminer, Yl, & Funk, R. (in press). Main Findings of the Cannabis Youth Treatment (CYT) Randomized Field Experiment. *Journal of Substance Abuse Treatment*.

Dennis, M. L., Titus, J. C., Diamond, G., Donaldson, J., Godley, S. H., Tims, F., et al. (2002). The Cannabis Youth Treatment (CYT) experiment: Rationale, study design, and analysis plans. *Addiction, 97*, S16-S34.

Donovan, D. (1998). Continuing care: Promoting the maintenance of change. In W. Miller & N. Heather (Eds.), *Treating Addictive Behaviors* (2nd ed.pp317–336), New York: Plenum Press.

DuRant, R. H., Smith, J. A., Kreiter, S. R., & Krowchuk, D. P. (1999). The relationship between early age of onset of initial substance use and engaging in multiple health risk behaviors among young adolescents. *Archives of Pediatric and Adolescent Medicine, 153*, 286–291.

Fergusson, D. M., Lynskey, M. T., & Horwood, L. J. (1996). The short-term consequences of early onset cannabis use. *Journal of Child Psychology, 24*(4), 499–512.

Friedman, A. S., & Glickman, N. W. (1986). Program characteristics for successful treatment of adolescent substance abuse. *Journal of Nervous and Mental Disease, 174*, 669–679.

Friedman, A.S. & Beschner, G.M., (Eds.) (1985) *Treatment Services for Adolescent Drug Abusers* (DHHS Publication No. ADM 85–1342m), Rockville, MD: National Institute on Drug Abuse.

Gamso, R. and Mason, P. (1958). A hospital for adolescent drug addicts. *Psychiatric Quarterly, Supplement, 32*, 99–109.

Garner, B. R., Godley, S. H., & Funk, R. (2002). Evaluating admission alternatives in an outpatient substance abuse treatment program for adolescents. *Evaluation and Program Planning, 25*, 287–294.

Godley, M. D., Godley, S. H., Dennis, M., Funk, R., & Passetti, L. (2002). Preliminary outcomes from the assertive continuing care experiment for adolescents discharged from residential treatment. *Journal of Substance Abuse Treatment, 23*, 21–32.

Godley, M. D., Kahn, J. H., Dennis, M. L., Godley, S. H., & Funk, R. R. (in press). The stability and impact of environmental factors on substance use and problems after adolescent outpatient treatment for Cannabis abuse or dependence. *The Psychology of Addictive Behaviors*.

Godley, S. H., Godley, M.D., Pratt, A., & Wallace, J.L. (1994). Case management services for adolescent substance abusers: A program description. *Journal of Substance Abuse Treatment, 11*, 309–317.

Grant, B. F., & Dawson, D. A. (1997). Age at onset of alcohol use and its association with DSM-IV alcohol abuse and dependence. *Journal of Substance Abuse, 9*, 103–110.

Henggeler, S.W., Borduin, C.M., Melton, G.B., Mann, B.J., Smith, L., Hall, J.A., Cone, L., & Fucci, B.R. (1991). Effects of a multisystemic therapy on drug use and abuse in serious juvenile offenders. A progress report from two outcome studies. *Family Dynamics of Addiction Quarterly, 1*, 40–51.

Hingson, R. W., Heeren, T., Jananka., A., & Howland, J. (2000). Age of drinking onset and unintentional injury involvement after drinking. *Journal of the American Medical Association, 284*, 1527–1533.

Hingson, R. W., Heeren, T., & Zakocs, R. (2001). Age of drinking onset and involvement in physical fights after drinking. *Pediatrics, 108*(4), 872–877.

Hoffman, N., & Miller, N. (1992). Treatment outcomes for abstinence-based programs. *Psychiatric Annals, 22*(8), 402–408.

Hoffman, N., Mee-Lee, D., & Arrowood, A. (1993). Treatment issues in adolescent substance use and addictions: Options, outcome, effectiveness, reimbursement, and admission criteria. *Adolescent Medicine, 4*(2), 371–390.

Hubbard, S. (1920). The New York City Narcotic Clinic and different points of view on narcotic addiction. *Monthly Bulletin of the Department of Health of New York, 10*(2):33–47.

Hser, Y.I., Grella, C. E., Hubbard, R. L., Hsieh, S., Fletcher, B. W., Brown, B. S., et al. (2001). An evaluation of drug treatments for adolescents in 4 U.S. cities. *Archives of General Psychiatry, 58*, 689–695.

Jainchill, N. (1997). Therapeutic communities for adolescents: The same and not the same. In G. DeLeon (Ed.), *Community as method: Therapeutic communities for special population and special settings*, (pp. 161-177). Wesport, CT: Praeger Publishers/Greenwood Publishing Group.

Johnson, A. (2003). *Customized data analysis for authors using 1995–2001 National Treatment Center Study data/Institute for Behavioral Research*. Athens: The University of Georgia.

Keller, M., Lavori, P., Beardslee, W., Wunder, J., Drs., D., & Hasin, D. (1992). Clinical course and outcome of substance abuse disorders in adolescents. *Journal of Substance Abuse Treatment, 9*, 9–14.

Kessler, R. C., Aguilar-Gaxiola, S., Berglund, P., Caraveo-Anduaga, J., DeWitt, D., Greenfield, S., et al. (2001). Patterns and predictors of treatment seeking after onset of a substance use disorder. *Archives of General Psychiatry, 58*(11), 1065–1071.

Kreichbaun, N., & Zering, G. (2000). Adolescent patients. In G. Zering (Ed.), *Handbook of Alcoholism* (pp. 129–136). Boca Raton, LA: CRC Press.

McLellan, A.T. (2003). *What's wrong with addiction treatment?* Washington DC: Author. Retrieved from http://www.tresearch.org/manuals_pubs/manuals_pubs.htm

Mosher, J. (1980). The History of Youthful-drinking Laws: Implications for Current Policy. In: Wechsler, H. *Minimum-Drinking Age Laws* Lexington, Massachusetts: Lexington Books.

Muck, R, Zempolich, K.A., Titus, J.C., Fishman, M., Godley, M.D., & Schwebel, R. (2001). An overview of the effectiveness of adolescent substance abuse treatment models. *Youth and Society, 33,* 143–168.

Musto, D. (1973). *The American Disease: Origins of Narcotic Controls.* New Haven: Yale University Press.

National Institute on Alcohol Abuse and Alcoholism. (2003). Underage drinking: A major public health challenge. *Alcohol Alert, 59,* 1–7.

National Institute on Drug Abuse. (1999). *National Survey Results on Drug Use From the Monitoring the Future Study, 1999.* Rockville, MD: Author. Retrieved from www.monitoringthefuture.org

Northrup, D. & Heflinger, C.A. (2000). *Substance Abuse Treatment Services for Publicly Funded Adolescents in the State of Mississippi.* Nashville, TN: Author. Retrieved from www.vanderbilt.edu/VIPPS/CMHP/pdfs/MSSubstance.pdf.

Office of Applied Studies (OAS). (2000). *Treatment Episode Data Set (TEDS) 1992–1997: National admissions to substance abuse treatment services.* Rockville, MD: Author. Retrieved from http://www.icpsr.umich.edu/SAMHDA.html

Office of Applied Studies. (2002). *The DASIS Report: Drug and Alcohol Treatment in Juvenile Correction Facilities,* Rockville, MD: Author. Retrieved from: http://www.samhsa.gov/oas/2K2/YouthJusticeTX/YouthJusticeTX.cfm

Office of Applied Studies (OAS). (2003). Alcohol and Drug Services Study (ADSS). *The National Substance Abuse Treatment System: Facilities, Clients, Services, and Staffing.* Retrieved from http://www.samhsa.gov/oas/ADSS/ADSSorg.pdf

Presley, C. A., Meilman, P. W., & Lyerla, R. (1991). *Alcohol and Drugs on American College Campuses: Volume 1: 1989–91.* Carbondale, IL: Southern Illinois University Student Health Programs (The Core Institute).

Roman, P., & Blum, T. (1997, January). *National Treatment Center Study: Summary Report.* Athens, GA: Institute for Behavioral Research, University of Georgia.

Roman, P., Blum, T., Johnson, A., & Neal, M. (2002, August). *National Treatment Center Study Summary Report (No. 5): Third Wave On-Site Results.* Athens, GA: Institute for Behavioral Research, University of Georgia.

Sobell, M. B., Sobell, L. C., Cunningham, J. C., & Agrawal, S. (1998). Natural recovery over the lifespan. In E. L. Gomberg, A. M. Hegedus, & R. A. Zucker (Eds.), *Alcohol Problems and Aging* (NIAAA Research Monograph No. 33, pp. 397–405). Bethesda, MD: National Institute on Alcohol Abuse and Alcoholism.

Stoltenberg, S. F., Hill, E. M., Mudd, S. A., Blow, F. C., & Zucker, R. A. (1999). Birth cohort differences in features of antisocial alcoholism among men and women. *Alcoholism: Clinical & Experimental Research, 23*(12), 1884–1891.

Substance Abuse and Mental Health Services Administration. (1999). *National Household Survey on Drug Abuse: Main Findings 1997.* Rockville, MD: Author.

Substance Abuse and Mental Health Services Administration, (SAMHSA) Office of Applied Studies. (2003). *Survey of Substance Abuse Treatment Services (N-SSATS): Data on Substance Abuse Treatment Facilities,* DASIS Series: S-19. DHHS Publication No (SMA) 03–3777. Rockville, MD.

Temple, M. T., & Fillmore, K. M. (1985–1986). The variability of drinking patterns and problems among young men, age 16–31: A longitudinal study. *International Journal of the Addictions, 20,* 1595–1620.

Terry, C. E. and Pellens, M. (1928). *The Opium Problem,* Montclair, New Jersey: Patterson Smith.

U.S. Department of Justice, Bureau of Justice Statistics. (1994). *Drugs and Crime Facts, 1994.* Retrieved from http://www.ojp.usdoj.gov/bjs/dcf/contents.htm

Warren, C. W., Kann, L., Small, M. L., Santelli, J. S., Collins, J. L., & Kolbe, L. J. (1997). Age of initiating selected health-risk behaviors among high school students in the United States. *Journal of Adolescent Health, 21,* 225–231.

White, W. (1998). *Slaying the Dragon: The History of Addiction treatment and Recovery in America.* Bloomington, Illinois: Chestnut Health Systems.

White, W. L. (1999). A history of adolescent alcohol, tobacco and other drug use in America. *Student Assistance Journal, 11*(5), 16–22.

White, W., Dennis, M. and Tims, F. (2002) Adolescent treatment: Its history and current renaissance. *Counselor* 3(2):20–23.

Williams, R.J., Chang, S.Y., & Addiction Centre Adolescent Research Group. (2000). A comprehensive and comparative review of adolescent substance abuse treatment outcome. *Clinical Psychology in Scientific Practice, 7,* 138–166.

Winters, K.C. (1999). Treating adolescents with substance use disorders: An overview of practice issues and treatment outcome. *Substance Abuse, 20,* 203–225.

Winters, K. C., Stinchfield, R.D., Opland, E. O., Weller, C. & Latimer, W.W. (2000). The effectiveness of the Minnesota Model approach in the treatment of adolescent drug abusers. *Addiction, 94*(4), 601–612.

Williams, R. J., Chang, S. Y., & Addiction Centre Adolescent Research Group. (2000). A comprehensive and comparative review of adolescent substance abuse treatment outcome. *Clinical Psychology: Science and Practice, 7,* 138–166.

Yahr, H. T. (1988). National comparison of public- and private-sector alcoholism treatment delivery system characteristics. *Journal of Studies on Alcohol, 49*(3), 233–239.

18

Evidence-Based Cognitive-Behavioral and Family Therapies for Adolescent Alcohol and Other Substance Use Disorders

Yifrah Kaminer and Natasha Slesnick

Although the research on adolescent substance abuse treatment is increasing, it still lags far behind that of adults. In comparison to over 1,000 alcohol treatment outcome studies with adults (Miller et al., 1995), Williams and Chang (2000) were able to locate and review only 53 empirical studies investigating the relative effectiveness of treatments for adolescents. Family Therapies (FT) and Cognitive Behavioral Therapy (CBT) has demonstrated repeatedly to be effective in randomized trials since the 1970s for adult alcohol and other substance use disorders (AOSUD). CBT has been an active ingredient in a variety of intervention conditions including FT. In comparison, while the evidence supporting FT and CBT use either independent or jointly in youth is promising, controlled clinical efficacy and effectiveness trials have only begun to emerge in 1990s.

Latest innovations in the management of treatment protocols for adolescent AOSUD and the recent completion of several randomized clinical trials examining manualized FT and CBT, have established the empirical support for these approaches in youth (Dennis et al., in press; Kaminer et al., 2002; Liddle, 2002; Waldron et al., 2001). The purpose of this chapter is to review: 1) theoretical models underlying FT and CBT, 2) evidence-based literature on FT and CBT for AOSUD in youth, and 3) mechanisms and therapeutic processes of FT and

Yifrah Kaminer • University of Connecticut Health Center, Alcohol Research Center and Department of Psychiatry, Farmington, CT 06030-2103.
Natasha Slesnick • Department of Psychology, University of New Mexico, Albuquerque, New Mexico 87131.

CBT associated with change are examined and future research directions and treatment implications wrap up the chapter.

1. Family Therapy Outcome for Adolescent Substance Use Problems Theoretical Rationale and History

Family systems researchers consider the behavior of a person to be best understood in terms of the individual's family interactions. According to Jacob (1987) the family systems theoretical and methodological perspective has two goals: 1) to identify family patterns and processes that are precursors to disordered behavior, and 2) to integrate this knowledge with the genetic, sociocultural and personality factors found to affect the development and perpetuation of psychopathology.

For this review, we will first define family and family treatment. Gladding (2000) utilizes the definition of family being "a group of two or more persons related by birth, marriage, or adoption and residing together in a household" (Statistical Abstracts of the United States, 1991, p. 5). This definition is flexible enough to encompass non-traditional family situations, as well as divorce or death. In addition, some interventions may involve the family but are not considered family therapy (Liddle & Dakof, 1995). These interventions might include the family in a psychoeducational intervention but do not focus on changing family interactions or relational patterns. To help clarify, Carr (2000) summarizes effective family therapy as helping "families clarify communication, family rules and roles, routines, hierarchies and boundaries; resolve conflicts; optimize emotional cohesion, develop parenting and problem-solving skills, and manage life-cycle transitions" (p. 42).

Family systems theory purports that adolescent problem behaviors, including substance abuse, running away and other externalizing problems are symptoms of maladaptive family interaction patterns (Jacob, 1987). In order to understand and address these problems, the therapist must work with the entire family to improve family functioning. Even so, given that the individual problem is often considered a symptom of broader systemic problems, the tendency among researchers is still to discuss the individual problem (adolescent substance use) as primary rather than the underlying systemic issue of which it is a symptom (Carr, 2000).

Dating nearly thirty years ago, the adult literature has shown that the adult alcoholic exhibits unique relationship patterns that are repetitive and identifiable and are relevant to the emergence and perpetuation of alcoholism (e.g., Steinglass, 1980). The literature continues to show that the family plays a role in the development, maintenance and recovery from substance use disorders (Hops et al., 1996; Stanton, Todd & associates, 1982). This research on family factors that influence addiction has been influential in developing intervention strategies for distressed marriages and family situations.

Adolescent and Family Research. Few interactional process studies have been completed with adolescents who are alcohol or drug addicted and their families. Those involving family-based treatments are even fewer with Stanton and Shadish (1997) identifying nine studies.

Family-based treatment approaches for adolescents have derived primarily from theories of family functioning and clinical experience rather than as an outgrowth of empirical study (Bry, 1988). However, researchers have observed unique family characteristics associated with adolescent substance use supporting the utility of including the family in intervention efforts. As children develop into adolescence other influences (e.g., peer) increase, but the family remains the major agent of socialization (Gecas & Seff, 1990). Parenting practices and psychopathology have been associated with adolescent alcohol and drug use. Poor parental monitoring and inconsistent discipline have been identified as key parenting practices related to negative child outcomes including substance use (e.g., Forehand, Miller, Dutra, & Chance, 1997). Parental depression, anxiety, substance use and stress is associated with substance use disorder, depression and conduct problems among youth (e.g., Downey & Coyne, 1990; Hops et al., 1996).

Even though the importance of the family in the socialization and developmental process of children has been noted, the family is not the only vehicle for healthy socialization. There are some situations in which working with the family may not be possible or advisable. For example, some researchers argue that running away may be a fundamentally healthy reaction to a pathological situation (Adams & Adams, 1987), that life on the streets may be perceived as more safe than life at home. In these and similar situations, substance use and related problem behaviors might be best addressed outside the family context.

Many note that even with an increase in the focus on family therapy with substance abusing youth, many studies lack the methodological rigor to allow definitive statements regarding the efficacy or effectiveness of family therapy (Liddle & Dakof, 1995). Cottrell and Boston (2002) note small sample sizes, wide age ranges and a lack of true randomization. Some family treatments are not specified, and control groups are not feasible treatments. Few studies conduct follow-up assessment past the post-treatment evaluation, and the assessment measures used do not have strong psychometric support.

Despite these limitations, several methodologically strong studies are available that lend support for a moderate effect of family therapy for individual and family change outcomes. Three reviews, Ozechowski and Liddle (2000), Liddle and Dakof (1995) and Waldron (1997), in addition to the meta analysis by Stanton and Shadish (1997) on controlled clinical trials of family based treatments for substance abuse, conclude that family therapy is more effective at engaging and maintaining substance abusing adolescents in treatment and reducing substance use than non family-based interventions. These reviewers concluded that studies found no significant difference in the reduction of adolescent problem behaviors (other than substance use) or family functioning between family and non-family-based interventions at post

Table 1. Overview of Recent Randomized Clinical Trials

Study	Treatment Groups	Sample Characteristics	Follow-up Points	Findings
Azrin et al. 2001	1.Behavioral Family therapy (N = 27) 2. Individual cognitive problem solving (N =29)	Youth aged 12–17, met DSM criteria for substance use and conduct disorder, 82% male, 21% minority status.	Post-treatment and 6 months.	Both treatments were equally effective in reducing substance use, and related problems and increasing satisfaction and problem-solving skills.
Henggeler et al. 1999, 2002	1. MST (N = 58 and at 4 years, N = 43) 2. Usual Communitu Services (N = 60 and at 4 years, N = 37)	Youth aged 12–17, met DSM criteria for substance abuse or dependence, 79% male, 53% minority status.	Posttreatment, 6 and 12 months and 4 years post treatment termination.	Significant reductions in substance use at posttreatment for MST, though findings did not maintain to any other time point. At 6 months, youths in MST had fewer days out of home placement and at 4 years MST clients showed significant reductions in aggressive criminal behavior compared to usual services.
Liddle et al., in press	1. MDFT (N = 112) 2. Individual Cognitive-Behavioral Therapy (N = 112)	Youth aged 13 to 17, met DSM criteria for drug use or dependence, 81% male, 82% minority status.	Posttreatment, 6 and 12 months.	Both treatments were equally effective in reducing substance use and related problems. These improvements continued to the 12 month follow-up for MDFT, but not for ICBT.
Liddle et al. 2001	1. MDFT (N = 33) 2. Multifamily Education Group (N = 34) 3. Adolescent Group Therapy	Youth aged 13 to 18, 51% polydrug users, 49% marijuana and alcohol users, 80% male, 49% minority status.	Posttreatment, 6 and 12 months.	Although all conditions showed improvement, MDFT showed greatest improvement from pretreatment to 12 months on overall drug use and related problem behaviors followed by adolescent group therapy and multifamily education group.

Santisteban et al. 2003	1. BSFT (N = 80) 2. Group (N = 46)	Youth aged 12 to 18, 52% reported alcohol or other drug use in the past month, 75% male, 100% Hispanic.	Posttreatment only.	Significant reductions in substance youth in both BSFT and group therapy were found. BSFT showed significantly greater improvements in family functioning than group therapy.
Waldron et al. 2001	1. FFT (N=30) 2. CBT (N = 31) 3. FFT + CBT (N = 29) 4. Group (N = 30)	Youth aged 13 to 17, met DSM criteria for substance use disorder, 80% male, 64% minority status.	Four and 7 months following intake assessment.	At 4 months, FFT and FFT + CBT showed significantly reduced frequency of marijuana use. At 7 months, significant reductions in frequency of use were found only in FFT + CBT and group.

treatment or follow-up. Proposed reasons for these lack of findings include treatment effects, insensitive measurement instruments or lack of significant statistical power.

This section of the chapter will review recent studies that have been published or are in press that evaluated at least one family-based intervention for adolescent substance use. Each study reviewed includes a comparison condition and random assignment of clients to conditions. Several of these studies follow from a programmatic line of research, which will be briefly summarized. Many of the earlier studies have been tabled and reviewed elsewhere (e.g., Ozechowski & Liddle, 2000), refer to Table 1 for a summary of recent clinical trials.

2. Ecologically Based, Family Systems Studies

Multisystemic Therapy. Multisystemic Therapy (MST) is described in detail (Henggeler et al., 1998) with a review of all MST publications in Henggeler (1999). Briefly, the intervention focuses on the individual, family, peer, school and social network variables linked with identified problems as well as on the interface of these systems (Henggeler, Clingempeel, & Brondino, 2002). Pickrel and Henggeler (1996) note the consensus regarding the multidetermined nature of substance use which provides the rationale for a multisystemic approach. MST views engagement and overcoming family resistance as the therapist's and program's responsibility (Pickrel & Henggeler, 1996), and virtually all services are provided in the natural environment of the youth and family, and may include up to 60 hours of intervention.

Recent Studies. Henggeler, Pickrel and Brondino (1999) examined outcomes from a randomized clinical trial of MST was compared with usual community services through the Department of Juvenile Justice. Youth were followed at posttreatment, and 6 and 12 months posttreatment. Although significant treatment effects for substance use were reported at posttreatment for those in the MST condition, those findings were not maintained at the 6-month follow-up. Youths in the MST condition received 50% fewer days of out of home placement at the 6 month followup than those in the service as usual condition. No other treatment by time effects (including 12 months posttreatment) were obtained.

Henggeler, Clingempeel and Brondino (2002) reported the findings from the four-year follow-up of this trial. The study did not obtain significant MST effects for reduced property crimes, biological indices of drug use or Internalizing and Externalizing behaviors. Self-report indications of substance use at this follow-up did not differentiate conditions. However, MST was associated with significant reductions in aggressive criminal behavior. The findings for adolescents with diagnosed substance use problems were not as favorable as Henggeler's earlier trials of MST with chronic and violent juvenile offenders who did not necessarily have substance abuse problems (e.g., Henggeler et al., 1992). The authors conclude that treatment fidelity was relatively low and that an increased focus in the intervention on drug use and the promotion of treatment integrity might improve MST outcomes for substance-abusing adolescents. The authors called for the study of mediational processes to advance the field and themselves examined mediated processes associated with outcome in MST (Huey et al., 2000).

Brief Strategic Family Therapy. Jose Szapocznik and his colleagues, through a series of clinical research studies over the past thirty years, have refined the Brief Strategic Family Therapy (BSFT) approach for Hispanic families with behavior problem youth. The approach draws upon the structural orientation of Minuchin (1974) and the strategic approach of Haley (1976) and Madanes (1981) and is manualized (Szapocznik, Hervis, & Schwartz, 2002). Research has shown positive impact of BSFT on adolescents with problems pertaining to conduct, delinquency and drug and alcohol use (e.g., Santisteban et al., 1997; Szapocznik et al., 1986).

Recent Studies. Santisteban et al. (2003) randomly assigned participants (N = 126) to BSFT or group therapy, both offered once weekly in the office (range 4 to 20 weeks). Substance use was not required for inclusion in the study, although 52% of participants reported either alcohol (35%) or other drug use during the past month. Findings showed that BSFT was more efficacious than group therapy for all three of the presenting problems—conduct problems, peer-based delinquency, and self-reported drug use using both parent and youth reports. Results showed, however, that BSFT was no more effective in reducing alcohol use than the group treatment condition. Additionally, BSFT was more efficacious than group therapy in improving family functioning, the hypothesized mediator of behavior change in BSFT. Although this study had several strengths, including the use treatment adherence manual and checklist, random assignment, a relatively large sample, the study analyses were not based on an intent to treat model and outcome was assessed only at posttreatment which does not allow conclusions to be drawn regarding treatment effectiveness once treatment attendance has stopped.

Multidimensional Family Therapy. Multidimensional family therapy (MDFT) is an outpatient, family-based treatment developed for multiproblem youth (Liddle, 1999) that has been tested and developed since 1985 in randomized clinical trials and treatment development and process studies (Liddle, 1999). A manual is available (Liddle, 2001) and other versions of the manual are available that vary by treatment length, treatment intensity, intervention (home vs. clinic) and inclusion of adjunct treatment methods. MDFT targets the multiple ecologies of adolescent development and the circumstances and processes that continue problem behavior including substance use (Liddle, 2001).

Recent Studies. Liddle et al. (2001) randomly assigned 182 marijuana and alcohol-abusing adolescents to one of three treatments: MDFT, Multifamily Education Group or Adolescent Group Therapy. Youth were followed at posttreatment and 6 and 12 months posttreatment. Youth showed improvement in all three treatments with MDFT showing the greatest improvement overall on measures of drug use, grade point average, and family functioning. Even at one year follow-up, youths assigned to MDFT showed continued improvement in school performance and family functioning and these youth maintained their substance use reduction at both 6 and 12 months.

In another study, Liddle, Dakof, Turner, and Tejeda (in press) randomly assigned 224 youth to MDFT or individual Cognitive Behavioral Therapy. Treatment integrity ratings were completed and follow-ups included posttreatment and 6 and 12 months. The sample of youth were reported to be urban, low-income, primarily African-American (72%), with significant co-morbidity and family dysfunction. Both treatments were efficacious with youths showing reduced drug use, externalizing and internalizing problems from intake to termination. However, those assigned to MDFT continued to show improvements up to 12 months posttreatment while improvement leveled off for those assigned to Cognitive Behavioral Therapy. Thus, it appears that the difference between the two efficacious treatments is that MDFT was able to retain the effects of treatment beyond the treatment phase. Although this study had a 20% treatment refusal rate, one strength of this work is that the referred sample was dually diagnosed from disadvantaged backgrounds, suggesting that each approach is effective in working with this challenging group.

Behavioral Family Systems Treatment. Functional Family Therapy (FFT; Alexander & Parsons, 1982), is a multisystemic approach that integrates and conceptually links behavioral and cognitive intervention strategies to the ecological formulation of the family disturbance. Similar to other behavioral family systems models, problems with drugs are viewed as behaviors which occur in the context of and have meaning for family relationships. It was initially developed and empirically supported for crisis intervention with juvenile offenders, including runaway adolescents, and their families (Alexander, 1971).

Recent Studies. One study found that FFT can lead to positive synergistic outcomes when combined with other individually based approaches. Waldron, Slesnick, Brody, Turner and Peterson (2001) compared FFT, individual cognitive behavioral therapy (CBT), a joint combination of FFT and CBT, and group psychoeducational therapy. Adolescents (N = 114) were randomly assigned to one of the four conditions and were followed at 4 and 7 months. At 4 months, youth showed significant reductions of marijuana use in the FFT and joint FFT + CBT intervention. At 7 months the joint and group therapy conditions showed significant reductions in use. The authors concluded that all interventions demonstrated some degree of treatment efficacy with differences only in the speed in which changes emerged and in the maintenance of change over time. Overall, the findings supported the efficacy of family-based treatment for both short and longer term changes. However, this study only analyzed youth's marijuana use even though youth were not recruited for primary marijuana abuse. Also, those in the joint treatment condition received twice the number of treatment contact hours as those in the other treatment conditions, limiting conclusions that can be drawn regarding the relative effectiveness of the joint condition compared to other conditions.

3. Behavioral Family Treatment

Behavioral family treatment (BFT) is not usually considered a family systems approach (Gladding, 2002). This intervention is based upon the theoretical foundations of behavioral therapy that all behaviors are learned and maintained by environmental consequences. Thus ineffective behaviors, including those between family members, can be extinguished and replaced with new behaviors.

Recent Studies. Azrin et al. (2001) evaluated the effectiveness of BFT compared to individual cognitive problem solving in a sample of adolescents who were dually diagnosed with conduct disorder and substance dependence. The primary intervention included behavioral contracting, stimulus control, urge control and communications training. Followup was completed at post treatment and at 6 months posttreatment and independent raters coded treatment fidelity. Results showed that both interventions were equally effective at the follow-up points in reducing the frequency of alcohol and illicit drug use and reducing conduct problems, depression and increasing problem-solving, life satisfaction and satisfaction with parents. This study had several strengths including a viable comparison condition, equal duration and frequency of sessions between the two treatment conditions, treatment reliability and validity measures, and standardized self-report and objective measures. However, the sample size was small, making conclusions regarding differences or lack of differences suspect as they may be attributable to lack of sufficient power given group heterogeneity.

4. Summary of Family Therapy

Seven randomized trials which evaluated substance use outcomes were reviewed. All studies showed significant pre to posttreatment reductions in substance use for the family-based intervention utilized. Findings were primarily for illicit drug use including marijuana and cocaine (Henggeler et al., 2002), marijuana alone (Waldron et al., 2001), and marijuana, alcohol and hard drugs (Azrin, 2001, Liddle et al., 2001; Liddle et al., in press). Two studies examined alcohol use specifically among the substances used at outcome (Azrin et al., 2001; Santisteban et al., 2003). Although earlier work showed that alcohol use was differentially and significantly impacted by the family intervention (Azrin, 1994a), Azrin et al. (2001) found no impact of either behavioral family therapy or individual cognitive therapy on alcohol use. Santisteban et al. (2003) also showed no differential impact of BSFT on alcohol use compared to group therapy. To date, conclusions regarding the effectiveness of family therapy for adolescent problem drinkers are difficult to make because of the void of treatment effectiveness studies with this population.

The long-term effects of family therapy for adolescent substance use are listed as one of the unknowns in Ozechowski and Liddle's review (2000).

Only one study reports findings beyond 12 months (Henggeler et al., 2002). However, several recent studies (Liddle et al., 2001; Liddle et al., in press; Waldron et al., 2001) suggest that substance use outcomes not only endure but continue to improve up to 7 and 12 months compared to the control conditions. Those findings combined with similar findings from earlier studies (Friedman, 1989; Henggeler et al., 1992; Szapocznik et al.,1986) provide support to the powerful effect of family therapy to intervene in the substance use trajectory during adolescence.

Results from the studies reviewed here provide further support for prior findings that family therapy may be especially effective at reducing related problems including low school attendance and poor scholastic performance (Henggeler, Pickrel, & Brondino, 1999; Liddle et al., 2001), arrests and aggressive behavior (Henggeler, Clingempeel, & Brondino, 2002), internalizing and externalizing problems (Liddle et al., in press) conduct problems and peer based delinquency (Santisteban et al., 2003). Observer and self report ratings of family functioning, considered a mechanism of change in family therapy, has shown differential improvement (Liddle et al., 2001; Santisteban et al., 2003).

Perhaps ironically, the inclusion requirement for family therapy to involve more than one person (with the exception of unilateral family therapy) does not represent a limitation of the approach. In fact, Stanton and Shadish (1997) concluded that family therapies, compared to other approaches for treating substance abusers showed relatively higher rates of engagement and retention. Recent studies continue to show this trend (Donohue et al., 1998; Henggeler et al., 1999, 2002; Liddle et al., 2001) although several other studies showed comparable rates of engagement and retention in non-family based interventions (Azrin et al., 2001; Liddle et al., in press; Santisteban et al., 2003; Waldron et al., 2001). As Ozechowski and Liddle (2001) conclude, these data suggest that alternative manualized, empirically validated treatments can also be successful at engaging and retaining youth and their families, utilizing assertive recruitment strategies.

In summary, this brief review provided an overview of empirically-based and manualized interventions commonly utilized with adolescent substance abusers. Recent developments in family-based treatment for adolescent substance abuse continue to build support for the efficacy of family therapy. For example, to facilitate the process of integrating family therapies into community settings, MST (Henggeler, Pickrel & Brondino, 1999), MDFT (Liddle et al., 2002) and BSFT (Robbins, Bachrach, & Szapocznik, 2002) are beginning to focus on transportability of these interventions into community-based programs. Family studies are including cost benefit analyses such as in the Cannabis Youth Treatment experiment (Dennis et al., 2002). Research continues to evaluate mechanisms of change (e.g., Huey et al., 2000; Schmidt, Liddle, & Dakof, 1996) which, supported by process studies, can further illuminate family change beyond self-report mechanisms. These exciting developments continue to pave the way for future research.

5. Cognitive Behavioral Therapy

5.1. *Theoretical Models Underlying CB Intervention Approaches*

Cognitive-behavioral intervention approaches are varied, with most approaches integrating strategies derived from classical conditioning, operant, and social learning perspectives. Each of these perspectives view substance use and related problems as learned behaviors that are initiated and maintained in the context of environmental factors. Yet, experimental research within each theoretical perspective has focused on unique aspects of substance use behavior, resulting in the development of distinct interventions techniques that are often combined into a multicomponent cognitive behavioral intervention. (Dimeff & Marlatt, 1995; Monti et al., 1995). Such interventions typically involve identifying contextual factors, such as the setting, time, or place, which may serve as potential "triggers." Strategies to manage urges and cravings, once stimulus cues have been identified, may involve techniques from different learning perspectives, such as self-control, reinforcers for competing behaviors, or other coping- skills training. Operant perspectives view alcohol and drug use behaviors in the context of the antecedents and consequences surrounding the behavior. In addition to the powerful reinforcement associated with the physiological effects of drugs that serve to maintain use, reinforcers can also include the reduction of tension, attenuation of negative affect, or enhancement of social interactions. Intervention strategies based on operant learning often include identifying alternative reinforcers that compete with drug use and other applications of contingency management (Higgins et al., 1995; Stitzer et al., 1979). The social learning model incorporates the influence of environmental events on the acquisition of behavior, but also recognizes the role of cognitive processes (e.g., how environmental influences are perceived and appraised) in determining behavior (Bandura, 1977; 1986). Within this perspective, substance use can be influenced through a variety of cognitive and behavioral factors including modeling parents, siblings, or peers, social reinforcement, the expectation of the effects of drug use, self-efficacy beliefs about one's ability to refrain from use, and physical dependence (Abrams & Niaura, 1987).

Multicomponent CBT approaches for substance abuse often include such components as self-monitoring, avoidance of stimulus cues, altering reinforcement contingencies, and coping-skills training to manage and resist urges to use. Drug and alcohol refusal skills, communication skills, problem solving skills, assertiveness, relaxation training, anger management, modifying cognitive distortions, and relapse prevention are often incorporated to promote sobriety (Marlatt & Gordon, 1985; Monti et al., 1989; Monti et al., 1993). Therapy sessions characteristically include modeling, behavior rehearsal, feedback, and homework assignments. Specific targets of change, however, such as negotiating privileges or identification of contingencies, must take into account the age and developmental level of the adolescent. Moreover, many youth may not have had sufficient opportunity to acquire certain social and coping skills normally developed during adolescent because of their heavy drug use and components may need to be incorporated to address basic skill deficits.

5.2. *Randomized Clinical Trials for Adolescent Substance Abuse Treatment*

Early treatment outcome research on cognitive behavioral interventions for adolescent substance use disorders, while providing an important impetus for later efficacy and effectiveness trials, was limited in a variety of ways. Methodological limitations such as small samples, inadequate control or comparison conditions, nonrandomized assignment to treatment, poor measures of variables of interest, absence of attrition data, limited descriptions of treatments, and the absence of treatment manuals and fidelity measures (Catalano et al., 1990–91; Kaminer, 2000; Waldron, 1997). Wide variations in selection criteria, measures of substance use outcome, and number and latency of follow-up assessments also characterized the research. The mixed findings in the literature likely derived from this methodological variability across studies. The emergence of formal randomized controlled trials and field experiments, however, has added significantly to the base of empirical support for CBT. These recent studies have employed more rigorous designs, with larger samples, random assignment, direct comparisons of two or more active treatments, improved measures of substance use and other variables, manual-guided interventions, and longer-term outcome assessments (Dennis et al., in press; Kaminer et al., 1998a; 2002; Kaminer & Burleson, 1999; Waldron et al., 2003). These findings, taken together, establish the foundation for the effectiveness of CBT for adolescent substance use disorders.

Azrin and his colleagues (1994a; 1994b) conducted two studies comparing a behavioral intervention to a process-oriented, nondirective (supportive) adolescent group therapy intervention. The first study involved a mixed sample of adults and fourteen adolescent substance abusers whose average age was16 years. The behavioral-therapy condition utilized role-playing, response rehearsal, home assignments, and diary keeping. The supportive counseling comparison condition involved a process-oriented, nondirective group intervention. Treatment for each group was delivered for one hour per week for 12 months. The behavioral treatment was shown to be superior to supportive counseling in terms of reducing drug use and drug-related problems at treatment completion. Azrin and his colleagues followed with a replication study involving adolescents only (N=26). Analysis of the differential efficacy of these interventions revealed that adolescents in the behavioral therapy condition reported less frequent substance use than those in supportive counseling and had fewer positive urine screens.

A few studies have also focused on the hypothesized mechanisms of change underlying CBT. Most notably, Brown and her colleagues have found that among adolescents treated for substance-use disorders, abstainers and minor relapsers were more likely to utilize problem-solving coping strategies than were major relapsers (Myers & Brown, 1990a; 1990b). Moreover, coping factors have been identified as significant predictors of treatment outcome (Myers, Brown, & Mott, 1993).

Kaminer and his colleagues (1998a) have conducted several studies evaluating a group CBT intervention for outpatient adolescent substance abusers. The intervention was originially developed in the context of a patient-treatment matching study for adults (Cooney et al., 1991; Kadden et al., 1989). In this adolescent patient-treatment matching study, youth (n=32) between the ages of 13 and 18 years of age were randomly assigned to 12 sessions of CBT or to a similar number of interactional group therapy sessions. Youth were all dually diagnosed. No patient-treatment matching effects between psychopathologies (i.e. externalizing, internalizing disorders) and treatment modalities (i.e. CBT, Interactional Therapy) were found (Kaminer et al., 1998b). However, the short-term efficacy of CBT was significant. Adolescents assigned to CBT showed a greater short-term improvement than those assigned to interactional therapy. As in other adolescent treatment-outcome studies, however, relapse was a problem for many youth and differences between the groups were no longer significant a year later (Kaminer & Burleson, 1999).

In a larger-scale controlled, randomized trial, Kaminer et al. (2002) compared the efficacy of CBT to Psychoeducational Therapies (PET) for adolescent substance abusers. It was hypothesized that participants in both conditions would improve from pretreatment to 3- and 9-month post-treatment follow-up, but that youth assigned to the CBT condition would have better retention rates in treatment and follow-up and superior short- and long-term outcomes, relative to the PET condition. The 88 predominantly dually diagnosed adolescents were randomly assigned to one of the two 8-week group interventions. Participants were between the ages of 13 and 18 years (mean 15.4, SD 1.3 years), and included 62 males and 26 females. The majority (n=79) were white. For older youth and for males, the CBT group showed significantly lower rates of positive urinalysis than the PET group at 3-month follow-up. Moreover, self-report drug use measures revealed significant improvement from baseline to 3- and to 9-month follow-up across conditions. There was also a trend toward improvement for adolescents who received CBT at the 3-month follow-up, with significant improvement for males and older subjects. Similar patterns were not found for PET. Contrary to hypotheses, CBT did not produce any long-term differential relapse rate compared to PET, due to an increase in relapse among CBT participants at the 9-month follow-up. However, most of the participants improved substantially in a variety of domains. The majority of the substance-use related problems assessed showed improvements at 3-month post-treatment follow-up and continued to improve at 9-month follow-up, relative to baseline, regardless of assigned treatment condition.

Waldron et al. (2003) evaluated the efficacy of individual CBT for youth (n=31) who were initially treatment refusers, but later entered treatment as a result of a parent-focused engagement intervention. The CBT intervention was the same as in the previous trials (Waldron et al., 2001). Adolescents in this study completed an average of five therapy sessions, half the number of sessions completed by youth in the earlier studies, but were using drugs or alcohol an average of 80.39% of the days in the past 3 month period. CBT was associated with a significant decrease in percent days of substance use from pre- to pretreatment ($F(1, 27) = 9.42, p < .005$). Although reduction in use was statistically significant, adolescents' continued heavy use at post-treatment suggests that more intensive engagement and intervention strategies may be needed to increase the dose of treatment received and enhance the impact of the intervention for this difficult treatment-resistant population.

The Cannabis Youth Treatment (CYT) study was a randomized field experiment which compared a total of five interventions, in various combinations, across four implementation sites (Dennis et al., 2002). The study was designed to address the differential efficacy of the treatments implemented and the effect of treatment dose on outcome. A total of five interventions were evaluated across the four sites. Two group CBT interventions were offered. Both began with two individual motivational-enhancement sessions, followed by either 3 CBT sessions (MET/CBT-5; (Sampl and Kadden, 2001) or 10 CBT sessions (MET/CBT-12; Webb et al., 2002). A third intervention represented a family-based add-on intervention involving MET/CBT-12 plus a 6-week family psychoeducational intervention (Hamilton et al., 2002). In addition, a 12-session individual adolescent Community Reinforcement Approach (ACRA; Godley, Meyers, & Smith, 2002), and a 12-week family therapy condition (Liddle et al., 2001) were included. The five treatment models were evaluated in two arms, in a community-based program and an academic medical center. Although all five models were not implemented within treatment sites, the replication of the MET/CBT5 intervention across all four sites made it possible to study site differences and conduct quasi-experimental comparisons of the interventions across study arms.

Overall, a total of 600 adolescents were randomly assigned to one of three interventions. The average age of the adolescents was 16, with 83% male and 61% Caucasian non-Hispanic. With follow-up rates of 98% at 3 months and 94% at 12 months, Dennis and his colleagues (in press) reported that all five interventions produced significant reductions in cannabis use and negative consequences of use from pretreatment to the 3-month follow-up, and that these reductions were sustained through the 12-month follow-up. In addition, changes in marijuana use were accompanied by reductions in behavioral problems, family problems, school problems, school absences, argumentativeness, violence, and illegal activity.

Although not entirely expected, some initial differences were found across conditions. For example, the 12-session CBT produced initially poorer outcomes, while the CBT plus support produced initially better outcomes, relative to the briefer CBT intervention, findings that are inconsistent with a simple dose-response relationship. Also, despite considerable support for family interventions in the literature, the individual (ACRA) and individual/group

(MET/CBT5) behavioral interventions produced better outcomes than the family approach (MDFT) in terms of days of substance use at 3 months. Nevertheless, these initial differences were not sustained, and the best predictor of long-term outcomes was initial level of change. In terms of cost effectiveness ratio MDFT was found to be higher than the other interventions (French et al., 2002).

5.3. *Treatment Modality: Group vs. Individual Intervention*

Questions have also been raised as to whether CBT is best implemented with groups of adolescents or individually. Taken together, studies conducted by the authors and their colleagues provide support for the benefits of behavioral group therapy, with modest additional support for the efficacy of individual CBT in reducing youth substance abuse and related problems in outpatient settings. The empirical support for the efficacy of CBT with adolescents is also similar to evidence found for treatment studies for adult drinking and drug use (Graham, et al., 1996; Kadden et al., 1989; Marques & Formigoni, 2001; PROJECT MATCH, 1997; Woody et al., 1983).

The results of the recent clinical trials for adolescents are particularly important because of their enhanced design and methodological features that represent significant improvements over previous studies. Although the absence of untreated control groups represents a limitation in the recent clinical trials, the differential efficacy of treatments across multiple studies provides compelling evidence that the reductions in substance use were a direct function of the treatments clients received, rather than an artifact of the passage of time or involvement in a clinical trial.

It is important to note, however, that despite the advances of recent clinical trials over previous studies, none of these interventions sufficiently addressed the adolescents' problems. Relapse was a consistent problem for youth across studies. In the CYT study, for example, approximately a third of the adolescents were in a state of early recovery (i.e., in the community without any marijuana use or problems) during the follow-up period, but another third of CYT clients received additional treatment during the rest of the year. The single best predictor of 12-month outcomes was not baseline client characteristics or components of the intervention, but whether the adolescent initially responded to treatment at 3 months.

This consistent empirical support of group CBT for substance-abusing adolescents stands in contrast to the iatrogenic "Deviant" peer-group effects reported for group interventions (Ang & Hughes, 2001; Dishion et al., 1999; Dishion et al., 2002). Dishion's publications expressed concern and not an ultimate judgement against group therapy including youth manifesting antisocial behavior. To summarize his position "Based on the studies reviewed, there is a reason to be cautious and to avoid aggregating young high-risk adolescents into intervention groups. Age of the child and format of the peer aggregation may impact the risk of producing negative effects on problem behavior"

(Dishion et al., 1999). Research with older adolescents (e.g., high school) has shown mixed results (Eggert et al., 1994).

Neither the CYT study group interventions nor Waldron (2001) and Kaminer studies in outpatient settings that included a significant number of adolescents with conduct disorders (39%; Kaminer et al., 2002) have experienced any severe or unmanageable problems conducting group therapy (i.e. need to eject subjects, discontinue a session, physical abuse etc).It appears that diverse referral sources allow for a mix of adolescents that are manageable in a group setting once a clearly communicated and signed behavioral contract for ground rules is introduced. Experienced therapists can competently address inappropriate behavior and other "trouble shooting" particularly in a manual driven treatment.

A number of features associated with group approaches to treatment may facilitate cognitive, affective, and behavioral changes. These factors include the realization that others share similar problems, the development of socializing techniques, modeling, rehearsal, and peer/therapist feedback. The opportunity to try out new behaviors in a social environment and the development and enhancement of interpersonal learning and trust may also be influential. Teens typically use alcohol or drugs when in the company of other users, and they are easily influenced in group settings (Myers & Brown, 1996), group treatment has the benefit of mirroring their daily experience. Role-playing, an effective component employed in CBT, takes advantage of the group setting by allowing the participants to practice scenes of high-risk experience.

5.4. *Mechanism of Change in Cognitive Behavioral Therapy for Youth and Adults with AOSUD*

Establishing support for CBT is complicated by the wide variations in treatment components comprising different CBT models. These variations also make the identification of mechanisms of change more difficult. That is, intervention approaches often include a diverse array of modules and can range from those involving a select few components to those with a full complement of distinct components. While research aimed at elucidating mechanisms of change of therapy process variables associated with adolescent outcomes has been virtually nonexistent, researchers have begun to wrestle with the mechanisms and therapeutic processes of CBT associated with change in adults with substance-use disorders (Litt et al.,2003; Morgentstern & Longabaugh, 2000; Maisto et al., 2000;Wilson, 1999). This research may point the way to similar research for adolescent substance abuse treatment.

A central role for cognitive and behavioral coping is the hypothesis that deficits in the ability to cope with life stress in general and substance cues in particular serve to maintain substance use or lead to relapse. Therefore, all CBT packages use a standard set of techniques to teach coping skills that include identification of high-risk situations where these skills should be employed (Morgenstern & Longabaugh, 2000). It has been suggested that treatment works at least partially through non-specific effects (Wampold et al., 1999). Similarly, Wilson (1999), addressed the renewed attention to the "nonspecifics" of therapy as mediators of rapid response to CBT. Rapid response to CBT with alcohol abusers resulted in 64% of total improvement evident during the first four weeks of treatment (Breslin et al., 1997). This pattern appears to be a general phenomenon that might emerge before the presumed specific impact of CBT affects the client. Furthermore, rapid response is not limited to any specific disorder (e.g. depression, substance use disorders, bulimia nervosa). The rapid treatment effect of CBT cannot be dismissed as a placebo or a "nonspecific" response. CBT quickly becomes significantly more effective than equally credible, alternative psychological therapies including interpersonal psychotherapy for adults (Jones et al., 1993) and youth (Kaminer et al., 1998a) and supportive psychotherapy (Wilson, 1999).

Although little research addressing mechanisms of change associated with CBT has been conducted for the adolescent age group, Kaminer and colleagues (1998b) were able to identify several active ingredient characterizing CBT (i.e., problem solving, identification of high-risk situations, Skills training, and role-playing) and discriminate between them and ingredients characterizing interactional therapy. However, the efficacy of these components was not examined. In other research, Myers and Brown (1990a; 1990b) found that, following cognitive-behavioral treatment, problem solving coping strategies were more likely to be used by adolescent alcohol abstainers and minor relapsers than by major relapsers. Coping factors have also been identified as significant predictors of treatment outcome (Myers et al., 1993). Research has been challenged, however, by the lack adequate measures for assessing pre- to post-treatment change in coping skills.

5.5. *Clinical Implications and Future Research Directions*

Despite some prominent differences in design and methodology, the studies employing different treatment modalities in youth with substance use disorders including CBT and FT have reported remarkably similar outcomes. Taken together, the findings represent significant developments in treatment outcome research. Yet, many of the questions raised in this review are valid including the contribution of the 'Placebo-assessment effect," and other "non-specific" mediators that might be responsible to the similar results in outcome regardless of the specificity of interventions. Future research directions should focus on improving short- and long-term outcomes, including maintenance of treatment gain in aftercare programs (Kaminer, 2001), examine the transportability of CBT into other treatment modalities such as phone (Kaminer , 2003) or internet interventions as well as settings such as therapeutic communities, residential treatment, juvenile justice system facilities, enhancing motivation/ readiness to change, improving engagement strategies, increasing self-efficacy, and identifying mechanisms and processes associated with positive change, especially for youth with co-morbid conditions.

The two most important clinical implications are to determine when patients who have not improved will be unlikely to respond to more of the same treatment and should have their treatment changed and what alternative treatment to implement. Innovative, sequential intervention treatment design is needed to address these issues.

ACKNOWLEDGMENTS. This research was supported by grants to Dr Kaminer from the National Institute on Alcohol Abuse and Alcoholism—(K24 AA13442), and (RO1 AA12187–01A2)- and to Dr Slesnick from?

References

Abrams, D. B., & Niaura, R. S. (1987). Social learning theory. In H. T. Blane., & K. E. Leonard., (Eds.), Psychological theories of drinking and alcoholism (pp. 131–178). New York: Guilford Press.

Adams, P. R., & Adams, G. R. (1987). Intervention with runaway youth and their families: Theory and practice. In J. C. Coleman (Ed.), Working with troubled adolescents (pp. 281–301). Orlando, FL: Academic Press.

Alexander, J. F. (1971). Evaluation summary: Family groups treatment program. Report to Juvenile court, District 1, State of Utah, Salt Lake City.

Alexander, J. F., & Parsons, B. V. (1982). Functional family therapy: Principles and Procedures. Carmel, CA: Brooks/Cole.

Ang, R. P., & Hughes, J. N. (2001). Differential benefits of skills training with antisocial youth based on group composition: A meta-analytic investigation. School Psychology Review, 31, 164–185.

Arzin, N. H., Donahue, B., Teichner, G. A., Crum, T., Howell, J., & DeCato, L. A. (2001). A controlled evaluation and description of individual-cognitive problem solving and family-behavior therapies in dually-diagnosed conduct-disordered and substance-dependent youth. Journal of Child & Adolescent Substance Abuse, 11, 1–43.

Azrin, N. H., Donohue, B., Besalel, V. A., Kogan, E. S., & Acierno, R. (1994a). Youth drug abuse treatment: A controlled outcome study. Journal of Child and Adolescent Substance Abuse, 3, 1–16.

Azrin, N. H., McMahon, P., & Donohue, B. (1994b). Behavior therapy for drug abuse: a controlled outcome study. Behavior Research and Therapy, 32, 857–866.

Bandura, A. (1977). Social learning theory. Englewood Cliffs, NJ: Prentice Hall.

Bandura, A. (1986). Self foundations of thought and action: A social cognitive theory. Englewood Cliffs, NJ: Prentice Hall.

Breslin, F.C., Sobell, M. B., Sobell, L.C., Buchan, G., & Cunningham, J.A. (1997). Toward a stepped care approach to treating problem drinkers: The predictive utility of within treatment variables and therapist prognostic ratings. Addiction, 92, 1479–1489.

Bry, B. H. (1988). Family-based approaches to reducing adolescent substance use: Theories, techniques, and findings. National Institute on Drug Abuse: Research Monograph Series, 77, 39–68.

Carr, A. (2000). Evidence-based practice in family therapy and systemic consultation I Child-focused problems. Journal of Family Therapy, 22, 29–60.

Catalano, R. F., Hawkins, J. D., Wells, E. A., Miller, J., & Brewer, D. (1990–91). Evaluation of the effectiveness of adolescent drug abuse treatment, assessment of risks for relapse, and promising approaches for relapse prevention. The International Journal of the Addictions, 25, 1085–1140.

Cooney, N. L., Kadden, R. M., Litt, M. D., & Getter, H. (1991). Matching alcoholics to coping skills or interactional therapies: Two-year follow-up results. Journal of Consulting and Clinical Psychology, 59, 598–601.

Cottrell, D., & Boston, P. (2002). Practitioner Review: The effectiveness of systemic family therapy for children and adolescents. Journal of Child Psychology and Psychiatry, 43, 573–586.

Dennis, M. L., Godley, S.H., Diamond, G., Tims, F.M., Babor, T., Donaldson, J., Liddle, H., Titus, J.C., Kaminer, Y., Webb, C. & Hamilton, N. (in press). Main findings of the Cannabis Youth Treatment (CYT) randomized field experiment. Journal of Substance Abuse Treatment.

Dennis, M. L., Titus, J. C., Diamond, G., Donaldson, J., Godley, S.H., Tims, F.M., Webb, C., Kaminer, Y., Babor, T., Roebuck, M.C., Godley, M.D., Hamilton, N., Liddle, H., & Scott, C. K. (2002). The Cannabis Youth Treatment (CYT) experiment: Rationale, study design, and analysis plans. Addiction, 97: suppl 1, 58–69.

Dennis, M., Titus, J. C., Diamond, G., Donaldson, J., Godley, S. H., Tims, F. M. (2002). The Cannabis Youth Treatment (CYT) experiment: Rationale, study design and analysis plans. Society for the Study of Addiction to Alcohol and Other Drugs, 97, 16–34.

Dimeff, L. A., & Marlatt, G. A. (1995). Relapse prevention. In R. K. Hester., & W. R. Miller., (Eds.), Handbook of alcoholism treatment approaches: Effective alternatives pp. 176–194. Boston: Allyn and Bacon.

Dishion, T. J., McCord, J.,& Poulin, F. (1999). When interventions harm: Peer groups and problem behavior. American Psychologist, 54, 755–764.

Dishion, T. J., Poulin, F., & Barraston, B. (2002). Peer group dynamics associated with iatrogenic effects in group interventions with high-risk young adolescents. New Directions for Child and Adolescent Development, 91, 79–92.

Donahue, B., Arzin, N. H., Lawson, H., Friedlander, J., Teichner, G., & Rindsberg, J. (1998). Improving initial session attendance of substance abusing and conduct disordered adolescents: A controlled study. Journal of Child and Adolescent Substance Abuse, 8, 1–13.

Downey, G., & Coyne, J. C. (1990). Children of depressed parents: An integrative review. Psychological Bulletin, 108(1), 50–76.

Eggert, L. L., Thompson, E. A., & Herting, J. R. (1994). Preventing adolescent drug abuse and high school dropout through an intensive school-based social network development program. American Journal of Health Promotion, 8, 202–215.

Forehand, R., Miller, K. S., Dutra, R., & Chance, M. W. (1997). Role of parenting in adolescent deviant behavior: Replication across and within two ethnic groups. Journal of Consulting and Clinical Psychology, 65(6), 1036–1041.

French, M. T., Roebuck, C., Dennis, M. L., Diamond, G., Godley, S. H., Tims, F., Webb, C., Herell, J. M. (2002). The economic cost of outpatient marijuana treatment for adolescents:findings from a multi-site field experiment. Addiction, 97: suppl 1, 84–97.

Friedman, A. S. (1989) Family therapy vs. parent groups: Effects on adolescent drug abusers. The American Journal of Family Therapy, 17, 335–347.

Gecas, V., & Seff, M. A. (1990). Social class and self-esteem: Psychological centrality, compensation and the relative effects of work and home. Social Psychology Quarterly, 53(2). 165–173.

Gladding, S. T. (2002). Family therapy: History, theory, and practice. Upper Saddle River, NJ: Prentice-Hall.

Godley, S. H., Meyers, R. S., & Smith, J. E. (2002). The adolescent community reinforcement approach for adolescent cannabis users. Substance Abuse and Mental Health Services Administration; Cannabis Youth Treatment (CYT) Manual Series, 4. Rockville, MD: Center for Substance Abuse.

Graham, K., Annis, H. M., & Brett, P. J. (1996). A controlled field trial of group versus individual cognitive-behavioral training for relapse prevention. Addiction, 91, 1127–1139.

Haley, J. (1976). Problem-solving therapy. San Francisco, CA: Jossey-Bass.

Hamilton, N., Brantly, L., Tims, F., Angelovich, N., & McDougall, B. (2002). Family support network (FSN) for adolescent cannabis users. Substance Abuse and Mental Health Services Administration; Cannabis Youth Treatment (CYT) Manual Series, 4. Rockville, MD: Center for Substance Abuse.

Henggeler, S. W. (1999). Multisytemic Therapy: an overview of clinical procedures, outcomes, and policy implications. Child Psychology & Psychiatry Review, 4, 2–10.

Henggeler, S. W., Clingempeel, W. G., & Brondino, M. J. (2002). Four-year follow-up of multisystemic therapy with substance-abusing and substance-dependent juvenile offenders. Journal of the American Academy of Child and Adolescent Psychiatry, 41, 868–874.

Henggeler, S. W., Melton, G. B., & Smith, L. A. (1992). Family preservation using multisystemic therapy: An effective alternative to incarcerating serious juvenile offenders. Journal of Consulting and Clinical Psychology, 60(6), 953–961.

Henggeler, S. W., Pickrel, S. G., & Brondino, M. J. (1999). Multisystemic treatment of Substance-Abusing and Dependent Delinquents: Outcomes, treatment, fidelity, and transportability. Mental Health Services Research, 1, 171–184.

Henggeler, S. W., Schoenwald, S. K., Borduin, C. M., Rowland, M. D., & Cunningham, P. B. (1998). Multisystemic treatment of antisocial behavior in children and adolescents. New York, NY: Guilford Press.

Higgins, S. T., Budney, A. J., Bickel, W. K., Badger, G. I, Foerg, F. E., & Ogden, D. (1995). Outpatient behavioral treatment for cocaine dependence: One-year outcome. Experimental Clinical Psychopharmacology, 3, 205–212.

Hops, H., Duncan, T. E., Duncan, S. C., & Stoolmiller, M. (1996). Parent substance use as a predictor of adolescent use: A six-year lagged analysis. Annals of Behavioral Medicine, 18, 157–164.

Huey, S. J., Henggeler, S. W., Brondino, M. J., & Pickrel, S. G. (2000). Mechanisms of change in multisystemic therapy: Reducing delinquent behavior through therapist adherence and improved family and peer functioning. Journal of Consulting and Clinical Psychology, 68, 451–467.

Jacob, T. (Ed). (1987). Family interaction and psychopathology: Theories, methods, and findings. New York, NY: Plenum Press.

Jones, R., Peveler, R. C., Hope, R. A., & Fairburn, C. G. (1993). Changes during treatment for bulimia nervosa: A comparison of three psychological treatments. Behavior Research and Therapy, 31, 479–485.

Kadden, R. M., Cooney, N. L., Getter, H., & Litt, M. B. (1989). Matching alcoholics to coping skills or interactional therapies: Posttreatment results. Journal of Consulting and Clinical Psychology, 57, 698–704.

Kaminer, Y. (2003). Aftercare for Adolescents With Alcohol and other Substance Use Disorders (AOSUD): Feasibility and Acceptability of Phone Therapy. The 2nd Annual Meeting of the Society for Adolescent Substance Abuse Treatment Effectiveness (SASATE), June, Miami, FL.

Kaminer, Y., Haberek, R., Napolitano, C., & Burleson, J. (2003). Aftercare for Adolescents With Alcohol and other Substance Use Disorders: Feasibility and Acceptability of Phone Therapy. Presented at the 2nd Annual Meeting of the Society for Adolescent Substance Abuse Treatment Effectiveness (SASATE), June 20, Miami, FL.

Kaminer, Y. (2000). Contingency management reinforcement procedures for adolescent substance abuse. Journal of the American Academy of Child and Adolescent Psychiatry, 39, 1324–1326

Kaminer, Y. (2001). Adolescent substance abuse treatment: Where do we go from here? Psychiatric Services, 52, 147–149.

Kaminer, Y., & Burleson, J. (1999). Psychotherapies for adolescent substance abusers: 15-month follow-up. American Journal of Addictions, 8, 114–119.

Kaminer, Y., Blitz, C., Burleson, J., Sussman, J., & Rounsaville, B. J. (1998a). Psychotherapies for Adolescent Substance Abusers: Treatment outcome. Journal of Nervous and Mental Disease, 186, 684–690

Kaminer, Y., Blitz, C., Burleson, J.A., Kadden, R.M., & Rounsaville, B.J. (1998b). Measuring treatment process in cognitive-behavioral and interactional group therapies for adolescent substance abusers. Journal of Nervous and Mental Disease, 186, 407–413.

Kaminer, Y., Burleson, J., & Goldberger, R. (2002). Psychotherapies for adolescent substance abusers: Short- and long-term outcomes. Journal of Nervous and Mental Disease, 190, 737–745.

Liddle, H. A. (1999). Theory development in a family-based therapy for adolescent drug abuse. Journal of Clinical Child Psychology, 28, 521–532.

Liddle, H. A. (2001). Multidimensional Family Therapy Treatment (MDFT) for the adolescent cannabis users. Cannabis Youth Treatment (CYT) Manual series (Vol. 5). Rockville, MD: CSAT, SAMHSA.

Liddle, H. A. (2002). Advances in family-based therapy for adolescent substance abuse: Findings from the Multidimensional Family Therapy research program. In L.S. Harris (Ed.), Problems of Drug Dependence 2001: Proceedings of the 63rd Annual Scientific Meeting (pp. 113–115), NIDA Research Monograph No. 182, NIH Publication NO. 02–5097. Bethesda, MD: National Institute on Drug Abuse.

Liddle, H. A., & Dakof, G. A. (1995). Efficacy of family therapy for drug abuse: promising but not definitive. Journal of Marital and Family Therapy, 21, 511–543.

Liddle, H. A., Dakof, G. A., Diamond, G. S., Parker, G. S., Barrett, K., & Tejeda, M. (2001). Multidimensional family therapy for adolescent substance abuse: Results of a randomized clinical trial. American Journal of Drug and Alcohol Abuse, 27, 651–687.

Liddle, H. A., Dakof, G. A., Parker, K., Diamond, G. S., Barrett, K., & Tejeda, M. (2001). Multidimensional family therapy for adolescent drug abuse: Results of a randomized clinical trial. American Journal of Drug Alcohol Abuse, 27, 651–688.

Liddle, H. A., Dakof, G. A., Turner, R. M., & Tejada, M. (in press). Treating adolescent substance abuse: a comparison of individual and family therapy interventions. NIDA Monograph on the June 2001 CPDD Conference (paper presented at Symposium on Adolescent Drug Abuse Treatment).

Liddle, H. A., Rowe, C. L., Quille, T. J., Dakof, G. A., Mills, D. S., Sakran, E. (2002). Transporting a research-based adolescent drug treatment into practice. Journal of Substance Abuse Treatment, 22, 1–13.

Litt, M. B., Kadden, R. M., Cooney, N. L., & Kabela, E. (2003). Coping skills and treatment outcomes in cognitive-behavioral and interactional group therapy for alcoholism. Journal of Consulting and Clinical Psychology, 71, 118–128.

Madanes, C. (1981). Strategic family therapy. San Francisco, CA: Jossey Bass.

Maisto S. A., Connors, G. J., & Zywiak, W. H. (2000). Alcohol treatment , changes in coping skills, self-efficacy, and levels of alcohol use and related problems 1 year following treatment initiation. Psychology of Addictive Disorders, 14, 257–266.

Marlatt, G. A. & Gordon, J. R. (Eds.). (1985). Relapse prevention: Maintenance strategies in the treatment of addictive behaviors. New York: Gilford Press.

Marques, A. C., & Formigoni, M. F. (2001). Comparison of individual and group cognitive-behavioral therapy for alcohol and/or drug dependent patients. Addiction, 96, 835–846.

Miller, W. R., Brown, J. M., Simpson, T. L., Handmaker, N. S., Bien, T. H., Luckie, L. F., Montgomery, H. A., Hester, R. K., & Tonigan, J. S. (1995). What works? A methodological analysis of the alcohol treatment outcome literature. In R. K. Hester & W. R. Miller (Eds.), Handbook of alcoholism treatment approaches (2nd ed.) (pp. 12–44). Needham Heights, MA: Allyn & Bacon.

Minuchin, S. (1974). Families and family therapy. Cambridge, MA: Harvard University Press.

Monti, P. M., Abrams, D. B., Kadden, R. M., & Cooney, N. L. (1989). Treating alcohol dependence. London: Gilford Press.

Monti, P. M., Rohsenow, D. J., Colby, S. M., & Abrams, D. B. (1995). Coping and social skills training. In W. R. Miller., & R. K. Hester., (Ed.), Handbook of alcoholism treatment approaches: Effective alternatives (2nd ed., pp. 221–241). New York: Allyn & Bacon.

Monti, P. M., Rohsenow, D. J., Rubonis, A. N., Niaua, R. S., Sirota, A. D., & Colby, S. M. (1993). Cue exposeure with coping skills treatment for male alcoholics: A preliminary investigation. Journal of Consulting and Clinical Psychology, 61, 1011–1019.

Morgenstern, J., & Longabaugh, R. (2000). Cognitive-behavioral treatment for alcohol dependence: A review of evidence for its hypothesized mechanisms of action. Addiction, 95, 1475–1490.

Myers, M. G., & Brown, S. A. (1996). The adolescent relapse coping questionnaire: psychometric validation. Journal of Studies on Alcohol, 57, 40–46.

Myers, M. G., Brown, S., & Mott V. (1993). Coping as a predictor of adolescent substance abuse treatment outcome. Journal of Substance Abuse, 5, 15–29.

Ozechowski, T. J., & Liddle, H. A. (2000). Family-based therapy for adolescent drug abuse: Knowns and unknowns. Clinical Child and Family Psychology Review, 3, 269–298.

Pickrel, S. G., & Henggeler, S. W. (1996). Multisystemic therapy for adolescent substance abuse and dependence. Adolescent Substance Abuse and Dual Disorders, 5, 201–211.

Project MATCH (1997). Matching alcoholism treatments to client heterogeneity: Project MATCH post-treatment drinking outcomes. Journal of Studies on Alcohol, 58, 7–29.

Robbins, M. S., Bachrach, K., & Szapocznik, J. (2002). Bridging the research-practice gap in adolescent substance abuse treatment: The case of brief strategic family therapy. Journal of Substance Abuse Treatment, 23 ,123–132.

Sampl, S., & Kadden, R. (2001). Motivational Enhancement Therapy and Cognitive Behavioral Therapy for Adolescent Cannabis Users:5 sessions. Cannabis Youth Treatment Series Volume 1. Center for Substance Abuse Treatment, Rockville, MD.

Santisteban, D. A., Coatsworth, J. D., Perez-Vidal, A., Mitrani, V., Jean-Gilles, M., & Szapocznik, J. (1997). Brief structural/strategic family therapy with African American and Hispanic high-risk youth. Journal of Community Psychology, 25, 453–471.

Santisteban, D. A., Perez-Vidal, A., Coatsworth, J. D., & Kurtines, W. M. (2003). Efficacy of brief strategic family therapy in modifying Hispanic adolescent behavior problems and substance use. Journal of Family Psychology, 17, 121–133.

Schmidt, S. E., Liddle, H. A., & Dakof, G. A. (1996). Changes in parenting practices and adolescent drug abuse during multidimensional family therapy. Journal of Family Psychology, 10, 12. 27.

Stanton, M. D., & Shadish, W. R. (1997). Outcome, attrition, and family-couples treatment for drug abuse: A meta-analysis and review of the controlled, comparative studies. Psychological Bulletin, 122, 170–191.

Stanton, M. D., Todd, T. C., & Associates (1982). The family therapy of drug abuse and addiction. New York, NY: Gardner Press.

Steinglass, P. (1980). Assessing families in their own homes. American Journal of Psychiatry, 137, 1523–1529.

Stitzer, M. L., Bigelow, G. E., & Liebson, I. (1979). Reinforcement of drug abstinence: A behavioral approach to drug abuse treatment. Rockville, MD: NIDA.

Szapocznik, J., Hervis, O. E., & Schwartz, S. (2002). Brief strategic family therapy for adolescent drug abuse. Rockford, MD: National Institute on Drug Abuse.

Szapocznik, J., Kurtines, W. M., Foote, F. H., Perez-Vidal A., & Hervis, O. (1986). Conjoint versus one-person family therapy: Further evidence for the effectiveness of conducting family therapy through one person with drug-abusing adolescents. Journal of Consulting and Clinical Psychology, 54, 395–397.

US Bureau of the Census (1991). Statistical abstracts of the United States 1991 (111th ed.). Washington DC: US Government printing office.

Waldron, H. B. (1997). Adolescent substance abuse and family therapy outcome: A review of randomized trials. In T. H. Ollendick, & R. J. Prinz (Eds.). Advances in clinical child psychology (pp.199–234). New York, NY: Plenum Press.

Waldron, H. B., Slesnick, N., Brody, J. L., Turner, C. W., & Peterson, T. R. (2001). Treatment outcomes for adolescent substance abuse at 4- and 7-month assessments. Journal of Consulting and Clinical Psychology, 69, 802–813.

Waldron, H. B., Slesnick, N., Brody, J. L., Turner, C. ., & Peterson, T. R. (2001). Treatment outcomes for adolescent substance abuse at 4- and 7-month assessments. Journal of Consulting and Clinical Psychology, 69, 802–813.

Waldron, H. B. (1997). Adolescent substance abuse and family therapy outcome: A review of randomized trials. In T. H. Ollendick., & R. J., Prinz (Eds.), Advances in Clinical Child Psychology, Volume 19 (pp. 199–234). New York: Plenum.

Wampold, B.E, Mondin, G.W., Moody, M., & Hyun-Nie, A. (1999). Meta-analysis of outcome studies comparing bona fide psychotherapies: empirically, "all must have prizes." Psychological Bulletin, 122, 203–215.

Webb, C., Scudder, M., Kaminer, Y., & Kadden, R. (2002). Motivational enhancement therapy and cognitive behavioral therapy for adolescent cannabis users: 7 sessions. Cannabis Youth Treatment Series Volume 1. Rockville, MD: Center for Substance Abuse Treatment.

Williams, R. J., & Chang, S. Y. (2000). A comprehensive and comparative review of adolescent substance abuse treatment outcome. Clinical Psychology: Science and Practice, 7(2), 138–166.

Wilson, G. T. (1999). Rapid response to cognitive behavior therapy. Clinical Psychology: Science and Practice, 6, 289–292.

Woody, G. E., Luborsky, L., & McLellan, A. T. (1983). Psychotherapy for opiate addicts: Does it help? Archives of General Psychiatry, 40, 639–645.

19

Assessment Issues in Adolescent Drug Abuse Treatment Research

Ken Winters and Tamara Fahnhorst

Abstract. Experimentation with alcohol and other drugs (AOD) is commonplace among American adolescents. Despite reduction efforts, the use of AOD by adolescents has increased over the past decade. A number of youth experience significant negative personal, societal, economic, and health ramifications, but continue to abuse AOD and develop substance use disorders (SUD). Accurate assessment of adolescent AOD use is essential in determining the prevalence of SUDs, the development of effective interventions, and the implementation of beneficial prevention initiatives. Developmental considerations are significant factors in the validity of youth AOD assessment and are detailed in this chapter.

1. Introduction

Adolescent use of alcohol and other drugs (AOD) is seemingly omnipresent and may be part of the "normal developmental trajectory for adolescents" (Shedler & Block, 1990). The National Institute on Drug Abuse (NIDA), in collaboration with Monitoring the Future, reported that despite a reduction or stabilization of the use of some drugs, a rise in AOD use among American adolescents since 1992 is largely evident (Johnston, O'Malley, & Bachman, 2003). Of 43,000 students surveyed, over one-third of eighth graders and three-quarters of twelfth graders drank in the past year. In regards to prior month usage, 19.6% of eighth graders and 48.6% of twelfth graders reported consuming alcohol.

Ken C. Winters and Tamara Fahnhorst • Center for Adolescent Substance Abuse Research, University of Minnesota, Minneapolis, Minnesota 55455.

Beyond experimentation, adolescent AOD use behaviors can progress to a substance abuse or dependence disorder. Of 74,000 students surveyed in Minnesota who used AOD over the past year, 13.8% of ninth graders and 22.7% of twelfth graders met substance abuse criteria (Diagnostic and Statistical Manual of Mental Disorders-IV; DSM-IV; Harrison, Fulkerson, & Beebe, 1998). In this same study, 8.2% of ninth graders and 10.5% of twelfth graders met criteria for substance dependence. Data from the recent National Survey on Drug Use and Health revealed that of 12–17 year olds, eight percent of this extensive epidemiological sample met criteria for either substance abuse or dependence (Substance Abuse and Mental Health Services Administration; SAMHSA, 2001).

Personal, as well as societal, ramifications of adolescent drug abuse are profound. School failure, risky sexual behavior (MacKenzie, 1993), delinquency, incarceration, suicidality (Kaminer, 1994; Shedler & Block, 1990), motor vehicle injuries/fatalities (Kokotailo, 1995), and significant health care costs (DAWN, 1996) are all highly correlated with adolescent AOD use. Accurate assessment of adolescent AOD use is therefore crucial to understanding the prevalence, proliferation, and exacerbation of teen substance abuse and ensuing treatment and prevention initiatives. The following chapter will outline the issues surrounding the assessment of adolescent AOD use and substance use disorders (SUD). Specifically, the chapter will discuss developmental considerations of AOD use; the types of instruments in the field; key AOD problem severity and psychosocial factors measured by instruments in the field; and methods and sources of data collection.

2. Developmental Considerations in AOD Use Assessment

Pediatricians and general practitioners have come to understand and emphasize the complexities involving the physical health assessment and treatment of adolescents. Issues regarding physical, cognitive, and emotional development, confidentiality, and emerging reproductive health are factors that differentiate adolescent physical health care from child and adult prevention and intervention initiatives. Like physicians, mental health professionals can benefit from applying developmental considerations to the psychological domains that pertain to the accurate assessment and treatment of adolescent drug abuse and much needed prevention initiatives.

Unfortunately, the foundation for AOD use disorders is rooted in longstanding beliefs centered around adult characteristics; thus, the applicability to adolescents has been questioned (Martin & Winters, 1998). Whereas much is known about factors involving adult use and SUDs, research reveals that adolescents manifest behavioral, psychological, and physiological characteristics differently than adults (Kaminer, 1991). For example, patterns of use differ between the age groups, as does the development of an SUD. We discuss below seven significant developmental dimensions of adolescent AOD involvement that require attention in the assessment process.

2.1. *AOD Involvement*

We begin with the important issue of adequately distinguishing normative and developmental roles played by drug use in this age group. It is difficult to determine when adolescent drug use has negative long-term implications versus short-term effects and social payoff. In a strict sense, a "normal" trajectory for adolescents is to experiment with the use of psychoactive substances. As described in the seminal work by Kandel and colleagues (Kandel, 1975; Yagamuchi & Kandel, 1984), experiences by adolescents with substance use most often first take place in a social context with the use of "gateway" substances such as alcohol and cigarettes, which are legal for adults and readily available to minors. While almost all adolescents experiment with gateway drugs, progressively fewer of them advance to later and more serious levels of substance use, including the use of marijuana and other illicit drugs (Kandel, 1975). Moreover, the presence of some abuse symptoms is not all that rare among adolescents who use substances, even if not at heavy levels (Harrison et al., 1998). Also, it has been observed that moderate alcohol users reveal relatively high rates of personal consequences associated with such use (Kaczynski & Martin, 1995).

Thus, it is important to conceptualize AOD use along a continuum. Center for Substance Abuse Treatment (CSAT, 1999) offers this continuum for heuristic purposes: 1) *Abstinence;* 2) *Experimental Use:* Minimal use, typically associated with recreational activities; often limited to alcohol use; 3) *Early Abuse:* More established use; often involving more than one drug; greater frequency; adverse consequences begin to emerge; 4) *Abuse:* Regular and frequent use over an extended period; several adverse consequences emerge; 5) *Dependence:* Continued regular use despite repeated severe consequences; signs of tolerance; adjustment of activities to accommodate drug-seeking and drug use; failed attempts to reduce or discontinue use.

Early, accurate, and ongoing assessment of adolescent AOD use is important in distinguishing typical use from problematic AOD use behaviors. Unfortunately, there are several factors that make this challenging. Of significant concern is the fact that AOD use can progress rapidly from experimentation to abuse or dependence for teens. Martin and colleagues (1995) reported that some adolescents can be diagnosed with abuse or dependence in as little as 12 months after their initial use. This is in contrast to adults whereby the development of an SUD typically takes much longer. Furthermore, it has been documented that teens often underestimate or ignore severe potential consequences. A growing evidence of health outcomes are often minimized (Lewinsohn, Rohde, & Seeley, 1996) while teens engage in a risky lifestyle riddled with significant AOD use that they inaccurately feel they can control (Botvin & Tortu, 1988). Other factors that may hinder early assessment include the common adolescent that reveal lack of respect for authority, are egocentric, and carryout risk-taking behaviors. Moreover, adolescents demonstrate delays in social and emotional functioning (Noam & Houlihan, 1990) and may lack the necessary insight to accurately report their use of AOD (Winters, 2001).

Despite these obstacles, there are several AOD use behaviors that are associated with the likelihood of progression toward the end of the AOD use continuum. Perhaps none is more predictive than age of onset. It has been replicated many times in studies that the earlier the use, the greater likelihood that an adolescent will progress toward abuse and dependence (Winters, 1994). Additional important factors to consider include: a) regular use of a drug increases the likelihood of development an SUD; b) polydrug assessment is crucial because the use of more than one drug increases the odds of meeting criteria for an SUD for one of the used drugs (Winters, 1994); c) preadolescent cigarette use predicts early adolescent marijuana use (Clark, Kirisci, & Moss, 1998) and; d) marijuana use during early adolescence predicts the progression of involvement with other illicit substances (Kandel & Davies, 1996).

2.2. *Abuse and Dependence*

AOD use that goes beyond experimentation and evolves into problematic involvement is formally delineated by the DSM-IV (1994) into two categories: *abuse* and *dependence.* Substance abuse is characterized by negative health and social consequences whereby one or more of the following are endorsed: a) school, home, or work status is compromised; b) substances are used in physically hazardous situations (e.g., driving under the influence); c) recurrent substance-related legal problems; and d) exacerbation of social and interpersonal problems due to AOD use. Whereas abuse symptoms are expected to be associated with clinically significant impairment or distress, they are meant to occur prior to and fall short of dependence symptoms on a severity spectrum. The method is variably successful in fulfilling these intentions (Martin & Winters, 1998).

In contrast to abuse, psychological and physiological factors play a substantial role in the life of an individual who meets criteria for substance dependence. These people continue to use AOD despite significant negative psychosocial ramifications while biological factors cause significant health consequences. Specifically, criteria for dependence is met if an individual meets three or more of the following: a) an individual either requires more of a substance for a similar effect or experiences a reduction in the effect produced by the use of the same amount of a substance (tolerance); b) withdrawal symptoms are experienced (e.g., shakes, dizziness, confusion, etc.); c) larger quantities of the substance are taken or it is used for longer periods than intended; d) efforts to cut down or control use are unsuccessful; e) substantial amount of time is spent getting, using, or recovering from use; f) leisure activities are reduced or eliminated; and g) use of AOD is continued despite the knowledge that it may have caused or exacerbated physical or psychological problems. In DSM-IV, substance abuse and substance dependence are mutually exclusive, and the diagnoses of abuse and dependence are hierarchically arranged (i.e., a dependence diagnosis precludes an abuse diagnosis).

The applicability of SUD criteria for the adolescent developmental period has been called into question (Martin & Winters, 1998). There is evidence that symptoms of abuse do not always precede symptoms of dependence, contrary to the notion that abuse should be a prodromal category with respect to dependence (Martin, Kacyzniski, Maisto & Tarter, 1996). Some adolescents as well as adults "fall through the cracks" of the DSM-IV system. That is, some individuals meet criteria only for one or two of the seven dependence symptoms (three or more symptoms are required for a diagnosis), and no abuse symptoms, and therefore do not qualify for any diagnosis (Hasin & Paykin, 1998; Pollock & Martin, 1999). These "diagnostic orphans" have been found to range from 10–30% among adolescents in clinical settings (Lewinsohn et al., 1996; Harrison et al., 1998; Pollock & Martin, 1999).

In addition to the diagnostic orphans, other questionable applications of SUD criteria arise in the assessment of adolescent AOD use. One such application is an important criteria for dependence, tolerance, which appears to have low specificity because the development of tolerance for drugs is likely a normal developmental phenomena which happens to most adolescents; this is particularly the case for alcohol (Chung, Martin, Winters, & Langenbucher, 1991). Withdrawal has limited utility because it occurs at very low base rates in the adolescent population, even in clinical samples (Martin et al., 1995; Winters, Latimer, & Stinchfield, 1999). Also, the criteria for DSM-IV substance abuse produces a great deal of heterogeneity because these symptoms cover a broad range of problems and only one symptom is required to meet the criteria.

Nonetheless, the application of formal diagnostic criteria for youth clinical samples is necessary in several settings, such as when researchers need to categorically describe their study participants in a language familiar to other researchers, and when clinicians have to assess and record a valid diagnosis to justify the need for treatment. Fortunately, several comprehensive structured and semi-structured interviews for evaluating SUDs have been developed for use with adolescent populations (CSAT, 1999). Further discussion pertaining to the tools utilized in adolescent AOD assessment is outlined later in this chapter.

2.3. *Psychological Benefits*

One factor that may entice adolescents to experiment with AOD involves the psychological benefits they may receive from substance use. Social acceptance, elevated mood, recreational enjoyment, and stress reduction are all outcomes adolescents may experience from AOD use (Petraitis, Flay, & Miller, 1995). An important finding in one study revealed that of these psychological benefits, social conformity and mood enhancement were found to be more important to adolescents who have a substance use dependence disorder than to those who use AOD infrequently (Henly & Winters, 1988). The impact these psychological benefits may have on the allurement and exacerbation of AOD use among adolescents emphasizes the importance of effective prevention and early intervention efforts. These initiatives need to underscore the detrimental psychological and physical ramifications AOD use can have on teens in an attempt to outweigh the enticing benefits substance use appears to have on youth.

2.4. *Psychosocial Factors*

Contrary to the benefits adolescents may experience from AOD use, they can also can experience numerous psychosocial ramifications. Measurement of these dimensions provides beneficial information regarding the extent of the AOD use, aids in treatment planning, and provides data to monitor treatment efficacy. The protocol should include the assessment of an adolescent's history of legal problems, evidence of deteriorated relationships with family and friends, status of school and employment experiences (e.g., dropping grades, suspension, being fired), extent of sexual promiscuity, and quality and quantity of leisure or extracurricular activities.

Peer issues are often recognized as one of the most important psychosocial factors in the onset and maintenance of AOD use. Peer influence has been a factor in the quantity of AOD consumed as well as in the types of substances used. Higher rates of AOD use were found among adolescents whose friends used substances compared to those who friends did not (Farrell & Danish, 1993; Winters, Latimer, Stinchfield, & Henly, 1999). Guo and colleagues (2002) found that high levels of peer involvement with antisocial behavior predicted higher risk of initiation of illicit drug use among adolescents. Other researchers found a nearly 6-fold increase in drug use risk among children who associated with peers who used drugs verses those who did not (Chilcoat & Breslau, 1999). Additional factors related to peer influences on adolescent AOD use include peer attitudes and expectancies pertaining to substance use, and peer attachment (Dishion, Capaldi, Spracklen, & Fuzhong, 1995; Hawkins, Catalano, & Miller, 1992; Patterson, Forgatch, Yoerger, & Stoolmiller, 1998). Understanding the complexities involved in the specific aspects by which peers influence adolescent AOD is most likely complex, nonetheless. In fact, a culturally diverse, three-year study of over 6,000 sixth through ninth grade youth reported a bidirectional relationship between levels of adolescents' alcohol use and levels of alcohol use among their peers (Bray, Adams, Getz, & McQueen, 2003).

2.5. *Co-existing Mental Health Disorders*

Adolescents who are involved with AOD often have co-existing psychological disorders (Clark & Bukstein, 1998). Rohde and colleagues (1996) reported that among adolescents who were either abusing or dependent on alcohol, 80 percent also had some other form of psychopathology. Therefore, AOD use assessment should not only address the problems the teen is experiencing with alcohol and other drugs, but also identify comorbid psychiatric disorders. Doing so may be a key element in the projected success of an SUD intervention and subsequent relapse prevention.

Mental health disorders that commonly co-occur with SUDs in adolescents include ADHD, conduct disorders, depressive disorders, and anxiety disorders. Some researchers have found ADHD to be predictive of AOD use and related problems (Mannuzza, Klein, Blessler, Malloy, & LaPadula, 1993; Milberger, Beiderman, Faraone, Chen, & Jones, 1997). Some controversy over this association exits however, for other studies have found that conduct disorder comorbid with ADHD was the mediating factor that predicted AOD use or abuse (Biederman, Wilens, Mick, Farone, Weber, Curtis, Thornell, Pfister, Jetton, & Soriano, 1997; Clark, Parker, & Lynch, 1999; Lynskey & Fergusson, 1995). Yet others have found an independent correlation between ADHD and SUD beyond that attributed to conduct disorder (Thompson, Riggs, Mikulich, & Crowley, 1996). Determining the independent or conjoint impact ADHD and conduct disorder has in regards to the onset of AOD misuse for adolescents remains unclear and further research is needed.

In addition to disruptive behavior disorders, mood disorders such as depression and anxiety have been found to be correlated with AOD disorders. Clark & Sayette (1993) reported that emotional dysregulation, which is associated with depression and anxiety, may pose risk factors associated with AOD use disorders. Other studies reported that early use of alcohol was found to significantly predict later major depressive disorder (Brook, Brook, Zhang, Cohen, & Whiteman, 2002), diagnosis of an SUD was predictive of later major depressive disorder in adolescents females, (Rao, Daley, & Hammen, 2000) and adolescents with an SUD reported higher rates of affective disorders and sympotmology, especially for females (Deykin, Levy, & Wells, 1987; Martin, Lynch, Pollock, & Clark, 2000).

Clearly, causal relationships between SUDs and psychological disorders are yet to be fully during determined. Thus, it is vital to consider the potential influences of both SUDs and other psychological disorders during assessment. Of importance is the need to carefully pinpoint the onset and course of possible psychological symptoms and differentiating these behaviors from the onset and course of AOD involvement and resultant symptoms of abuse and dependence. A carefully constructed, temporally-oriented interview is necessary in order to validly distinguish bonafide symptoms of psychological disorders and the mental and behavioral effects of AOD involvement (Winters, 1994).

2.6. *Family Factors*

Another developmental element associated with adolescent AOD use is that of familial risk factors. These parental risk factors involve both genetic and environmental characteristics that elevate a child's risk for AOD use. Parental modeling of drinking and drug use can be powerful catalysts for adolescent SUD (Moss, Clark, & Kirisci, 1997). McGue (1999) reported that children whose parents suffered from an SUD were at increased risk for the development of an SUD. Furthermore, parental psychopathology can also exacerbate risk for early and problematic drug use by teens (Rose, 1998). Researchers have also reported higher rates of affective disorders and related symptomology in children of parents who had an SUD (Clark, Moss, Kirisci, Mezzich, Miles, & Ott, 1997; Earls, Jung, & Cloninger, 1988; Hill & Muka, 1996). Finally, antisocial behavior and related disorders are commonly found in children whose parents had an SUD (Clark et al., 1997; Earls et al., 1988; Zucker, Fitzgerald, & Moses, 1995).

2.7. *Neurobiology*

AODs do more than affect the behavior of adolescents; they also have a direct impact on brain functioning in the young person. The adolescent brain, by not being fully developed until early adulthood (e.g., some parts of the brain undergo 50% transformations during adolescence) is vulnerable to the effects of AOD. For example, adolescents with a history of extensive alcohol use have been reported to have a smaller hippocampus, the brain region responsible for converting information into memory, and to reveal memory deficits and other neuropsychological impairments resulting from reduced brain activation during memory tasks (Spear, 2000). Work in laboratory animals provides confirming evidence that adolescent exposure to drugs can influence later neural behavioral functioning. For instance, alcohol exposure during adolescence has been shown to result in long-term disruptions in brain electrical activity in the hippocampus and in other brain areas. After chronic exposure during adolescence, rats have been reported to exhibit greater cognitive disruptions and a greater sensitivity to later alcohol-induced memory disruptions than animals receiving equivalent exposure in adulthood (Markwiese, Acheson, Leven, Wislosn, & Swartzwelder, 1998).

Research using laboratory animals has also shown adolescents to differ considerably from adults in their initial responsiveness to alcohol. Adolescent rats show a *decreased* sensitivity to the adverse effects of alcohol when compared to older rats. Adolescent rats also appear to require a higher initial amount of alcohol to reduce anxiety then to adults (Varlinskaya & Spear, in press). These findings, which suggest that adolescent rats are less sensitive to alcohol than mature individuals, serve to promote higher alcohol consumption. That is, moderation in drinking by adults occurs as the individual experiences the compounding adverse effects of alcohol. The decreased sensitivity to alcohol in adolescents would, therefore, minimize the dampening effect that serves to alert the user that he or she is intoxicated.

3. Basic Instruments for Determining AOD Involvement and Related Problems

Significant contributions by researchers over the past decade have provided clinicians and researchers with numerous instruments to accurately assess adolescent drug use behaviors (Lecesse & Waldron, 1994). Many measures have been normed on adolescents of varying ages, are limited in length, and written conducive to young people's comprehension levels. Some tools are designed to quickly identify youth at risk for AOD problem behavior, while the purpose of other measures is to provide extensive information that allows diagnostic assessment of SUD as well as other coexisting psychiatric disorders. A summary of several adolescent screening and comprehensive assessment measures is provided in Table 1. Inclusion in the table required that the instrument was developed specifically for adolescents and that its psychometric properties has been reported in a peer-reviewed publication. Several extensive summaries of such measures are available via web sites, such as the Screening Assessment of Adolescents with a Substance Use Disorder (Treatment Improvements Protocol Series: TIPS #31) (CSAT; www.samhsa.gov/csat/csat.htm) and the National Institute on Drug Abuse (NIDA; www.nida.nih.gov). Printed reviews of adolescent AOD assessment measures included journal articles (Lecesse & Waldron, 1994; Martin & Winters, 1998), and chapters in a handbook (Winters, 2001).

3.1. *Screening Measures*

A wide range of school personnel, health professionals, clinicians, and researchers can benefit from screening instruments that quickly and accurately identify adolescents who may be abusing AOD and may be at risk for developing a SUD. These screening tools are typically administered in a self-report paper-pencil format and can measure a single dimension or briefly assess multiple areas of risk. Screening instruments can be organized into four categories: alcohol use only, non-alcohol drug use, non-specific drug use including alcohol, and "multi-screen." Instruments in the latter category, in addition to AOD involvement, quickly survey a teenager's level of functioning in areas such as fulfillment of educational goals, recreational activities, social skill development, delinquent behavior, physical health, and relationships with family and peers.

3.2. *Comprehensive Measures*

In contrast to the brief screening instruments, comprehensive measures provide a thorough evaluation of multiple domains and can clarify status on indicators that were flagged on screening instruments. Comprehensive measures not only render extensive information pertaining to the types of AOD used, the pattern of use, and extent of drug involvement, but also ascertain information on the psychosocial factors that may precipitate, exacerbate, and sustain AOD use problems. Comprehensive measures can be organized into three categories: diagnostic interviews, problem-focused interviews, and multi-scale questionnaires, all of which are detailed below.

Diagnostic Interviews. These DSM-based tools typically adhere to a structured format whereby the administrator uses standardized questions and follow-up queries guided by a decision tree configuration. The individual conducting the interview should be thoroughly trained in the administration of the measure, as well as have adequate knowledge in psychopathology. While some of the diagnostic interviews are developed for the adolescent client, others are designed for the parent. These interviews ascertain diagnostic information pertaining to multiple psychological domains including AOD abuse and dependence.

Problem-Focused Interviews. In contrast to the diagnostic interview, the problem-focused interview not only measures AOD use history but also addresses the ramifications of AOD use and other aspects of psychosocial functioning that may perpetuate or exacerbate AOD use. Relationships with parents and peers, leisure activities, school and employment status, involvement with criminal or other rebellious activity against authority, and medical status are assessed by this type of comprehensive measure. The problem-focused interview was adapted from the well-known adult Addiction Survey Index (ASI; McLellan, Luborsky, Woody, and O'Brien, 1980). These measures typically utilize a severity rating scale to indicate the extent to which the client is experiencing problems associated with each domain.

Multi-scale Questionnaires. The third type of comprehensive measure is the multi-scale questionnaire. These self-administered measures assess the severity of drug use involvement and the psychosocial risk factors associated with AOD use. Although administration time ranges in length from 20 to 60 minutes, multi-scale questionnaires are easily administered by individuals with minimal training, can be completed by hand or via the computer, and some even have the benefit of computerized scoring. In addition, many of these tools provide methods for determining inconsistent or distorted responses, are normed on a clinical sample, can be scored via the computer, and maintain favorable psychometric properties (Winters, 2001)

3.3. *Assessment of AOD Use Patterns*

An accurate historical account of all categories of substance use can be difficult to ascertain from screening or comprehensive measures. The Time Line Follow-back (TLFB) method is a useful approach for documenting AOD use patterns. Sobell and Sobell (1992) developed this tool that employs a day-by-day account of alcohol use over the past year. Rather than lumping AOD use into time frames such as a year or a month as other measures do, the TLFB allows a more accurate chronological assessment of an individual's use and is beneficial in illustrating drug use patterns. Fairly extensive reliability and validity data for this method has been reported in the adult literature (Sobell & Sobell, 1992), and more recently psychometric data has supported its use with adolescents (Winters, 2001).

4. Methods of Data Collection and Sources of Information

There are several types of data collection that when combined, can provided a thorough and accurate account of a young person's AOD use history. Parents, peers, professionals and adolescents themselves can all contribute important information that will assist in determining whether an SUD is present.

4.1. *Self-Report*

The approach that renders the most comprehensive information pertaining to an adolescent's AOD use experiences is self-report. However, the validity of self-report has been called into question by a number of researchers. Some adolescents in clinical and legal settings have been found to deliberately minimize or exaggerate their drug use behaviors (Babor, Stephens, & Marlatt, 1987; Harrison, 1995; Magura & Kang, 1997). In addition, inconsistent reports of drug use pertaining to substances that were used infrequently by adolescents were found by Single, Kandel, & Johnson (1975). Stinchfield (1997) recognized that adolescents completing treatment for AOD dependence generally reported considerably more past AOD use and consequences compared to reports at the start of intervention.

Despite these concerns, a substantial amount of research does support the use of self-report as a valid and accurate measure for adolescent AOD assessment. Four major findings supporting the validity include: a) only a very small proportion of teenagers in treatment endorse questions that are highly improbable such as the use of a fictitious drug; b) the majority of youth endorse the use of illicit drugs on surveys, and youth in drug treatment settings endorse the use of drugs at a significantly higher rate than those not in a treatment setting; c) adolescent account of drug use remains consistent over time (however, this is less so for drugs used infrequently) and; d) information provided by the adolescent as a rule is in agreement with corroborating sources of information including archival record and, for the most part, urinalysis (Johnston & O'Malley, 1997; Maisto, Connors, & Allen, 1995; Winters, Anderson, Bengston, Stinchfield, & Latimer, 2000; Winters, Stinchfield, Henly, & Schwartz, 1990–91). Furthermore, two factors have been shown to improve the validity of self-report: the assurance of confidentiality (Harrell, 1997) and the utilization of urinalysis (Wish, Hoffman, & Nemes, 1997).

4.2. *Laboratory Testing*

The type of laboratory testing most familiar to researchers and clinicians to detect AOD use and validate self-report is urinalysis. The utility in the identification of drugs in the urine, particularly THC found in marijuana and hashish, can be beneficial. The most valuable aspect of urinalysis however, may not be so much the identification of drugs in the urine, but rather may lie in the message the administration of the test sends regarding a means of "revealing the truth" (CSAT, 1999).

Unfortunately, urinalysis is riddled with inaccuracies. Researchers have generally found a low correlation between adolescent self-report of AOD use and urinalysis (McLaney, Del-Boca, & Babor, 1994). Factors including quantity of drug used, time between sample collection and use of drug, alteration of the output with the ingestion of diuretics or water, adding large quantities of salt to the sample, and the use of some over-the-counter medications all contribute to inaccurate results (CSAT, 1999). A sample that has shown dilutement or high salt content, however, can provide valuable information in and of itself by sending a clear message to the clinician, employer, or researcher that the sample has been adulterated, indicating a possible attempt to conceal the truth.

4.3. *Direct Observation*

In addition to self-report and urinalysis, direct observation by a clinician or researcher for behavioral and psychological symptomology can be an objective and useful supplement to adolescent AOD use assessment. A simple checklist of items such as the presence of needle marks, unsteady gate, slurred or incoherent speech, shaking of hands or twitching of eyelids, etc., can indicate problem use.

4.4. *Parent Report*

Although parent report is critical in the identification of many mental health problems such as ADHD and conduct problems, it is not possible for parents to provide the detailed reports about the types, frequency, and quantity of AODs used by the teenager necessary for accurate SUD assessment. Winters and colleagues (2000) found, not surprisingly, that parents tended to underreport the extent to which their adolescent child experimented with AOD. Parental reports may be helpful however, in providing valuable information on risk factors associated with SUDs such as medical history, family environment, and psychosocial stressors that may have contributed to the AOD use status of the adolescent and impact subsequent treatment outcome.

4.5. *Peer Report*

Although not crucial, collecting information from friends could prove to be a valuable resource especially if the peers are not currently using AOD or are in recovery. Peers may be able to detail a change in an adolescent's recent behavior or provide information substantiating the drug use behaviors in which they had witnessed or collaboratively participated.

4.6. *Archival Records*

Data collected from sources other than family and friends can help to document the severity of an adolescent's AOD use and outline the consequences of use the teen has experienced. Following client consent, obtaining information from government documents, school data, police reports, employment files, medical records, and other data that document behaviors such as noncompliance with authority, can augment self-report data and clarify important assessment and treatment information. In addition, archival record information can provide beneficial information useful in the development of treatment initiatives and subsequent recovery maintenance.

4.7. *Additional Assessment Issues*

Assessment of AOD involvement is multifacited and can be enhanced by the utilization of some additional factors. It is beneficial to clearly identify the specific categories of drugs used by the teen such as beer, hard liquor, crack, crank, and especially the currently popular "club drugs" such as Ecstacy, Rohypnol, and GHB. With this, interviewers need to have thorough knowledge of all drug categories and the numerous slang terms young people use to reference the various drugs. Furthermore, in order to increase the accuracy in the documentation of amount of alcohol used, it is important to utilize standardized units of measurement such as one drink equals a 12 oz. glass of beer, a four oz. glass of wine, or one oz. of hard liquor (Martin & Nirenberg, 1991). Furthermore, for marijuana and some of the other illicit drugs, the utilization of non-standardized units of measurement can also be helpful to understand the general quantity and progression of use (i.e., hit, joint, blunt, gram, etc.). Finally, issues that should also be addressed during AOD assessment pertain to the age at which the adolescent first used each substance regularly, (e.g., on a monthly basis), how frequently each substance is used in a particular period (e.g., evening, 24 hours, weekend), and the number of months or years the individual has used each of the substances.

5. Assessment of Outcomes

Drug treatment programs have generally received intensive scrutiny, perhaps more so than other healthcare services, because of the nature of addiction and the visibility of its effects. Adolescent drug treatment programs and models have recently been subject to similar scrutiny (Williams and Chang, 2000; Winters, 1999). Treatment outcome information is thus invaluable to the field; such documentation provides a clearer picture of the types of clients served and helps programs determine the effectiveness and cost offsets of different strategies, and improve program performance. Many of the standardized instruments included in Table 1 are worthy of consideration as an appropriate tool when measuring treatment outcome. What parameters are relevant when choosing outcome measures? Newman, Ciarlo, and Carpenter (1999) enumerated eleven guidelines for instrument selection and they are listed below:

1. Relevance to target group
2. Simple, teachable methods
3. Use of measures with objective referents
4. Use of multiple respondents
5. More process-identifying outcome measures
6. Psychometric strengths
7. Low measure costs relative to its uses
8. Understanding by nonprofessional audiences
9. Easy feedback and uncomplicated interpretation
10. Useful and clinical services
11. Compatibility with clinical theories and practices

The value of any standardized questionnaire as a measure of change is an important statistical and clinical question (Collins & Horn, 1991). Some investigators use difference scores, but they tend to be less reliable than the scores used to compute them, and the value of the Time-1 score introduces a bias into the difference score calculation (Allen & Yen, 1979). Dividing the simple difference score by the Time-1 score provides a partial correction for this bias. From a clinical standpoint, the important question is how many clients got better, how many got worse, and how many did not change. Along these lines, Jacobson and Truax (1991) have proposed using the concept of "clinically significant change," which refers to a score change from the abnormal to the normal range. They have statistically operationalized this concept with the Reliable Change Index (RCI). The RCI yields a change score that is corrected for the amount of measurement error inherent in the instrument. This is done by computing the difference between pre-test and post-test scores and dividing by the standard error of difference for the measure (which is estimated from the measure's temporal stability). We regard the RCI analysis as quite appealing because it addresses the practical needs of the treatment service provider while still maintaining statistical standards of significance. Thus, it can be argued that for an instrument to have utility as an outcome measure, it must demonstrate satisfactory measurement error and provide meaningful information to treatment providers and researchers.

6. Summary

Adolescents use and abuse AOD at an alarming rate in this country and experience devastating consequences because of it. AOD use also has a substantial impact on society as well. Therefore, it is critical to quickly and accurately identify those adolescents who are abusing AOD and possibly suffering from an SUD. Distinguishing adult SUD assessment from youth assessment is very important and therefore, developmental considerations are among the most significant factors that need to be considered in the assessment of adolescent AOD use/abuse. Fortunately, research over the past decade has provided health professionals, school personnel, and clinicians with various tools to properly identify those teens who may abusing AOD and suffer from a SUD. However, continued research in the assessment field is still necessary to further improve the their validity of tools for identification, referral, and treatment of adolescent AOD involvement.

References

Allen, M. J., & Yen, W. M. (1979). *Introduction to measurement theory.* Monterey, CA: Brooks/Cole.

American Psychiatric Association. (1994). *Diagnostic and statistical manual of mental disorders* (4th ed.). Washington, DC.: Author.

Babor, T. F., Stephens, R. S., & Marlatt, G. A. (1987). Verbal report of methods in clinical research on alcoholism: Response bias and its minimization. *Journal of Studies on Alcohol, 48,* 410–424.

Biederman, J., Wilens, T., Mick, E., Farone, S. V., Weber, W., Curtis, S., Thornell, A., Pfister, K., Jetton, J. G., & Soriano, J. (1997). Is ADHD a risk factor for psychoactive substance use disorders? Findings from a four-year prospective follow-up study. *Journal of the American Academy of Child and Adolescent Psychiatry, 36,* 21–29.

Botvin, G. J., & Tortu, S. (1988). Peer relationships, social competence, and substance abuse prevention: Implications for the family. In R. H. Coombs (Ed.), *The family context of adolescent drug use* (pp. 245–273). New York, NY: Haworth Press.

Bray, J., Adams, G., Getz, G., & McQueen, A. (2003). Individuation, peers, and adolescent alcohol use: A latent growth analysis. *Journal of Consulting and Clinical Psychology, 71*(3), 553–564.

Brook, D. W., Brook, J. S., Zhang, C., Cohen, P., & Whiteman, M. (2002). Drug use and the risk of major depressive disorder, alcohol dependence and substance use disorders. *Archives of General Psychiatry, 59* (11), 1039–1044.

Center for Substance Abuse Treatment. (1999). Screening and assessing adolescents for substance use disorders. *Treatment Improvement Protocol (TIP) Series #31.* Rockville, MD: Substance Abuse and Mental Health Services Administration.

Chilcoat, H., & Breslau, N. (1999). Pathways from ADHD to early drug use. *Journal of the American Academy of Child & Adolescent Psychiatry, 38*(11), 1347–1354.

Chung, T., Martin, C. S., Winters, K. C., & Langenbucher, J. W. (2001). Assessment of alcohol tolerance in adolescents. *Journal of Studies on Alcohol, 62,* 687–695.

Clark, D. B., & Bukstein, O. G. (1998). Psychopathology in adolescent alcohol abuse and dependence. *Alcohol Health & Research World, 22(2),* 117–121.

Clark, D. B., Kirisci, L., & Moss, H. B. (1998). Early adolescent gateway drug use in sons of fathers with substance use disorders. *Addictive Behaviors, 23,* 561–566.

Clark, D. B., Moss, H., Kirisci, L., Mezzich, A. C., Miles, R., & Ott, P. (1997). Psychopathology in preadolescent sons of substance abusers. *Journal of the American Academy of Child and Adolescent Psychiatry, 36,* 495–502.

Clark, D. B., Parker, A., & Lynch, K. (1999). Psychopathology and substance-related problems during early adolescence: A survival analysis. *Journal of Clinical Child Psychology, 28,* 333–341.

Clark, D. B., & Sayette, M. A. (1993). Anxiety and the development of alcoholism: Clinical and scientific issues. *The American Journal on Addictions, 2,* 59–76.

Collins, L. M., & Horn, J. L. (Eds.) (1991). *Best methods for the analysis of Change.* Washington, DC: American Psychological Association.

DAWN (Drug Abuse Warning Network). (1996). *1996 DAWN report*. Washington, D.C.: Substance Abuse and Mental Health Services Administration.

Dennis, M.L. (1999). *Global Appraisal of Individual Needs (GAIN): Administration Guide for the GAIN and Related Measures*. Bloomington, IL: Lighthouse Publications.

Deykin, E. Y., Levy, J. C., & Wells, V. (1987). Adolescent depression, alcohol and drug abuse. *American Journal of Public Health, 77*, 178–182.

Dishion, T. J., Capaldi, D., Spracklen, K. M., & Fuzhong, L. (1995). Peer ecology and male adolescent drug use. *Development and Psychopathology, 7*, 803–824.

Earls, F., Reich, W., Jung, K. G., & Cloninger, C. R. (1988). Psychopathology in children of alcoholic and antisocial parents. *Alcoholism: Clinical and Experimental Research, 12*, 481–487.

Farrell, A. D., & Danish, S. J. (1993). Peer drug associations and emotional restraint: Causes and consequences of adolescents' drug use? *Journal of Consulting and Clinical Psychology, 61*, 327–334.

Friedman, A.S., & Utada, A. (1989). A method for diagnosing and planning the treatment of adolescent drug abusers. Adolescent drug abuse diagnosis instrument. *Journal of Drug Education*, 19: 285–312.

Grisso, T., & Barnum, R. (2000). *Massachusetts Youth Screening Instrument—2: User's Manual and Technical Report*. Worcester, MA: University of Massachusetts Medical School.

Guo, J., Hill, K. G., Hawkins, J. D., Catalano, R. E., & Abbott, R. D. (2002). A developmental analysis of sociodemographic, family, and peer effects on adolescent illicit drug initiation. *Journal of the American Academy of Child and Adolescent Psychiatry, 41*, 838–845.

Harrell, A. V. (1997). The validity of self-reported drug use data: The accuracy of responses on confidential self-administered answered sheets. *National Institute on Drug Abuse (NIDA) Research Monograph, 167*, 37–58.

Harrison, L. D. (1995). The validity of self-reported data on drug use. *Journal of Drug Issues, 25*, 91–111.

Harrison, P. A., Fulkerson, J. A., & Beebe, T. J. (1998). DSM-IV substance use disorder criteria for adolescents: A critical examination based on a statewide school survey. *American Journal of Psychiatry, 155*, 486–492.

Hasin, D., & Paykin, A. (1998). Dependence symptoms but no diagnosis: Diagnostic orphans in a community sample. *Drug and Alcohol Dependence, 50*, 19–26.

Hawkins, J. D., Catalano, R. F., & Miller, J. Y. (1992). Risk and protective factors for alcohol and other drug problems in adolescence and early adulthood: Implications for substance abuse prevention. *Psychological Bulletin,112*, 64–105.

Henly, G. A., & Winters, K. C. (1988). Development of problem severity scales for the assessment of adolescent alcohol and drug abuse. *The International Journal of the Addictions, 23*, 65–85.

Hill, S. Y., & Muka, D. (1996). Childhood psychopathology in children from families of alcoholic female probands. *Journal of the American Academy of Child and Adolescent Psychiatry, 31*, 1024–1030.

Inwald, R.E., Brobst, M.A., & Morissey, R.F. (1986). Identifying and predicting adolescent behavioral problems by using a new profile. *Juvenile Justice Digest, 14*, 1–9.

Jacobson, N. S., & Truax, P. (1991). Clinical significance: A statistical approach to defining meaningful change in psychotherapy research. *Journal of Consulting and Clinical Psychology, 59*, 12–19.

Johnston, L. D., & O'Malley, P. M. (1997). The recanting of earlier reported drug use by young adults. *NIDA Research Monograph, 167*, 59–80.

Johnston, L. D., O'Malley, P. M., & Bachman, J. G. (2003). *Monitoring the Future national survey results on drug use, 1975–2002*. Volume 1: Secondary School Students (NIH Publication No. 03–5375). Bethesda, MD: National Institute on Drug Abuse.

Kaczynski, N. A., & Martin, C S. (1995). Diagnostic orphans: Adolescents with clinical alcohol symptomology who do not qualify for DSM-IV abuse or dependence diagnosis. Paper presented at the annual meeting of the Research Society on Alcoholism, Steamboat Springs, CO, June, 1995.

Kaminer, Y. (1991). Adolescent substance abuse. In R. J. Frances & S. I. Miller (Eds.), *The clinical textbook of addictive disorders* (pp. 320–346). New York: Guilford Press.

Kaminer, Y. (1994). *Adolescent substance abuse*. New York: Plenum Publishing Corporation.

Kaminer, Y., Bukstein, O. G., & Tarter T. E. (1991). The Teen Addiction Severity Index (T-ASI): Rationale and reliability. *International Journal of Addiction, 26*, 219–226.

Kandel, D. B. (1975). Stages in adolescent involvement in drug use. *Science, 90*, 912–914.

Kandel, D. B., & Davies, M. (1996). High school students who use crack and other drugs. *Archives of General Psychiatry, 53*, 71–80.

Knight, J., Sherritt, L., Harris, S.K., Gates, E., & Chang, G. (2003). Validity of brief alcohol screening tests among adolescents: A comparison of the AUDIT, POSIT, CAGE and CRAFFT. *Alcoholism: Clinical & Experimental Research, 27*, 67–73.

Kokotailo, P. (1995) Physical health problems associated with adolescent substance abuse. In E. Rahdert & D. Czechowicz (Eds.). *Adolescent drug abuse: Clinical assessment and therapeutic interventions* (pp.112–129). NIDA Research Monograph No. 156, NIH Publication No. 95-3908. Rockville, MD: National Institute on Drug Abuse.

Leccese, M., & Waldron, H. B. (1994). Assessing adolescent substance use: A critique of current measurement instruments. *Journal of Substance Abuse Treatment, 11*, 553–563.

Lewinsohn, P. M., Rohde, P., & Seeley, J. R. (1996) Alcohol consumption in high school adolescents: Frequency of use and dimensional structure of associated problems. *Addiction, 91*, 375–390.

Lynskey, M. T., & Fergusson, D. M. (1995). Childhood conduct problems, attention deficit behaviors, and adolescent alcohol, tobacco, and illicit drug use. *Journal of Abnormal Child Psychology, 23* (3), 281–302.

Mackenzie, R. G. (1993). Influence of drug use on adolescent sexual activity. *Adolescent Medicine: State of the Art Reviews, 4*(2). Philadelphia, PA: Herley & Belfus.

Maisto, S. A., Connors, G. J., & Allen, J. P. (1995). Contrasting self-report screens for alcohol problems: A review. *Alcoholism: Clinical and Experimental Research, 19*, 1510–1516.

Magura, S., & Kang, S. Y. (1997). The validity of self-reported cocaine use in two high-risk populations. *National Institute on Drug Abuse (NIDA) Research Monograph, 167*, 227–246.

Mannuzza, S., Klein, R. G., Bessler, A., Malloy, P., & LaPadula, M. (1993). Adult outcome of hyperactive boys' educational achievement, occupational rank, and psychiatric status. *Archives of General Psychiatry, 50*, 565–576.

Markwiese, B. J., Acheson, S. K., Leven, E. D., Wislosn, W. A., & Swartzwelder, H. S. (1998). Differential effects of ethanol on memory in adolescent and adults rats. *Alcoholism: Clinical and Experimental Research, 22*, 416–421.

Martin, C. S., Kaczynski, N. A., Maisto, S. A., Buckstein, O. M., & Moss, H. B. (1995). Patterns of DSM-IV alcohol abuse and dependence symptoms in adolescent drinkers. *Journal of Studies on Alcohol, 56*, 672–680.

Martin, C. S., Kaczynski, N. A., Maisto, S. A., & Tarter, R. E. (1996). Poly drug use in adolescent drinkers with and without DSM-IV alcohol abuse and dependence. *Alcoholism: Clinical and Experimental Research, 20*, 1099–1108.

Martin, C. S., & Nirenberg, T. D. (1991). Alcohol content variation in the assessment of alcohol consumption. *Addictive Behaviors, 16(6)*, 555–560.

Martin, C. S., & Winters, K. C. (1998). Diagnosis and assessment of alcohol use disorders among adolescents. *Alcohol Health and Research World, 22(2)*, 95–105.

Martin, C. S., Lynch, K. G., Pollock, N. K., & Clark, D. B. (2000). Gender differences and similarities in the personality correlates of adolescent alcohol problems. *Psychology of Addictive Behaviors, 14*, 121–133.

Martino, S., Grilo, C.M., & Fehon, D.C. (2000). The development of the drug abuse screening test for adolescents (DAST-A). *Addictive Behaviors, 25*, 57–70.

McGue, M. (1999). Behavioral genetics models of alcoholism and drinking. In K. E. Leornard, & H. T. Blane, (Eds.), *Psychological Theories of Drinking and Alcoholism* (2nd Ed). New York: Guilford, (pp. 372–421).

McLaney, M. A., Del-Boca, F., & Babor, T. (1994). A validation study of the Problem Oriented Screening Instrument for Teenagers (POSIT). *Journal of Mental Health- United Kingdom, 3*, 363–376.

McLellan, A. T., Luborsky, L., Woody, G. E., & O'Brien, C. P. (1980). An improved diagnostic evaluation instrument for substance abuse patients: The Addiction Severity Index. *Journal of Nervous and Mental Disease, 186*, 26–33.

Milberger, S., Biederman, J., Faraone, S. V., Chen, L., & Jones, J. (1997). ADHD is associated with early initiation of cigarette smoking in children and adolescents. *Journal of the American Academy of Child and Adolescent Psychiatry, 36,* 37–44.

Miller, G. (1985). *The Substance Abuse Subtle Screening Inventory-Adolescent Version.* Bloomington, IN: SASSI Institute.

Moss, H. B., Clark, D. B., & Kirisci, L. (1997). Developmental timing of paternal substance use disorder offset and the severity of problem behaviors in their prepubertal sons. *The American Journal on Addictions, 6,* 30–37.

Meyers, K., McLellan, A.T., Jaeger, J.L., & Pettinati, H.M. (1995). The development of the Comprehensive Addiction Severity Index for Adolescents (CASI-A): An interview for assessing multiple problems of adolescents. *Journal of Substance Abuse Treatment, 12,* 181–193.

Noam, G. G., & Houlihan, J. (1990). Developmental dimensions of DSM-III diagnoses in adolescent psychiatric patients. *American Journal of Orthopsychiatry, 60,* 371–378.

Newman, F.L., Ciarlo, J.A., & Carpenter, D (1999). Guidelines for selecting psychological instruments for treatment planning and outcome. In M. E. Maruish (Ed), *The use of psychological testing and treatment planning for outcomes and assessment, second edition* (pp. 153–170). Mahwah, New Jersey: Lawrence Erlbaum Associates.

Patterson, G. R., Forgatch, M. S., Yoerger, K. L., & Stoolmiller, M. (1998). Variables that initiate and maintain an early-onset trajectory for juvenile offending. *Development and Psychopathology, 10,* 531–548.

Petraitis, J., Flay, B. R., & Miller, T. Q. (1995). Reviewing theories of adolescent substance abuse: Organizing pieces in the puzzle. *Psychological Bulletin, 117,* 67–86.

Pollock, N. K., & Martin, C. S. (1999). Diagnostic orphans: Adolescents with alcohol symptoms who do not qualify for DSM-IV abuse or dependence diagnoses. *American Journal of Psychiatry, 156,* 897–901.

Rahdert, E. (Ed.) (1991). *The Adolescent Assessment/Referral System Manual.* Rockville, MD: U.S. Department of Health and Human Services, ADAMHA, National Institute on Drug Abuse, DHHS Pub. No. (ADM) 91–1735.

Rao, U., Daley, S., & Hammen, C. (2000). Realtionship between depression and substance use disorders in adolescent women during the transition to adulthood. *Journal of the American Academy of Child & Adolescent Psychiatry, 39*(2), 215–222.

Rohde, P., Lewinsohn, P. M., & Seely, J. R. (1996). Psychiatric comorbidity with problematic alcohol use in high school students. *Journal of the American Academy of Child and Adolescent Psychiatry, 35*(1), *101–109.*

Rose, R. (1998). A developmental behavioral-genetic perspective on alcoholism risk. *Alcohol Health and Research World, 22,* 131–143.

Shaffer, D., Fisher, P. & Dulcan, M. (1996). The NIMH Diagnostic Interview Schedule for Children (DISC 2.3): Description, acceptability, prevalences, and performance in the MECA study. *Journal of the American Academy of Child and Adolescent Psychiatry, 35,* 865–877.

Shedler, J., & Block, J. (1990). Adolescent drug use and psychological health. *American Psychologist, 45,* 612–630.

Single, E., Kandel, D., & Johnson, B. D. (1975). The reliability and validity of drug use responses in a large-scale longitudinal survey. *Journal of Drug Issues, 5,* 426–443.

Sobell, L. C., & Sobell, M. B. (1992). Time-line Follow-back: A technique for assessing self-reported alcohol consumption. In R. Z. Litten & J. P. Allen (Eds.), *Measuring Alcohol Consumption* (pp. 73–98). Totowa, NJ: Humana Press.

Spear, L. P. (2000). The adolescent brain and age-related behavioral manifestations. *Neuroscience and Biobehavioral Reviews, 24,* 417–463.

Stinchfield, R. D. (1997). Reliability of adolescent self-reported pretreatment alcohol and other drug use. *Substance Use and Misuse, 32,* 63–76.

Substance Abuse and Mental Health Services Administration. (2001). 2001 National Household Survey on Drug Abuse. Retrieved July 30, 2003,from http://www.samhsa.gov/oas/nhsda/2k1nhsda/vol1/toc.htm

Tarter, R. E., Laird, S. B., Bukstein, O., & Kaminer, Y. (1992). Validation of the adolescent drug use screening inventory: Preliminary findings. *Psychology of Addictive Behaviors, 6,* 322–236.

Thompson, L. L., Riggs, P. D., Mikulich, S. K., & Crowley, T. J. (1996). Contribution of ADHD symptoms to substance problems and delinquency in conduct-disordered adolescents. *Journal of Abnormal Child Psychology, 24(3),* 325–347.

Varlinskaya, E.I., & Spear, L.P. (in press). Acute effects of ethanol on social behavior of adolescent and adult rats: Role of familiarity of the test situation. *Alcoholism: Clinical and Experimental Research.*

Wanberg, K. (1992). *Adolescent Self-Assessment Profile.* Arvada, CO: Center for Addictions Research and Evaluation.

Welner, Z., Reich, W., Herjanic, B., Jung, K., & Amado, K. (1987). Reliability, validity and parent-child agreement studies of the Diagnostic Interview for Children and Adolescents (DICA). *Journal of American Academy of Child Psychiatry, 26,* 649–653.

White, H. R., & Labouvie, E. W. (1989). Towards the assessment of adolescent problem drinking. *Journal of Studies on Alcohol, 50,* 30–37.

Williams, R.J., & Chang, S.Y. (2000). Comprehensive and comparative review of adolescent substance abuse treatment outcome. *Clinical Psychology: Science and Practice, 7,* 138–166.

Willner, R. (2000). Further validation and development of a screening instrument for the assessment of substance misuse in adolescents. *Addiction, 95,* 1691–1698.

Winters, K.C. (1992). Development of an adolescent alcohol and other drug abuse screening scale: Personal Experience Screening Questionnaire. *Addictive Behaviors, 17,* 479–490.

Winters, K. C. (1994). Assessment of adolescent drug abuse: A handbook. Los Angeles, CA: Western Psychological Services.

Winters, K. C. (2001). Adolescent assessment of alcohol and other drug use behaviors. In J. P. Allen & V. Wilson (Eds.), *Assessing alcohol problems: A guide for clinicians and researchers* (2nd ed.). Rockville, MD: National Institute on Alcohol Abuse and Alcoholism.

Winters, K. C., Anderson, N., Bengston, P., Stinchfield, R. D., & Latimer, W. W. (2000). Development of a parent questionnaire for the assessment of adolescent drug abuse. *Journal of Psychoactive Drugs, 32,* 3–13.

Winters, K. C., & Henly, G. A. (1989). *Personal Experience Inventory and Manual.* Los Angeles: Western Psychological Services.

Winters, K.C., & Henly, G.A. (1993). *Adolescent Diagnostic Interview Schedule and Manual.* Los Angeles: Western Psychological Services.

Winters, K. C., Latimer, W., & Stinchfield, R. D. (1999). The DSM-IV criteria for adolescent alcohol and cannabis use disorders. *Journal of Studies on Alcohol, 60(3),* 337–344.

Winters, K. C., Latimer, W. W., Stinchfield, R. D., Henly, G. A. (1999). Examining psychosocial correlates of drug involvement among drug clinic-referred youth. *Journal of Child & Adolescent Substance Abuse, 9(1), 1–17.*

Winters, K. C., Stinchfield, R. D., Henly, G. A. & Schwartz, R. (1990–1991). Validity of adolescent self report of substance involvement. *The International Journal of the Addictions, 25,* 1379–1395.

Wish, E., Hoffman, A., & Nemes, S. (1997). The validity of self-reports of drug use treatment admission and at follow-up: Comparisons with urinalysis and hair analysis. *National Institute on Drug Abuse (NIDA) Research Monograph, 167,* 200–226.

Yamaguchi, K., & Kandel, D. B. (1984). Patterns of drug use from adolescence to young adulthood-III: Patterns of progression. *American Journal of Public Health, 74,* 673–681.

Zucker, R. A., Fitzgerald, H. E., & Moses, H. D. (1995). Emergence of alcohol problems and the several alcoholisms: A developmental perspective on etiologic theory and life course trajectory. In D. Cicchetti, & D.J. Cohen (Eds.), *Developmental Psychopathology Vol. 2: Risk, Disorder, and Adaptation* (pp.677–711). New York: Wiley.

Contents of Previous Volumes

Volume 1

Volume 2

Volume 3

Volume 5

Volume 6

Volume 7: Treatment Research

Volume 10: Alcohol and Cocaine

Volume 11: Ten Years of Progress

Volume 12: Alcoholism and Women

Volume 13: Alcohol and Violence

Volume 14: The Consequences of Alcoholism

Index